Maureen Lawlor

# OBSTETRICAL NURSING

THE MACMILLAN COMPANY
NEW YORK • CHICAGO
DALLAS • ATLANTA • SAN FRANCISCO
LONDON • MANILA
IN CANADA
BRETT-MACMILLAN LTD.
GALT, ONTARIO

# OBSTETRICAL NURSING

---

Carolyn Conant Van Blarcom, R. N.

*Revised by*

Erna Ziegel, R. N., B. S.

Instructor of Clinical Nursing and Supervisor of Obstetric and Gynecologic Services, University of Wisconsin School of Nursing and Hospitals, Madison, Wisconsin

FOURTH EDITION

NEW YORK · THE MACMILLAN COMPANY · 1958

Published simultaneously in Canada.



Printed in the United States of America

THIRD PRINTING, 1959



Library of Congress Catalog card number: 57-5029

# Foreword to the Fourth Edition

This textbook has been completely rewritten because obstetric nursing, like medicine as a whole, is ever changing. New advances in medical science necessitate revision, additions, and deletions to achieve a modern textbook. It is significant that this book on obstetric nursing has been written by a nurse reflecting her practical experience as a supervisor and instructor of obstetric nursing in a service associated with a medical and a nursing school and in a large general hospital. The author obtained authoritative information for her revision from obstetricians, pediatricians, and practitioners in allied branches of medicine.

Normal obstetrics and its complete nursing care have been emphasized; in addition, the obstetric complications have been given adequate discussion. Basic anatomy, physiology, and fetal development have been covered thoroughly, as well as physiologic changes during pregnancy, labor, and the puerperium. Prenatal care has been presented well with especial emphasis on the nursing aspects. Nutrition of the pregnant woman has been given the attention that the subject now merits.

Important and ancillary considerations, such as education for childbirth, mental hygiene, social and economic factors, and community health services, have been given appropriate coverage.

The section on care of the fetus and newborn has been enlarged and extended in all its aspects from the standpoint of both the normal and abnormal.

The organization of the book is excellent and indicates considerable thought, time, and preparation. The select illustrations throughout the book will aid understanding and teaching. I am sure that this textbook will be of value to medical students and doctors, as well as to the nurse.

Miss Ziegel and her collaborators are to be commended, and it is my opinion that this textbook will have wide acceptance and continued success.

Ralph E. Campbell, M.D.
Professor of Obstetrics and Gynecology, University of Wisconsin School of Medicine

# Preface to the Fourth Edition

The purpose of this revision is to present in a modern and comprehensive form the many recent advances in obstetrics and obstetric nursing. With such complete coverage the nurse can acquire an understanding of her role in all phases of care to be given to the mother, the newborn infant, and the family during and following pregnancy. This is a textbook for student nurses, and it should, because of its enlarged scope, also serve as a reference for graduate nurses.

Nursing practice is the main theme, and its presentation is based on the underlying principles of obstetric care. To clarify these principles, essential scientific information regarding physiologic processes, pathologic conditions, and therapy has been included. Because the emotional aspect of care during pregnancy and childbirth is important, the discussion includes subjects such as parents' classes during the prenatal period and the experience of rooming-in after delivery. Care of the newborn infant is emphasized, because I believe that the nurse's responsibility in the first few days of life is of particular importance.

Medical practice is described according to information obtained from authoritative sources, and with the advice of obstetricians, pediatricians, and members of allied medical sciences. Of necessity, only certain generally recognized medical practices have been presented, since the basic purpose of this text precluded more detailed description. Current nursing practice has been presented in more detail, and, in important ways, it reflects my own experience and my ever-continuous evaluation of obstetric nursing. It is my hope that the nurse reading this book will be stimulated to think through the total care she gives each patient, to make adaptations of care with insight, and to be always aware of further advances in scientific knowledge as they relate to, and influence, her professional responsibilities.

Changes in the obstetric regimen have affected the nursing care given to mothers and newborn babies, and have necessitated some reorganization of Miss Van Blarcom's book. For example, in Part IV, "The Birth of the Baby," I have added Chapter 13, "Analgesia and Anesthesia"; the subject of nutrition for both the mother and baby has been incorporated into Chapter 6, "Prenatal Care," and Chapter 17, "The Nursing Mother," where this subject can be more properly presented as part of the total care given. Since so many women are now being admitted to hospitals for childbirth, the material on "The Preparations for Home Delivery" is included in the Appendix rather than Part VI, "The Maternity Patient in the Community." To Part VII, "The Care of the Baby," has been added Chapter 23, "The Premature Infant: Characteristics and Nursing Care"; Chapter 24, "Abnormalities and Diseases of the Newborn Infant—Medical Aspects and Nursing Care," has been expanded to include a full discussion of respiratory disturbances at birth and of erythroblastosis fetalis.

Because I am in agreement with Miss Van Blarcom's philosophy—the importance of the nurse "adopting a sympathetic, understanding attitude toward the patient"—I have made every effort to weave this belief throughout the text discussion. I have also continued the emphasis that Miss Van Blarcom placed on the nurse's function of *teaching* patients, as well as the role the nurse plays in assisting the doctor on the medical team in striving for the safety and well-being of mothers and babies.

In the individual chapter "Bibliography and Student References," I have included a majority of the articles on maternal and child care that have appeared in the *American Journal of Nursing* and *Nursing Outlook* for the past five years; by so doing, I felt this comprehensive listing would give the student ample opportunity to know the scope and coverage that these two journals have to offer. I have included other articles from obstetric and pediatric journals because I felt this would help the student become acquainted with material in medical libraries. In order to present a complete over-all coverage of bibliographic material, there are also suitable textbooks for reference.

Madison, Wisconsin
March 12, 1957

Erna Ziegel, R.N.

# Acknowledgments

As in the first three editions of this book, valuable assistance was given by the late Dr. John W. Harris. During many years of association with Dr. Harris, I came to appreciate his interest and skill in teaching nurses, and I was pleased to undertake this revision with his assistance. Dr. Harris' interest in promoting the welfare of mothers and babies and his genuine concern for each patient as an individual were an inspiring influence. Through this influence and his interest in teaching nurses he was able to give the same help and encouragement in this revision that he gave to the original preparation of this text and its subsequent revisions. His generous guidance and wise counsel were a continuous source of encouragement.

I acknowledge the assistance I received from faculty members of the University of Wisconsin Medical School and School of Nursing. I express my appreciation to Dr. William Kiekhofer for his valuable assistance and advice regarding many aspects of obstetric care, and to Dr. H. Kent Tenney for his critical reading and counsel with Part VII, "The Care of the Baby." My long-continued association with the late Dr. John E. Gonce resulted in an understanding of the newborn infant and his care which contributed immeasurably to the content of this book. I wish to thank Dr. Karl Siebecker for reading Chapter 13, "Analgesia and Anesthesia," and for his helpful suggestions. I gratefully acknowledge the assistance I received from my nursing colleagues in the preparation of this text. Miss Margaret Crump gave valuable help in various sections and especially with Part VII, "The Care of the Baby." Miss Eugenia Schoen made helpful suggestions regarding Chapter 7, "Mental Hygiene of the Expectant Mother," and Mrs. Signe Cooper read many portions of the manuscript and generously gave constructive advice.

Many of the illustrations in this edition are new. All new photographs were made by Mr. Homer Montague, photographer, University Hospitals, Madison, Wisconsin. I express my appreciation for his expert photography and for his cooperation in obtaining the desired illustrations. I also thank the patients who were willing to assist, and the administration of University Hospitals, Madison, Wisconsin, for the use of available facilities.

I especially wish to express my gratitude to Mr. W. Holt Seale and Miss Barbara Russell of the Medical-Public Health Department, The Macmillan Company, for their assistance throughout the preparation of this text.

E.Z.

# Contents

*Chapter*

CONTENTS

PART XII. THE CARE OF THE BABY

# OBSTETRICAL NURSING

# PART I. ANATOMY AND PHYSIOLOGY

*Chapter 1*

## Anatomy of the Female Pelvis and Reproductive Organs

### THE BONY PELVIS

Detailed knowledge of the anatomy of the female pelvis has resulted in an enormous reduction in injury and death among obstetric patients and their babies. This knowledge of the pelvic anatomy, relating as it does to both normal and malformed pelves, has made possible a system of measurements, termed *pelvimetry,* which gives the obstetrician a fair idea of the size and shape of the patient's pelvis. Such data, coupled with observations upon the size of the child's head, provide the obstetrician with information upon which to base his expectation of the ease or difficulty with which the approaching delivery is likely to be accomplished.

Since each patient's pelvic measurements are considered from the standpoint of their comparison with normal dimensions, it is manifestly important that the obstetric nurse have a clear idea of the structure of the normal female pelvis, and also of its commonest variations.

The obstetric significance of pelvic measurements may be more apparent to the nurse if we pause for a moment and mention the factors concerned in labor, "powers, passenger, and passage," as described by Matthews Duncan, a Scotch obstetrician, who wrote over 75 years ago. The "powers" that force the child through the birth canal are supplied by contractions of the uterine muscle and muscles of the abdomen. The "passenger" is the baby who must travel through the "passage," or bony pelvis and soft parts, during the process of labor. In the following pages we shall study the passage through which the infant passenger must make his way. It will be seen that the shortest diameters of the "passage" must accommodate the greatest diameters of the "passenger" if delivery is to take place safely through the birth canal.

## NORMAL PELVIS

Viewed in its entirety, the pelvis is an irregularly constructed, two-storied, bony cavity or canal situated below and supporting the movable parts of the spinal column, and resting upon the femurs or thigh-bones (Fig. 1).

Four bones enter into the construction of the pelvis: the two hip-bones, or *ossa innominata,* on the sides and in front, with the *sacrum* and *coccyx* behind.

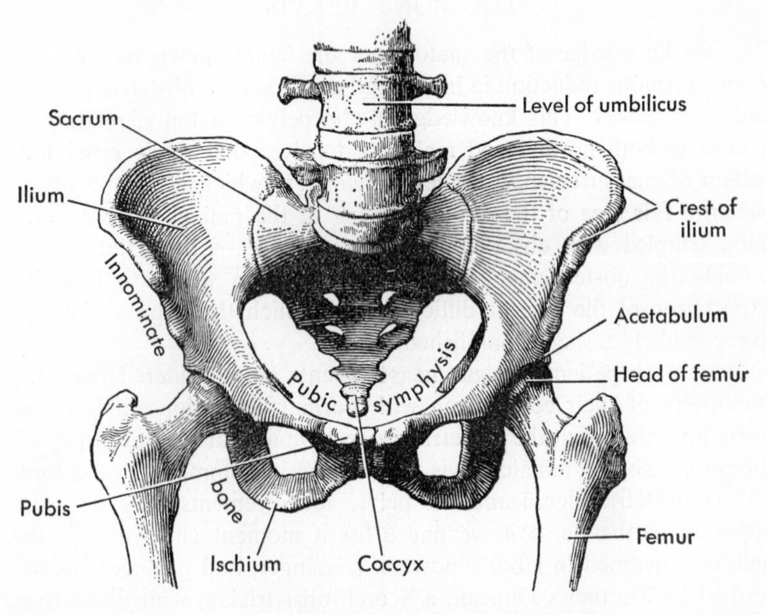


**Fig. 1.** The bony pelvis. It has the shape of a ring and is made up of four bones—the two innominate bones, the sacrum, and the coccyx. Each innominate bone consists of three parts—the ilium, ischium, and pubis. (Brady, L.; Kurtz, E.; and McLaughlin, E.: *Essentials of Gynecology,* 2nd ed. The Macmillan Company, New York, 1949.)

**The innominate bones** (ossa innominata), symmetrically placed on each side, are broad, flaring, and scoop-shaped. Each bone consists of three main parts, which are separate bones in early life, but firmly welded together in adults: the *ilium, ischium,* and *pubis* (Fig. 1). The ilia are the broad, thin, plate-like sections above; their upper, anterior prominences, which may be felt as the foremost angles of the hipbones, are the *anterior superior spinous processes* sometimes used in pelvic measurements. The margins extending backward from these points are termed the *iliac crests.*

The ischia are below, and it is upon their projections, known as the *tuberosities,* that the body rests when in the sitting position, and which also serve as landmarks in pelvimetry. The two pubic bones unite in the median line by means of heavy cartilage to form the *symphysis pubis* (Fig. 1).

**The sacrum and coccyx** behind are really the termination of the spinal column, the sacrum usually consisting of five rudimentary vertebrae which have fused into one bone (Fig. 1). It sometimes consists of four bones, sometimes six, but more often of five. It has both a vertical and lateral concavity. The sacrum completes the pelvic girdle behind by uniting on each side with the innominate bones by means of strong cartilages, thus forming the *sacroiliac joints* (Fig. 2). The spinal column rests upon the upper surface of the sacrum. The coccyx is a little wedge-shaped, tail-like appendage, which is the vestige of the tail seen in the early embryo. Ordinarily it has but slight obstetric importance. It extends in a downward curve from the lower margin of the sacrum, to which it has a cartilaginous attachment, the *sacrococcygeal joint.* This joint between the sacrum and coccyx is much more movable in the female than in the male.

We find, therefore, that although the pelvis constitutes a rigid, bony, ring-like structure, there are four joints: the symphysis pubis, the sacrococcygeal, and the two sacroiliac articulations. As the cartilages in these joints become somewhat softened and thickened during pregnancy, because of the increased blood supply, they all permit of a certain, though limited, amount of motion at the time of labor. This provision is of considerable obstetric importance, since the sacrococcygeal joint allows the child's head to push back the forward-protruding coccyx, as it passes down the birth canal, thus removing what otherwise might be a serious obstruction.

The normal *male pelvis* is deep, narrow, rough, and massive as compared with the female structure (Figs. 2 and 3), and the angle of the pubic arch, formed by the two pubic bones, is deeper and more acute in the male than in the female skeleton. The normal female pelvis, on the other hand, is light, broad, shallow, smooth, and large.

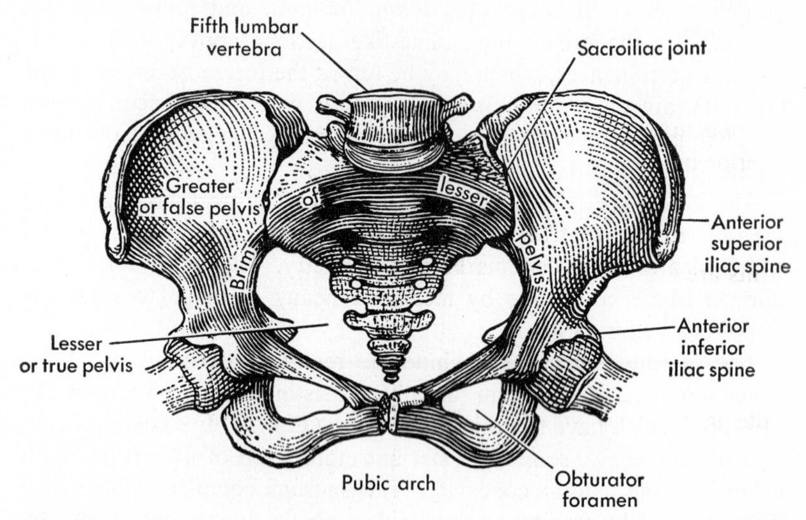


**Fig. 2.** The female pelvis, ventral view. The disk of fibrocartilage which unites the pubic bones is not shown in order that the end of the coccyx may be seen. (Kimber, D.; Gray, C.; Stackpole, C.; and Leavell, L.: *Textbook of Anatomy and Physiology,* 13th ed. The Macmillan Company, New York, 1955.)

**The pelvic cavity** as a whole is divided into the *true* and *false pelvis* by a constriction of the entire structure known as the *linea terminalis, brim,* or *inlet.* As the pelvis occupies an oblique position in the body (the degree of inclination is greater in the female than in the male), the plane of this brim is not horizontal, but slopes up and back from the symphysis pubis to the promontory of the sacrum. Being swung upon the heads of the femurs, the relation of the pelvis to the entire body differs in the sitting and standing positions. When a woman stands upright, her pelvis is so markedly oblique in its position that she would tip backward but for strong tendons attached to the pelvis and running down the front of the thighs. Added strain upon these tendons during pregnancy may account for some of the apparently undue fatigue experienced by the expectant mother.

**The false, or large, pelvis** is the shallow, expanded portion above the brim or linea terminalis. Its walls are formed by the lumbar vertebrae behind, the fan-like flare of the ilia on each side, and in the anterior portion this bony wall is filled in by abdominal muscles. It ordinarily serves simply as a support for the abdominal viscera.

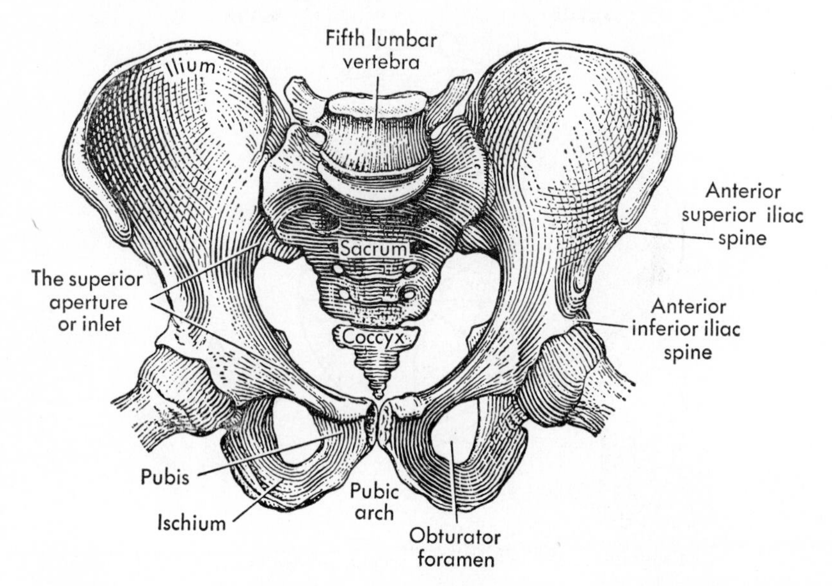


**Fig. 3.** The male pelvis, ventral view. The disk of fibrocartilage which unites the pubic bones is not shown in order that the end of the coccyx may be seen.

Note the broad, shallow, light construction of the female pelvis, Fig. 2, as compared with the more massive male pelvis, Fig. 3. The true pelvis of the female is shallower, wider, and has a greater capacity than the true pelvis of the male which is deep and narrow. (Kimber, D.; Gray, C.; Stackpole, C.; and Leavell, L.: *Textbook of Anatomy and Physiology,* 13th ed. The Macmillan Company, New York, 1955.)

The false pelvis is of little obstetric importance, its function during pregnancy being to support the enlarged uterus, while at the time of labor it acts as a funnel to direct the child's head into the true pelvis below.

**The true pelvis,** on the other hand, is of greatest possible obstetric importance since it constitutes the "passage" through which the "passenger," or child, must be forced by the "powers" of muscular contraction during birth. It lies below and somewhat behind the brim; is an irregularly shaped, bottomless basin; and contains the reproductive organs, the rectum, and the bladder. Its bony walls are more complete than those of the false pelvis, and are formed by the sacrum, coccyx, and innominate bones.

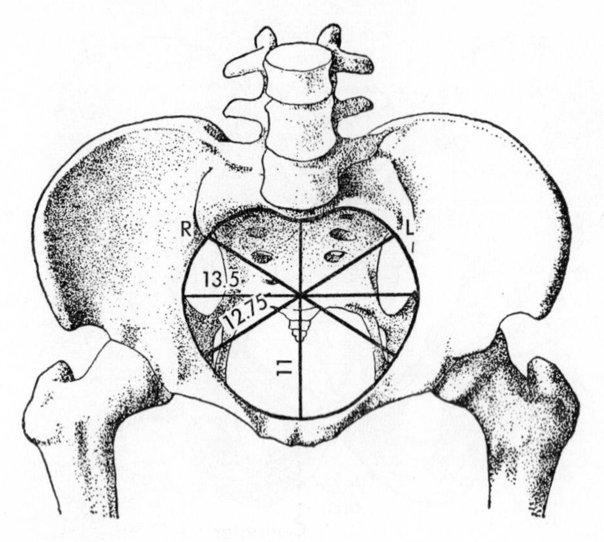


**Fig. 4.** Diagram of the pelvic inlet, seen from above, with most important diameters.

**The inlet and outlet** of the true pelvis are smaller than the middle part and are called the *superior* and *inferior strait* respectively. The *inlet,* or *superior strait,* is bounded by the pubic bones in front, the linea terminalis on the sides, and the body of the first sacral vertebra, known as the *promontory of the sacrum,* in the back. The inlet may be round, or its anteroposterior diameter may be shortened by the promontory of the sacrum which gives the opening a blunt, heart-shaped outline (Fig. 4).

The lower margin of the true pelvis, which has a diamond-shaped appearance, constitutes the *outlet,* or *inferior strait;* and being longer in the anteroposterior dimension than in its transverse measurement, its long axis is at right angles to the long axis of the inlet (Fig. 5). A baby's head, accordingly, must twist, or rotate, in making its descent through this bony canal, because the long diameter of the head must first conform to one of the long diameters of the inlet, either transverse or oblique, and then turn so that the length of the head is lying anteroposteriorly, in conformity to the long diameter of the outlet, through which it next passes.

The posterior wall of the pelvis, consisting of the sacrum and

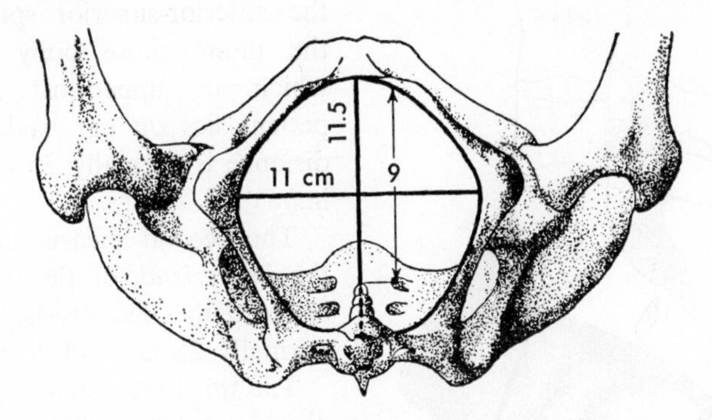


**Fig. 5.** Diagram of pelvic outlet, seen from below, with most important diameters.

coccyx, forms a vertical curve and is about three times as deep as the anterior wall formed by the narrow symphysis pubis. The structure as a whole, therefore, curves upon itself, resembling a bent tube with its concavity directed forward (Fig. 6).

Thus it becomes apparent that the structure of the pelvis requires the child's head not only to rotate in its passage through the birth canal, but also to describe an arc, since the part of the head which passes down the posterior wall travels farther in a given time than the part which passes under the symphysis pubis. This twisting and curving of the birth canal must be appreciated in order to understand the mechanism of labor.

## PELVIC MEASUREMENTS

Pelvimetry is done by measuring the distance between certain points on the pelvis with a pair of calipers, known as a pelvimeter (Fig. 7), or by means of x-ray. In considering the question of pelvimetry we find that both *external* and *internal measurements* may be taken for the purpose of estimating as accurately as possible the size of the passage through which the passenger must advance.

**External Inlet Measurements.** According to some systems of mensuration the external inlet measurements are taken first with the patient lying flat on the examining table and her knees close together for the first three measurements and on her side for the fourth.

The first measurement is the *interspinous,* the distance between the anterior-superior spines of the ilium, those bony points which are uppermost as the patient lies on her back. This distance is normally 25 cm (10 in.).

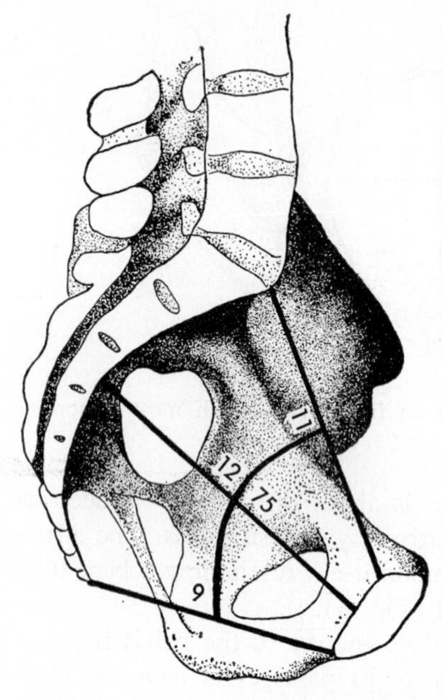


**Fig. 6.** Diagram of sagittal section of the pelvis showing curve of the bony canal, with most important diameters.

The second measurement is the *intercristal,* or the distance between the iliac crests, and is normally 28 cm (11.2 in.).

The third measurement is the distance between the *great trochanters,* or heads of the femurs, and is normally 31 cm (12.4 in.).

*Baudelocque's diameter* is the fourth measurement and is taken with the patient lying on her side. This diameter is the distance from the top of the symphysis pubis to a depression between the last lumbar vertabra and the top of the sacrum. This depression is easily located as it also marks the upper angle of a space just above the buttocks, known as Michaelis' rhomboid, which in normal pelves is quadrilateral. In certain malformed pelves this quadrangle may be so misshapen as to become almost a triangle with the apex directed either up or down. This dimension is sometimes called the *external conjugate* and ordinarily measures 20 cm (8 in.).

These external measurements, which are only an estimate of the size of the pelvic inlet, are merely of relative importance. Therefore, their only value is that they may give an indication of some type of pelvic contraction, if they depart a considerable degree from normal. Shortening of Baudelocque's diameter may be considered a danger sign because the length of the true conjugate may then also be shortened. Because these external pelvic diameters give very little useful information many doctors have eliminated taking these measurements.

**Internal Inlet Measurements.** There are four internal inlet measure-

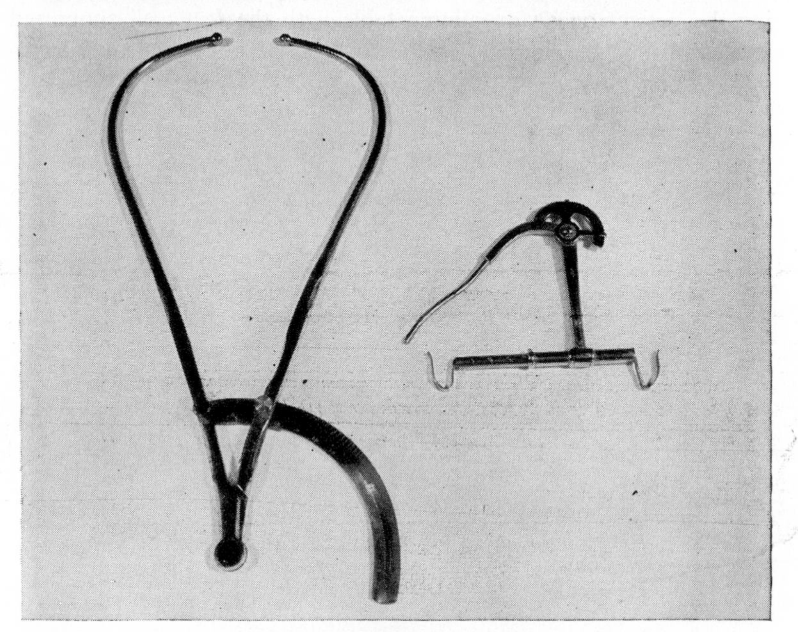

**Fig. 7.** Two types of pelvimeters frequently used in taking pelvic measurements. *Left,* Martin; *right,* Thom.

ments (Fig. 4) of obstetric importance: the *anteroposterior* or *true conjugate,* which is the distance from the top of the symphysis pubis to the promontory of the sacrum and is normally 11 cm (4.4 in.); the *transverse diameter,* which is at right angles to the true conjugate and is the greatest width of the inlet, measuring from a point on one side of the brim to the corresponding point on the other, and is normally 13.5 cm (5.4 in.); and the two diagonal measurements, known respectively as the *right* and *left oblique diameters,* using the sacroiliac joints as denominators, which are normally 12.75 cm (5.1 in.).

Although it is very important to the expectant mother that all of these dimensions be of normal length, the length of the true conjugate, or *conjugate vera,* is of the greatest importance because it is the shortest diameter of the inlet. If it is shorter than normal, the channel may be too constricted for the full-term baby's head to pass through.

The length of the all-important true conjugate is estimated by placing the patient on an examining table with the feet well supported in stirrups and the buttocks to the edge of the table, and then intro-

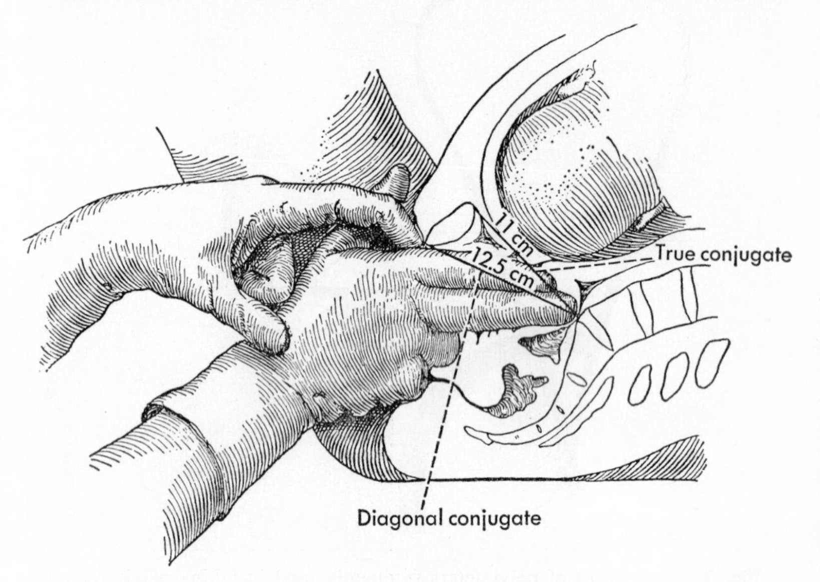


**Fig. 8.** Diagram showing method of estimating the true conjugate by measuring the length of the diagonal conjugate.

ducing the first two fingers of one hand into the vagina until the tip of the second finger touches the promontory of the sacrum (Fig. 8). The point at which the lower margin of the symphysis pubis then rests upon the forefinger is marked, and the distance from this point to the tip of the second finger measured, thus giving the length of the *diagonal conjugate.* Since normally it measures 12.5 cm (5 in.) or more, and is 1.5 to 2 cm (.6 to .8 in.) longer than the true conjugate, the length of the latter may be obtained by subtracting 1.5 to 2 cm (.6 to .8 in.) from the diagonal conjugate. The other internal inlet measurements cannot be made on the living woman clinically and for all practical purposes are not necessary.

While the diagonal conjugate is being measured the motility of the coccyx may also be determined, the vertical and lateral concavities of the sacrum palpated, and the prominence of the ischial spines determined. The ischial spines extend from the middle of the posterior margin of each ischium and are of great obstetric importance because the distance between them is the shortest diameter of the pelvic cavity. They can readily be felt on vaginal and rectal examina-

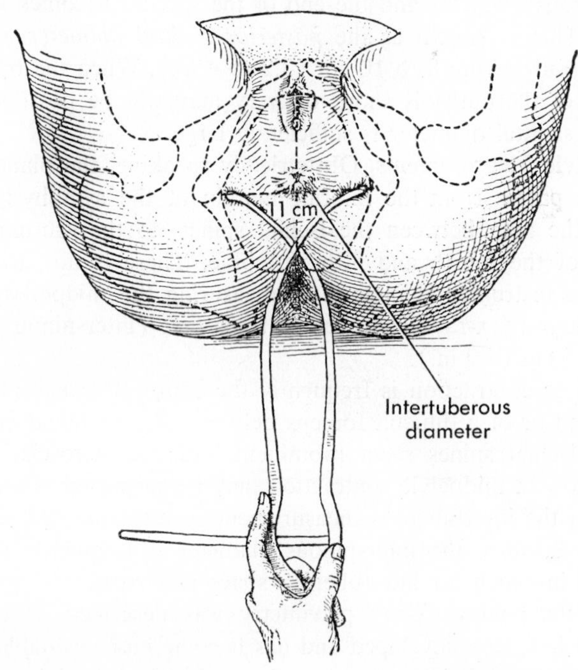


**Fig. 9.** Diagram showing method of measuring the intertuberous diameter.

tion and serve as valuable landmarks in determining the descent of the presenting part of the fetus into the pelvis.

**Outlet Measurements.** While the patient is on the examining table with her feet in stirrups, the size of the pelvic outlet also may be determined. By palpation of the descending rami of the pubic bones the acuteness of the angle of the *pubic arch* can be determined. Then the distance between the tuberosities of the ischia, the *intertuberous diameter,* is measured. This is the most important measurement of the outlet because it is the shortest diameter through which the child must pass in the inferior strait, and normally measures between 10 and 11 cm (4 and 4.4 in.) (Fig. 9). The narrower the pubic arch, the shorter the intertuberous diameter will be. Since this is true, it becomes apparent that the shorter the intertuberous diameter is, the less space there is for the baby's head to pass directly under the symphysis pubis. If the head must stem itself lower down along the pubic arch in passing through the outlet the distance between the intertuberous diameter and the end of the sacrum becomes very important. This is known as the *posterior sagittal diameter* and normally measures from 8 to 10 cm (3.2 to 4 in.). When the transverse diameter of the outlet is short, delivery may still be possible if the posterior sagittal diameter is sufficiently large.

**Midpelvic Measurements.** Obstetrically speaking, the plane of the midpelvis passes from the inferior margin of the symphysis pubis, through the area between the ischial spines, to the sacrum at the juncture of the fourth and fifth vertebrae. There is no satisfactory manual or instrumental method of measuring the midpelvis; it can only be done by x-ray. The average transverse (interspinous) diameter is 10.5 cm (4.2 in.).

Midpelvic contraction is frequently the cause of transverse arrest of the head or of a difficult forceps delivery. If on vaginal examination the ischial spines seem prominent and the sacrosciatic notch feels narrow, a midpelvic contraction may be suspected. This is also true when the intertuberous measurement seems small, 8.5 cm (3.4 in.) or less, since the interspinous diameter is frequently small in the pelvis in which the intertuberous space is narrow.

**X-ray Pelvimetry.** X-ray pelvimetry was described as early as 1900, but has been developed and has become more valuable during the past 20 years. It is now commonly used to make pelvic measurements which are otherwise impossible to obtain and to verify those which have been obtained by means of the pelvimeter and the finger. With the x-ray there is then a method of measuring diameters which previously could not be made clinically, such as the transverse diameter of the inlet and the interischial spinous dimension. The x-ray also makes it possible to visualize the birth canal as a whole, to view the general architecture of the pelvis, and to determine the size and shape of the fetal head and its relation to the various pelvic diameters (Figs. 10 and 11). When standing films are taken during labor, especially if they are repeated one or two times, definite evidence is obtained as to whether or not there is descent of the biparietal plane

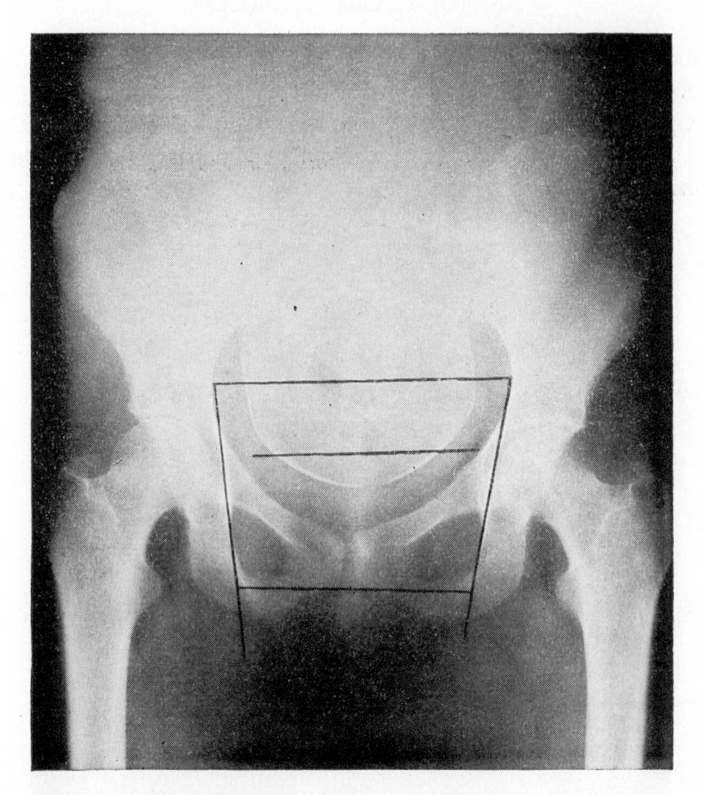

**Fig. 10.** Anteroposterior view of a roentgenogram of a pelvis taken to determine the size of the pelvis, its general architecture, and the relationship of the size of the fetal head to the size of the pelvis. This x-ray was taken on a primigravida near term whose measurements by clinical pelvimetry seemed to be within normal limits, but in whom the fetal head had not engaged.

The horizontal black lines on the film designate the diameters measured. The uppermost horizontal line indicates the transverse diameter of the inlet which measured 12.2 cm (4.88 in.). The center horizontal line runs between the ischial spines and measures the transverse diameter of the midpelvis; this measured 10.1 cm (4.04 in.). The lowermost horizontal line lies between the ischial tuberosities and thus measures the transverse diameter of the pelvic outlet; this was found to be 10.2 cm (4.08 in.). (After the distances had been measured on the film a correction factor was applied to make adjustment for magnification and other technical considerations.)

This x-ray shows the presentation to be cephalic with the occiput anterior; the back lies anteriorly and slightly to the right. The fetal head is small as compared to the size of the pelvis.

of the head. With elongation of the head during labor this is difficult to determine manually by palpation of the presenting part.

X-ray pelvimetry is not used routinely on all obstetric patients because the usual methods of clinical pelvimetry give valuable information on the size and shape of the pelvis and the x-ray pro-

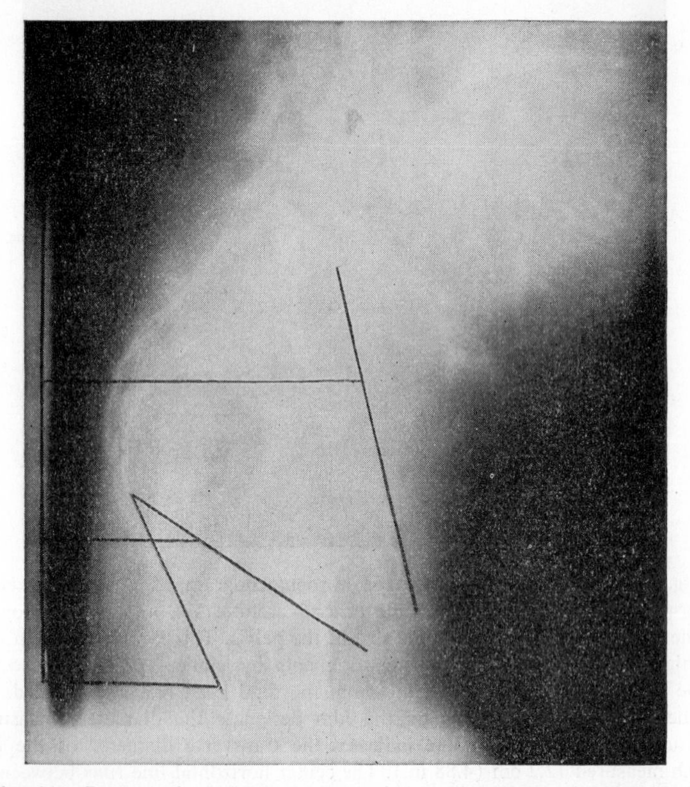

**Fig. 11.** Lateral view roentgenogram of the pelvis shown in Fig. 10. This x-ray was taken with the patient in an upright position, and shows that the head is engaged just within the pelvis. The oblique black lines designate the diameters measured. The anterior line is the A-P diameter of the pelvic inlet which measured 13.1 cm (5.24 in.); the center line indicates the A-P diameter of the midpelvis which measured 10.7 cm (4.28 in.); and the posterior line shows the posterior sagittal diameter which measured 7.8 cm (3.12 in.). (These measurements are the readings after the application of the correction factor.)

The conclusion that was drawn from the x-rays shown in Figs. 10 and 11 was that the pelvic diameters are adequate for the size of this baby and that if the woman delivers near the expected time there is no apparent reason for difficulty due to disproportion between the fetal head and the bony pelvis.

cedure involves some specialized technic and added expense. Roentgenograms are valuable, however, in all cases in whom pelvic contraction is suspected: when the ischial spines are prominent, the pubic arch is narrow, the sacral promontory is easily reached, or the diagonal conjugate measures below 11.5 cm (4.6 in.). It is also wise to use the findings of the x-ray in making a prognosis of labor when there is a history of previous difficult forceps delivery, cesarean section, or stillbirth; when the presentation is other than vertex; when the head does not engage in the pelvis in the primigravida at term; or when the head does not descend during labor.

Although the x-ray is very valuable in determining the size and shape of the pelvis it should be only one of several factors taken into consideration when a decision is made upon the method of delivery. All other clinical factors such as the presentation and position of the fetus, the size and moldability of the head, and the forces of labor are very important and will to a large extent determine the final outcome. The main purpose of x-ray pelvimetry, then, is to measure accurately the size of the pelvis, even those diameters which can be obtained with the pelvimeter, and to measure diameters which previously were not obtainable; however, it must be remembered that it subjects the baby in utero to some radiation exposure.

## CONTRACTED PELVES

A pelvis is considered contracted when one, or more, of its diameters is shortened enough to affect the mechanism of labor, but not necessarily the delivery of the baby. Delivery may be, and frequently is, accomplished through a pelvis which is not entirely normal in size or shape, but the obstetrician of today is closely observant of the patient whose pelvic measurements depart from the normal by more than the accepted margin of safety, and he plans for labor in accordance with the indications in each case. Disproportion between the measurements of the mother's pelvis and the size of the child's head must be considered in this connection. A small pelvis may permit of the spontaneous delivery of a small child, but be too small for the passage of a full-sized baby, while a woman with a normal pelvis may have an extremely difficult labor because of an unusually large child. In short it is a question of ascertaining whether or not the passage is large enough for the passenger.

A history of a previously normal delivery does not always indicate a normal pelvis, but a history of a difficult delivery should suggest the possibility of a contracted pelvis.

The size and shape of the pelvis is found to vary among different races, in different individuals, and with various pathologic and environmental conditions. Rickets or other nutritional diseases; congenital defects; diseases or trauma of the spine, the pelvis, or the lower extremities may considerably alter the size and contour of the pelvis. One readily sees the importance to the patient of having such variations discovered before labor begins.

The various kinds of abnormally small or contracted pelves may be classified as generally contracted; flat; funnel; generally contracted funnel; and the rachitic pelves, both flat and generally contracted. There may be a contracted inlet; a contracted midplane; or a contracted outlet; or any combination of these contractions may occur in the same pelvis.

In the generally contracted pelves all of the external measurements are shorter than normal, and the diagonal conjugate measures 11.5 cm (4.6 in.) or less. In simple flat pelves, on the other hand, the external measurements are normal, except Baudelocque's diameter, which is shortened, and the diagonal conjugate is 11 cm (4.4 in.) or less. These shortened measurements indicate contraction of the pelvic inlet.

If the distance between the tuberosities is only 8 cm (3.2 in.) or less, the patient has a pelvic outlet contraction (funnel pelvis). Whether or not delivery of the baby can safely take place through this narrowed outlet will depend upon the length of the posterior sagittal diameter. If the sum of the intertuberous and posterior sagittal diameters is below 15 cm (6 in.), difficulty may be anticipated. Since a contracted outlet is frequently accompanied by a midpelvic contraction the narrowed midpelvis may interfere with passage of the baby's head even before it reaches the contracted outlet. In order to discover midpelvic contraction x-ray pelvimetry is indicated whenever the intertuberous diameter is 8.5 cm (3.4 in.) or less.

Rachitic pelves are not frequent among white women, but are more common among Negro women. This greater frequency in the Negro race is due to the fact that a rachitic pelvis is one of the many manifestations of rickets, a disease of malnutrition that is more widespread among Negroes. The rachitic pelves present certain characteristic features; of these a peculiar deformity of the sacrum is the most characteristic abnormality. The concavity from above downward is markedly increased, in some cases almost forming an angle, while the horizontal concavity is nearly or almost obliterated. The commonest type of a rachitic pelvis is one in which all of the inlet measurements are shortened, the intertuberous distance normal, and the sacrum characteristically deformed. This is called the generally contracted, rachitic pelvis.

## FEMALE ORGANS OF REPRODUCTION

The female organs of reproduction are divided into two groups, the *internal* and the *external genitalia.* With them are usually considered certain other structures; the *ureters, bladder, urethra, rectum,* and the *perineum,* because of their close proximity, and the *breasts* because of their functional relation to the reproductive organs.

### INTERNAL GENITALIA

The internal organs of reproduction are contained in the true pelvic cavity and comprise the *uterus* and *vagina* in the center, an *ovary* and *fallopian tube* on each side, together with their various ligaments, membranes, nerves, lymph supply, and blood vessels and a certain amount of fat and connective tissue (Fig. 12).

The *uterus* is the largest of these organs (Fig. 12). In its nonpregnant state it is a hollow, flattened, pear-shaped organ about 7.5 cm (3 in.) long, 5 cm (2 in.) wide at its broadest point, 2.5 cm (1 in.) thick, and weighs about 60 gm (2 oz). It is made up of three layers: the serous, the muscular, and the mucous. Ordinarily it is a firm, hard mass, consisting of irregularly disposed, involuntary (nonstriated) muscle fibers, connective tissue, elastic fibers, nerves, and blood vessels. The *muscular,* or middle, layer makes up the largest part of the uterus. The arrangement of the uterine muscle fibers is unique, since they run up and down, around and crisscross, forming a veritable network. The contraction of these unusually arranged muscle fibers is the chief factor in preventing hemorrhage after delivery. The uterus is covered, front and back, by a fold of the *peritoneum* which is the *serous* layer, except along the lower part of the anterior wall where the peritoneum is reflected up over the bladder (Fig. 13). The *mucous* layer, which lines the uterine cavity, is a thick, velvety, highly vascular mucous membrane, the *endometrium,* the surface of which is covered with ciliated columnar epithelium.

Embedded in the endometrium are small tubular glands which project down from the surface and are known as *uterine glands*.

The uterus as a whole is comprised of two parts: the upper tri-

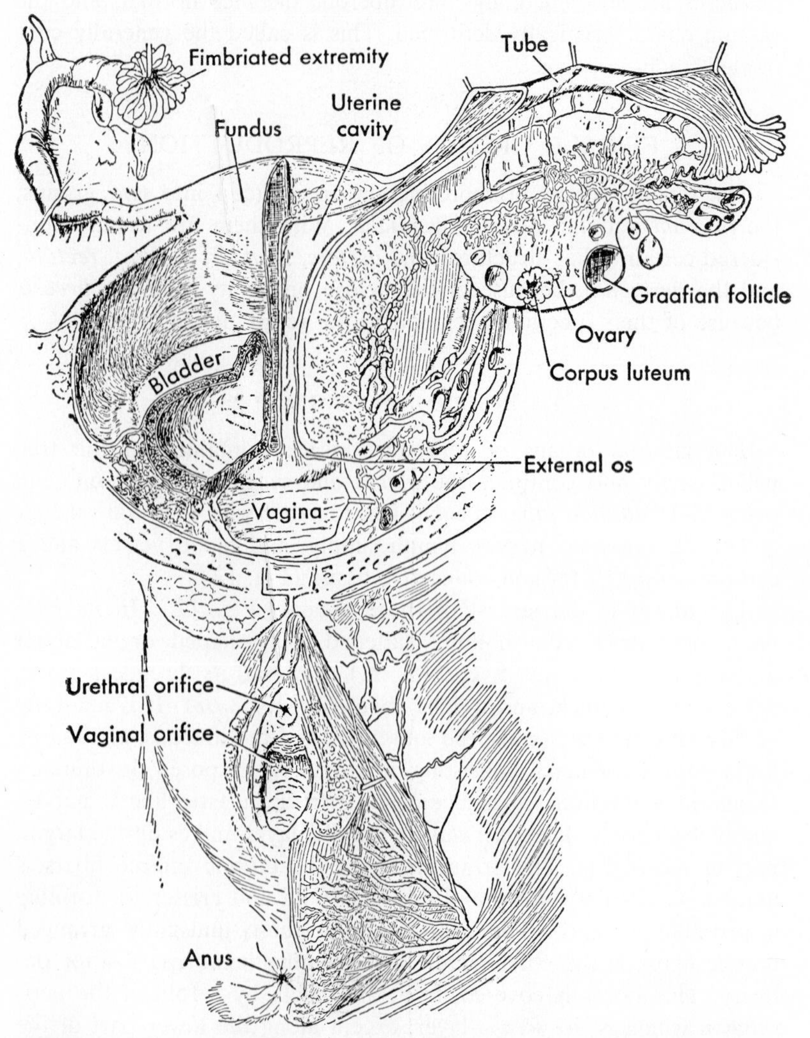


**Fig. 12.** Female reproductive tract, showing both external and internal organs. The internal organs are represented as laid out flat, parallel with the external organs. (Kimber, D.; Gray, C.; Stackpole, C.; and Leavell, L.: *Textbook of Anatomy and Physiology,* 13th ed. The Macmillan Company, New York, 1955.)

angular part known as the *corpus,* or *body,* and the lower cylindrical part called the *cervix*. The upper, rounded portion of the corpus between the points of insertion of the fallopian tubes is called the

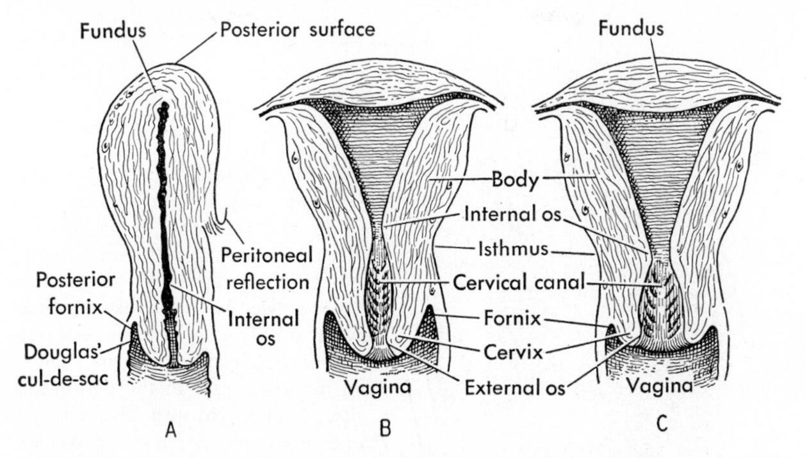


**Fig. 13.** Diagrams of sections of virgin and multigravidous uteri. (*A*) Anteroposterior section; (*B*) lateral section of a virgin uterus; and (*C*) lateral section of a multigravidous uterus.

Since Douglas' cul-de-sac lies behind the upper portion of the posterior wall of the vagina it is through the posterior fornix that pathology in the cul-de-sac can often be determined by palpation, by cul-de-sac puncture, or by insertion of a culdoscope for visualization.

*fundus uteri,* and the lower, narrowed portion where it meets the cervix is called the *isthmus* (Fig. 13). It is in the body and cervix that we find the long, narrow uterine cavity divided by a constriction into two parts. The cavity of the body is little more than a vertical slit, being so flattened from before backward that the anterior and posterior surfaces are nearly if not quite in contact. It is somewhat triangular in shape with an opening at each angle. The lower of these openings leads into the cavity of the cervix through a constriction termed the *internal os,* while at the *cornua,* or two upper angles, are the openings into the fallopian tubes (Fig. 13). Besides connective tissue and nonstriated muscle fibers the cervix contains elastic tissue which allows it to distend during childbirth.

The cervical canal is lined with a single layer of ciliated columnar epithelium and contains branching *racemose glands* which dip into the stroma of the cervix and secrete a thick mucus. The cavity of the cervix is spindle-shaped, being expanded between its two constricted openings, the internal os above and the *external os* below, which opens into the vagina (Fig. 13). The external os is a small round opening in the virgin, but has a ragged outline in women who

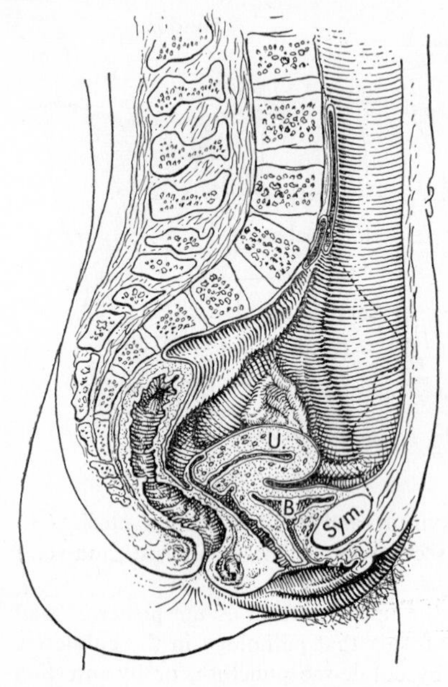


**Fig. 14.** Sagittal section through the female body showing the normal position and relation of the uterus, bladder, rectum, and abdominal walls. The dotted line represents the outline of the pelvic bones. This drawing shows that only a small layer of tissue separates the upper part of the vagina from the lower part of the peritoneal cavity. (Kelly, Howard A.: *Operative Gynecology,* courtesy of Appleton-Century-Crofts, Inc.; in Brady, L., et al.: *Essentials of Gynecology,* 2nd ed., The Macmillan Company, New York, 1949.)

have borne children and then appears as a small transverse opening which is bounded in front by the *anterior lip* and posteriorly by the *posterior lip* of the cervix.

The uterus has an excellent blood, lymph, and nerve supply. Its abundant blood supply merits a word. It is derived from the uterine arteries, arising from the internal iliacs, and the ovarian arteries from the aorta. The arteries from the two sides of the uterus are united by a branch where the neck and body of this organ meet, thus forming an encircling artery. A deep cervical tear during labor may break this vessel, and a profuse hemorrhage occur as a result.

This oblong, muscular body, the uterus, is suspended obliquely in the center of the pelvic cavity by means of ligaments. In its normal position the entire organ is curved slightly forward and the cervix points down and back. This position is affected by a distended bladder or rectum, and also by postural changes in the body as a whole. The cervix protrudes into the vagina for about 1.3 cm (½ in.) and almost at a right angle (Figs. 13 and 14).

The upper part of the uterus is held in position by means of ligaments, the lower part being embedded in fat and connective tissue between the bladder and the rectum. This more or less of a floating position makes possible the enormous increase in size and upward push or extension of the uterus during pregnancy. The pregnant uterus becomes soft and elastic as it grows. At term it is about 20 to 25 cm (8 to 10 in.) wide, 30 to 35 cm (12 to 14 in.) long from top to bottom, and reaches up to 2.5 cm (1 in.) from the sternum. This growth is due in part to the development of new muscle fibers and in part to a growth of the fibers already existing in the uterine wall. After labor the uterus returns almost, but never entirely, to its former size, shape, and general condition (Fig. 13).

**The fallopian (uterine) tubes** are two tortuous, muscular tubes, 7 to 14 cm (2.8 to 5.6 in.) long, extending laterally in an upward curve from the cornua of the uterus and within the folds of the upper margin of the *broad ligament* by which they are covered (Fig. 12). Through them the ova gain access to the uterine cavity. The part of the tube passing through the muscular wall of the uterus is known as the *uterine portion,* the *isthmus* is the part immediately adjoining the uterus, the *ampulla* is a wider lateral portion, and the wide outer funnel-shaped orifice, which opens directly into the peritoneal cavity, is called the *fimbriated end.* At their juncture with the uterus the diameter of these tubes is so small as to admit the introduction of only a fine bristle, but they gradually increase in size toward their termination. They sometimes contain diverticulae. Finger-like projections, called *fimbriae,* fringe the margins of these openings. The mucous lining of the tubes is covered with cilated epithelium.

Here it will be well to say a word about the peritoneum because of the possibility of its becoming infected during labor and the puerperium, and the very grave consequences of such infection. It is a delicate, highly vascular, serous membrane which both lines the abdominal cavity and covers the abdominal and pelvic organs, which press into its outer surface and are covered much as one's fingers would be covered by pushing them into the outer surface of a child's toy balloon. The continuity of this membrane is broken only where it is entered by the fallopian tubes.

**The ovaries,** the sex glands of the female, are small, tough, ductless glands 4 to 5 cm (1.6 to 2 in.) long and 2 cm (.8 in.) wide, or about the size and shape of an almond. They are dull white in color and present a more or less irregular, dimpled surface. An ovary is suspended on either side of the uterus, in the posterior fold of the broad ligament, by which it is partly covered (Fig. 12). The margin which is attached to the ligament is nearly straight and is called the *hilum*. The free margin is convex. The outer end of the ovary is usually attached to the longest of the fimbriated extremities of the fallopian tube, the *fimbria ovarica,* which has the form of a shallow gutter, or groove. The inner end is attached to the *ovarian ligament* which in turn is attached to the uterus below and behind the tubal entrance.

The ovary consists of two parts: the central part or *medulla,* composed of connective tissue, nerves, and blood and lymph vessels; and the *cortex,* in which are embedded both *primordial follicles* and vesicular *graafian follicles* containing the ova. At birth each ovary contains at least 100,000 of these ova, the germ cells concerned with reproduction.

The ovaries perform two vital functions: in addition to their prime function of producing and maturing the germinal cell of the female, they elaborate internal secretions which exercise an immeasurably important, though imperfectly understood, influence upon the general well-being of the entire organism and upon the reproductive organs in particular.

**The vagina** is an elastic, muscular canal, from 7 to 9 cm (2.8 to 3.6 in.) long, lying behind the bladder and urethra and in front of the rectum. It leads interiorly up and backward from the vulva to the cervix, which it encases for about 1.3 cm (½ in.) The space between the outer surface of the cervix that extends into the vagina and the surrounding vaginal walls is called the *fornix* (Fig. 13). For convenience of description, this is divided into four sections or fornices: the anterior, posterior, and the two lateral fornices. The posterior fornix is considerably deeper than the anterior because the vagina is about 2 cm (¾ in.) longer posteriorly than anteriorly and is attached higher up on the posterior wall of the cervix than on its anterior wall. Between the posterior wall of the vagina and the rectum a fold of the peritoneum drops down and forms a blind pouch in the peritoneal cavity, known as *Douglas' cul-de-sac* (Fig. 13). At this point the peritoneum is separated from the vagina by only a thin muscular wall.

The bore of the vaginal canal ordinarily permits of the introduction of one or two fingers. It is somewhat flattened from before backward, and on cross section resembles the letter H. Because of its remarkable elasticity this canal is capable of great dilatation, and accordingly during labor it is stretched into a tube 10 to 12.5 cm (4 to 5 in.) in diameter, which permits the passage of the full-term child.

The vagina possesses an abundant blood supply and is lined with a thick, heavy, mucous membrane which normally lies in small transverse folds or corrugations called *rugae* (Fig. 14). These folds are obliterated and the lining is stretched into a smooth surface as the canal dilates during labor. There are no glands in the vagina.

Attention must be drawn to the fact that the vagina, cervix, uterus, and tubes form a continuous canal from the vulva to the easily infected peritoneum, a fact which makes absolute asepsis in obstetrics essential in the prevention of peritoneal infection. This muscular tube is lined throughout its entire length with continuous mucous membrane. Along this variously constructed canal, at different periods in the life of the individual, pass the matured ovum, the menstrual flow, the uterine secretions, the fetus, the placenta, and the lochia (the discharge which occurs during the puerperium).

Although the bladder and rectum are not organs of reproduction, they are contained in the pelvic cavity and lie in such close proximity to the internal genitalia that at least a brief discussion of their description is indicated.

**The bladder** is a musculomembranous sac which serves as a reservoir for the urine and is situated behind the symphysis pubis and in front of the uterus and vagina (Fig. 14). Urine is conducted into the bladder by the *ureters,* two slender tubes running down on each side from the basin or pelvis of the kidney, across the brim of the bony pelvis, to the posterior part of the bladder, which they enter somewhat obliquely, at about the level of the cervix. It is thought that pressure of the enlarged pregnant uterus upon the ureters at this point may be one factor in the causation of pyelitis, sometimes a complication of pregnancy. The bladder empties itself through the *urethra,* a short tube about 3.8 cm (1½ in.) long which terminates in the *urinary meatus,* a tiny opening situated in the midline of the vestibule between the clitoris and the vaginal orifice.

**The rectum,** the lowest segment of the intestinal tract, is situated in the pelvic cavity behind and to the left of the uterus and vagina (Fig. 14). It extends downward from the sigmoid flexure of the colon to its termination in the anal opening. The anus is a deeply pigmented, puckered opening situated 3.8 to 5 cm (1½ to 2 in.) below the vaginal orifice. It is provided with bands of circular muscles, the *internal* and *external sphincter ani.* The normal contraction and relaxation of these muscles makes possible the retention and expulsion of the rectal contents. The skin covering the surface of the body extends upward into the anus where it becomes highly vascular and merges into the mucous lining of the rectum. Pressure exerted during pregnancy by the enlarged uterus is felt in both the rectum and bladder, frequently causing a good deal of discomfort and an almost painful desire to evacuate their contents.

The blood vessels in the anal lining just within the external sphincter sometimes become engorged and inflamed, even bleeding during pregnancy, as a result of the pressure exerted by the greatly enlarged uterus. The distended blood vessels, which are called hemorrhoids, not infrequently protrude from the anus and become very painful.

## UTERINE LIGAMENTS

After having considered the structure and relative positions of the pelvic organs, one is able to picture more clearly the arrangement and disposition of the *uterine ligaments,* all of which are formed by folds of the peritoneum. They are 12 in number, namely: two *broad,* two *cardinal,* two *round,* two *uterosacral,* one *anterior,* one *posterior,* and two *ovarian.*

**The broad ligaments** are in reality one continuous structure that is formed by a fold of the peritoneum, which drops down over the uterus, investing the fundus, body, part of the cervix, and part of the posterior wall of the vagina. It unites on each side of the uterus to form a broad, flat membrane which extends laterally to the pelvic wall, dividing the pelvic cavity into an anterior and posterior compartment, containing respectively the bladder and rectum. Between the folds of the broad ligament are situated the ovaries and ovarian ligaments, the fallopian tubes, the round ligaments, the cardinal ligaments, and a certain amount of muscle and connective tissue, blood vessels, lymphatics, and nerves.

**The cardinal ligaments,** one on each side, make up the lower borders of the broad ligament. They are bands of dense connective tissue which attach to the supravaginal part of the cervix and run to the lateral wall of the pelvis. These ligaments along with the pelvic diaphragm and the perineum keep the uterus from prolapsing by supporting it from below.

**The round ligaments,** one on each side, are narrow, flat bands of connective tissue, derived from the peritoneum, and muscle prolonged from the uterus, and contain blood and lymph vessels and nerves. They pass upward and forward from their uterine origin just below and in front of the tubal entrance, pass through the inguinal canal, and merge in the mons veneris and labia majora, which are described below.

**The uterosacral ligaments,** of which there is one on each side, arise in the uterus and, extending backward, serve to connect the cervix and vagina with the sacrum and aid in keeping the uterus in its normal position by exerting traction on the cervix.

**The anterior ligament** is a portion of the peritoneum which forms a fold between the bladder and the uterus.

**The posterior ligament** is formed in the same manner by a deep fold of peritoneum between the uterus and the rectum.

**The ovarian ligaments,** as previously described, are attached to the uterine wall and to the inner end of the ovary, one on each side.

## EXTERNAL GENITALIA

**The vulva,** or external genitalia, are situated in the *pudendal crease* which lies between the thighs at their junction with the torso, and extend posteriorly from the symphysis pubis to the anus (Fig. 15).

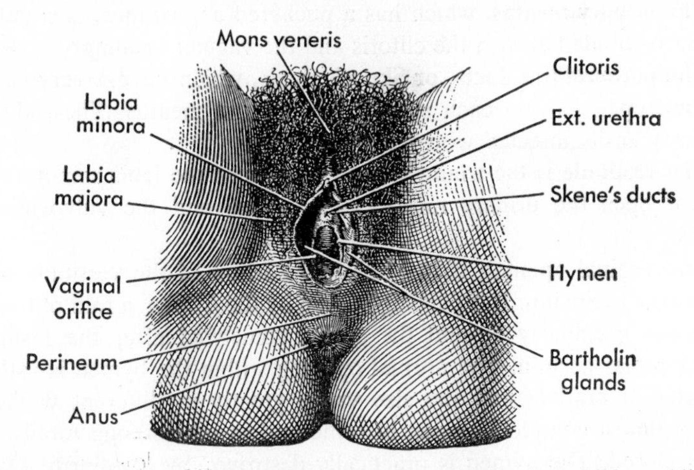


**Fig. 15.** The external genitalia of a woman who has had children. All that remains of the hymen are a few fleshy projections at the orifice of the vagina. (Brady, L.: Kurtz, E.: and McLaughlin, E.: *Essentials of Gynecology,* 2nd ed. The Macmillan Company, New York, 1949.)

**The mons veneris** is a firm cushion of fat and connective tissue, just over the symphysis pubis. It is covered with skin which contains many sebaceous glands and after puberty is abundantly covered with hair.

**The labia majora** are heavy ridges of fat and connective tissue, prolonged from the mons veneris and extended down to the perineum on each side, forming the lateral boundaries of the groove. They become narrower as they approach the perineum. On their inner surface they are moist and have a mucous-membrane appearance and on the outer aspect are covered with skin and hair, the latter growing thinner toward the perineum.

**The labia minora** are two small cutaneous folds lying between the labia majora on each side of the vestibule. Like the larger folds they taper toward the back and practically disappear into the vaginal wall. Their attentuated posterior ends are joined together behind the vaginal opening by means of a thin, flat fold called the *fourchette.* The labia minora divide for a short distance before joining at an angle in front, thus forming a double ridge anteriorly. The upper ridge, which forms a hood-like covering for the clitoris, is known as the *prepuce.*

**The clitoris,** a small sensitive projection composed of erectile tissue, nerves, and blood vessels, and covered with mucous membrane, is found in the depression between these ridges.

**The urinary meatus,** which has a puckered appearance, is situated in the vestibule between the clitoris and the vaginal opening.

**The paraurethral ducts, or Skene's ducts,** which have a very small caliber, open just on each side of the urethral meatus. These ducts are very easily infected with the gonococcus.

**The vestibule** is the triangular space between the labia minora and into it open the urinary meatus, the vagina, and the vulvovaginal glands.

**The vaginal opening** is in the lower portion of the vestibule and above the perineum. It is partially closed by the *hymen,* a fold of tissue disposed irregularly around the outlet, somewhat after the fashion of a circular curtain. The normal opening within the hymen is rather circular in outline, and the size varies greatly in different women, being almost completely open in some and in others congenitally almost closed. The hymen is practically destroyed by childbirth.

**The fossa navicularis** is a depressed space between the hymen and fourchette, so named because of its boat-like shape.

**The Bartholin glands,** probably the largest and most important of the vulvovaginal glands, are situated one on each side of the vagina and open just outside its lateral margins. These are mucous-secreting glands. An infection of these glands may occur and may lead to a gland abscess or cyst formation.

**The perineum** is a pyramidal structure of connective tissue, fascia, and muscle which occupies the space between the rectum and vagina, and by forming the floor of the pelvis serves as a support for the pelvic organs. The lower and outer surface of this mass, representing the base of the pyramid, lies between the vaginal opening and the anus and is covered with skin. As the anterior part of the perineum is incorporated in the posterior wall of the vagina, the entire structure becomes stretched and flattened when the vagina is dilated during labor by the passage of the child's head. Unless very carefully guarded at the time of delivery, and often even then, the perineum gives way under the great tension undergone at that time, and a tear is the result. The injury may be only a slight nick in the mucous membrane which is termed a first-degree tear; it may extend to the *levator ani,* the most important muscle of the perineal body, and is then termed a second-degree tear; or it may extend all the way through the perineum and completely through the sphincter ani, resulting in a third-degree or complete tear. Such a tear, which breaks the continuity of the ring-shaped sphincter muscle surrounding the anal opening, results in loss of bowel control unless it is repaired. In order to prevent tearing and to facilitate the birth of the baby the perineum is often cut at the time of delivery. A cut or an injury of any extent must be repaired to re-establish the sling-like support to the pelvic floor that this structure provides.

## BREASTS

The breasts are large, specially modified skin glands of the compound racemose or grape-cluster type, embedded in fat and connective tissue and abundantly supplied with nerves and blood vessels. They are situated quite remotely from the pelvic organs, but because of the intimate functional relation between the two, the breasts of the female may be regarded as accessory glands of the reproductive system. They exist in the male, also, but only in a rudimentary state.

Although the breasts sometimes contain milk during infancy, their true function is to secrete, in the parturient woman, suitable nourishment for the human infant during the first months of its life.

These glands are symmetrically placed, one on each side of the chest, and occupy the space between the second and sixth ribs, extending from the margin of the sternum almost to the midaxillary line. A bed of connective tissue separates them from the underlying muscles and the ribs (Fig. 16). They vary in size and shape at different ages, and with different individuals, particularly in women who have borne and nursed children, when they tend to become pendulous. But in general they are hemispherical or conical in shape with the nipple protruding from .6 to 1.3 cm (¼ to ½ in.) from the apex. The nipples are composed largely of sensitive, erectile tissue and become more rigid and prominent during pregnancy and at the menstrual periods. Their surfaces are pierced by the orifices of the milk ducts, which are 15 to 20 in number (Fig. 17).

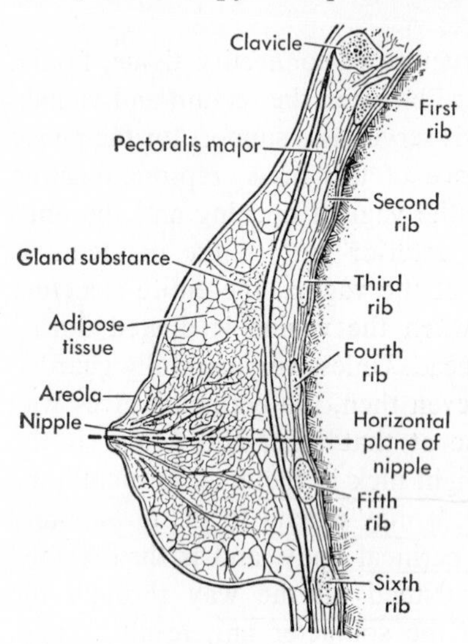


**Fig. 16.** Right breast in sagittal section, inner surface of outer segment. (Gerrish.) (Kimber, D.; Gray, C.; Stackpole, C.; and Leavell, L.: *Textbook of Anatomy and Physiology,* 13th ed. The Macmillan Company, New York, 1955.)

The breasts are covered with very delicate, smooth, white skin, excepting for the *areolae,* those circular, pigmented areas 2.5 to 10 cm (1 to 4 in.) in diameter, which surround the nipples. The areolae are darker in brunettes than in blonds, and in all women grow darker during pregnancy, gradually becoming paler after labor. The surface of the nipples and of the areolae is roughed by small, shot-like lumps or papillae known as the *tubercles of Montgomery* (Fig. 17). This roughness becomes more marked during pregnancy, since the papillae then grow larger. These tubercles are sebaceous glands that secrete a lipoid material which lubricates the nipples and thus helps to protect them during nursing.

The secretory apparatus of the breasts is divided into 15 to 20 lobes, these in turn being divided into clusters of lobules. The lobules in turn are composed of a collection of circularly arranged secreting cells about a small duct, this structure constituting an *acinus,* in which

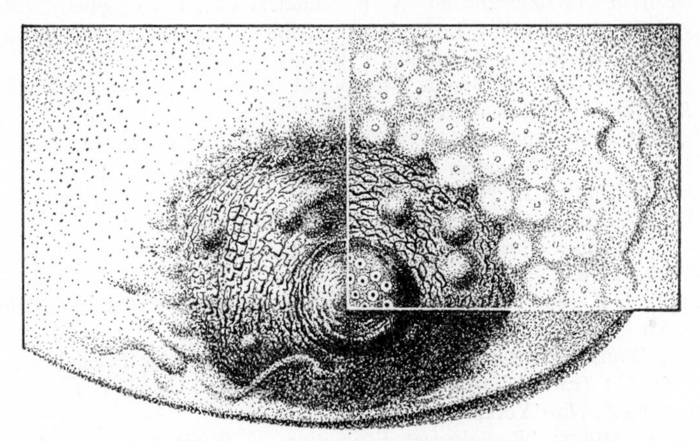

**Fig. 17.** Front view of breast showing areola, tubercles of Montgomery, and orifices of milk ducts.

the milk is elaborated from the blood. Tiny ducts carry the milk from the acini to the main duct of the lobule, around which the acini cluster. These ducts empty the milk into the larger duct of the lobe, which runs straight to the nipple and opens upon the surface. Just before reaching the surface, each of these lactiferous sinuses expands into an *ampulla,* a minute reservoir for collecting the milk, which is secreted during the periods between nursings.

These clusters of acini, uniting to form lobules with tiny ducts leading into the main duct of each lobule, closely resemble a bunch of grapes. The separate grapes correspond to the acini, their small stems correspond to the tiny ducts of the glands which lead to a larger one, and the central stem of the grape cluster, to the milk duct that opens upon the nipple.

The secretory tissue really constitutes a small part of the breasts until they begin to function, but during lactation the acini become enormously developed and enlarged. After lactation ceases the secreting tissues of the breast atrophy markedly.

## BIBLIOGRAPHY AND STUDENT REFERENCES

Bookmiller, Mae M., and Bowen, George L.: *Textbook of Obstetrics and Obstetric Nursing,* 2nd ed. W. B. Saunders Co., Philadelphia, 1954.

Brady, Leo; Kurtz, Ethna L.; and McLaughlin, Eileen: *Essentials of Gynecology,* 2nd ed. The Macmillan Company, New York, 1949.

Curry, Robert W.: "A Simple Method of Roentgen Pelvimetry," *Am. J. Roentgenol.,* **69**:638–46, (Apr.) 1953.

Davis, M. Edward, and Sheckler, Catherine E.: *DeLee's Obstetrics for Nurses,* 15th ed. W. B. Saunders Co., Philadelphia, 1951.

Eastman, Nicholson J.: "Pelvic Mensuration: A Study in the Perpetuation of Error," *Obst. & Gynec. Surv.,* **3**:301–29, (June) 1948.

———: *Williams Obstetrics,* 11th ed. Appleton-Century-Crofts, Inc., New York, 1956.

Greenhill, J. P. (ed.): *Obstetrics,* 11th ed. W. B. Saunders Co., Philadelphia, 1955.

Kimber, Diana C.; Gray, Carolyn E.; Stackpole, Caroline E.; and Leavell, Lutie C.: *Textbook of Anatomy and Physiology,* 13th ed. The Macmillan Company, New York, 1955.

Weinberg, Arthur: "Radiological Estimation of Pelvic Capacity," *Obst. & Gynec. Surv.,* **7**:455–81, (Aug.) 1952.

Woodward, H. L.; Gardner, B.; Bryant, R. D.; and Overland, Anna E.: *Obstetric Management and Nursing,* 5th ed. F. A. Davis Co., Philadelphia, 1955.

Zabriskie, Louise, and Eastman, Nicholson J.: *Nurses Handbook of Obstetrics,* 9th ed. J. B. Lippincott Co., Philadelphia, 1952.

*Chapter 2*

# Physiology of the Female Reproductive Organs

## PUBERTY

Puberty is that period during which childhood develops into sexual maturity, and the individual becomes capable of reproduction. The age at which puberty occurs varies greatly even in individuals of the same status. The more the subject is studied the less significance is attached to such influences as race and climate. Individual factors such as environment, social status, nutrition, and general health appear to be the most important factors. Although the entire process of puberty is rather gradual, the first menstrual period is commonly accepted as evidence of sexual maturity or puberty. It is found that 13 years is the average age at which the first menstruation occurs among girls in the United States. Boys usually mature between the ages of 12 and 16.

At this time there are many physical and psychic manifestations of the maturing changes in the internal female reproductive organs. The undeveloped girl grows rapidly at this stage. Her entire body rounds out and assumes a more graceful contour, her breasts increase in size, her hips broaden, the external genitalia enlarge, and hair appears on the external genitalia and in the axillae. As this physical maturity progresses, there is a developing sex consciousness, and the maturing girl becomes shy, modest, retiring, and introspective. She is very likely to be emotional and to display a lack of stability and nervous control which are not in accord with her usual temperament. A formerly dependable child may become capricious, erratic, and perplexingly inconsistent. One day she may be quite her normal, little-girl self and the next show inexplicably mature qualities; or she may display a bewildering number of moods and fancies in the span of one short day.

Too much cannot be said of the importance of wise supervision and guidance of the girl's physical, mental, and emotional life at this critical period. Many gynecologic, obstetric, and emotional difficulties in her later life may be averted by understanding and wise guidance of her physical and mental health needs.

Vigorous and regular out-of-door exercise; a simple, nourishing, and well-balanced diet; adequate sleep in a well-ventilated room; regular bathing; and correction of any discoverable physical defects are essential.

Of equal, or even greater, importance is an understanding and sympathetic oversight of the girl's mental and emotional life, a steadying sort of comradeship. Her extreme sensitiveness and impressionability should be recognized and borne in mind, and every effort made to save her from strain and shock. Her nervous forces should be sedulously conserved by protecting her against experiences which would be unduly stimulating or irritating; nor should demands be made upon her uncertain nervous endurance which she is able to meet only by great strain, if at all. It is important to her future poise and health that her confidence be courted and, when it is won, that all of her outpourings be received with a respect and seriousness commensurate with their great importance to her. Ridicule or even unresponsiveness or indifference to her interests may, and often do, result in a harmful repression of one form or another. The logical consequence of such repression is an increasingly damaging neurosis later on in her life, capable of greatly impairing her health, happiness, and usefulness. In short, all phases of the life of the adolescent girl should be made as wholesome, tranquil, and free from stress and strain as is possible. This must not, however, be done by protection from all frustrating experiences, but rather by offering intelligent support and guidance through such experiences in order to give ample opportunity for emotional growth.

These comments upon the importance of mental hygiene at puberty may seem irrelevant to a discussion of obstetric nursing. But the preparation of the entire female organism for its supreme function—

that of childbearing—is of concern to the obstetric nurse and should be understood by her. Moreover, every nurse is inevitably a health teacher, either by precept or example, or both. An awareness on her part of the maturing girl's needs will fit her to help many perplexed mothers of girls to a happy solution of their grave and important problem.

The occurrence of puberty marks the establishment of *ovulation* and *menstruation.* These two functions are usually performed once a month, except during the first year or two after menstruation begins, when it may occur irregularly, with several months of amenorrhea, and may not always be preceded by ovulation.

## OVARIAN CYCLE

**Primordial Follicle.** The formation of each woman's full quota of ova is complete before birth. These *primary* or *primordial oöcytes,* as they are called, are single cells scattered throughout the connective tissue of the ovary. As the ovary continues to develop, these ova are surrounded by a single layer of flattened cells and they are then called *primordial follicles* (Fig. 18). It is estimated that at birth each ovary contains at least 100,000 primordial follicles closely packed together and separated by thin bands of connective tissue, but many of these ova disappear in early life by an atretic process, so that perhaps only 30,000 to 40,000 are present in each ovary when puberty is reached. The remaining ova continue to disappear during the fertile period. At birth the ovary is largely cortex, but the cortex becomes thinner and thinner with advancing years and the disappearance of the ova.

**Graafian Follicle.** The primordial follicles are constantly in the process of development from birth until the end of sexual life, although they rarely rupture before puberty. Whenever a follicle begins to mature, remarkable changes take place in both the surrounding cells and the enclosed ovum (Fig. 18). The cells which surround the egg change in character and proliferate rapidly, with the result that the ovum is surrounded by several layers of epithelial cells instead of one. Some of the inner cells degenerate and liquefy, and the fluid formed by this degeneration of cells plus some exudate from surrounding vessels fills the cavity of the follicle and surrounds the ovum. This fluid, known as *liquor folliculi,* contains the ovarian follicular hormone known as *estrogen.* This endocrine secretion is responsible for the growth and development of the reproductive organs, the development of the female secondary sexual characteristics, and the proliferation of the endometrium during the first stages of the menstrual cycle (Fig. 18). The epithelium surrounding the follicle which has not degenerated and now encloses the ovum and liquor folliculi is still of several-layers' thickness and is known as the *membrana granulosa.*

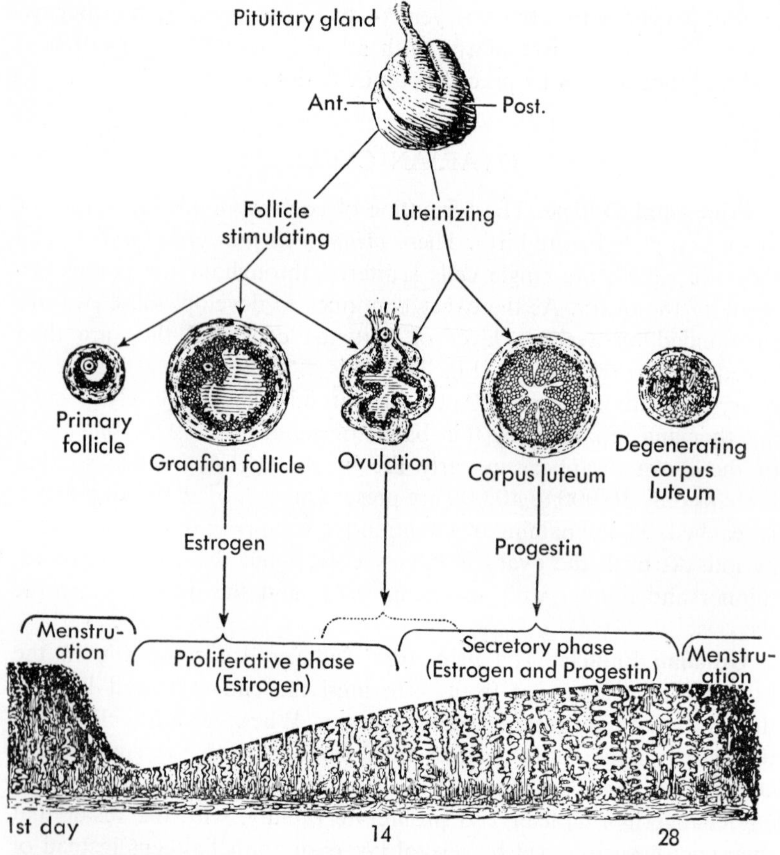


**Fig. 18.** Diagram showing phases of menstruation and the relationship of menstruation to ovulation. This also shows how the anterior lobe of the pituitary gland indirectly controls menstruation through its hormones acting on the ovaries. (Brady, L.; Kurtz, E.; and McLaughlin, E.: *Essentials of Gynecology,* 2nd ed. The Macmillan Company, New York, 1949.)

The ovum is pushed to one side of the follicle, and at one point in the enveloping membrana granulosa the cells proliferate into a pyramidal mass in which the ovum is included. Surrounding the membrana granulosa is a connective-tissue covering, the *theca folliculi,* which is formed from the stroma surrounding the primordial follicle, and this serves as the outermost layer of the matured follicle. As soon as the primordial follicle begins to develop, the cells surrounding it increase

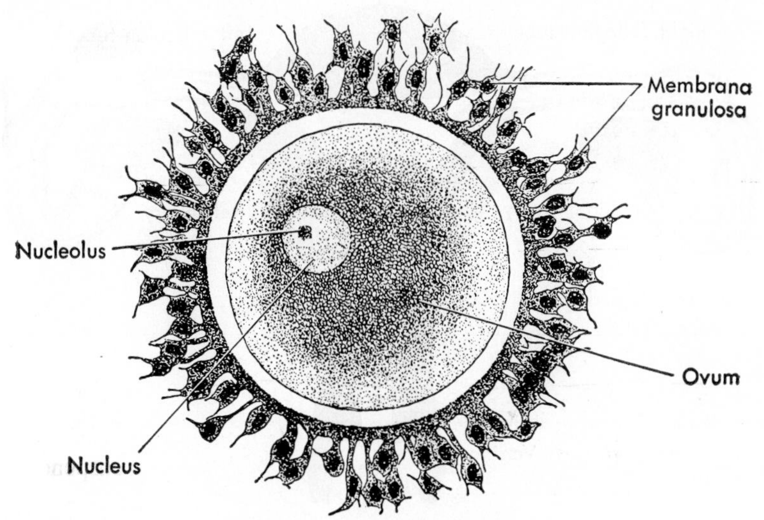


**Fig. 19.** Diagram of human ovum.

in number and size, and develop a granular appearance due to fat and a yellow pigment. These cells, known as *theca lutein cells,* are important in the degeneration of follicles which do not rupture. The structures described above constitute a *graafian follicle,* named for Dr. DeGraaf who first described it, which in the course of its maturation expands toward the surface of the ovary where it presents more or less the appearance of a clear blister. When fully developed and about to rupture, this blister-like protrusion on the surface of the ovary measures about 1 cm (roughly ½ in.) in diameter.

While these changes are going on in the follicle, the *ovum* itself has increased in size until it has become the largest single cell in the entire body, measuring about ⅕ mm in diameter. The mature ovum differs from the primordial ovum by its increase in size and by the presence of yolk granules, known as *deutoplasm,* which push the nucleus to one side. The nucleus undergoes changes and prepares for the formation of a polar body, and the nucleolus also increases greatly in size (Fig. 19).

Usually, for some strange reason, one and only one ovum ripens regularly each month during the years from puberty to the meno-

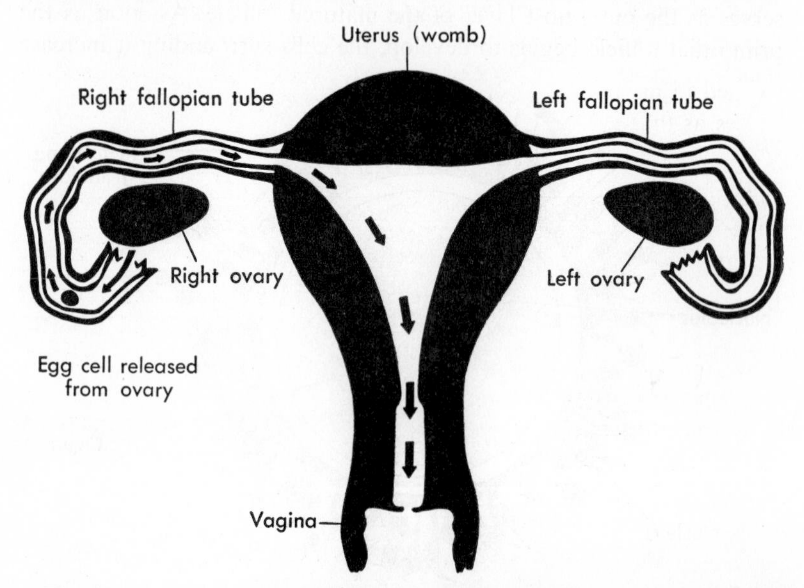


**Fig. 20.** Menstrual physiology. (Printed by permission of the makers of Modess.)

pause, excepting during pregnancy, when this function is suspended. Occasionally, however, more than one ovum matures at the same time, double-ovum twins resulting from double ovulation and triple-ovum triplets from triple ovulation.

**Ovulation.** When a graafian follicle, containing a matured ovum, reaches the surface of the ovary, its wall becomes thinner and finally it ruptures and its contents are gradually extruded. The ovum in this state, with some adherent epithelial cells, is discharged into the peritoneal cavity near the fimbriated end of the tube where it may enter the opening of the nearby tube or float about in the peritoneal cavity (Figs. 12 and 20). In the latter case, it may enter the tube on the opposite side of the body or disintegrate and be absorbed. This process of extrusion of the mature ovum from the ovary through the rupture of a graafian follicle is called *ovulation.*

Ovulation apparently occurs in most cases between the twelfth and sixteenth days after the onset of the previous menstrual period. Human ova have been recovered from the fallopian tubes at this time; a fact which fits in satisfactorily with the fertility curve. It has been found that conception is likely to occur anywhere between the eighth and twentieth days after the onset of the previous menstruation, the twenty-first to twenty-eighth days being relatively sterile. In cycles that vary from the average 28-day cycle the postovulatory period tends toward a fairly uniform length of 14 to 16 days while the preovulatory period is more variable. Various attempts have been made to estimate by some indirect way the exact time of ovulation. One of these methods, which is often employed in cases of sterility, is to carefully record the basal body temperature each day. The woman is instructed to take her temperature rectally each morning before arising. There is a rather abrupt rise in body temperature of 0.6 to 0.8° F (0.16 to 0.27° C) immediately after ovulation; the temperature then remains at this higher level until just before the next menstrual period when it again drops.

**Corpus Luteum.** The torn wall of the follicle which remains in the cortex of the ovary after extrusion of the ovum becomes filled with clotted blood. This clot is surrounded by some of the granulosa cells which continue to adhere to the follicle wall after ovulation. These granulosa cells grow in size and number and assume a yellowish tint. They are now called *lutein cells*. These lutein, or yellow, cells, as the Latin name implies, invade the follicle to form a solid mass of cells and to push the blood clot to the center. The ruptured follicle has now become the *corpus luteum* (Figs. 12 and 18). Connective tissue arising from the theca folliculi grows into the follicle between the lutein cells.

The corpus luteum reaches its greatest development in about 10 days after rupture of the follicle. It is then larger than the original follicle, measuring from 10 to 20 mm in diameter. It produces a hormone known as *progestin* or *progesterone* (Fig. 18), which prepares the endometrium for implantation and nourishment of a fertilized ovum, suppresses ovulation during pregnancy and lactation, and relaxes the smooth muscle of the uterus. Although progesterone is the main hormone, some estrogenic substance is also elaborated by the corpus luteum.

If the discharged ovum becomes fertilized, the corpus luteum continues to develop and may occupy as much as one-third or even one-half of the ovary. It is then termed the *corpus luteum of pregnancy,* or the *true corpus luteum,* and continues to exist throughout pregnancy and until after delivery when it is soon absorbed and replaced by normal ovarian tissue. Despite the fact that the corpus luteum persists throughout pregnancy, its important activity seems to be confined to the first three months, since, after this time, some retrogessive changes take place and pregnancy will proceed normally even though both ovaries are removed. Some observations have demonstrated that pregnancy may continue normally even if the ovary which contains the corpus luteum must be removed after the first month of pregnancy; the placenta then elaborates hormones which take over the function of the corpus luteum.

If fertilization does not occur, the corpus luteum in the ovarian cortex, which is then termed the *corpus luteum of menstruation* or *false corpus luteum,* undergoes rapid degenerative changes and is almost wholly absorbed within a few weeks. By means of a rather complicated procedure of absorption the ovary is saved from becoming a steadily enlarging mass of scar tissue, and consequently devoid of reproductive powers, which would be the case if the wound made by the rupturing of each graafian follicle were to heal by the usual formation of scar tissue.

**Follicular Atresia.** The very large number of ova that do not mature disappear by means of a process termed *atresia.* Many of the follicles develop to a certain stage but do not fully mature and rupture. When partially grown there occur within the follicles the atretic changes that cause complete dissolution and final disappearance of the cells. The membrana granulosa degenerates, is cast off into the liquor folliculi, and is eventually absorbed. The ovum undergoes cytolysis. The theca lutein cells proliferate and form many layers around the follicle. When the fluid in the follicle has been absorbed it collapses, the theca lutein cells undergo changes, and the whole structure appears much like a corpus luteum which has undergone certain degenerative changes. The follicle is then finally replaced by new connective tissue. This atretic process goes on from intrauterine life of the individual until the menopause and is particularly active before puberty and during pregnancy.

The reason for nature's lavish provision of at least 100,000 ova for each woman who uses only a few hundred in the course of her life is not known. But whatever the purpose of this enormous supply, its presence makes possible the removal of all but a small fragment of ovarian tissue, in case of disease, since between one-fifth and one-eighth of the amount of ovarian tissue normally present is sufficient to preserve the reproductive capacity providing the remaining tissue is normal.

## MENSTRUATION

**Menstruation,** which is the evidence of sexual maturity, is a periodic discharge of blood from the uterus which escapes through the vagina, normally recurring throughout the entire childbearing period, except during pregnancy and lactation. The duration of this childbearing period, or sexual activity, is about 30 years and continues from puberty to the menopause.

The frequency of the menstrual period varies in different women from 21 to 32 days, but the normal interval between periods is usually considered to be 28 days. There are many variations from this, not only in different women, but also in the individual person. The time elapsing between the beginning of one menstrual period to the be-gining of the next is called the *menstrual cycle.* Since it is usually four weeks, or a lunar month, from the beginning of one period to the beginning of the next, there are usually 13 menstrual periods during each calendar year.

Menstruation cannot be considered an entirely pelvic phenomenon since it is quite clear that the pituitary gland plays an important role in stimulating the production of hormones in the ovary which in turn stimulate the endometrium. The anterior lobe of the pituitary gland produces two hormones which stimulate the ovary, the *follicle-stimulating hormone* and the *luteinizing hormone,* known as *gonadotropic hormones* (Fig. 18). The follicle-stimulating hormone is responsible for the development of the graafian follicle and thereby makes possible the production of estrogen, and the luteinizing hormone, which appears shortly before ovulation, stimulates the development of the corpus luteum and thus the production of progesterone. The interaction of the two gonadotropic principles and the two ovarian hormones produces the changes which occur in the endometrium during the menstrual cycle (Fig. 18).

The menstrual cycle is usually divided into four stages: the *postmenstrual,* the *interval,* the *premenstrual,* and the *menstrual.* The first two phases, which are the proliferative phases of the endometrium, coincide with the period of development of the graafian follicle and its hormone estrogen, and the last two phases, sometimes known as the secretory phases, occur after ovulation and are under the influence of the corpus luteum hormone, progesterone (Fig. 18).

**The postmenstrual phase** is the stage which immediately follows a menstrual period and lasts from four to five days. At the beginning of this phase the endometrium is from 1 to 2 mm thick; the glands are straight, narrow, and collapsed; and the surface and the glandular epithelium are cuboidal. At the end of this phase there is some increase in the height of the endometrium and a change from cuboidal to columnar epithelium.

**The interval phase,** which lasts approximately 10 days, is manifested by a great increase in thickness of the endometrium, by more abundant and more vascular stroma, and by an increase in the size of the uterine glands. Toward the latter part of this phase there is some evidence of glandular secretion.

The changes described in the above two phases, which represent the proliferative period, occur after the completion of a menstrual period when the follicles, which have been held in abeyance by progesterone from the corpus luteum of the previous cycle, are released from the inhibition due to retrogression of the corpus luteum. They begin to develop and mature under the influence of the follicle-stimulating hormone which is given off in increasing amounts by the anterior pituitary gland. As these follicles grow and develop they give off increasing amounts of estrogen which produces the growth of the endometrium described in these first two phases and is manifested by increased thickness and vascularity of the mucosa and increased size and tortuosity of the glands. Usually only one of the follicles which begins to develop reaches complete maturity.

Ovulation takes place when maturity is reached. This usually occurs at about the middle of the menstrual cycle. After ovulation the luteinizing gonadotropic hormone becomes dominant and stimulates the development of the corpus luteum which then produces progesterone and some estrogen. The changes described in the premenstrual, or secretory, phase now take place under the influence of the progesterone.

**The premenstrual phase** is of approximately 10-days' duration. The endometrium now measures from 4 to 6 mm in thickness and it is soft, velvety, and edematous; the glands become wide and tortuous; and the nuclei of the glandular cells recede to the base of the cell. These glands now contain large quantities of glycogen. The blood vessels, especially the coiled arterioles, become more conspicuous. Toward the end of this phase the degenerative changes which precede menstruation begin to occur.

All this preparation of the endometrium is for the reception of a fertilized ovum. If pregnancy occurs the corpus luteum continues to function, and the endometrium continues to develop into the decidua of pregnancy; but if the ovum remains unfertilized, which is usually the case, it does not attach itself to this elaborately prepared lining, but passes out with the uterine discharges.

**The menstrual phase,** which lasts from four to five days, is the period during which the newly developed tissues are sloughed off and the menstrual discharge occurs (Fig. 18). About four days before this phase starts, the corpus luteum begins to retrogress, and, due to the withdrawal of its hormones, retrogressive changes begin to take place in the endometrium. This results in stasis of the coiled arterioles with prolonged spasm of these arterioles. Because of this vasoconstriction the endometrium around the arterioles degenerates, and bleeding and desquamation of tissue occur in numerous areas. Tissue loss and bleeding are usually scant on the first day, increase in amount on the second day, and then diminish steadily until cessation. There is usually desquamation of the entire upper layer of the endometrium. Regeneration takes place in the lower layer and in the gland stumps even before desquamation is complete. It will be seen that the duration of the menstrual period is about five days, but it is entirely within normal bounds if it varies in length from two to seven days.

The menstrual discharge is a dark red color and consists of blood, fragments of endometrium, mucus, and bacteria. It does not coagulate. The normal, rather offensive, odor of the discharge is due to decomposition of the blood and also to the increased secretions of the sebaceous glands of the vulva.

The average amount of blood loss is from 30 to 60 ml (1 to 2 oz), but it varies greatly among women who are otherwise normal and in good health. Some women lose so little blood that they are scarcely aware of their menses. Others lose what appears to be a large quantity at each period without suffering any ill effect. Since the discharge is greatly diluted by secretions from the uterine glands, the amount of blood lost is less than it appears. The quantity may be affected by living conditions or by mental or physical excitement or stimulation.

A shock or great grief, any severe emotional experience, or a long trip may bring on a period before it is due, while the regularity of the periods may be much disturbed, temporarily, by a marked change of climate or altitude, a serious illness, or a decided change in one's daily regime. The function may be entirely suspended for several months or a year in women who suddenly take up hard work or begin a new occupation and persist with it regularly. In such cases the periods gradually recur and finally become normal and regular.

The menstrual period may be preceded and attended by a certain amount of *mental and physical disturbance.* Premonitory signs, such as abdominal distention, headache, backache, breast fullness, a state of depression or of anxiety, all of which are grouped together under the term of premenstrual tension, are frequently noticed a few days before bleeding begins. While the average woman may notice little or no change during menstruation there are many who, though in good health in other respects, are more or less uncomfortable at this time. They may be tired and may have less endurance and resistance than usual. Headaches, with a sense of fullness, dizziness, and heaviness are common accompaniments. Backache is a frequent source of distress. Abdominal discomfort may vary from an uncomfortable sense of dragging heaviness to rather severe pain. There may be pain in the hips and thighs as well. This discomfort is sometimes increased by a loss of appetite, nausea, and even vomiting. At the same time there are changes in the breasts which are much the same as, though slighter than, those occurring during pregnancy. They are firmer and may be somewhat increased in size, and many women experience a burning, tingling sensation, soreness, and even pain. The nipples are turgid and prominent, and the pigmented areas grow darker for the time being. The skin over the rest of the body sometimes changes in appearance, circles under the eyes and pimples being common; some women are pale and others are flushed during their periods. Slight bladder irritability and a tendency to constipation are sometimes noted.

In addition to the physical discomfort which may be coincident with menstruation, there are sometimes evidences of mental and nervous instability. These often show themselves in the form of irritability, in lack of poise and control, and in a state of depression or a state of tension. Drowsiness and mental sluggishness are not uncommon.

These disturbances accompanying menstruation vary so widely in different women, and in the same woman at different times and under different conditions, that it is not possible to draw a classical picture, but all of the symptoms described above will persist with more or less severity throughout the entire menstrual life of one woman, while perhaps only one or two of them will occasionally disturb another. Whatever discomfort there may be usually begins from one day to a week before the discharge appears, is at its height during the following day, and from that time subsides steadily, until the normally comfortable state is regained. In fact, many women feel better at the end of their menstrual period and during the days immediately following than at any other time during the cycle.

An understanding of the premenstrual tension is essential to good *mental hygiene. Physical hygiene* during menstruation is not necessarily different from the ordinary daily hygiene. Frequent bathing and frequent changes of the perineal pads are necessary. The vaginal tampon has become increasingly popular during the past few years, due to certain advantages over the perineal pad, and in most instances there is no objection to its use. The tampon is comfortable, does not cause irritation to the vaginal mucous membrane, and does not interfere with the flow of the blood from the uterine cavity. Its use eliminates the bulk and irritation of the external pad and overcomes the problem of odor accompanying the menstrual flow, since the menstrual discharge is almost entirely odorless unless it is exposed to the air. Exercise in moderation and all other normal activities may be carried on as usual.

Heat applied to the abdomen and lumbar region during the period of discomfort and warm baths, rest and quiet, and good posture will usually give great relief, as might be expected when there is local congestion and general nervous irritability. In this connection it is worth mentioning that the discomfort of some women is needlessly increased by their heeding the widespread, but fallacious, belief that bathing during menstruation is injurious. Warm baths at this time, as at any other, are usually restful and soothing, and there is no known reason why they should not be taken. Cold bathing is not advisable during painful menstruation simply because it may increase the discomfort. The general tendency is to get away from the influence of old-wives' tales concerning menstruation and to regard this occurrence as a normal physiologic process. A healthy mental attitude reduces the discomforts of menstruation. Abnormalities require attention, but under ordinary conditions it is seldom necessary to depart markedly from one's usual mode of living. Aside from other considerations it is of obstetric importance for a woman to ascertain if the cause of her discomfort is due to an anomaly or disease of the pelvic organs, since an abnormality may also be causing sterility or if conception does take place, it may later be a cause of an interrupted pregnancy.

### IRREGULARITIES OF MENSTRUATION

**Dysmenorrhea** is painful menstruation.

**Menorrhagia** is an abnormally copious menstrual flow.

**Metrorrhagia** is bleeding between the menstrual periods.

**Amenorrhea** is absence of menstruation. The commonest causes are pregnancy, lactation, and endocrine disturbances, especially those associated with obesity.

## MENOPAUSE

**The menopause,** also termed the climacteric and "change of life," is the period of life at which ovarian function stops and menstruation ceases permanently. It occurs ordinarily between the ages of 45 and 50. There is a wide variation, however, in the time at which the menopause may occur, and in some women menstruation normally ceases before the age of 45 while in others it continues until after the age of 50. Just as puberty is a normal developmental process during which ovarian activity begins, so the menopause is a normal retrogressive change in which there is a physiologic cessation of ovarian activity. It is at this time that the childbearing period ends. Menstrual periods may stop suddenly, but this "change of life" is more apt to be a gradual process in which periods of fairly regular menstrual cycles alternate with periods of amenorrhea. Although the term menopause, which means cessation of menstruation, is commonly applied to this period of life, the word climacteric is often considered a better term for this transitional phase which may take from six months to three years, or even longer, to be completed.

As the menopause approaches, menstruation occurs irregularly; the discharge sometimes increases slightly, but usually diminishes in amount and finally disappears altogether, while the reproductive organs all undergo atrophic changes. This change is a normal physiologic process, and the entire organism—mental, emotional, and physical—is gradually prepared for the cessation of the internal secretion of the ovary. As the transition is made slowly it should not be greatly disturbing. It is true that many women suffer a certain amount of nervous instability at the menopause, they tire easily, have "hot flashes" and possibly headaches; but under ordinary conditions the discomfort is not great, and after the function has entirely ceased and they become physiologically adjusted, these women often enjoy better health than before.

The vasomotor symptoms—hot flushes of the face and neck, sweats, and flashes of heat which involve the whole body—are the most characteristic symptoms of the menopause. The severity of these symptoms varies, being almost absent in some, moderate in others, and very severe in a few. It has been shown that whenever ovarian function is increased the pituitary function is decreased, and when ovarian function is diminished there is an increase in pituitary function. At the menopause there is an increase in pituitary function due to the cessation of ovarian function, and it is this increased activity of the pituitary that may be responsible for the vasomotor phenomena. The majority of women pass through this transitional period without much discomfort and without treatment. In cases where the symptoms are severe, estrogenic preparations may be given which will replace the patient's estrogen deficiency and thereby inhibit the production of an excessive amount of gonadotropic principle. This treatment will relieve the symptoms temporarily and aid the patient in gradually adjusting to the changes in endocrine function.

Unfortunately, wide currency has been given to exaggerations concerning the symptoms of the menopause. The result is that serious organic diseases which are in no way related to the climacteric are not infrequently attributed to it. For this reason excessive bleeding or heart symptoms, for example, are all too often accepted as a matter of course, and accordingly neglected until the patient is beyond medical aid. This is particularly and tragically true of cancer of the uterus. It is a wise precaution, therefore, to regard with apprehension an increase in the amount of the menstrual flow of any woman past thirty, and not to accept it as a normal forerunner of the menopause. Any bleeding, no matter how slight, occurring after the menopause, should be brought to the attention of a doctor. By this means an early diagnosis of cancer, if present, may be made and a cure effected through prompt treatment.

## BIBLIOGRAPHY AND STUDENT REFERENCES


Bickers, William, and Woods, Maribelle: "Premenstrual Distress and What to Do about It," *Am. J. Nursing* **52**:1087–88, (Sept.) 1952.

Blake, Florence G.: *The Child, His Parents and the Nurse.* J. B. Lippincott Co., Philadelphia, 1954.

Bookmiller, Mae M., and Bowen, George L.: *Textbook of Obstetrics and Obstetric Nursing,* 2nd ed. W. B. Saunders Co., Philadelphia, 1954.

Brady, Leo; Kurtz, Ethna L.; and McLaughlin, Eileen: *Essentials of Gynecology,* 2nd ed. The Macmillan Company, New York, 1949.

Cottrell, Lillian: "Understanding the Adolescent," *Am. J. Nursing,* **46**:181–83, (Mar.) 1946.

Davis, M. Edward, and Sheckler, Catherine E.: *DeLee's Obstetrics for Nurses,* 15th ed. W. B. Saunders Co., Philadelphia, 1951.

Eastman, Nicholson J.: *Williams Obstetrics,* 11th ed. Appleton-Century-Crofts, Inc., New York, 1956.

Fulton, John F. (ed.): *A Textbook of Physiology,* 17th ed. W. B. Saunders Co., Philadelphia, 1955.

Greenhill, J. P. (ed.): *Obstetrics,* 11th ed. W. B. Saunders Co., Philadelphia, 1955.

Kimber, Diana C.; Gray, Carolyn E.; Stackpole, Caroline E.; and Leavell, Lutie C.: *Textbook of Anatomy and Physiology,* 13th ed. The Macmillan Company, New York, 1955.

Mayers, Lawrence H.: "Coming of Age," in *Educational Material on Menstruation.* Tampax, Inc., New York.

Newton, Niles: *Maternal Emotions.* Paul B. Hoeber, Inc., New York, 1955.

Novak, Emil: *The Woman Asks the Doctor,* 2nd ed. Williams & Wilkins Co., Baltimore, 1944.

Novak, Emil, and Novak, Edmund R.: *Textbook of Gynecology,* 4th ed. Williams & Wilkins Co., Baltimore, 1952.

Oed, Minnie K.: "Helping the Bewildered Adolescent," *Am. J. Nursing,* **50**:298–301, (May) 1950.

Potter, Edith L.: *Fundamentals of Human Reproduction.* McGraw-Hill Book Co., New York, 1948.

Spock, Benjamin: *The Common Sense Book of Baby and Child Care.* Duell, Sloan & Pearce, Inc., New York, 1946.

Stone, Abraham: "Infertility," *Am. J. Nursing,* **47**:606–8, (Sept.) 1947.

Tampax, Inc.: *Educational Material on Menstruation.* Tampax Inc., New York.

TeLinde, Richard W.: "The Menopause," *Am. J. Nursing,* **54**:950–52, (Aug.) 1954.

Werner, August A.: "The Menopause," *Am. J. Nursing,* **42**:1373–80, (Dec.) 1942.

Woodward, H. L.; Gardner, B; Bryant, R. D.; and Overland, Anna E.: *Obstetric Management and Nursing,* 5th ed. F. A. Davis Co., Philadelphia, 1955.

# PART II. THE DEVELOPMENT OF THE BABY

*Chapter 3*

## Development of the Embryo and Accessory Structures

As was learned in the last chapter, most of the ova discharged from the graafian follicles enter the fimbriated end of the tube nearby, where they either perish or continue their development, depending upon whether or not they are fertilized (Fig. 21). Occasionally the ovum is not discharged into the funnel formed by the erect, finger-like processes of the fimbriae but is expelled directly into the abdominal cavity. Such an ovum either may be absorbed like any other cell cast off into the peritoneal cavity or may find its way, eventually, into the end of the tube near which it was expelled or migrate across the body and into the other tubal opening. This migration of the ovum, as it is termed, has been demonstrated in cases in which pregnancy has followed removal of the ovary on one side and the fallopian tube on the other. There are various theories as to how and why an occasional migrating ovum, floating around in a relatively large cavity, ever enters the tubal opening, which, after all, is not large. The most widely accepted belief is that the motion of the cilia lining the tubes, combined with peristalsis, creates a suction which draws the microscopic cell into the opening, these two forces being the means by which the ovum is later propelled downward through the tube to the uterus.

The journey of the ovum through the tube is of enormous consequence, for during its course occur the events which decide whether the ovum shall, like most others, be simply swept along to no end and lost, or whether by chance it is to meet a male germinal cell and begin the development of a new human being. The amazing

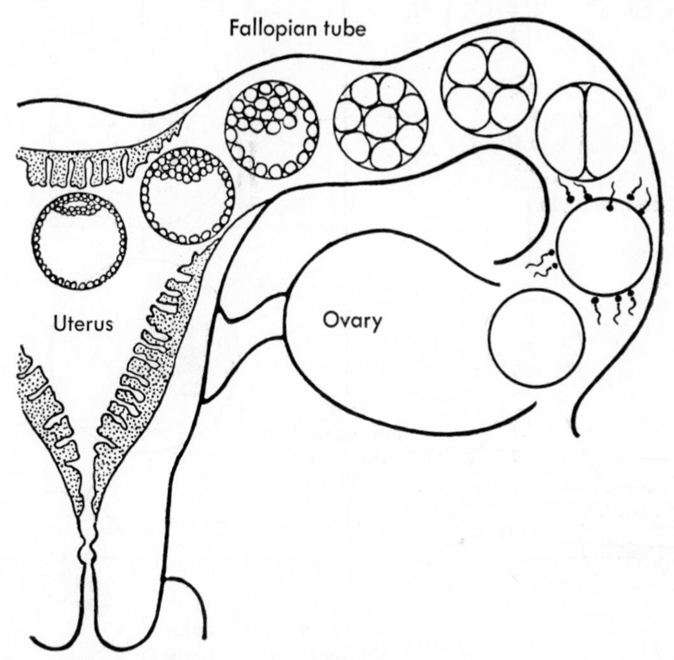


**Fig. 21.** The egg escapes from a follicle in the ovary, enters the fallopian tube, and is fertilized in the terminal portion of the tube. It moves slowly down through the tube and over the lining of the uterus, usually coming to rest seven or eight days after fertilization. During this interval, the zygote develops first into a ball of cells and then becomes a fluid-filled sphere with a small mass of cells persisting in one area on the inner surface. Indications of the amniotic cavity and a two-layered embryonic disk become visible as implantation in the uterus begins. (By permission from *Fundamentals of Human Reproduction,* by Edith L. Potter. Copyright, 1948, McGraw-Hill Book Company, Inc.)

power which enables this cell to reproduce itself, and to develop with unbelievable complexity, is acquired somewhere in the tube by meeting and fusing with a spermatozoon, the germinal cell of the male.

The spermatozoa look very much like microscopic tadpoles, with their flat, oval heads, tapering bodies, and long tails (Fig. 23). The

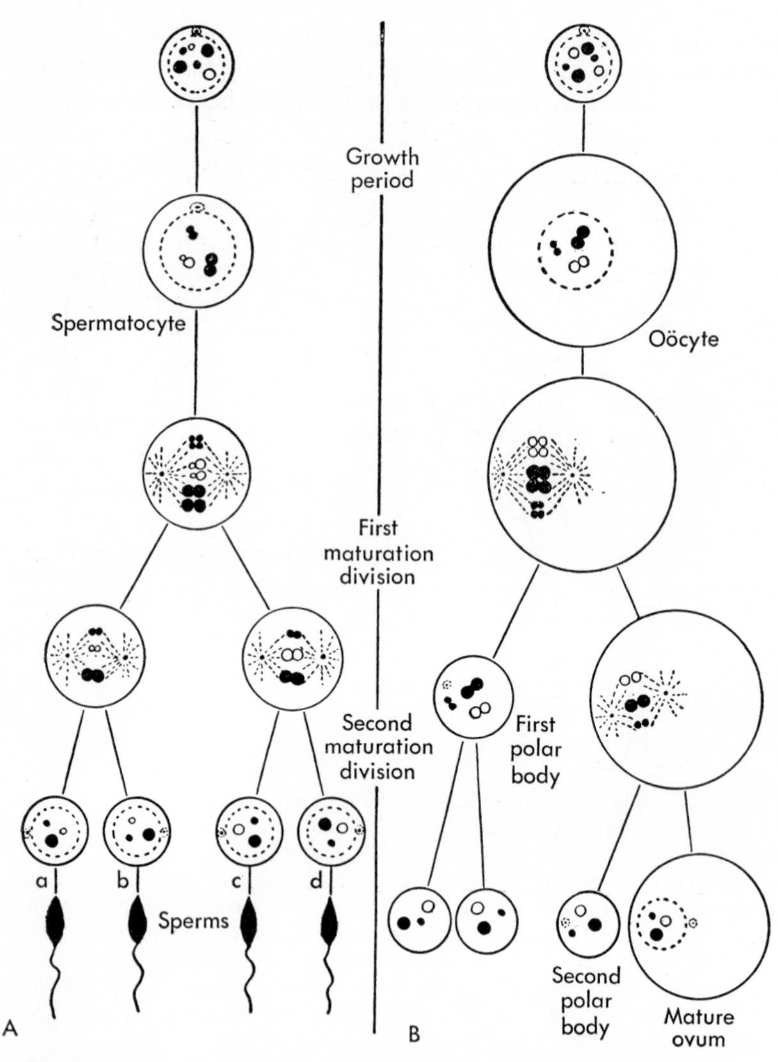


**Fig. 22.** Diagram to show maturation of reproductive cells. This process consists of meiosis (meiotic, or reduction, division) and mitosis. *A,* sperm cells; *B,* ova. In *A* each of these four cells is a functional sperm. In *B* only one of the cells is a functional ovum; the other three usually disappear. The spermatocyte and oöcyte are shown with two pairs of autosomes (black) and one pair of sex chromosomes (white). In the oöcyte the two sex chr are alike (white circles of same size)—the two *x* chr referred to in the text. It is evident

entire cell is approximately 1/600 in. in length and the head 1/6000 in. in diameter. As these tails serve somewhat as propellers, the male cells are capable of very rapid motion, being observed under the microscope to swim the distance of 2.5 cm (1 in.) in eight minutes. In spite of their strange appearance, they are cells after all and resemble the female cells in that each one contains a nucleus.

An almost inconceivably large number of spermatozoa, floating in the seminal fluid, is deposited in the vagina at the time of intercourse, the estimated number being something over 300,000,000. Nature evidently supplies both the male and female cells with lavishness, in order to provide for the large number of both kinds which must inevitably be lost and still have enough survive to accomplish creation. A very considerable number of spermatozoa enter the uterus, and are enabled, through their peculiar ability to swim upstream, to travel up into the tubes against the downward current created by the cilia and peristalsis. In the tube, usually in the upper end, about two hours after entering the vagina, they meet a recently discharged and matured ovum which is being swept downward. The meeting may be due to random movements or the result of an attraction (Fig. 21). An ovum is fertilizable for about 12 hours after extrusion from the ovary while the fertilizing power of a spermatozoon may last for as long as 48 hours. Although the ovum which is destined to be fertilized is surrounded by several spermatozoa, only one actually enters and fuses with it.

Before an ovum is ready for fertilization, it must undergo certain developmental changes, known as *maturation,* a process which probably begins just before rupture of the graafian follicle and continues in the outer one-third of the fallopian tube. The chromatin in the germ cells, as well as in all general body cells, appears in bodies of different size and shape, known as *chromosomes;* the human cell has 48, which appear as 24 pairs. There are 23 pairs of ordinary

---

that in *B* all possible ova will be alike in having one *x* chr. In the spermatocyte the two sex chr are not alike (a large white circle and a small white circle)—the *x* and *y* chr referred to. There are in *A,* therefore, two possible kinds of sperm cells—(*c*) and (*d*) containing an *x* chr and (*a*) and (*b*) containing a *y* chr. (Modified from *Essentials of Human Embryology,* by G. S. Dodds, John Wiley and Sons, Inc., New York.) (Kimber, D.; Gray, C.; Stackpole, C.; and Leavell, L.: *Textbook of Anatomy and Physiology,* 13th ed. The Macmillan Company, New York, 1955.)

chromosomes and one pair of sex chromosomes, usually known as the *x* chromosomes. Maturation is the process by which the number of chromosomes in the cell is reduced to one-half of the original number, so that, when a matured ovum is fertilized, the chromosomes from the male cell can be introduced without changing the number characteristically found in the human cell. The male cell must, therefore, undergo the same reduction process before it unites with the ovum (Fig. 22).

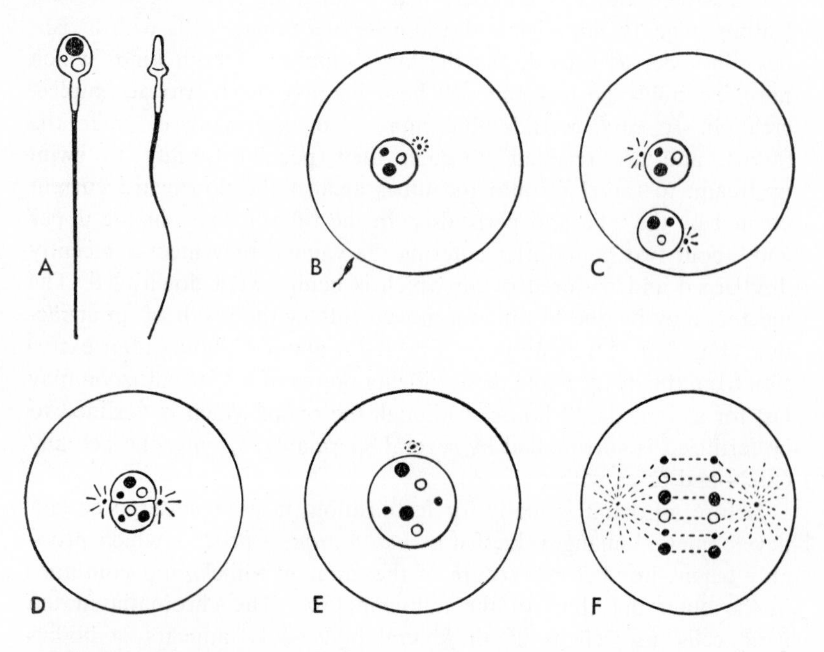


**Fig. 23.** Diagram to show fertilization. *A,* human sperm cell, face and side views. Note the head containing the chromosomes, the middle piece, and the tail. *B,* sperm entering ovum. *C,* sperm nucleus within ovum, showing chromosomes. *D,* the sperm nucleus approaches the ovum nucleus. *E,* the two nuclei fuse, and fertilization is complete; the zygote formed in *E* has six chromosomes—two pair of autosomes (black) and one pair of sex chromosomes (white). Since the two sex chromosomes are alike (*x* chromosomes), the zygote would develop into a female. *F,* first embryonic cell division, which when complete would give a two-celled embryo. (Modified from *Essentials of Human Embryology,* by G. S. Dodds, John Wiley and Sons, Inc., New York.) (Kimber, D.; Gray, C.; Stackpole, C.; and Leavell, L.: *Textbook of Anatomy and Physiology,* 13th ed. The Macmillan Company, New York, 1955.)

The first step in the maturation process is the formation and casting off of a *polar body*. This process occurs by typical cell division, in which the chromosomes also divide; therefore, the nucleus of both the ovum and the polar body contain 48, or the typical number of, chromosomes for the human species. The only difference in the two cells is that of size; the polar body being much smaller. The next division of the ovum occurs without preliminary cleavage of the chromosomes and the two cells formed, the mature ovum and the second polar body, each contains only 23 ordinary and one *x* chromosome, or one-half of the original number (Fig. 22).

The fusion of the ovum and spermatozoon, which brings the chromosomes of both maternal and paternal origin together into one cell and restores the original number, is termed *impregnation, fertilization,* or in lay parlance *conception,* and the instant at which it occurs marks the beginning of pregnancy (Fig. 23). Establishment of this fact is of considerable importance, since it does away with any possible controversy concerning the time at which a new life begins. The origin of the child is exactly coincident with the fusion of the male and female germinal cells; furthermore, the sex of the child and any inherited traits and characteristics are established at this decisive instant. This fact has been ascertained as a result of long, painstaking study in the field of human heredity. It is now known that the chromosomes in the nucleus of the ovum and the spermatozoon, these tiny microscopic particles, are directly decended from the nuclear substance of the parents and their ancestors and carry all the intricate and elaborate material which the child inherits from its parents, grandparents, and yet more distant progenitors.

Within each chromosome there are large numbers of chromatin particles called *genes;* these are too small to be separately identified, but are believed to be thousands in number. These genes carry the factors, within the chromosomes, that are responsible for the characteristics of an individual. Just as the chromosomes are arranged in pairs so the genes are also arranged in pairs within the chromosome. In the process of reduction division of the ovum and sperm, during which the number of chromosomes is reduced to one-half, the pairs of genes as well as the chromosomes divide. Although each chromosome always possesses the same number of genes, the genes within the chromosome pair may cross over from one chromosome in the pair to the other during this process of division. Each sex cell then, as it is ready for fertilization, has one chromosome of each pair and one set of genes in each chromosome, but there are many possible combinations of chromosomes, and genes within the chromosomes, and therefore a great variation in the characteristics that the cell carries. As the ovum and sperm unite, the new cell resulting from the fertilization has a complete set of 24 pairs of chromosomes and likewise a complete set of genes. One chromosome of each pair and one gene of each pair have been inherited from the mother and one from the father. All the body characteristics of the individual that will develop from this new cell are influenced by the combination of genes carried by the ovum and the sperm; all characteristics are present at the time of fertilization. Some genes carry recessive traits and some carry traits which are completely or partially dominant. The recessive trait may not appear in an individual who also has a gene which is dominant for the same characteristic. This recessive gene may, however, be carried to another generation, and the trait may appear in an individual who lacks a dominant gene for that particular characteristic. For example, the gene for brown eyes is dominant to the gene for blue eyes. If one of the genes present is for brown eyes and one for blue eyes the eyes will be brown because the gene for brown eyes is dominant. The gene for blue eyes is present in the individual's cells, however, and when passed on to an individual in another generation who inherits two genes for blue eyes that individual's eyes will be blue. The inheritance of all characteristics is actually more complicated than this explanation, but it can be seen from this that there may be great variation in characteristics inherited by different children of the same parents. It is through certain combinations of factors that it is possible to apparently skip the inheritance of certain characteristics from parents, but inherit traits from grandparents or even more remote ancestors. After the ovum and sperm unite all further cell division results in duplication of chromosomes and genes. Every cell in the body contains the same chromosomes and the same genes as every other cell. There are two complete sets of chromosomes and genes, inherited from the mother and father, which govern body characteristics—anatomic and physiologic. The manner in which these inherited characteristics are finally developed, after fertilization has taken place, is determined by environmental conditions.

In any event, all the characteristics which are transmitted to the child from its parents and other ancestors are completely determined at the time of fusion of ovum and spermatozoon. At this decisive moment the entire contribution of inheritance from both parents has been made. After this the only contribution made to the child is in the form of nourishment that is derived from its mother's tissues. The foregoing facts make clear why the mother's thoughts or frame of mind during pregnancy cannot affect the child's character or disposition. They dispel the widespread, but erroneous, belief that maternal impressions may "mark" or deform the unborn infant.

Almost countless theories have been advanced to explain what it is that establishes the sex of the forthcoming child. Recent investigations show that the determining factor is found in the spermatozoon. There are 48 chromosomes in the spermatocytes as well as in the ovum, but the chromosomes in the sex pair differ in size and shape and are known as the *x* and *y* chromosomes. Therefore, reduction division will give rise to two varieties of spermatozoa; one-half will have 23 ordinary and one *x* chromosome and the other one-half will have 23 ordinary and a *y* chromosome (Fig. 22). Sex, then, is determined by the type of spermatozoon fertilizing the ovum. If it is fertilized by a spermatazoon with an *x* chromosome, it will have 23 pairs of ordinary chromosomes and one pair of *x* chromosomes and will produce a female. If the ovum is fertilized by a *y* chromosome, the sex chromosomes will be an *x* and *y* pair and will produce a male individual.

It is an interesting fact that more male than female babies are born, the usual proportion being about 106 boys to 100 girls. So far no accurate means has ever been found whereby it is possible to influence the development of, or discover, the sex of a child before its birth.

As soon as a spermatozoon enters an ovum, the nucleus of the spermatozoon and of the ovum fuse into a single cell and fertilization is complete. The result of this union is a cell which was previously nonexistent. This new cell is not only capable of reproduction by means of *segmentation,* or cell division, but in the course of its subdivision and proliferation, it forms groups of cells which develop into tissues and structures widely different from each other. The entire complex human body, in addition to the cord and membranes, and in part the placenta, arises from this single, extraordinary cell. It first divides into two; these two divide into four; the four into eight; and thus the process of division and subdivision continues until a solid mass is formed, shaped something like a mulberry, and called the *morula* (Fig. 24).

As the cellular activity continues within the morula, fluid appears in the center, with the result that the cells are rearranged and pushed toward the periphery, thus forming a sac. At this stage the embryo is called the *blastodermic vesicle* (Fig. 24). As fluid collects in the

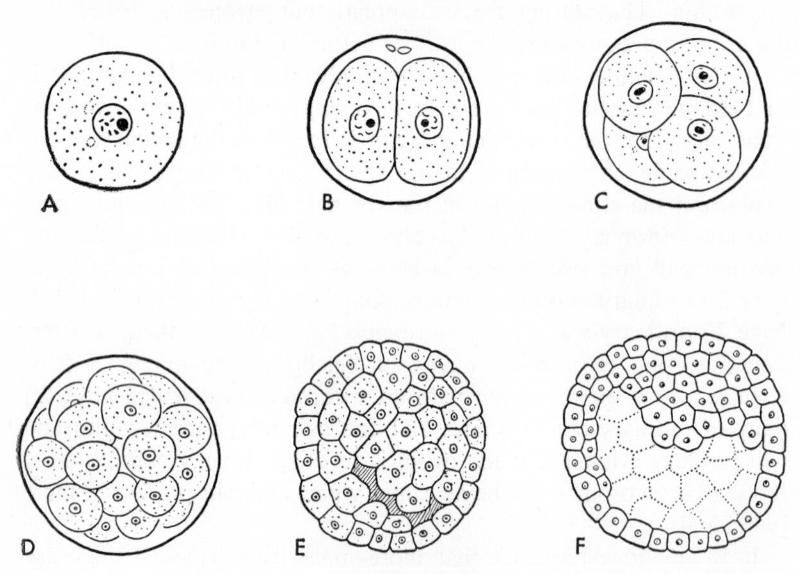


**Fig. 24.** Diagram to show very early stages of mammalian development. *A,* one-celled embryo; *B,* two-celled embryo; *C,* four-celled embryo; *D,* berry-like ball of cells, or *morula; E,* beginning the formation of the blastocyst; *F,* well-developed blastocyst, consisting of a hollow ball of *trophoblast* cells and an inner mass of cells known as *blastomeres.* (Kimber, D.; Gray, C.; Stackpoles, C.; and Leavell, L.: *Textbook of Anatomy and Physiology,* 13th ed. The Macmillan Company, New York, 1955.)

vesicle it crowds the cells to one side, where they form a mass which is sometimes called the internal cell mass, or *embryonic area.* A single layer of cells, known as the *primitive chorion,* comprises the remainder of the vesicular wall. The cells in this outer layer, or primitive chorion, are *trophoblastic cells* which have the ability to invade the endometrium for the implantation of the blastocyst.

While these developmental changes are taking place, the morula is being carried down the tube, toward the uterus, by the combined force of peristalsis and the sweeping motion of the ciliated membrane. The time consumed by this journey is believed to take about three to four days. Since the fertilized cell is free in the uterus for another two to three days, continuing its existence as a floating blastocyst, it quite evidently has no attachment to the mother and cannot, therefore, derive any appreciable nourishment directly from her. The development to this point, then, must be due chiefly to inherent powers within the mass of cells itself.

Thus, while still in the morula stage and about 1/200 in. in diameter, the embryo reaches the uterus and there implants when it has reached the blastocyst stage or on about the sixth to eighth day after fertilization (Fig. 21). There is little if any increase in size until after implantation in the endometrium, which has been prepared for reception of the ovum by the premenstrual swelling. After conception the hypertrophied endometrium of the premenstrual stage becomes even thicker, until it has reached its height, or a thickness of 10 mm (.4 in.) at the third or fourth month of pregnancy. This uterine lining, which is now known as *decidua,* is so thick it has deep furrows, its cells are large and oval with round vesicular nuclei, and the glands are distended, hyperplastic, and secretory. Just before implantation of the ovum the decidua undergoes some vascular changes similar to those occurring just previous to menstruation. Implantation depends upon these vascular changes and the power of the trophoblastic cells surrounding the blastodermic vesicle to invade and destroy tissue. These trophoblasts also have phagocytic power.

The point at which the embryo attaches itself is entirely a matter of chance. It usually rests somewhere in the upper part of the uterine cavity, promptly destroys the minute underlying area of tissue-capillaries, venous sinuses, glands, and stroma by digestive action and burrows into the decidua. Although this seems to imply extensive tissue destruction, it actually involves only the width of a few cells. As the margins of the opening thus made meet and fuse above the ovum, the embryo is completely encapsulated in a cavity of its own that has no connection with the uterine cavity (Fig. 25).

After this occurrence the decidua consists of three portions. (1) The hypertrophied membrane which lines the uterus as a whole is called the *decidua vera.* With the increasing distention of the uterus during the latter part of pregnancy, it becomes very thin. This layer is thrown off in part with the membranes during labor, and later in the uterine discharges. (2) The *decidua basalis,* or the *decidua serotina,* is that portion lying directly beneath the embryo which later enters into the formation of the placenta. (3) The *decidua capsularis,*

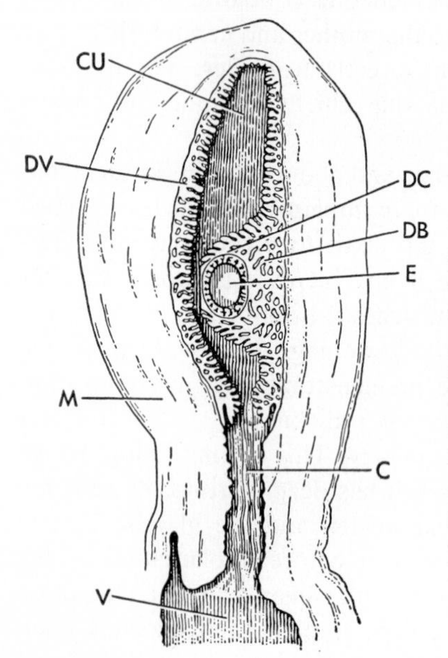


**Fig. 25.** Diagram of a longitudinal section of the gravid uterus, showing the relations of the implanted embryo and the uterine mucosa. *C,* cervix of uterus; *CU,* cavity of uterus; *DB,* decidua basalis; *DC,* decidua capsularis; *DV,* decidua vera; *E,* embryo about two weeks of age in chorion showing villi; *M,* muscle layers of wall of uterus; *V,* vagina. (Kimber, D.; Gray, C.; Stackpole, C.; and Leavell, L.: *Textbook of Anatomy and Physiology,* 13th ed. The Macmillan Company, New York, 1955.)

or *decidua reflexa,* which surrounds and covers the buried embryo, consists of the fused margins of mucosa that have grown over the embryo (Figs. 25 and 26).

The inner cell mass now begins segmentation and differentiation, and the cells in the mass are very early arranged in layers: the outer layer being termed the *ectoderm;* the inner layer the *entoderm;* while a third layer, which appears a little later between the other two, is called the *mesoderm.* Although these three primitive layers of cells have all developed from the single cell formed by the fused spermatozoon and ovum, they are even now very different in character. The differences steadily increase until finally all of the complex fetal organs and tissues, the membranes, the cord, and the placenta result from their further specialization and development.

**From the ectoderm** arises the skin with its appendages, and the salivary and mammary glands, the nasal passages and upper part of the pharynx, the anus, the crystalline lens, the external ear, the entire nervous system, the sense organs, and, in part, the fetal membranes.

**From the mesoderm** are derived the urinary and reproductive organs, the muscles, bones, and connective tissues, and the circulatory system.

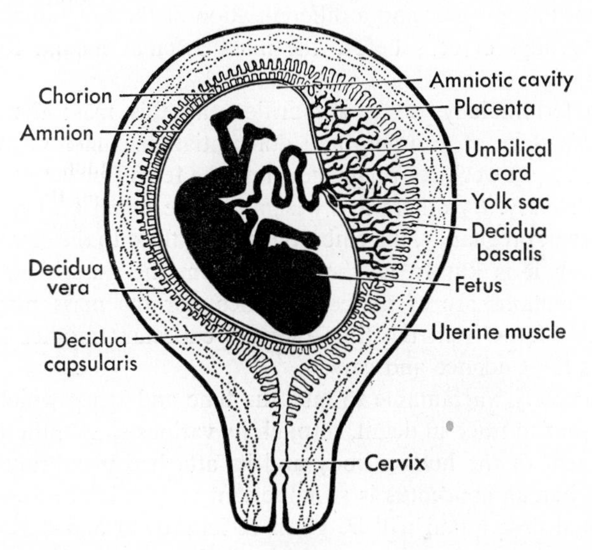


**Fig. 26.** Early in the fourth month of pregnancy the decidua capsularis fuses with the decidua vera, and the uterine cavity is obliterated. The villi disappear from the surface of the chorionic vesicle nearest the uterine cavity, and the placenta becomes well delineated. The space between the amnion and chorion disappears, and the two membranes form the wall of the sac within which the fetus develops. (By permission from *Fundamentals of Human Reproduction,* by Edith L. Potter. Copyright, 1948, McGraw-Hill Book Company, Inc.)

**From the entoderm** are developed the alimentary canal, the thymus, thyroid, liver, lungs, pancreas, bladder, and the various small glands and tubules.

It was formerly believed that the human being existed in miniature in the first cell and that its development during pregnancy was entirely a matter of increase in size. The microscope has disproved this, and we now know that embryonic development comprises both growth and evolution. Much of the information accepted today is, of course, speculative, having been deduced from observations made upon the reproductive processes of lower mammals. The youngest fertilized human ovum which has been discovered and examined was probably three days old, but the fourth-, fifth-, sixth-, and seventh-day human conceptus had not yet been seen. Evidence points quite convincingly to the belief that the early stages of development consist of proliferation of, and alterations in, the kinds of cells, their arrangement into groups, and a differentiation of the functional activity of these groups of cells before the mass assumes human form and develops organs.

As to terminology, some authorities call this mass the embryo during this stage of grouping and differentiation, which corresponds to the first eight weeks of pregnancy, and the fetus from then until the time of delivery. By others it is designated the ovum during the first two weeks of pregnancy, the embryo from the third to the eighth week, after which it is known as the fetus. From the nurse's standpoint these distinctions are of no consequence, for the mass may safely be called a fetus from the time that the expectant mother looks to the nurse for guidance and care.

It is scarcely warrantable to take the time and space which would be necessary to trace in detail, through its various stages, the intricate development of the human body and its attached membranes; however, the human conceptus is so important and so interesting that an abbreviated description will be given of its growth and development and of the accessory structures which are important to its existence.

Although the exact length of time required for the maturation of the fetus is not known, it is estimated that 280 days, or 10 lunar months, elapse between the beginning of the last menstrual period and the beginning of labor. In spite of the difference in size among mothers, it is found that the products of conception develop and grow at a fairly uniform rate of speed.

A new human being is the ultimate result of conception, but the chorion, amnion, placenta, and umbilical cord must also be created to serve as aids in building and protecting the developing child during its uterine life. The part played by these accessory structures is so vital, in spite of being temporary, that it will be well for us to look into their origin and functions before considering the fetus itself, which they serve.

## THE CHORION

The chorion or outer fetal membrane is derived from the ectodermal layer of cells growing within the blastodermal vesicle.

On about the twelfth or thirteenth day after ovulation, at least a few days after the actual implantation of the fertilized ovum in the uterine mucosa, primitive *chorionic villi,* tiny, thread-like projections, begin to develop. These villi soon cover the surface of the primitive chorion, giving it the shaggy appearance of a chestnut bur.

The chorion grows rapidly in size and thickness, and the villi upon its surface increase in size, number, and complexity by frequent branching. In so doing, the villi push their way farther into the maternal tissues surrounding them and destroy the capillary walls with which they come in contact. Maternal blood escapes through the destroyed walls, forming tiny hemorrhagic areas or "lakes of blood." Some of the villi, known as *fastening villi,* extend far enough into the decidua to attach the ovum to it, while the rest dip freely in these pools of maternal blood, which is constantly being refreshed by an inflow of arterial and an outflow of venous blood through the mother's blood vessels.

Blood vessels soon appear in these chorionic villi, and at about the fourth week fetal blood circulates through them (Fig. 27). It becomes apparent, therefore, that the maternal and fetal blood streams are in close relation, being separated by only the thin tissues which form the walls of the villi and the walls of the blood vessels within the villi. This arrangement makes it possible for the steadily proliferating villi to discharge one of their functions, which is to receive nourishment for the embryo from the maternal blood and give up to the parent waste products from the growing body. This exchange of nourishment and waste matter takes place by means of osmosis and by selective cell activity. Freely as the exchange of materials occurs, there is never any contact or mixing of maternal and fetal blood, nor does maternal blood at any time flow through fetal vessels.

The second function of the villi, particularly after they have developed to the placental stage, is to attach the embryonic sac to the uterine wall.

The villi are equally distributed over the chorion at first, *chorion frondosum,* but as the sac increases in size and pushes out into the uterine cavity they gradually atrophy and disappear, excepting over the relatively small area beneath the vesicle where the chorion is in contact with the decidua basalis (Fig. 26). At this site the villi become much more abundant, and it is here that the placenta eventually develops. After the greater part of the surface of the chorion, which is in contact with the decidua capsularis, has become denuded of villi, it is known as the *chorion laeve,* or bald chorion.

As pregnancy advances and the fetal sac enlarges, the chorion laeve, covered by the decidua capsularis, or decidua reflexa, is pushed farther out into the uterine cavity, until finally it reaches the opposite

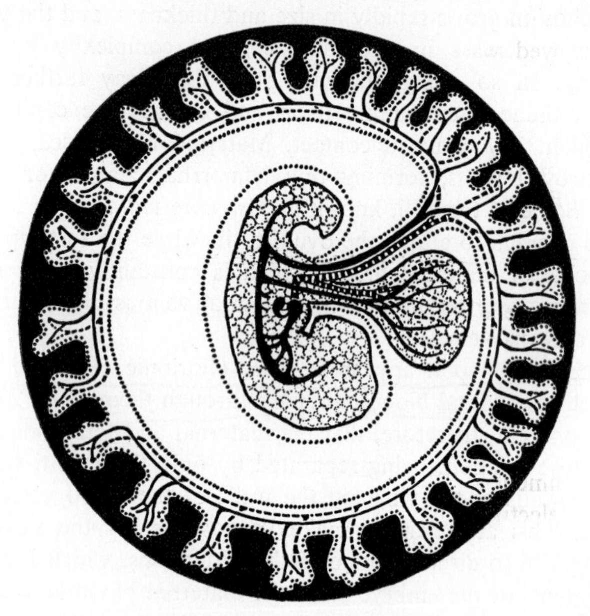

**Fig. 27.** Blood vessels form in the embryo, the yolk sac, and the villi simultaneously. They unite and establish a circulation that carries blood between the embryo and the yolk sac and between the embryo and the wall of the chorionic vesicle. Maternal blood surrounds the chorionic vesicle and circulates between the villi. (By permission from *Fundamentals of Human Reproduction,* by Edith L. Potter. Copyright, 1948, McGraw-Hill Book Company, Inc.)

wall, meets the decidua vera, and obliterates the entire space which had existed between the two membranes (Fig. 26). This means that instead of a uterine cavity lined with decidua and a tiny capsule somewhere off to the side lined with chorion, the latter has distended until it completely fills and really becomes the cavity within the uterine walls. The decidua capsularis and decidua vera fuse between the third and fourth months, and finally the decidua capsularis degenerates and almost entirely disappears.

## THE AMNION

The amnion begins to develop very early in embryonic life, and soon invests the fetus completely in a membranous sac. This sac is reflected up around the umbilical cord, thus forming its outer covering (Figs. 26 and 31).

The amnion, like the chorion, is derived from the ectoderm. At first there is an appreciable space with some fluid between the two membranes, but as the amnion increases in size with the advance of pregnancy, it comes in contact with, and is loosely adherent to, the chorion, the outer membrane.

Very early in its development the double-layered membranous sac formed by the amnion and chorion contains a slightly opaque fluid known as the *amniotic fluid,* or *liquor amnii,* in which the fetus floats (Fig. 26). This fluid increases in amount until the end of pregnancy when the normal quantity is about 600 ml (20 oz). The source of the liquor amnii is not definitely known. The theories are that it may be a maternal transudate, it may be secreted by the amniotic membrane, or it may be, in part, fetal urine. It is about 99 per cent water, containing particles of dead skin and *lanugo,* a soft downy hair cast off from the body of the fetus, and traces of albumin and both organic and inorganic salts.

The amniotic fluid serves a variety of purposes. Since the intestines of the fetus contain lanugo and particles of dead skin, it is evident that the child swallows some of this fluid during its uterine life, but the role that this fluid plays in the nutrition of the fetus is not known. The increasing bulk of the fluid serves to distend the fetal sac and surrounding uterus, and thus provides the fetus with room for growth and movement. It is believed by some authorities that it prevents adhesions between the child's skin and the amnion, which they think constitute a factor, when by mischance they do occur, in causing monstrosities and intrauterine amputations. On the other hand, Dr. G. L. Streeter, embryologist of the Carnegie Institution, who conducted extensive investigations in this connection, felt that the amniotic adhesions and bands did not cause monster formation, but that the adhesions were secondary to the primary fetal abnormalities. The fluid with which it is surrounded keeps the fetus at an equable temperature in spite of variations of temperature in the mother's environment and minimizes the danger of injury to the fragile body from pressure or blows on the mother's abdomen. By acting as a water wedge, forced down by uterine contractions at the time of labor, it may possibly aid in dilating the cervix to permit the expulsion of the full-term child.

## THE PLACENTA

Because the amount of yolk accompanying the human ovum is small, the fetus is soon dependent upon the mother for its nutrition. During the first few days it derives its nutritive material from the serum accompanying the edema of the decidua, the increased glandular secretion and glycogen content of the decidua, and the maternal tissues which have undergone necrosis. In about a week the *intervillous spaces* between the trophoblasts and the decidua become filled with blood, and the embryo is nourished by direct osmosis. Finally blood vessels appear in the villi, the placenta develops, and nutritive material is transmitted directly from the maternal blood in the spaces between the villi to the fetal blood which circulates in the villi.

The placenta, in lay parlance the afterbirth, is really a thickened, amplified portion of the fetal sac, which has developed at the site of the implantation of the ovum. It is partly fetal and to a smaller extent maternal in origin, being developed jointly from the chorion frondosum with its branching villi and the underlying decidua basalis (Figs. 26 and 28).

The chorionic villi, already referred to, grow and branch in a treelike fashion, and push their way farther and farther into the uterine tissues, the decidua basalis, creating the intervillous spaces which fill with maternal blood. From the time that the first fetal blood vessels appear in these floating villi until the child is born, there is a constant exchange of nutriment and waste material between the maternal and fetal blood; the arterial maternal blood in the intervillous spaces giving to the fetal blood in the villi the oxygen and other substances necessary to nourish and build the growing body, and receiving in return the broken-down products of fetal activity. The waste is carried by the maternal blood stream to the mother's lungs, kidneys, and skin, by which it is excreted. This exchange of substances is accomplished by osmosis, by selective powers of the cells in the villi, and by the power of these cells to alter some substances. Thus the placenta virtually serves the fetus as lungs, stomach, intestines, and kidneys throughout its uterine life.

The placenta also has an endocrine function since it takes over some of the ovarian function and produces the chorionic gonadotropic hormone.

In addition to the nutritive substances in the mother's blood—glucose, albumin, fat, minerals, vitamins, and gases, which pass through the placenta by direct osmosis or are so altered by cell action as to be absorbable through the villi—certain drugs and certain protective substances such as the antitoxins of diphtheria and tetanus are evidently transmitted from the maternal to the fetal circulation.

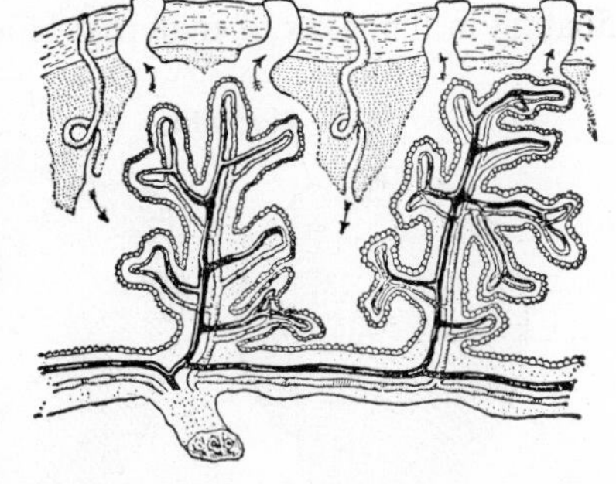

**Fig. 28.** Placenta with its blood supply. Cellular line separates maternal and embryonic portions. The embryonic portion is shown as two much-lobed villi enclosing blood vessels. Note umbilical cord containing umbilical vein and two arteries. Two uterine arteries and two uterine veins are indicated by the arrows. White area would contain maternal blood. (Kimber, D.; Gray, C.; Stackpole, C.; and Leavell, L.: *Textbook of Anatomy and Physiology,* 13th ed. The Macmillan Company, New York, 1955.)

It is claimed by some authorities that pathogenic organisms, for example, anthrax and tubercle bacilli, may be transmitted from mother to fetus, but the reported cases are so rare that the accepted belief is that organisms are seldom transmitted, if the placenta is healthy and intact. However, the viruses of certain diseases, such as smallpox and possibly rubella, do occasionally pass through the placenta.

When we examine this interesting structure, the placenta, after it is cast off, we find it to be a flattened, fairly round spongy mass 15 to 20 cm (6 to 8 in.) in diameter, and about 2 to 3 cm (1 in.) thick where the cord arises and thinning out toward the margin. Continued from the margin are the filmy fetal membranes. A rupture in these membranes during labor provides the opening through which the amniotic fluid escapes and the child passes during birth (Fig. 29).

The placenta weighs from 500 to 600 gm (about 1¼ lb) or one-sixth as much as the child and accordingly varies in size and weight with the baby. The maternal surface (Fig. 30A) having been detached from the uterine wall is rough and bloody and is irregularly divided into lobes, while the inner, or fetal, surface (Fig. 30B) is smooth and glistening and covered with the amnion. The fetal surface is traversed by a number of large blood vessels which converge toward the point of insertion of the umbilical cord, from the vessels of which they really arise (Figs. 28 and 30B). These vessels branch and divide until their termination in the innumerable chorionic villi floating in the lakes of maternal blood.

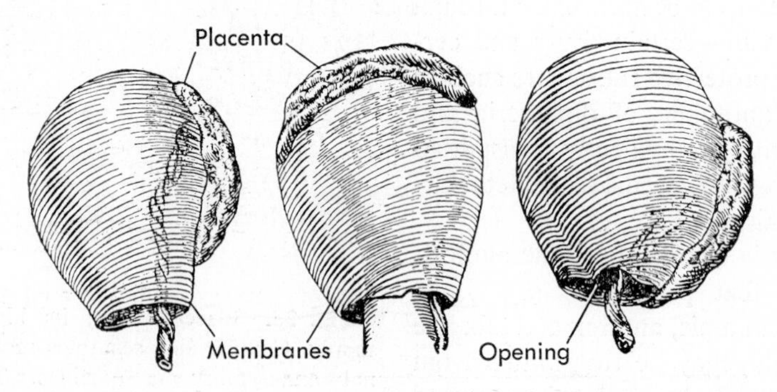


**Fig. 29.** Diagram showing general structure and relation of membranes, placenta, and umbilical cord.

## THE UMBILICAL CORD

The cord, or *funis* (Figs. 26 and 30B), is bluish white, about 2 cm (¾ in.) in diameter, and twisted and tortuous throughout its length of about 55 cm (22 in.). It is the one actual link between the mother and her unborn child, one end being attached to the abdomen of the fetus, about midway between the xiphoid process and symphysis pubis, and the other to the inner surface of the placenta. The cord is derived from the *abdominal pedicle*. It is covered with a layer of ectoderm, which is continuous with the ectodermal covering of the fetus.

The cord consists of a gelatinous mass known as *Wharton's jelly,* in the center of which are embedded three blood vessels; two arteries through which the vitiated blood flows to the placenta, where it gives up its waste products, and one vein which carries oxygenated, nourishment-bearing blood back to the fetus. The life of the fetus, therefore,

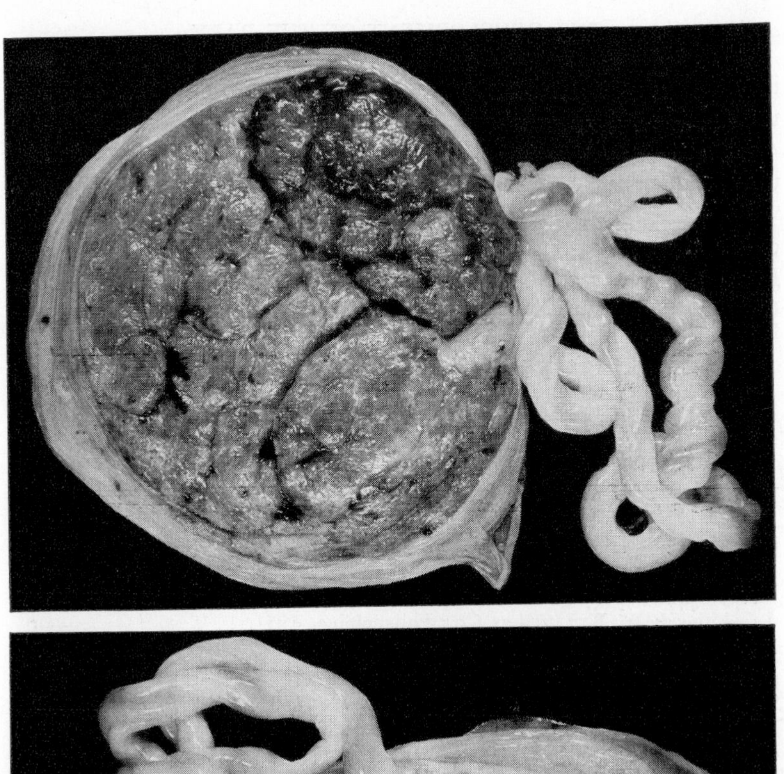

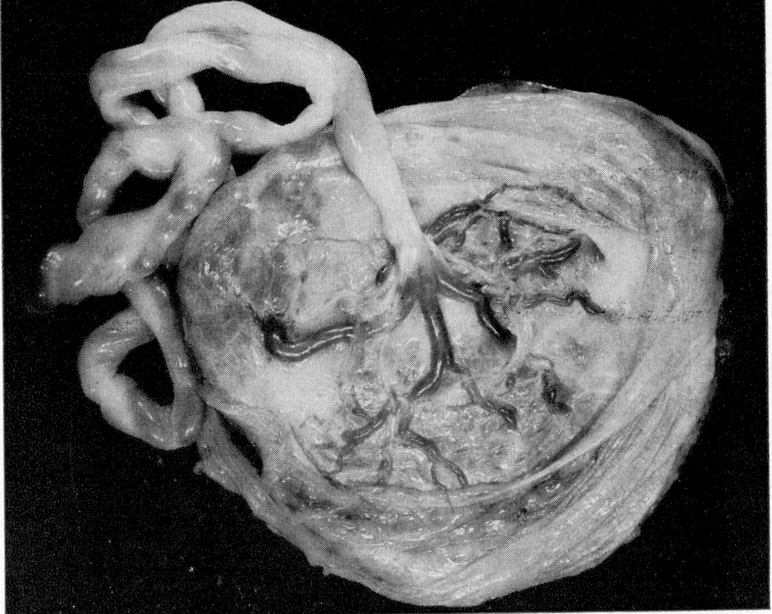

**Fig. 30A.** *(Top)* Maternal surface of the placenta, surrounded by the membranes. The umbilical cord arises from the fetal surface.

**Fig. 30B.** *(Bottom)* Fetal surface of the placenta, showing some of the membranes and the origin of the umbilical cord.

is absolutely contingent upon an uninterrupted, two-way flow of blood through the cord.

In tracing the development of the ovum after its implantation in the uterine lining, we begin, as previously stated, with a shaggy-looking vesicle, containing fluid and a clump of cells hanging toward the center from their point of attachment on the inner surface of the sac. From this clump develops the embryo, which will be discussed in Chapter 4.

## BIBLIOGRAPHY AND STUDENT REFERENCES

Arey, Leslie B.: *Developmental Anatomy,* 6th ed. W. B. Saunders Co., Philadelphia, 1954.

Bookmiller, Mae M., and Bowen, George L.: *Textbook of Obstetrics and Obstetric Nursing,* 2nd ed. W. B. Saunders Co., Philadelphia, 1954.

Corner, George W.: *Ourselves Unborn.* Yale University Press, New Haven, 1945.

Davis, M. Edward, and Sheckler, Catherine E.: *DeLee's Obstetrics for Nurses,* 15th ed. W. B. Saunders Co., Philadelphia, 1951.

Eastman, Nicholson J.: *Williams Obstetrics,* 11th ed. Appleton-Century-Crofts, Inc., New York, 1956.

Greenhill, J. P. (ed.): *Obstetrics,* 11th ed. W. B. Saunders Co., Philadelphia, 1955.

Kimber, Diana C.; Gray, Carolyn E.; Stackpole, Caroline E.; and Leavell, Lutie C.: *Textbook of Anatomy and Physiology,* 13th ed. The Macmillan Company, New York, 1955.

Maternity Center Association: "The Propitious Time," *Briefs,* **14**:6–7, (June) 1950.

———: "Three Centuries after Harvey," *Briefs,* **15**:8–11, (Sept.) 1951.

———: "The Umbilical Cord," *Briefs,* **16**:8–11, (Autumn) 1952. (Digest of article by Dr. Samuel R. M. Reynolds in *Scientific American,* July, 1952.)

Potter, Edith L.: *Fundamentals of Human Reproduction.* McGraw-Hill Book Co., New York, 1948.

Rock, John, and Hertig, Arthur: "The Human Conceptus during the First Two Weeks of Gestation," *Am. J. Obst. & Gynec.,* **55**:6–17, (Jan.) 1948. (Digest of this article under title "The First Days of Life" in *Briefs,* **12**:2–5, [May] 1948.)

Woodward, H. L.; Gardner, B.; Bryant, R. D.; and Overland, Anna E.: *Obstetric Management and Nursing,* 5th ed. F. A. Davis Co., Philadelphia, 1955.

*Chapter 4*

# Growth and Development of the Fetus

*During the first month* of pregnancy the embryo described in Chapter 3 increases in size and becomes somewhat elongated and curved upon itself with the two extremities almost in contact. The abdominal pedicle, which later becomes the umbilical cord, appears; the alimentary canal exists as a straight tube, and the thymus, thyroid, lungs, and liver begin to develop. The heart, eyes, nose, ears, and brain appear in rudimentary form, and the extremities begin to be evident as tiny, bud-like projections on the surface of the embryo (Fig. 31).

*By the end of the fourth week* the sac is about 20 mm (.8 in.) in diameter and has two walls. The outer wall, or chorion, as we have already seen, is covered with villi, and the amnion, or inner wall, is smooth; the contained embryo is surrounded by amniotic fluid and measures about 5 mm (.2 in.) from crown to rump.

*By the end of the second month, or eighth week,* the head end of the embryo has greatly increased in size and is about as large as the rest of the body (Fig. 32). Bone centers appear in the rudimentary clavicles, the kidneys and suprarenal bodies are formed, the limbs are more developed, webbed hands and feet are formed, and the external genitalia make their appearance. The amnion is distended with fluid, but it is not yet in contact with the chorion; the chorionic villi have become more luxuriant on that part of the chorion resting on the decidua basalis, the future site of the placenta (Fig. 25). The approxi-

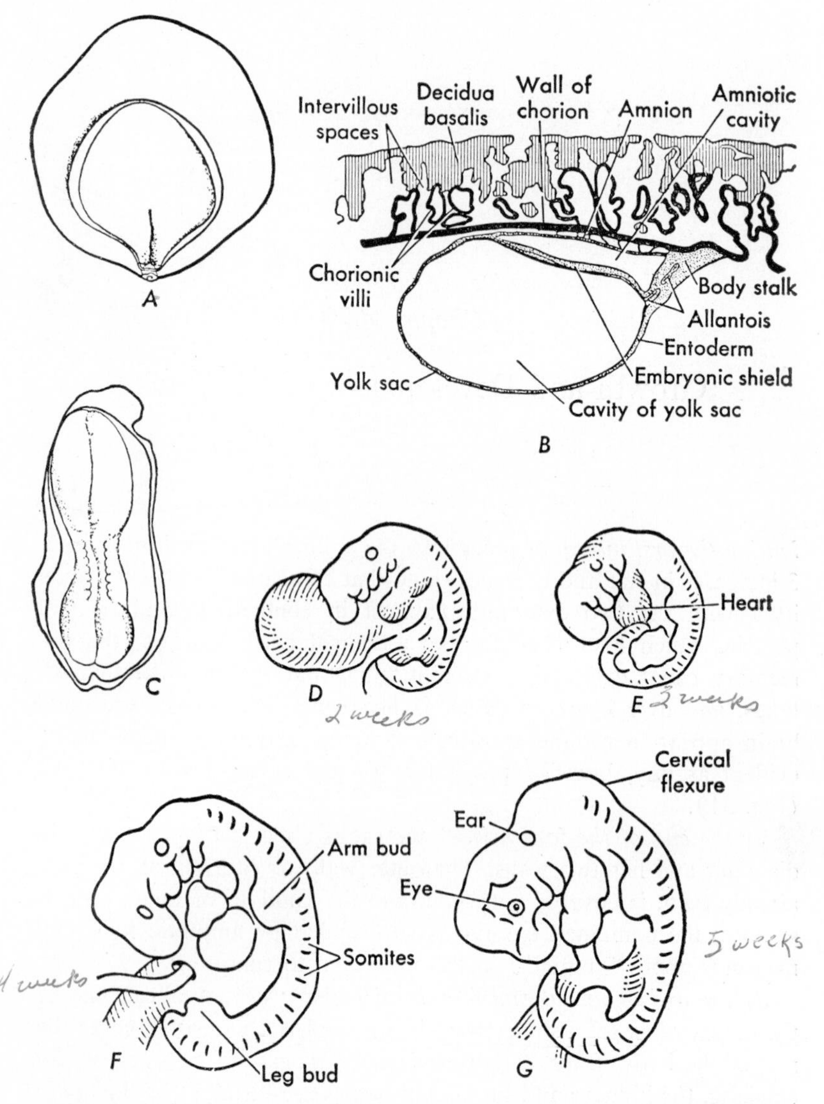


**Fig. 31.** Human embryos. *A, C,* dorsal view. *A* shows *primitive* streak. *B,* human embryo (Mateer) described by Streeter, estimated to be 17 days old and 0.92 mm long. Formation of the body stalk. The amnion is detaching itself from the chorion. (A. F. Huettner, *Fundamentals of Comparative Embryology of the Vertebrates,* 1st ed. Courtesy of The Macmillan Company.) *C* (1.38 mm long) shows primitive streak, *neural groove,* and the beginning of

mate weight of the embryo is 1 gm ($\frac{1}{30}$ oz), and its crown-heel length is about 30 mm (1.2 in.).

*By the end of the third month, or twelfth week,* centers of ossifica-

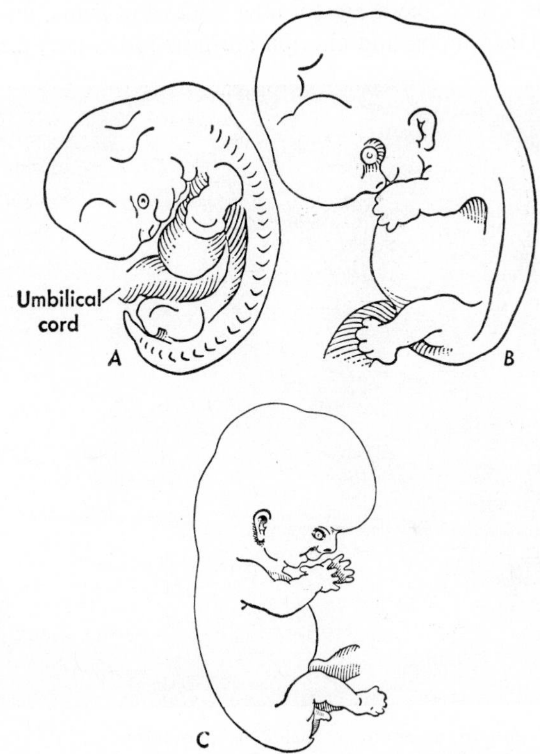


**Fig. 32.** Human embryos. Approximate age of *A* and *B*, 6 to 7 weeks. *C*, age about 2 months, length about 25 mm. Human form established, fetal period of development begun. Cervical flexure nearly gone; head, though still relatively large, lifted; body straightened. Neck well marked though short. Face developing; eyelids, nose, lips, external ears, cheeks appear. Ventral body wall formed, prominence due to the heart less conspicuous. Fore limbs have appearance of arms, thumbs well marked off from fingers, shoulders begin to appear. Legs smaller than arms; soles of feet close together. (Kimber, D.; Gray, C.; Stackpole, C.; and Leavell, L.: *Textbook of Anatomy and Physiology,* 13th ed. The Macmillan Company, New York, 1955.)

---

*somites.* Amnion has been cut away to show embryo, *D, E, F, G,* ages from 2 to 5 weeks. (Kimber, D.; Gray, C.; Stackpole, C.; and Leavell, L.: *Textbook of Anatomy and Physiology,* 13th ed. The Macmillan Company, New York, 1955.)

tion have appeared in most of the bones; the fingers and toes are separated and bear nails in the form of fine membranes; the umbilical cord has definite form, has increased in length, and begun to twist. The neck is longer, teeth are forming under the gums, and the eyes have lids. The amnion and chorion are now in contact, and the villi

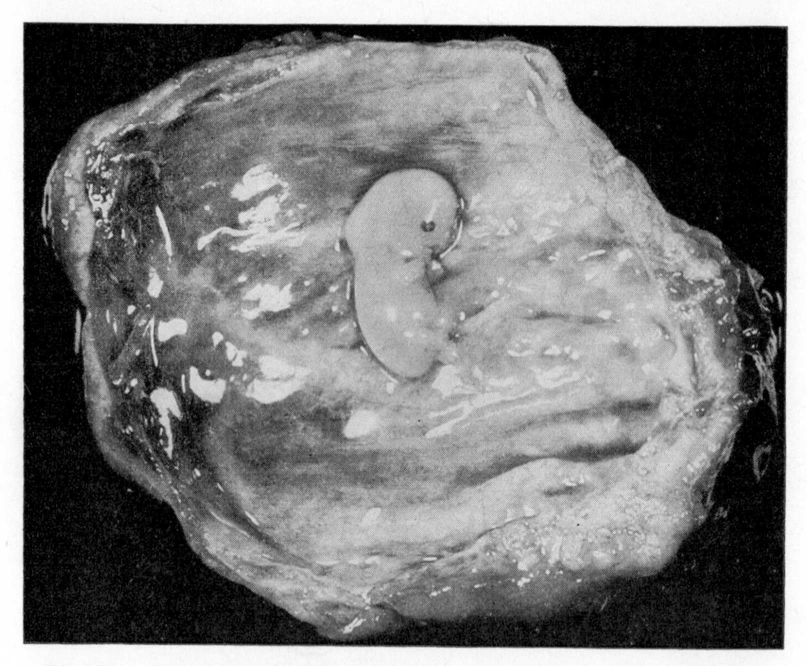

**Fig. 33.** Embryo in amniotic sac. This photograph is of a spontaneous complete abortion at 12 weeks of gestation. (Courtesy of Dr. Madeline J. Thornton.)

have disappeared except at one point where a small, but complete, placenta has developed. The embryo is about 6 cm (2.4 in.) long from crown to rump and weighs about 14 gm (½ oz) (Fig. 33).

*By the end of the fourth month, or sixteenth week,* all parts show growth and development; the external genitalia definitely show the sex; *lanugo,* a downy covering, appears over the body; and there is tarry fecal matter, called *meconium,* in the intestines. The placenta is larger, and the cord longer, more spiral, and also thicker because of the Wharton's jelly which is beginning to form. The fetus is about 15 cm (6 in.) long and weighs about 105 gm (3.5 oz).

*By the end of the fifth month, or twentieth week,* the fetus has both grown and developed markedly. The skin is less transparent, and has occasional patches of *vernix caseosa,* a greasy, cheesy substance consisting largely of a secretion of the sebaceous glands plus epithelial cells and lanugo hair. There is some fat beneath the skin, but the

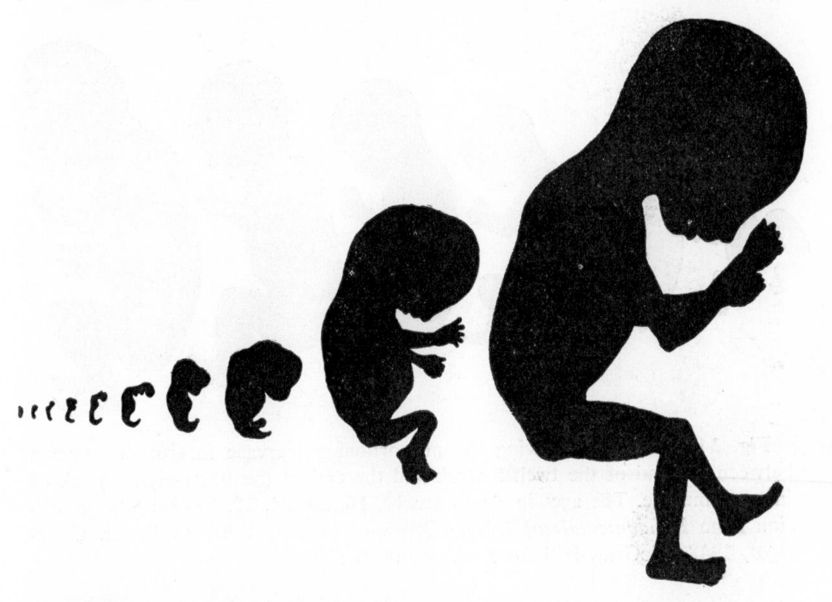

**Fig. 34A.** Embryos showing the proportionate increase in size that occurs between the end of the second week and the end of the twelfth week. The ages in days are 14, 16, 18, 20, 22, 25, 30, 42, 56, 84. (By permission from *Fundamentals of Human Reproduction,* by Edith L. Potter. Copyright, 1948, McGraw-Hill Book Company, Inc.)

face looks old and wrinkled. Hair has appeared upon the head, and the eyelids are opening. It is usually during the fifth month that the expectant mother first feels the fetal movements which are commonly referred to as "quickening." The body is about 24 cm (9.6 in.) long and weighs about 310 gm (10.3 oz).

*By the end of the sixth month, or twenty-fourth week,* the skin is markedly wrinkled, but fat begins to be deposited beneath it. The head is still comparatively large. A fetus born at this time will attempt to survive, but often dies shortly after birth. It is 28 to 34 cm (11.2 to 13.6 in.) long and weighs about 640 gm (1 lb, 6 oz).

*By the end of the seventh month, or twenty-eighth week,* the fetus still looks thin and scrawny, the eyelids are open, the skin is reddish and is well covered with vernix caseosa, and the intestines contain an increased amount of meconium. If born at this time the child will move quite vigorously and cry feebly. It is about 35 cm (14 in.)

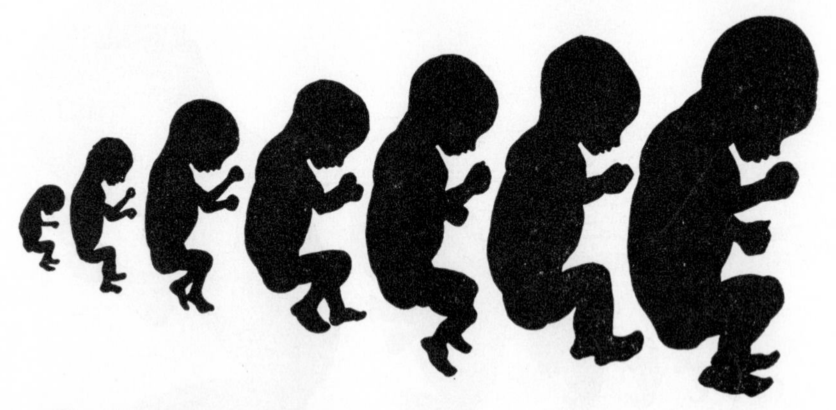

**Fig. 34B.** Fetuses showing the proportionate increase in size that occurs between the end of the twelfth week and the end of the thirty-eighth week of intrauterine life. The ages in weeks are 12, 16, 20, 24, 28, 32, 38. (By permission from *Fundamentals of Human Reproduction,* by Edith L. Potter. Copyright, 1948, McGraw-Hill Book Company, Inc.)

long and weighs about 1080 gm (2 lb, 6 oz). An infant this size is very immature, but its chances for survival are not entirely unfavorable if given expert care.

*By the end of the eighth month, or thirty-second week,* the child has grown to about 42 cm (16.8 in.) in length and 1680 gm (3 lb, 11 oz) in weight, but continues to look thin and old and wrinkled. The nails do not extend beyond the ends of the fingers, but are firmer in texture; the lanugo begins to disappear from the face, but the hair on the head is more abundant. If born at this stage, the baby will have a good chance to live, if given painstaking care. This is true in spite of the ancient superstition, still widely current, that a seven-month baby is more likely to live than one born at eight months (meaning calendar months). The fact is that after the eighth lunar month, a little more than seven calendar months, the probability of the child's living increases with each hour spent within the uterus.

*By the end of the ninth month, or thirty-sixth week,* the increased deposit of fat under the skin has given a plumper, rounder contour to the entire body; the aged look has passed, and the chances for life have greatly increased. The baby now weighs about 2400 gm (5¼ lb) and is about 45 cm (18 in.) long.

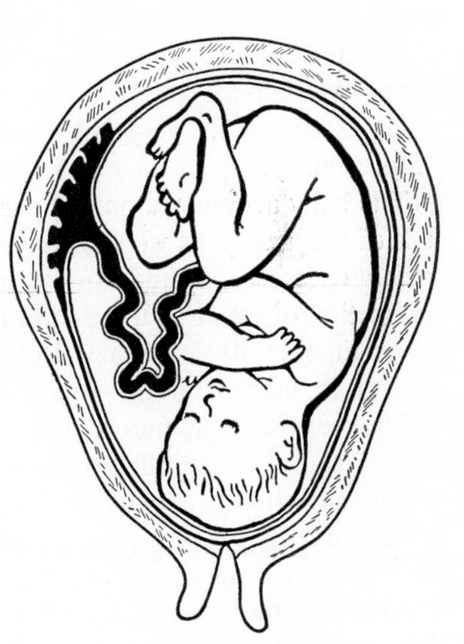

**Fig. 35.** Diagram of a section of uterus with well-developed fetus. The amnion is represented by a thin black line bounding the amniotic fluid in which the fetus lies. The heavy black line is the chorion. The fetal placenta and umbilical cord are shown at the left. (Kimber, D.; Gray, C.; Stackpole, C.; and Leavell, L.: *Textbook of Anatomy and Physiology,* 13th ed. The Macmillan Company, New York, 1955.)

*The end of the tenth month, or fortieth week,* usually marks the end of pregnancy (Fig. 35). The skin is now smooth with little or no lanugo hair, the fingers and toes have well-developed nails which extend beyond their tips, the eyes are a slate color, and the bones of the skull are well ossified and come close together at the suture lines. The average normally developed baby has attained a length of 50 cm (20 in.), and a weight of 3300 gm (about 7¼ lb), boys usually being about 90 gm (3 oz) heavier than girls. It must be remembered, however, that these figures merely represent the average drawn from a large number of cases, since there may be a variation in weight among entirely normal healthy babies from a minimum of 2500 gm (5½ lb) to as high as 5000 gm (11 lb), or more. In spite of this normal variation in birth weight, a baby weighing over 4500 gm (10 lb) is considered excessive in size.

The length of a normal baby is less variable than the weight. In fact, it is so nearly constant in its increase during the successive months of pregnancy that the age of a prematurely born fetus may be fairly accurately estimated from its length. There are two standards for the measurement of length, one being termed the *crown-rump* length, or sitting height, and the other the *crown-heel,* or total length. As it is difficult to maintain the legs in extension while the infant is measured, the crown-rump length may be a more accurate indication of the duration of intrauterine life. Chart I on page 77 shows the increase of the crown-rump and crown-heel length of the fetus, as well as its weight, by lunar months, from the second month of pregnancy.

The baby acquires about 90 per cent of its weight during the latter half of pregnancy, as well as a steadily increasing proportion of solids and a decrease of fluids in its tissues, since in its early days the proportion of water in the tissues of the embryo is larger than at any other time in its existence. But for all of that, its existence and growth in utero and the functioning of its heat-producing center, which keeps its temperature about $5/9°$ C (1° F) above the mother's, require surprisingly little oxygen and nourishment. The amniotic fluid keeps the fetus at a equable temperature, and as space within the uterine cavity permits only limited movement, there is very little combustion for the liberation of heat and energy.

Although the fetus at term is in many respects simply a diminutive, immature man, or woman, its anatomy and physiology present certain characteristics which have adapted it to a protected existence in a sac of fluid. Some of the fetal structures and functions become increasingly active after birth, while others subside and disappear.

We have seen that after the first month of pregnancy the placenta serves the fetus as a combined respiratory and digestive apparatus, not alone in supplying the oxygen and nourishment requisite for life and growth, but also in excreting the broken-down products of fetal life. Obviously, then, the fetus must possess a *circulatory mechanism* which is peculiar to itself alone, and not found in the independently existing human body, in which the lungs and alimentary tract are functioning as intended. This mechanism is provided by means of certain structures which exist in the fetal circulatory system and which automatically disappear shortly after birth. The structures which change or disappear after birth are the *foramen ovale,* a direct opening between the right and left atria, and four blood vessels: the *ductus arteriosus, ductus venosus,* and the two *hypogastric arteries.*

An understanding of the functions of these vessels involves an understanding of the course followed by the fetal blood currents, as indicated in Figure 36.

We see that there are three vessels within the umbilical cord: the umbilical vein and two arteries. In spite of its name, the vein conveys

RELATIONS OF AGE, SIZE, AND WEIGHT IN THE HUMAN EMBRYO

| *Age of Embryo* | *Crown-rump Length* (mm) | *Crown-heel Length* (mm) | *Weight in Grams* |
|---|---|---|---|
| Two lunar months | 23.0 | 30.0 | 1 |
| Three lunar months | 56.0 | 73.0 | 14 |
| Four lunar months | 112.0 | 157.0 | 105 |
| Five lunar months | 160.0 | 239.0 | 310 |
| Six lunar months | 203.0 | 296.0 | 640 |
| Seven lunar months | 242.0 | 355.0 | 1080 |
| Eight lunar months | 277.0 | 409.0 | 1670 |
| Nine lunar months | 313.0 | 458.0 | 2400 |
| Full term (38 weeks) | 350.0 | 500.0 | 3300 |

Chart I. A table showing relations of age, size, and weight in the human embryo. (From Arey, Leslie B.: *Development Anatomy*. 6th ed. W. B. Saunders Co., Philadelphia, 1954, p. 105.)

arterial blood from the placenta to the fetus. After piercing the baby's abdominal wall, it divides into two vessels; the larger one, called the ductus venosus, empties into the inferior, or ascending, vena cava, while the smaller branch joins the portal vein, which enters the liver. The relatively large amount of arterial blood sent directly to the liver may in part account for the large size of this organ in the fetus. Upon its emergence from the liver this blood stream flows into the inferior vena cava. The ascending vena cava, then, pours into the right atrium a mixture of arterial blood, directly from the placenta, and venous blood returned from the liver, intestines, and lower extremities.

The descending, or superior, vena cava, carrying blood returning from the head and arms, also empties into the right atrium, where the blood may mix with that entering from the ascending vena cava. The blood that enters the right atrium then passes into the left atrium and the right ventricle and on to other parts of the body. The eustachian valve, guarding the foramen ovale, deflects some of the blood through this opening from the right into the left atrium. It then pours into the left ventricle, is pumped into the arch of the aorta, from which most of the blood is sent to the head and upper extremities, although a small part carries nourishment to other parts of the body. The rest of the blood flows into the right ventricle by which it is pumped into the pulmonary artery. The circulation of blood through the lungs,

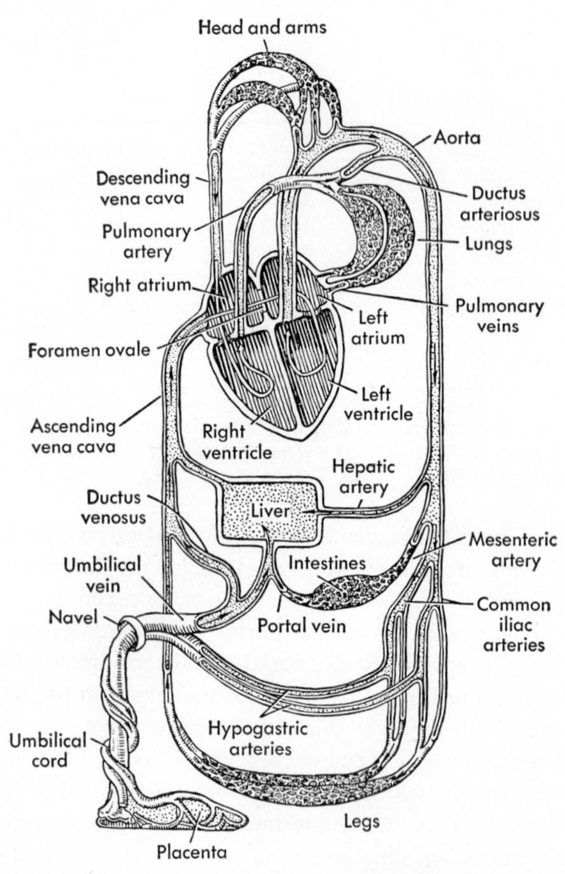


**Fig. 36.** Diagram showing course of fetal circulation through hypogastric arteries, ductus venosus, ductus arteriosus, and the foramen ovale. (Modified from *The American Textbook on Obstetrics.*) (Kimber, D.; Gray, C.; Stackpole, C.; and Leavell, L.: *Textbook of Anatomy and Physiology,* 13th ed. The Macmillan Company, New York, 1955.)

however, is for their own nourishment, and not for aeration as with the adult. For this reason most of the content of the fetal pulmonary artery empties into the aorta through the ductus arteriosus, one of the temporary fetal structures already referred to. From the aorta the stream is directed in part to the lower extremities and the pelvic and abdominal viscera, but most of it flows into the hypogastric arteries. These also are temporary arteries. They lead to the umbilical cord and, as the umbilical arteries, carry the venous or vitiated blood through the cord to the placenta where it is oxygenated, freed of its waste in the chorionic villi, and returned to the fetus through the umbilical vein.

The blood circulating in the fetus then is never entirely arterial or entirely venous, but that in the inferior, or ascending, vena cava is purer than that in the aorta.

As soon as the child is born and is obliged to obtain its oxygen from the surrounding air, its pulmonary circulation of necessity becomes immediately more important and is greatly increased in volume. In fact, the entire fetal circulation is readjusted to meet the needs of the new and independent functions which the body now assumes. The temporary structures are obliterated, since they are no longer needed, and the lungs and other excretory organs become more active in compensation (Fig. 37).

As the ductus venosus and hypogastric arteries terminate in blind ends and become useless as soon as the umbilical cord is cut, they begin to atrophy and are obliterated within a few days after birth. This means that less blood is poured into the right atrium from the ascending vena cava which naturally results in relatively less tension in the right side of the heart and an increased pressure on the left; this tends to close the foramen ovale. The foramen ovale thus closes functionally within a few minutes after birth, but anatomic obliteration occurs gradually. Occasionally it remains open permanently, and although some people have gone through life comfortably with a patent foramen ovale, its ultimate failure to close usually results in serious circulatory trouble. This is true also of the ductus arteriosus, which sometimes, but not often, fails to close. The rule is that as the lungs expand and an increased amount of blood is carried to them for aeration, the ductus arteriosus deflects a rapidly diminishing stream from the right ventricle to the arch of the aorta. Thus it quickly ceases functioning in most cases and disappears in the course of a few weeks. The abandoned vessels may degenerate and disappear in time or they may persist in the form of small fibrous cords.

Although the circulatory system shows the most elaborate adjust-

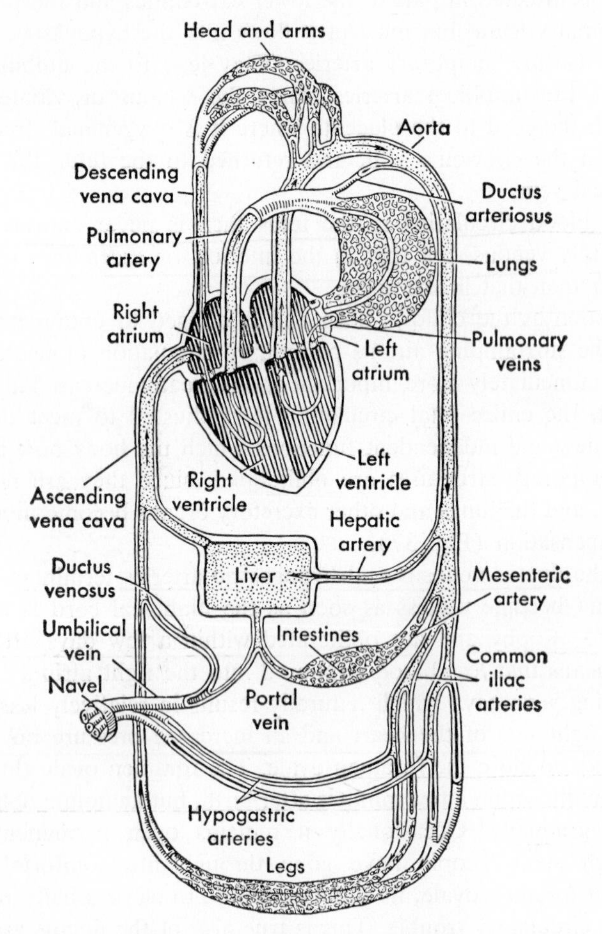


**Fig. 37.** Diagram showing circulation of the blood after birth, with hypogastric arteries, ductus venosus, ductus arteriosus, and foramen ovale *in process of obliteration* and pulmonary circulation greatly increased. The ductus arteriosus and the ductus venosus become the ligamentum arteriosus and the ligamentum venosus; the umbilical vein becomes the ligamentum teres. (Modified from *The American Textbook on Obstetrics.*) (Kimber, D.; Gray, C.; Stackpole, C.; and Leavell, L.: *Textbook of Anatomy and Physiology,* 13th ed. The Macmillan Company, New York, 1955.)

ments to the protection afforded by intrauterine life, there are also other adaptations made by the fetal organism.

**The kidneys** assume functional form at a very early fetal age, probably about the seventh week, and the presence of albumin and urea in the amniotic fluid suggests that small amounts of urine are voided, particularly during the latter part of pregnancy.

**The bowels,** on the other hand, are normally inactive; this in spite of the fact that the baby evidently obtains fluid, and possibly some nutriment, by swallowing amniotic fluid. The intestinal content of the fetus consists chiefly of meconium, a dark, tarry substance which is made up of bile pigment and cast-off hairs from the fetus' own body, which it swallows with the amniotic fluid. Normally, the fetus does not expel meconium until after birth. However, under abnormal conditions, some may be expelled and the amniotic fluid deeply stained by it. In a head presentation this may occur when the baby's life is endangered by some interference with its oxygenation, which in turn causes a relaxation of the anal sphincter muscles allowing the meconium to escape. Its presence, then, in the amniotic fluid in a head presentation is usually of grave significance. When the child presents by the buttocks, meconium is normally expelled because of pressure on its abdomen as it passes through the pelvis, and in this case meconium-stained amniotic fluid is not necessarily a sign of fetal distress.

**The respiratory system** shows some rapid superficial movements which begin after the first trimester of pregnancy. They are believed to be activated by the carbon dioxide in the blood.

**The head** is the most important part of the fetus, from the standpoint of delivery of the baby, since the process of labor is virtually a series of adaptations of the size, shape, and position of the fetal skull to the size and shape of the maternal pelvis. It is a question of the "passenger" being adapted to the "passage," and since the pelvis is rigid and inflexible the adjustment must all be made by the fetal head, which is moldable because of being incompletely ossified at birth. If the head passes through the pelvis safely, the rest of the delivery will usually be accomplished with comparative safety. A marked disproportion between the diameters of the head and the pelvis, or limited moldability of the head, constitutes a serious complication, which is discussed later in connection with obstetric operations (Chap. 14).

A baby's head is larger, in proportion to its body, than an adult's, while the face forms a relatively smaller part of the baby's than of the adult's head. The major portion is the dome, or vault-like structure, forming the top, sides, and back of the head, which in turn is made up of separate and as yet ununited bones. They are the two *frontal,* two *parietal,* two *temporal,* and the *occipital* bone, with which the wings of the *sphenoid* bone, though less important, may be included.

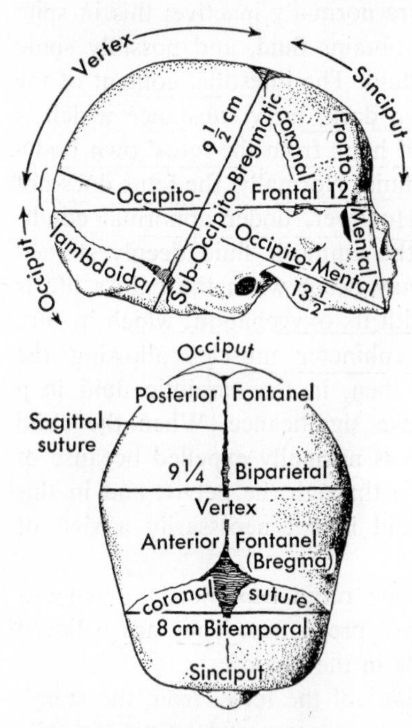


**Fig. 38.** Side and top views of fetal skull, giving average length of important diameters.

These bones are not joined in the fetal skull, but are separate structures, with soft, membranous spaces between their margins, called *sutures.* The irregular spaces formed by the intersection of two or more sutures are called *fontanels,* possibly so called by the early observers because the pulsation in the soft tissues beneath these spaces suggests the spurting of a fountain.

The sutures are named and situated as follows: the *frontal* lies between the two frontal bones, the *sagittal* extends anteroposteriorly between the parietal bones, the *coronal* lies between the frontal bones and the anterior margins of the parietals, while the *lambdoidal* suture separates the posterior margins of the parietals from the upper margin of the occipital bone (Fig. 38). There are also the temporal sutures between the upper margins of the temporal bones and the lower margins of the two parietals, but they are of no obstetric importance as they cannot be felt on vaginal examination.

There are two fontanels of obstetric significance (Fig. 38). The greater, or *anterior,* fontanel, also called the *bregma* or *sinciput,* is located at the meeting of the coronal, sagittal, and frontal sutures. It is diamond- or lozenge-shaped, about 2.5 cm (1 in.) in diameter, and is not obliterated during labor. The smaller, or *posterior,* fontanel, is the triangular space at the intersection of the sagittal and lambdoidal sutures, and may be obliterated as the surrounding bony margins approach each other during labor.

The coronal, frontal, lambdoidal, and sagittal sutures and the anterior and posterior fontanels are of great diagnostic value because they can be felt through the vagina during labor. It is by recognizing and locating these sutures and fontanels at this time that the obstetrician is enabled to determine the exact position and presentation of the fetus.

The fact that the skull is made up of separate bones, with soft membranous spaces interposed between them, permits its being compressed, or molded, to a considerable extent as it passes through the birth canal. Opposing margins may meet, or even overlap, to such a degree that the diameter of the head will be appreciably diminished and permit its passage through a relatively narrow canal. This moldability varies greatly, however, and the difference in the degree of compressibility of heads of approximately the same size may spell the difference between an easy and a difficult, or even an impossible, birth. A newborn baby's head may be so distorted and elongated by the molding process that its abnormal appearance gives the mother great concern, but the nurse can be quite confident in her assurances that the head will assume its normal outline in a very few days.

The five most important diameters of the newborn baby's head are (Fig. 38):

1. *The occipitofrontal* (abbreviation, O.F.), measured from the root of the nose to the occipital protuberance, is 11.75 to 12 cm (4.7 to 4.8 in.)

2. *The biparietal* (B.P.) is the greatest transverse diameter, being the distance between the parietal protuberances, and measures 9.25 cm (3.7 in.).

3. *The bitemporal* (B.T.) is the greatest distance between the temporal bones and measures 8 cm (3.2 in.).

4. *The occipitomental* (O.M.) is the greatest distance from the lower margin of the chin to a point on the posterior extremity of the sagittal suture, and measures 13.5 cm (5.4 in.).

5. *The suboccipitobregmatic* (S.O.B.) is measured from the under surface of the occiput, where it joins the neck, to the center of the anterior fontanel, a distance of 9.5 cm (3.8 in.).

Until the fetus weighs approximately 4500 gm (10 lb) the circumference of the head is greater than the circumference of the shoulders. At term, these circumferences are usually about the same, but if the child develops to an excessive size, the circumference of the shoulders is greater than that of the head.

The greatest circumference of the fetal head is at the plane of the fronto-occipital diameter and measures 34.5 cm (13.8 in.). The smallest circumference is at the plane of the suboccipitobregmatic diameter and measures 32 cm (12.8 in.).

These figures, however, like all of those which it is possible to give, simply represent averages taken from a large number of cases. Individual variations will be found among normal babies; boys' heads, for example, are usually larger than girls', while the head of the first child is likely to be smaller than the head of any born subsequently. The size of the baby is affected by race; Negro babies, for example, averaging a smaller weight than white babies. As might be expected, the size of the parents is likely to be reflected in the size of their infants, large parents tending to have large children and small parents to have small babies. The number of children which the mother has previously borne is also a factor, since the first child is usually the smallest; the size of those following showing an increase.

To sum up the normal pregnancy, we find that in the course of 10 lunar months, following the fertilization of an ovum, the uterus grows from a small, flattened, pelvic organ, 7.5 cm (3 in.) in length, to a large, globular, muscular sac, constituting an abdominal tumor between 30 and 35 cm (12 and 14 in.) long; it increases its weight 16 times, that is from 60 gm (2 oz) to 960 gm (2.1 lb), while the capacity of the uterine cavity is multiplied 500 times. Within the cavity is a child weighing about 3300 gm (7¼ lb), surrounded by about 600 ml (20 oz) of amniotic fluid. This fluid is contained in the sac composed of the fetal membranes, the amnion and chorion, which are excessively developed at one point into the placenta. The placenta, in turn, is attached to the child by means of the umbilical cord. The total weight of the uterus and its contents at term is usually about 5450 gm (12 lb).

After the mysterious and inexplicable development of these very complex structures from one tiny cell has reached the stage at which the new human being is ready to begin life as a separate entity, further changes occur within the mother's body which produce uterine contractions of such a character as to entirely empty the uterus of its contents.

### MULTIPLE PREGNANCIES

A multiple pregnancy is one in which the pregnant uterus contains two or more embryos, these being termed twins when there are two and triplets when there are three; quadruplets, or quintuplets, when there are four, or five embryos, respectively. Six are now the largest unquestionably accredited number on record.

Twin pregnancies may result from the fertilization of two separate ova or of a single ovum, giving rise respectively to double-ovum or fraternal twins and single-ovum or identical twins. In double-ovum or fraternal twins, both ova may come from the same ovary or one may come from each ovary; there are two placentas, although they may be fused, two amnions, and two chorions. The babies may or may not be of the same sex and do not resemble each other more than any other brothers and sisters. Biologically, double-ovum twins are not really twins, but simply the result of the maturation and fertilization of two ova at a single ovulation period.

Single-ovum or identical twins, on the other hand, are truly twins, the occurrence being thus defined by H. H. Newman: "Strictly speaking, twinning is twaining or two-ing—the division of an individual into two equivalent and more or less completely separate individuals." In the case of single-ovum twins there are one placenta, one chorion, and two amnions; the babies are always of the same sex and throughout life resemble each other closely, both physically and mentally. Their ears, for example, are alike as well as hair whorling and color of eyes and hair, and they have the same tendencies to disease. They are of the same type of intelligence, disposition, and personality. For this reason the general tenor of the lives of single-ovum or identical twins is strikingly similar.

There is apparently no one accepted explanation of the origin of single-ovum twins. It is usually believed that the embryonic portion of the developing ovum simply splits into two parts very early in its career. There is much evidence to show that this is probably due to an unexplained and transient retardation of its development.

The hereditary influence in the tendency toward multiple pregnancies is a moot question. The occurrence of a single pair of twins in a family where single pregnancies have been the rule does not suggest hereditary influence, but if several sets of twins occur in the same family the tendency is believed to be inherited and may come through either maternal or paternal transmission.

Triplets may derive from one ovum, as in the case of twins, or from two or three ova. Accordingly there may be single-, double-, or triple-ovum triplets. The same is true of quadruplets, the number being carried to four ova.

Multiple pregnancies seem to vary with race rather than with other factors. It is estimated that twins occur about once in every 86 pregnancies and triplets once in about every 7000 births; also that twins are born more frequently in the Negro than in the white race and are least common in the Mongolian race. The racial difference is apparently due to a variation in multiple ovulation.

Multiple pregnancies may give rise to more complications during the prenatal period and the delivery than single pregnancies, and the greater distention of the uterus will frequently lead to more discomfort of the patient.

Twins are often born prematurely, and each one is likely to be smaller than a baby resulting from a single pregnancy, but their combined weight is greater than that of one normal infant.

The prospect of twins or triplets living is affected by the same general factors as those influencing the outlook of a single baby, that is, the length of intrauterine life and the body weight at birth. The chances of all the babies of a quadruplet or quintuplet pregnancy surviving are rather small.

## BIBLIOGRAPHY AND STUDENT REFERENCES

Arey, Leslie B.: *Developmental Anatomy,* 6th ed. W. B. Saunders Co., Philadelphia, 1954.

Bookmiller, Mae M., and Bowen, George L.: *Textbook of Obstetrics and Obstetric Nursing,* 2nd ed. W. B. Saunders Co., Philadelphia, 1954.

Davis, M. Edward, and Sheckler, Catherine E.: *DeLee's Obstetrics for Nurses,* 15th ed. W. B. Saunders Co., Philadelphia, 1951.

Eastman, Nicholson J.: *Williams Obstetrics,* 11th ed. Appleton-Century-Crofts, Inc., New York, 1956.

Greenhill, J. P. (ed.): *Obstetrics,* 11th ed. W. B. Saunders Co., Philadelphia, 1955.

Kimber, Diana C.; Gray, Carolyn E.; Stackpole, Caroline E.; and Leavell, Lutie C.: *Textbook of Anatomy and Physiology,* 13th ed. The Macmillan Company, New York, 1955.

Potter, Edith L.: *Fundamentals of Human Reproduction.* McGraw-Hill Book Co., New York, 1948.

Woodward, H. L.; Gardner, B.; Bryant, R. D.; and Overland, Anna E.: *Obstetric Management and Nursing,* 5th ed. F. A. Davis Co., Philadelphia, 1955.

# PART III. THE EXPECTANT MOTHER

*Chapter 5*

## Signs, Symptoms, and Physiology of Pregnancy

The exact duration of pregnancy has never been ascertained, since there is no way of knowing when the ovum is fertilized, which is the moment that marks the beginning of pregnancy. It is obviously impossible, therefore, to foretell exactly the date of confinement, but labor usually begins about 10 lunar months, 40 weeks, or from 273 to 280 days after the onset of the last menstrual period.

### ESTIMATING THE PROBABLE DATE OF CONFINEMENT

The approximate date of confinement may be estimated by counting forward 280 days or backward 85 days from the first day of the last menstrual period. What is perhaps simpler, and gives approximately the same date is to add seven days to the onset of the last period and count back three months. For example, if the last period began on June third, the addition of seven days gives June tenth, while counting back three months indicates March tenth as the approximate date upon which the delivery may be expected. This is probably as satisfactory as any known method of computation, being accurate within 10 days before or after the estimated date in about two-thirds of all deliveries.

Another method sometimes employed by obstetricians is to estimate the month to which pregnancy has advanced by measuring the height of the fundus, and thus forecasting the probable date of confinement. It is generally agreed that the ascent of the fundus is fairly uniform and that at the fourth lunar month it is several fingerbreadths above the symphysis pubis; at the fifth lunar month, over halfway between the symphysis and umbilicus; at the sixth month, on a level with the umbilicus; at the seventh month, three fingerbreadths, and at the eighth month six fingerbreadths above the umbilicus; and at the ninth month, just below the xiphoid. At the tenth month, or term, the fundus in primigravidas sinks downward to about the position it occupied at the eighth month (Figs. 39 and 40.) This drop in waist line is more common among primigravidas because, as the head engages, the fetus descends a few inches into the pelvis. *Engagement* in primigravidas usually occurs in the last few weeks of pregnancy, but in multigravidas the head frequently remains unengaged until labor begins. By engagement is meant that the head enters the true pelvis and further movement of the head is strictly limited by the walls of the bony pelvis. This method, however, is measuring by months, not days, and leaves a wide margin for conjecture as to the exact date.

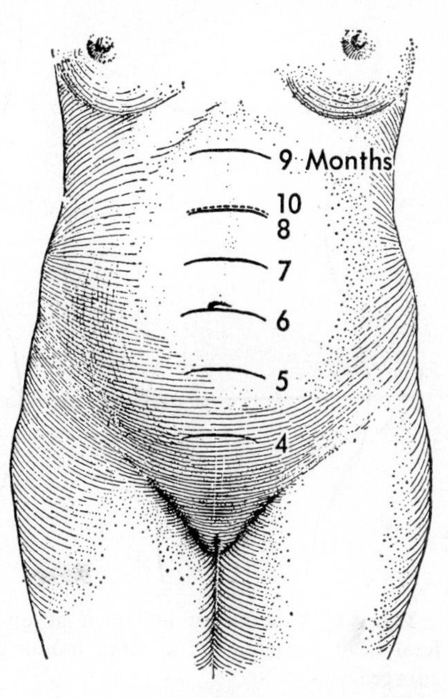


**Fig. 39.** Height of fundus at each of the ten lunar months of pregnancy.

Still another method is to count forward 20 to 22 weeks from the day upon which the expectant mother first feels the fetus move. As we shall see presently, this experience, termed "quickening," usually occurs about the eighteenth to twentieth week, but is so irregular that it is unreliable as a basis for computation.

The possibility of estimating the date of confinement is still further complicated by the fact that there are variations in the size of fetuses and amounts of amniotic fluid at the same periods of gestation, that the onset of the last normal menstrual period may be unknown, and that conception may have taken place during a period of amenorrhea as in the nursing mother.

## SIGNS AND SYMPTOMS OF PREGNANCY

Although the signs and symptoms of pregnancy have been observed throughout the ages by women who have borne children, and by the doctors at one time or another who have attended them, a positive diagnosis at an early stage of pregnancy is sometimes still difficult even for experienced obstetricians.

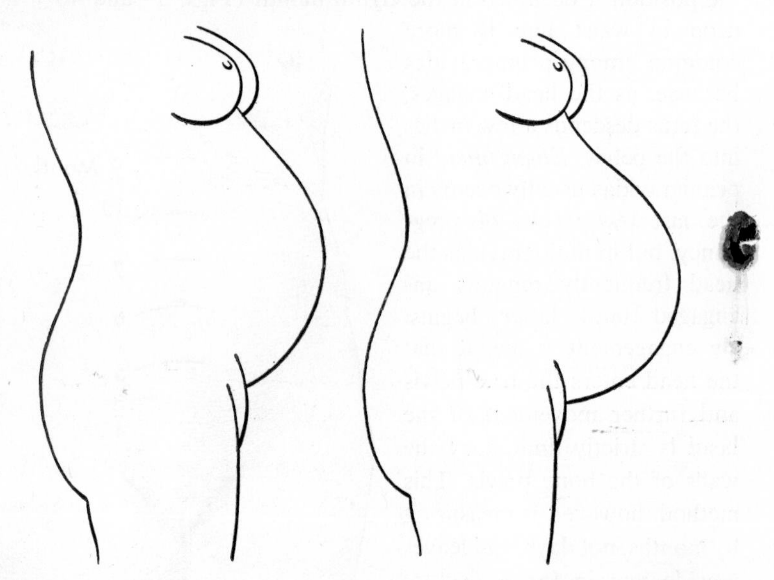

**Fig. 40.** Coutour of abdomen at ninth month of pregnancy, before the fetal head engages, and at tenth month of pregnancy, or after the head has engaged.

So many symptoms of pregnancy are known to women the world over, that an expectant mother frequently recognizes her pregnant state at a very early date. This is particularly true of women who have previously borne children. On the other hand, one hears of an occasional case in which a woman is entirely unaware of her pregnancy until she goes into labor.

The converse is also true, since women sometimes erroneously believe themselves pregnant because of the appearance of well-recognized symptoms, which are due to other causes. This condition is known as *pseudocyesis,* or spurious pregnancy, and is usually found in women approaching the menopause or in young women who intensely desire offspring. It is a pathetic occurrence, and the patient is usually so tenacious of her belief in her approaching motherhood that the obstetrician dispels it only with great difficulty.

For all of these and other reasons it is customary to divide the signs and symptoms of pregnancy into three groups, under self-explanatory headings, namely: *presumptive* signs and symptoms, *probable* signs, and *positive* signs. Although it is never within the province of a nurse to make a diagnosis, it is important that she be familiar with the symptoms. In obstetrics this seems to be particularly true if the nurse is engaged in prenatal work or in any branch of public health nursing that brings her in touch with possible or expectant mothers. The wider her grasp of obstetric knowledge, the more helpful and reassuring can be her relation to her patient. To this end, therefore, the most reliable signs and symptoms of pregnancy are discussed.

### PRESUMPTIVE SIGNS AND SYMPTOMS

The presumptive symptoms, which consist largely of subjective symptoms observed by the patient herself and which may be experienced at varying periods, are as follows:

**Cessation of Menstruation.** This is usually the first symptom noticed. A period may be missed from any one of several causes, as has been explained in Chapter 2, but in a healthy woman of the childbearing age, whose menses have previously been regular, the missing of two successive periods after intercourse is a strong indication of pregnancy.

**Changes in the Breasts.** These also occur early. The breasts ordinarily increase in size and firmness, and many women complain of throbbing, tingling, or pricking sensations and a feeling of tension and fullness. The breasts may be so tender that even slight pressure is painful. The nipples are larger and more prominent, while both they and the surrounding areolae grow darker. The veins under the skin are more apparent and the glands of Montgomery larger. If, in addition to these symptoms, it is possible to express a pale yellowish fluid from the nipples of a woman who has not had children, pregnancy may be strongly suspected. Practically all of these symptoms may be due to causes other than pregnancy, and, in the case of a woman who has borne children, milk may be present in the breasts for months, or even years, after the birth of a child.

**"Morning sickness,"** as the name suggests, is nausea, sometimes accompanied by vomiting, from which many pregnant women suffer immediately upon arising in the morning. It varies in severity from a mild attack when the patient first lifts her head to repeated and severe recurrences during the day, and even into the night. The morning nausea, lasting but a few hours, usually occurs daily for about six weeks when it gradually disappears. When the vomiting is very severe and not relieved by simple remedies, it is termed "pernicious vomiting" and is usually accepted as evidence of a toxic or neurotic condition, or both, all of which are discussed with the complications of pregnancy (Chap. 9). Morning sickness may begin immediately after conception, but as a rule it starts about the sixth week and continues until the third or fourth month. It occurs in about half of all pregnancies and is particularly common among women pregnant for the first time. Many women go throughout the entire period of gestation without nausea and vomiting, while others are entirely comfortable in the morning and nauseated only during the latter part of the day.

**Frequent Micturition.** There is usually a desire to void urine frequently during the first three or four months of pregnancy, after which the tendency disappears, but recurs during the later months. The inclination may be due in part to nervousness but is largely caused by reduction in the capacity of the bladder, due to crowding, by pressure exerted upon it from the outside by the enlarging uterus while both organs remain within the unyielding bony pelvis, and not to any functional disturbance of the kidneys, as is sometimes believed. Pressure on the outside of the bladder gives much the same sensation as is experienced when the bladder is distended with urine. After the uterus and bladder rise from the pelvic cavity into the abdomen, the uterus no longer crowds the bladder. During the last month or six weeks, it again presses upon the bladder and once more there is a desire to void frequently.

**Increased discoloration** of the pigmented areas of the skin and the appearance of *abdominal striae* are other presumptive signs. In addition to the deepened tint of the nipples and surrounding areolae, the *linea alba,* a pale, whitish line which divides the abdomen longitudinally from sternum to symphysis pubis, becomes darker and is then known as the *linea nigra.* This line grows progressively paler after delivery. There are also the brownish, irregularly shaped blotches which sometimes appear on the face and neck, known as *chloasma,* or "mask of pregnancy." Dark circles under the eyes are commonly seen.

**Chadwick's sign,** the dark bluish or purplish appearance of the vulval and vaginal lining, which is the result of a great increase in vascularity, is another early sign of pregnancy.

**"Quickening"** is the widely used term which designates the mother's first perception of the fetal movements, which occur about the eighteenth to twentieth week. The sensation is comparable to a very slight quivering or tapping, or to the fluttering of a bird's wings imprisoned in the hand. Beginning very gently, these movements increase in severity as time goes on; they may become very troublesome toward the latter part of pregnancy, amounting then to sharp kicks and blows. Women who have had children can usually be relied upon to distinguish between quickening and the somewhat similar sensation caused by the movement of gas in the intestines, but a woman pregnant for the first time may be deceived. Women often use the term "feeling life" when they feel the fetus move, and doctors and nurses frequently use this term when questioning the patient about the perception of fetal movements.

There are other possible symptoms of pregnancy, but their value is uncertain. Even the ones described above are not entirely dependable, but if two or more of them occur coincidently, they probably indicate pregnancy. Dr. J. Morris Slemons sums it up by saying:

> If, for example, menstruation has previously been regular and then a period is missed, the patient has good reason to suspect she is pregnant; if the next period is also missed, and meanwhile the breasts have enlarged, the nipple darkened, and the secretion of colostrum has begun, it is nearly certain that she is pregnant; whether morning-sickness and the desire to pass the urine frequently are present is of no importance.*

## PROBABLE SIGNS

The probable signs of pregnancy are chiefly discoverable by the physician after careful examination. They also are numerous and

* Slemons, J. Morris: *The Prospective Mother,* 4th ed. Appleton-Century-Crofts, Inc., New York, 1942, p. 13.

uncertain, but there are four which are considered fairly trustworthy.

**Enlargement of the abdomen,** which is first in order of importance, is apparent about the third month. At this stage, the growing uterus may be felt through the abdominal wall as a tumor which steadily increases in size as pregnancy advances. Rapid enlargement of the abdomen in a woman of childbearing age, therefore, may be taken as fair, but not positive, evidence of pregnancy. Too much reliance cannot be placed on this sign, as the abdomen may be enlarged by a tumor, fluid, or a rapid increase in fat.

**Changes in the size, shape, and consistency of the uterus** which take place during the first three months of pregnancy are very important indications. These are discoverable upon vaginal examination, which shows the uterus considerably enlarged, somewhat globular in shape, and of a soft, doughy consistency. About the sixth week, the so-called *Hegar's sign* is perceptible through bimanual examination. This is discovered when the fingers of one hand are pressed deeply into the abdomen, just above the symphysis pubis, and two fingers of the other hand are passed through the vagina until they rest in the posterior fornix, behind the cervix. The isthmus of the uterus, which may be felt between the finger tips of the two hands, is extremely soft and compressible. Occasionally the change in consistency is so marked that there appears to be no connection between the cervix which is felt below the finger tips and the body of the uterus which lies above them. This sign, named for the man who first described it, is one of the most valuable signs of early pregnancy.

**Softening of the cervix** occurs, as a rule, about the beginning of the second month. In some cases, such as certain inflammatory conditions and in carcinoma, this sign may not appear. This softening of the cervix is often called *Goodell's sign.*

**Painless uterine contractions,** called *Braxton-Hicks* contractions, from their first observer, begin during the early weeks of pregnancy and recur at intervals of 5 to 10 minutes throughout the entire period of gestation. The patient is not conscious of these contractions, but they may be observed during the early months by bimanual examination, and subsequently by placing the hand on the abdomen. One feels the uterus growing alternately hard and soft as it contracts and relaxes.

All of the probable signs of pregnancy, like the presumptive symptoms, may be simulated in nonpregnant conditions; hence the appearance of any one of them alone may not be deeply significant. Two or more occurring coincidently constitute strong evidence of pregnancy.

### POSITIVE SIGNS

The positive signs of pregnancy, of which there are four, are not apparent until the eighteenth to twentieth week, and all emanate from the fetus.

**Hearing and counting the fetal heartbeat** is unmistakable evidence of pregnancy. The sound of the fetal heartbeat is usually likened to the ticking of a watch under a pillow. The rate is from 120 to 140 beats per minute, being about twice as fast as the maternal pulse. So long as its rhythm is regular, however, the rate may drop to 100 or increase to 160 beats per minute without being considered abnormal or indicative of trouble in the fetus.

**Ability to palpate the outline of the fetus** is also a positive sign of pregnancy, if the head, breech, back, and extremities are unmistakably made out through the abdominal wall.

**Perception of active and passive movements of the fetus** is accepted as a third incontrovertible sign of pregnancy. If the fetal movements are perceptible by the obstetrician through the mother's abdominal wall or by vaginal examination, there can be no doubt about the diagnosis. The movements felt by placing the hand upon the abdomen are termed *active movements*, while the *passive movements* result from internal or external *ballottement*. Ballottement is accomplished by giving a sharp or sudden push to the head or an extremity, and feeling it rebound in a few seconds to its original position. Passive movements may be felt early in the fourth month, and active movements after the eighteenth to twentieth week.

**Ability to See the Skeletal Outline by X-ray.** This outline is not visible before the fourteenth week, or even later, but is valuable in obese women or when it is difficult to differentiate between a normal pregnancy and a tumor. Dr. William Snow states:

> . . . , with the advancement of x-ray technic we have been able to obtain valuable information relative to the fetus. The age may be determined from the size of the skull, appearance of epiphyses, the general size of the fetus, and the amount of visible subcutaneous fat. Fetal death may be detected as well as other pathologic states. Presentation, flexion, exten-

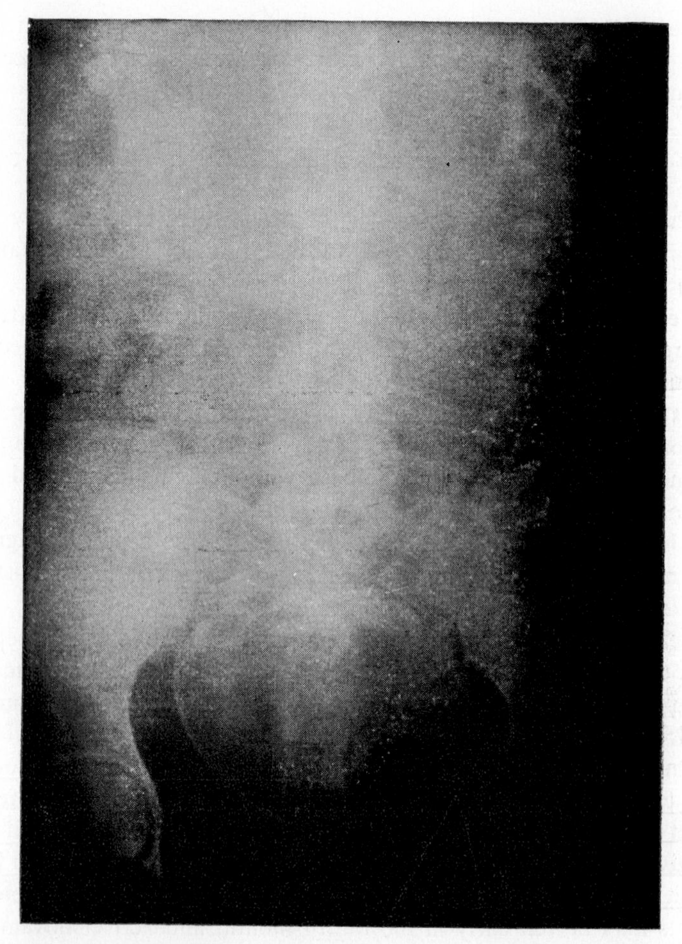

**Fig. 41.** An x-ray taken on a patient who was supposedly close to term. It had previously been determined that a cesarean section was indicated, but since the gestational age was not definitely known and palpation of the abdomen was difficult, a roentgenogram seemed indicated to determine fetal age and position.

This x-ray shows a single well-developed fetal skeleton with the head presenting at the inlet and with the back lying to the left and anteriorly. The fetal size and skeletal development corresponds to one in the last month of gestation. There is no evidence of fetal skeletal abnormalities.

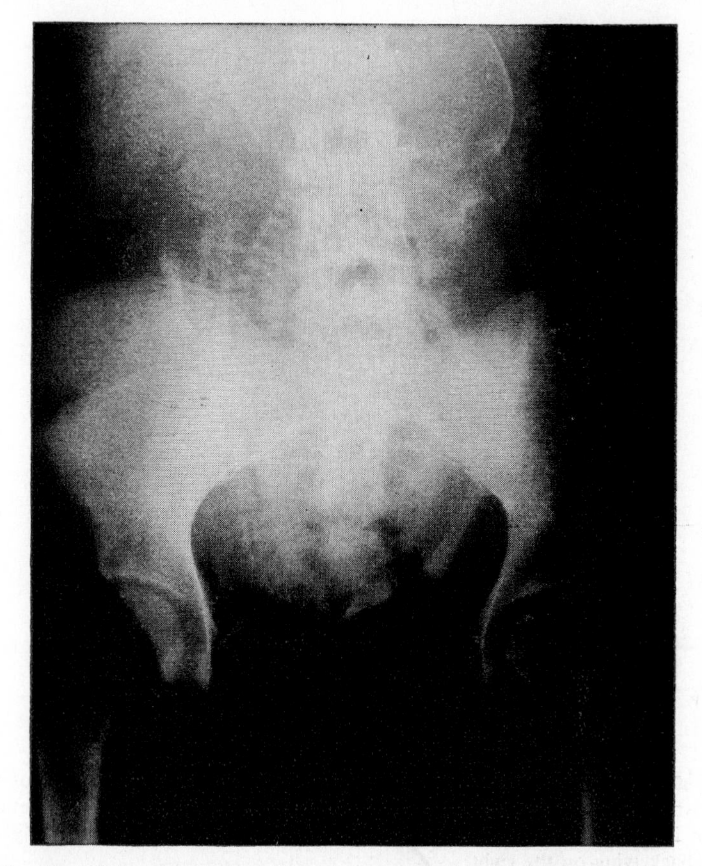

**Fig. 42.** This roentgenogram shows a well-developed fetus in a frank breech presentation with the sacrum to the right and anterior.

sion, deflection, and degree of engagement may be studied so that causes of abnormality may be more readily ascertained.*

## PREGNANCY TESTS

The idea that something in the urine of pregnant women would cause plants to grow or seeds to germinate has been held since ancient time, but it was not until the twentieth century that any real

* Snow, William: *Roentgenology in Obstetrics and Gynecology*. Charles C Thomas, Publisher, Springfield, Ill., 1952, p. 5.

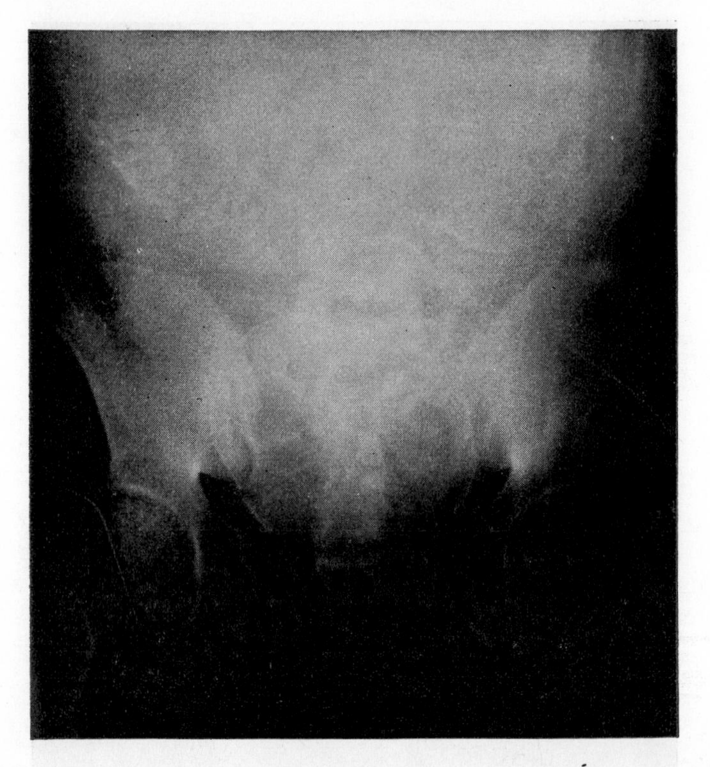

**Fig. 43.** Twin pregnancy. This roentgenogram shows that the head of one fetus is presenting at the inlet and with its back to the left. The other fetus is seen immediately above the first with the head lying somewhat anteriorly and the back lying on the right.

scientific research was carried out. Several men doing this work discovered that the urine of pregnant women contained large amounts of a hormone which would stimulate the ovaries of animals to ovulate. This hormone, now known as *chorionic gonadotropin,* is present in the blood and urine of pregnant women in fairly large concentration by the fifteenth day of pregnancy; this concentration increases until the thirtieth day, and it then begins to drop until the ninetieth day, after which it remains at a low level until separation of the placenta when it disappears. The chorionic gonadotropic hormone is elaborated by the chorionic villi.

As a result of this early research the first scientific test for pregnancy, known as the Aschheim-Zondek test, was demonstrated in 1928. The two German scientists, after whom the test is named, discovered that by injecting urine into immature female mice, they could determine whether or not the urine came from a pregnant woman with nearly 100 per cent accuracy. Although there are now other reliable tests which can be done in a shorter time its accuracy is still unsurpassed. In 1930 Dr. Friedman, of the University of Pennsylvania, modified the test by using the rabbit instead of the mouse as a test animal. The advantage of the rabbit over the mouse is that only one injection of urine is necessary instead of several, and the result can be determined within 48 hours instead of 100 hours which is required for the mouse test. This test has been used extensively, but is rather expensive.

For either test, the urine should be the first morning specimen, so that it will be concentrated, and must be kept in a refrigerator. For the *Aschheim-Zondek* test, 0.4 ml of urine is injected subcutaneously into 5 immature female mice for 6 times over a period of two days. One hundred hours after the first injection, the mice are killed, and the ovaries are examined for corpora lutea or hemorrhagic follicles. The test is considered positive if at least 1 of the 5 mice shows ovarian changes.

In the *Friedman test,* 15 ml of the urine are injected intravenously into a mature female rabbit which has previously been isolated for four weeks. Sixteen hours, or longer, after the injection, the ovaries are examined for hemorrhagic ruptured follicles. These follicles must be ruptured to indicate a positive reaction.

Another advancement in testing for pregnancy was to discover that the hormones present in the urine of pregnant women would stimulate ovulation in amphibian animals. Hogben, in 1930, demonstrated that the female of a certain species of South African toad could be stimulated to ovulate by injecting it with chorionic gonadotropic hormone. Since this toad was not available everywhere, tests were made with various other female toads in an effort to find a simple method.

Stimulation of the male gonads with the chorionic gonadotropin was next considered, and in 1947 C. G. Mainini published his work which was done with the male of a species of South American toad; a test which proved very reliable. Because this toad is not available everywhere, American workers looked for an amphibian native to North America. In 1948 papers were published by several investigators reporting work done with the male *Rana pipiens*, a common North American frog, which proved to be a very reliable test animal.

The *frog test* is easily carried out in the doctor's office. Frogs may be kept in the refrigerator at a temperature of 4.4° C (40° F) in a container with moss and ½ in. of water. They may be kept for several weeks under proper conditions, but it is not recommended that they be used after three months since they may become debilitated. They must not be allowed to become dry because this condition may give a false reaction.

To run the test the patient is asked to collect 60 ml (2 oz) of early morning urine into a clean bottle. It needs no special treatment, but should be refrigerated if it cannot be used within six to eight hours. The frog will react to the hormone more quickly when he is not cold. It is, therefore, advisable to remove him from the refrigerator and allow him to reach room temperature before use. Then 2.5 ml of urine are injected into the dorsal lymph sac with a hypodermic syringe and needle. The frog test is based on the fact that the chorionic gonadotropic hormone present in the urine of pregnant women causes a detachment and excretion of spermatozoa within a very short time after it is injected. The frog's testicles are attached to the kidneys by a ligament through which pass tubes that carry spermatozoa and empty them into the kidney glomeruli. The kidney tubules, the ureters, and the bladder are thus common channels for the excretion of both urine and sperm. Therefore, when sperm are found in the frog's urine there is evidence of detachment and excretion. It is on the basis of this knowledge that one hour following injection of the frog a drop of urine is removed from the bladder of the frog by means of a small pipette, is placed on a glass slide, and is examined for spermatozoa. If one or more sperm are found the test is positive; the number of sperm present is not important since there are no degrees of a positive reaction. The frog sperm are quite large and are easily recognized under the microscope. If sperm are not found on the first examination the frog's urine is reexamined every hour for five hours, and if at the end of that time none are found the test is negative. Serum is now often used in performing this pregnancy test. The level of chorionic gonadotropin is higher in serum than in urine, and the procedure of testing with serum is relatively short and simple.

Since these tests are accurate in most instances, especially between the fifteenth and ninetieth days of pregnancy, they are a means of diagnosing early pregnancy and are a particularly valuable aid in the diagnosis of complications in which it is essential to know whether or not conception has occurred. Tumors and cysts can simulate or mask pregnancy, and this test may help in making a final diagnosis. The test is one of several findings which may confirm or rule out the suspicion of an ectopic pregnancy when a tubal mass is discovered. When an abortion has threatened, the test may be valuable in determining whether or not the placenta has separated and may thus be important when a decision must be made upon further treatment. The pregnancy test is very strongly positive in such abnormal conditions as hydatidiform mole and choriocarcinoma and on this basis may be an aid in making the diagnosis and also in determining whether or not all abnormal tissue has been expelled or removed.

## PHYSIOLOGY OF PREGNANCY

A general understanding of the physiology of pregnancy is indispensable to an appreciation of the importance of observing the present-day teaching about the hygiene of pregnancy. Upon this, in turn, must rest intelligently administered prenatal care, one of the most important branches of obstetrics. The physiology of pregnancy really represents an adjustment of the various functions of the maternal organism, which are altered to meet the demands made upon the mother's organs by the body which is developing, growing, and functioning within hers. These adjustments are in the nature of an emergency service, since they come into existence and operate only while needed, which is during pregnancy, and promptly disappear when the need for them ceases with the birth of the child. The mother's body then begins to return to its normal, nonpregnant state, which, with the exception of the breasts that may function for several months if the mother nurses her baby, is accomplished in the course of approximately six weeks.

In addition to the normal changes in physiology during the course of pregnancy, there are sometimes abnormal changes, too, which may be symptoms of grave complications. The detection of these symptoms, as well as the employment of treatment which they indicate, constitutes one of the most valuable aspects of prenatal care.

Although, as might be expected, the alterations in the structure and functions of the maternal organism are most marked in the reproductive organs, there are definite changes in other and remote parts of the body as well. And there are adjustments in metabolism, which, although not wholly understood, are now widely recognized as important. There is also a changed hormone balance due to the persistence of the corpus luteum, some suppression in secretion of pituitary gonadotropic hormones, and the appearance of placental hormones—chorionic gonadotropin and increasing amounts of estrogen and progesterone.

At present, we know that in spite of the creation of an infant body weighing upward of 3178 gm (7 lb), a placenta weighing more than 454 gm (1 lb), together with an increase of over 908 gm (2 lb) in the weight of the uterine muscle, all in the short span of nine months, the expectant mother has to eat very little more during this period than she ordinarily does to maintain her own bodily functions. This suggests a highly developed economy in the use of nutritive material by the maternal cells.

We also know that the mother excretes waste materials for the fetus and we must assume that this requires an increased, or adjusted, functional activity of her excretory organs—the skin, lungs, and kidneys. Moreover, the secretory activity of the previously inactive mammary glands suggests a hormonal stimulation, which occurs only during pregnancy.

The changes in the **uterus** itself are unquestionably the most marked changes that take place during the period of gestation. Those that relate to the lining have been described in Chapter 3. The changes and growth in the muscle wall are amazing. New muscle fibers come into existence, those already there increase greatly in size, and there is a marked development of connective and elastic tissue, an increase in the size of the blood vessels, and a hypertrophy of the lymphatic and nervous tissue. The muscle fibers of the uterus are arranged as an interlacing network with blood vessels between them. Each fiber has a double curve and when any two interlace they form a figure of "8," which, when they contract after delivery, will constrict the blood vessels and control bleeding. The actual substance of the uterus is so increased that it is converted from an organ weighing 60 gm (2 oz) into one weighing over 908 gm (2 lb). From a firm, thick-walled, somewhat flattened body, in its nonpregnant state, the gravid uterus assumes a globular outline. After the first few weeks and later, due to a more rapid increase in length than width, it becomes oval in shape. At the end of pregnancy it is 30 to 35 cm (12 to 14 in.) long, from 20 to 25 cm (8 to 10 in.) wide, and 22 cm (8.8 in.) deep, and its capacity has increased 500 times. During the first few months the uterine walls increase in thickness, but later they grow progressively thinner, until by the end of pregnancy they are only about 5 mm (1/5 in.) thick and allow for easy palpation of the fetus through them. This early growth of the uterus is doubtless brought about by general systemic changes as well as by the presence of the contained embryo. Evidence of this is found in the case of tubal pregnancies when there is a definite enlargement of the uterus during the early weeks.

The **cervix** also undergoes radical changes during pregnancy which consist of a marked thickening of the mucous lining, an increase in the blood supply, and a proliferation of the glands near the external os. The connective tissue becomes looser, and the muscle fibers actually decrease in number, but those which remain hypertrophy. As a result, the cervix is softer, relatively shorter, more elastic, and larger in its diameter, and its glandular secretion is greatly increased.

The changes in the **vagina** are chiefly due to increased vascularity. The blood vessels actually become larger; this causes the normal pinkish tint of the mucous lining to deepen to red or even purple, the deepest color being termed "Chadwick's sign." The vaginal discharge is usually much more profuse during pregnancy. It is thick, white, and of a crumbly consistency and has a strong acid reaction due to lactic acid which, it is believed, helps to keep the vagina relatively free of pathogenic bacteria. To prepare the vaginal wall for the distention it must undergo during labor certain other changes take place. The mucosa increases in thickness, hypertrophy of the muscles takes place, and the connective tissue becomes looser.

**The perineal tissues** show similar changes; that is, increased vascularity, hypertrophy of the skin and muscles, and loosening of the connective tissues.

**The tubes and ovaries** show changes in their position because they are carried up by the enlarging uterus from the pelvis into the abdominal cavity, and, due to the traction, their long axis becomes nearly vertical instead of at right angles to the uterus. Because the enlargement of the uterus is more marked in the fundus, the tubes and the ovarian ligaments appear to be attached more nearly to the middle of the uterus during pregnancy than in its nonpregnant state. There is a great increase in vascularity, which is chiefly responsible for the large size of the corpus luteum during pregnancy. Ovulation does not occur during pregnancy; the follicles which begin to develop undergo atretic changes.

**The abdomen** as a whole changes in contour as it steadily enlarges, and the skin and underlying muscles are somewhat affected as a result. The tension upon the skin is so great that it may rupture the underlying elastic layers, which later atrophy and thus produce the familiar *striae* of pregnancy, known variously as the *striae gravidarum* and the *lineae albicantes.* It is believed by some that these striae are due more to hypertrophic changes occurring in the abdominal wall than to tension exerted by the enlarging uterus. Fresh striae are pale pink or bluish in color, but after delivery they take on the silvery, glistening appearance of scar tissue, which they really are. In a woman who has borne children, therefore, we find both new and old striae; those resulting from former pregnancies being silvery and shining, while the fresh striae are pink or blue. Striae may be found also on the breasts, hips, and upper part of the thighs. Abdominal striae in nonpregnant women may occasionally result from a stretching of the skin by ascites, a marked increase in fat, or an abdominal tumor, while those on the hips and thighs may be due to normal postpubertal changes.

The abdominal distention sometimes causes a separation of the *recti muscles.* This separation, known as *diastasis,* is sometimes slight but occasionally very marked, the space between the muscles being easily felt through the thinned abdominal wall.

**The umbilicus** is deeply indented during about the first three months of pregnancy. But during the fourth, fifth, and sixth months the pit grows steadily shallower, and by the seventh month it is level with the surface. After this it may protrude, in which state it is described as a "pouting umbilicus."

The increased pigmentation at the umbilicus and in the median line is scarcely to be classified among the abdominal changes, as certain other areas of the skin previously mentioned present the same discolored appearance. The degree of pigmentation varies with the complexion of the individual, as blonds may be but slightly tinted while the discolored areas on a brunette may be dark brown, sometimes almost black.

The changes in the **breasts** during pregnancy were practically all included in the enumerated signs and symptoms of pregnancy. They increase in size and firmness and become nodular, the nipples are more prominent and together with the surrounding areolae grow much darker, the glands of Montgomery are enlarged, striations frequently appear, the superficial veins grow more prominent, and after the third month a thin, yellowish fluid can be expressed from the nipples. This fluid, called *colostrum,* consists largely of serum albumin, fat, epithelial cells, and colostrum corpuscles (epithelial cells which have undergone fatty degeneration) and differs from milk, in its yellowish color, which is due to a pigment, and in the fact that it coagulates like the white of an egg when boiled. Very early in pregnancy the previously quiescent mammary glands develop an ability to select from the blood stream the necessary materials to produce a secretion. Colostrum is the product of their activity until about the third day after delivery, when milk appears. The mammary hyperplasia which occurs during pregnancy depends upon an interaction of the ovarian, placental, and anterior pituitary gland hormones.

**Cardiovascular System.** As pregnancy progresses the heart may tend to increase in size, its rate increases, and the amount of blood expelled with each beat, or cardiac output, is increased. These changes, plus an increase in blood volume, are necessary to supply the demands of the enlarging uterus and its contents and to help supply the fetus with a good exchange of oxygen and carbon dioxide. There is an actual increase in the amount of maternal blood, in both cells and plasma, during pregnancy. In spite of this the erythrocyte count and hemoglobin level often drop below normal as pregnancy progresses. This apparent decrease in the number of red blood cells is due to the dilution of the blood and does not indicate a true anemia since the number of cells is actually increased. Anemia may, however, occur in pregnancy due to the demands of the fetus for blood-building substances and due to dietary deficiencies. A slight leukocytosis and an increase in the sedimentation rate are also found during pregnancy.

The changes in the **respiratory system** are a result of the upward pressure of the enlarging uterus that gradually shortens the height of the thoracic cavity, but the cavity grows sufficiently wide in compensation so that there is actually a considerable increase in the amount of air inspired. The larynx is somewhat congested and edematous, a fact which explains the adverse effects which pregnancy may have upon the voice of singers.

Changes in the **digestive tract** during pregnancy are the morning sickness, already described, and constipation. The latter is present in at least one-half of all pregnant women and is due partly to pressure of the uterus on the intestines, and partly to decreased gastrointestinal tract motility during pregnancy. This condition is most troublesome during the latter part of pregnancy. There may also be gastric indigestion causing acidity, flatulence, and heartburn, and intestinal indigestion giving rise to diarrhea and cramp-like pains. The appetite may be very capricious during the early weeks, but it soon improves, and the pregnant woman is able to eat a well-balanced diet.

Changes in the **urinary apparatus** include frequency of micturition, mentioned among the symptoms of pregnancy, due to pressure of the uterus on the bladder. This is relieved when the uterus rises and carries the bladder into the abdominal cavity with it. The kidneys are under an increased strain, and it has been shown that there is a normal dilatation of the ureters during pregnancy which will be referred to later in connection with pyelitis (Chap. 9).

The changes in the **bony structures** of the pregnant woman are characterized by a softening of the pelvic cartilages, due to a temporarily increased blood supply.

**The skin changes** consist chiefly of the appearance of striae and the increased pigmentation to which reference has already been made. There is also an increased activity of the sebaceous and sweat glands and the hair follicles, the latter sometimes resulting in the hair becoming much more abundant during the period of gestation. On the other hand, the reverse is sometimes true, and the pregnant woman may lose a good deal of hair during this period. Although the pigmented areas on the breasts and abdomen never quite return to their original hue, the *chloasma,* which is frequently called the "mask of pregnancy," practically always disappears and leaves no trace, a fact that is frequently a comfort to an expectant mother.

**The carriage** is somewhat affected during pregnancy because the increased size and weight of the abdominal tumor shifts the center of gravity forward. This is the cause of the tripping and falling forward so common among pregnant women. In an effort to preserve an upright position the woman throws back her head and shoulders and finally assumes a gait that may be described as a waddle, particularly noticeable in short women.

**Mental and emotional changes** are usually included among the alterations which occur during pregnancy; however, the present status of psychiatry suggests that this may not be altogether sound. It is a fact that some pregnant women show marked mental and emotional imbalance, but there seems to be no evidence that these states are inherently due to pregnancy, although the same condition may recur in the same woman each time that she is pregnant. We shall consider this important subject more at length in Chapter 7, "Mental Hygiene of the Expectant Mother"; therefore, it may be enough simply to say at this juncture that, in a somewhat unstable and easily disturbed woman, the state of being pregnant may be merely the last straw, so to speak, that upsets her equilibrium; and that some other experience, which would be an equal strain upon her ability to make adjustments, would result in exactly the same mental or emotional upset, just as certain physical signs in pregnancy may be produced also in the nonpregnant woman, and are not, therefore, necessarily inherent to the gravid state.

**The Endocrine Glands.** With the steady advance of knowledge concerning the *endocrine* or *ductless glands,* it becomes apparent that they undergo a profound physiologic alteration during the course of pregnancy. Everyone is familiar with the fact that the pregnant woman's neck may increase in size due to changes in the thyroid gland. Increased basal metabolic rate and an increase in the iodine content of the blood are also associated with the changes in this gland. The parathyroid glands, which affect calcium metabolism, are also hypertrophied. Increased pigmentation in pregnancy may be due to changes in endocrine glands. Another evidence of alteration of gland function is the coarsening in features which some pregnant women show. These are believed to be acromegaloid in character and, as is the case in acromegaly, are probably associated with changes in the anterior pituitary body. The effects of the ovarian, the anterior pituitary gland, and the placental hormones on gestation and lactation have been mentioned.

**General Metabolism.** Taking the condition as a whole, pregnancy is usually characterized by an improved state of health. During the first few months there may be lassitude and loss of weight, but the latter part of the period is notable for an unusual degree of general well-being. The average weight gain during pregnancy, due to metabolic changes in the body as well as to the fetus and accessory structures, is 11 kg (24 lb). This amount of increase is perhaps not desirable, and many obstetricians prefer to hold the weight gain under 9 kg (20 lb). About 5 kg (11 lb) of the increased weight are lost at the time of delivery and a still further reduction occurs during the succeeding weeks, when the mother's body returns approximately to its original condition, but it sometimes happens that some of the weight acquired during pregnancy becomes permanent. One of the metabolic alterations of late pregnancy is an increased tendency of the body to retain water in all its tissues. Release of this fluid, and a return to normal of the water metabolism during the first few days following delivery, results in a greater weight loss during the first week of the puerperium than in the succeeding weeks.

To facilitate the growth of the fetus and placenta and an increase in her own tissues without too great a strain on herself, the mother shows a highly developed economy in her general metabolism; as yet we do not know how much of this is accomplished.

## BIBLIOGRAPHY AND STUDENT REFERENCES

Beck, Alfred C.: "Advances in the Physiology of Pregnancy during the Past Quarter Century," *Am. J. Obst. & Gynec.*, **68**:97–109, (July) 1954.

Bookmiller, Mae M., and Bowen, George L.: *Textbook of Obstetrics and Obstetric Nursing,* 2nd ed. W. B. Saunders Co., Philadelphia, 1954.

Bruehl, Frances S.: "The Development of Pregnancy Tests," *Am. J. Nursing,* **52**:591–93, (May) 1952.

Davis, M. Edward, and Sheckler, Catherine E.: *DeLee's Obstetrics for Nurses,* 15th ed. W. B. Saunders Co., Philadelphia, 1951.

Eastman, Nicholson J.: *Williams Obstetrics,* 11th ed. Appleton-Century-Crofts, Inc., New York, 1956.

Greenhill, J. P. (ed.): *Obstetrics,* 11th ed. W. B. Saunders Co., Philadelphia, 1955.

Woodward, H. L.; Gardner, B.; Bryant, R. D.; and Overland, Anna E.: *Obstetric Management and Nursing,* 5th ed. F. A. Davis Co., Philadelphia, 1955.

Zabriskie, Louise, and Eastman, Nicholson J.: *Nurses Handbook of Obstetrics,* 9th ed. J. B. Lippincott Co., Philadelphia, 1952.

*Chapter 6*

# Prenatal Care

The day is long since past when the doctor's concern for his patient began when she went into labor. The obstetrician of today watches and cares for his patient throughout pregnancy, since he knows that by so doing he greatly increases her chance of surviving pregnancy and childbirth and the baby's prospect of living through the perilous first year. The aim of good prenatal care is to have the mother come to the end of her pregnancy in as good or better health than she had at its beginning and to have a healthy baby that she and her husband are well prepared to care for and enjoy. Although conditions that result in illness or death sometimes occur during labor or the puerperium, they may have their beginning during pregnancy. Their prevention, or their early recognition, followed by prompt and efficient treatment, will avert many of the dreaded complications and emergencies associated with childbearing.

The prevention of these disasters is accomplished in the vast majority of cases by supervising, teaching, and caring for the expectant mother throughout pregnancy. Complete premarital and preconceptional examinations would many times reveal, even earlier, defects which are potential sources of trouble during pregnancy, and such examinations should be encouraged whenever possible. Defects can then frequently be either corrected before pregnancy or observed and treated appropriately during pregnancy. There is a narrower borderline between health and disease in the pregnant woman than in the nonpregnant, and a seemingly mild disorder may become a major problem under the strain of pregnancy. Although pregnancy is a normal physiologic process, it may readily become pathologic, especially in the patient who is not entirely normal physically. It is of utmost importance, therefore, that the patient consult a doctor as soon as she suspects that she is pregnant. This is true even though previously she may have had safe and uncomplicated deliveries. Such care and supervision during pregnancy comprise prenatal care, which may be divided into examination, instruction, and observation, as follows:

**1. Examination.** The doctor's initial examination consists of a complete history and physical examination including the heart, lungs, breasts, abdomen, and pelvis and recording the height, weight, temperature, and blood pressure. The complete pelvic examination includes a study of the size and shape of the pelvis as well as the examination of the reproductive organs. Certain laboratory studies are done, which usually include chest x-ray, urinalysis, complete blood count, serologic test for syphilis and smears for gonorrhea, the determination of the Rh factor, and any others indicated by physical findings.

It is desirable to see the expectant mother for the first time as early as possible for this initial examination and to follow a fairly uniform plan in the kind and frequency of subsequent observations.

Thus, it has become generally customary to see the patient once a month during the first five to seven lunar months, then every two to three weeks, and finally once a week during the last month or until the onset of labor. At each of these visits the usual procedure is to take the temperature, pulse, blood pressure, and weight, to do a urinalysis, to palpate the abdomen to determine the size and position of the fetus, listen to the fetal heart tones, give the patient instructions, and discuss any questions or problems with her. These periodic examinations keep the physician constantly informed about his patient's condition and frequently disclose, very early, signs of a complication which might prove serious if allowed to progress unchecked. Albumin in the urine, for example, an increase in blood pressure, puffiness of face, fingers, or eyelids, or a rapid increase in the body weight (1 kg [2.2 lb] or more per week) during the latter part of pregnancy will inform the doctor of a developing toxemia and indicate the necessity of immediate treatment toward the prevention of eclampsia. An elevation of temperature, even though the patient is not uncomfortable, might lead to the early discovery of tuberculosis, pyelitis, or some infection not otherwise apparent.

**2. Instruction.** The expectant mother must be taught to adapt the principles of personal hygiene to her needs, to understand the normal changes of pregnancy, and to recognize the symptoms of any complications.

**3. Observation.** The physician and the nurse are alert to the recognition of early signs of the complications of pregnancy so that treatment can be instituted as these signs appear. They observe the patient for some of the common discomforts of pregnancy and give advice as to their relief.

Prenatal care of this character is essentially preventive for both the mother and the newborn baby. We gain a faint impression of what it may prevent when we learn that year after year at least 2000 young women in the United States die from causes associated with childbirth which are known to be largely preventable and that each year many babies are born dead. About 160,000 babies die before, during, or soon after birth. Of this number about 85,000 die prior to, or during, birth, some because of conditions that are largely controllable and others from causes as yet obscure.

This is not all. There are also the unrecorded and uncounted instances of mothers who have received little or no obstetric care and as a result may not be on the best level of health. Adequate care during pregnancy and childbirth would have helped to keep them on this level. The effect of the mother's impairment reaches far beyond her own illness, because sick women are not as well able to rear and care for their children satisfactorily as are well mothers. Whatever makes for good obstetrics, therefore, makes for a better race. As we shall see later, measures that tend to improve the health of the race tend to lessen the hazards of childbearing.

Ideal prenatal care would really begin during the expectant mother's own infancy, but we must be content here with a description of the care that is advisable for expectant mothers from the beginning of pregnancy. The most painstaking obstetrician requires the cooperation of his patient in innumerable ways if she is to have the fullest benefits of his skill. It is not so much what the doctor advises that counts as how the patient follows his instructions. It is at this point that nurses have an opportunity for performing immensely gratifying service. A private patient who is in the care of an obstetrician may be supervised and instructed solely by her doctor. Many doctors, however, like to have expectant mothers in their care attend classes in preparation for childbearing that are conducted by many maternity center associations. This work was inaugurated in this country by the Brooklyn Maternity Center Association in 1924. But there are other patients—women who cannot afford individual care—who need care nonetheless. It is these expectant mothers that nurses are helping the doctors to instruct in the principles of prenatal care, and to observe for danger signs, through visiting nurse agencies, outpatient departments of hospitals, and prenatal clinics, as well as in physicians' offices.

The character and extent of the instruction and supervision given by the nurse is, of course, decided by the medical board of her organization, and is often affected by the conditions under which the work is conducted. The nurses in a rural community, for example, may take blood pressure and test urine for albumin, while in cities, rich in doctors and medical institutions, these observations might not be among their duties.

In addition to this definite relation to expectant mothers, nurses are meeting them unofficially and informally; women who are not receiving care from a doctor or an organization; women who are puzzled or troubled over their condition, but do not know where or how to obtain advice; women who could employ a physician but do not appreciate the importance of his care. Every nurse should recognize it as her duty to advise an unsupervised pregnant woman to place herself under medical care, no matter under what conditions she meets her.

In the discharge of her duties the nurse will sometimes need no little ingenuity to adapt the plan for prenatal care, as prescribed by her organization, to the mentality, traditions, and varied demands of the daily lives of her patients, but this will have to be done. Although in a general way the needs of all expectant mothers are the same, their circumstances and personalities are infinitely varied.

It may require undreamed-of tact and resourcefulness to convince a patient that details of care, which seem wholly unrelated to her or her baby's welfare, will actually increase their chances for life and health. Moreover, the personal application of unfamiliar practices may be very confusing to a woman who has had neither time nor inclination to care for herself. It is wise, therefore, for the nurse to make her teaching and explanations as simple as possible and to show the patient just how to do each thing that is advised and not rely solely upon verbal instruction. In order to help her, the nurse must make conscious but unobtrusive effort to win her patient's friendship and confidence. She will then scarcely realize that she is being taught, but will do and continue to do as she is advised because of an almost insensible reliance upon the judgment and sincerity of her counselor.

It is not the single examination of a specimen of urine that counts, nor the exercise taken with pleasure and enthusiasm during the first few days of its novelty. It is not the rest, fresh air, or proper food, taken according to rule for a week or two, that will protect her and her baby. It is the repetition of details that make up the expectant mother's mental and physical life during 24 hours in each day, seven days a week, through 40 long weeks, that grow longer and more monotonous as pregnancy advances; it is the mosaic that she makes out of the minutiae of her daily life that counts. Paradoxical as it seems, she must shape her days to meet her own and her baby's needs with such steady persistence that she finally lives them almost unconscious of what she is doing, and without introspection.

Obviously, then, the expectant mother's mental attitude is of considerable importance. She should understand that childbearing is a normal function, but, like other normal functions, may become abnormal if neglected, and that a sick pregnancy is not a normal one. She should in general continue the diversions, work, and amusements that she is accustomed to and enjoys, if they are not contraindicated. She should cultivate a cheerful, hopeful frame of mind, guard against being self-centered and overwatchful of symptoms, and at the same time not adopt the dangerous habit of uncomplainingly ascribing to pregnancy all of the discomforts and unfamiliar conditions which may arise. In short, to forget that she is pregnant insofar as that is consistent with the care that she should take of herself.

## PARENTS' CLASSES

To facilitate the teaching which should accompany the physical care given in the prenatal period, many communities have of recent years offered parents' classes in both physical and psychologic preparation for childbearing.

The purposes of these classes are:

1. To teach both parents the anatomy and physiology of pregnancy and labor and the development of the baby so that they will understand the changes that are taking place in the mother's body
2. To teach the hygiene of pregnancy in such a manner that there will be a good understanding of the reasons for the instructions that are given and an appreciation of how both mother and baby will benefit from them
3. To give an understanding of the emotional aspects that accompany pregnancy and to prepare for parenthood in the broadest possible sense
4. To teach relaxation technics and muscle-training exercises which prepare the mother for a comfortable pregnancy, labor, delivery, and puerperium

The mother is thus aided in overcoming any fear that she may have of pregnancy and labor through a knowledge of the normal processes, both physical and emotional, that are taking place, and is given an understanding of how she can help to have a healthy and comfortable pregnancy. The father is given an opportunity to share his wife's experiences and so can be of much greater help to her because he has a better understanding of the changes during pregnancy and the reasons for the instruction she has been given to follow. This gives him a much better opportunity to take an active part in preparing for a family before the actual birth of the baby. These classes should develop confidence and a sense of security in both parents, help them to make the necessary adjustments in their lives with ease, and develop attitudes which will help them in the future. Another advantage of parents' classes is the strengthening of the patient-doctor-nurse relationship that comes through this close association.

These classes may be given in connection with a hospital prenatal clinic for patients attending the clinic or as a community project through a city or county health department or a community nursing service. Classes are taught by a physician or a nurse or in most instances both. The classes may be set up in any way that serves the best interests of the group, but a common arrangement is to devote a number of hours, depending upon the amount of material to be taught, to the mothers alone and two to three hours for the fathers alone and/or two to three hours for mothers and fathers together.

Included in these classes may be some or all of the following material:

1. Changes during pregnancy—physical and emotional
2. Development of the baby
3. Stages of labor and birth of the baby
4. Procedure for admittance to the hospital and preparation for delivery
5. Hygiene of pregnancy
6. Care of the baby—physical and emotional, layette planning, formula making
7. Relaxation technics and exercises to promote good muscle tone for improvement of posture and for use during labor

The subject matter is usually divided into that which is suitable for large groups and that which is more easily given to small groups. The material for the larger group, which frequently includes both parents, may consist of lectures on certain phases of pregnancy and labor and family relationships, and movies and slides on human reproduction, labor, and birth. A pediatrician may be asked to give a lecture on child care, and a psychiatrist may be asked to discuss with the group the emotional aspects of childbearing and also certain other phases of family relationships. A nutritionist will often be asked to discuss the diet of the pregnant woman and lactating mother. It is usually easier to present certain aspects of the hygiene of pregnancy and the care of the baby, as well as the practice of the exercises, to a small group than to the larger one.

Insofar as possible all of the classes should be small enough to make it feasible to conduct them on an informal basis, thus giving the parents an opportunity to ask questions. The classes will serve their purpose best if the needs of the group are given first consideration.

A reading list may be prepared from the large number of excellent books and pamphlets that have been written on prenatal care, infant care, and natural childbirth for those parents who wish to obtain information beyond that which can be discussed in the classes.

A visit to the hospital is frequently arranged to acquaint the mother with the maternity unit. This tour is usually conducted by a member of the obstetric staff who can explain hospital procedure and answer questions the mothers may have about its policies and customs. There is the added advantage of acquainting the mother with at least one or more of the nursing staff who will be caring for her while she is in the hospital.

## RELAXATION TECHNICS AND EXERCISES

Training for childbirth classes often includes breathing and relaxation technics, rest positions, and exercises. These are designed to help the mother carry her baby easily during pregnancy and to prepare her for labor and a comfortable postpartum period. They help to develop an ability to relax, improve body posture, increase the mobility of the pelvic joints, and strengthen the muscles which are used during labor by increasing their elasticity and improving their tone.

These classes should be kept small, preferably 8 to 10 participants, in order to allow for adequate space for practice and to provide sufficient time to guide each member. They should be started around the sixteenth week, but even a little practice late in pregnancy is beneficial. The consent of the patient's physician is usually necessary for acceptance into the class. It should be understood by the expectant mothers that these exercises are not designed to produce a painless labor, but to make them active participants in the delivery of the baby.

Only a general discussion of the technics and some suggestions as to when they can be applied follow in these pages. For a complete description the student is referred to some of the books and pamphlets on this subject.

The expectant mothers are taught the fundamentals of relaxation and controlled breathing so that they will get the rest they need during pregnancy, be able to use these valuable technics in labor, and be able to apply them for rest periods and for nursing the baby during the puerperium. Everyone, not only expectant mothers, can benefit from applying these technics which promote rest, relaxation, and good posture, and the mothers will find them useful the rest of their lives.

The relaxation and breathing technics teach (1) the proper positions to assume for resting, (2) how to relax all of the muscles in the body while in these positions, and (3) how to control breathing.

The positions for rest and relaxation which are suggested to the mothers are lying either flat on the back with a pillow under the head and the knees (Fig. 44), or lying on the side with all joints slightly bent and the hips rotated sufficiently to allow the abdomen to rest on the bed (Fig. 45). While assuming these positions the mothers learn how to check all of their muscles to make certain that none of them are under tension. The back position is ordinarily very comfortable early in pregnancy and with proper relaxation it is also the position which may be the most comfortable one to assume during the latter part of the first stage of labor. The side position becomes necessary in the latter half of pregnancy and is probably the most comfortable for most of the first stage of labor, at least until the transition period.

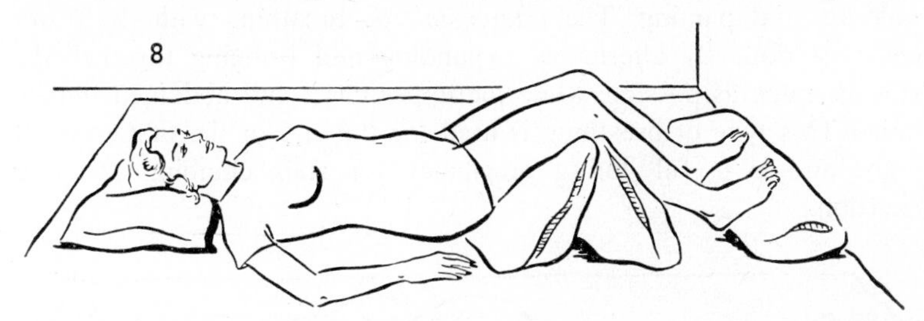


**Fig. 44.** Early in pregnancy—lying on back with all skeletal muscles loose and limp and concentrating attention on quiet, natural rhythmic breathing. (Reproduced from the *Reminder Sheets for Exercises, Rest Positions, Breathing and Relaxing Techniques,* published by Maternity Center Association, New York City, with their permission.)

*Abdominal breathing* (Fig. 46) is one of the most important and also one of the most difficult breathing exercises to be learned. While breathing gently and slowly, the abdominal wall is made to rise as far as possible and then slowly allowed to fall. If breathing is entirely abdominal the chest does not move; breathing is diaphragmatic. Abdominal breathing must be practiced every day to develop skill in prolonging the breath and controlling the speed and the depth. The aim is to learn to do it so slowly and deeply that it will take approximately 30 seconds to take the breath in and 30 seconds to let it out. Abdominal breathing is used to promote relaxation during pregnancy, but it should also be learned so well that it can be used during most of the first stage of labor, when it will preclude painful spasm of the abdominal wall muscles. Very long slow breaths should be taken during contractions—one or two will suffice. Abdominal breathing can then be resumed at a somewhat faster rate in the intervals between contractions. This breathing can usually be practiced before the afternoon rest period and before going to sleep at night, after having assumed a good resting position. Conscious effort must be made to think of the breathing only and put all other thoughts out of mind while it is practiced. After abdominal breathing has been learned in the recumbent position it can also be practiced while sitting or standing. All of this may take considerable practice, but the mother should try to become so adept at it that it can be done at will and controlled under stress.

Other controlled breathing exercises which are useful during labor are intercostal, sternal, a combination of intercostal and sternal, breath holding, and panting. The *intercostal,* or breathing with the lower chest, is done by alternately expanding and bringing together the ribs as much as possible while the upper chest and abdomen remain quiet. This type of breathing is used for the end of the first stage of labor and is useful during pregnancy for stair climbing or other exertion.

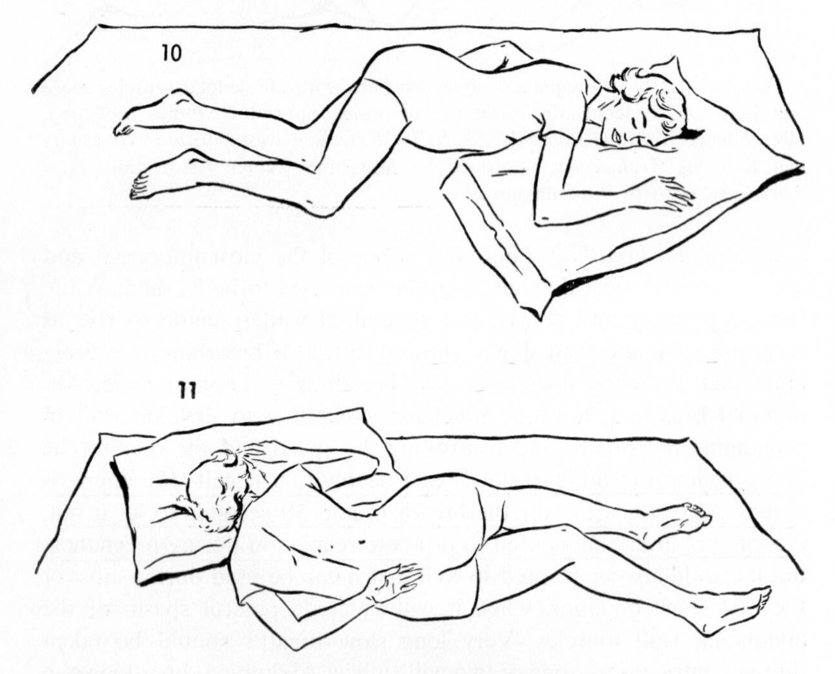


**Fig. 45.** Relaxing later in pregnancy and during some first-stage contractions.

*Lying on side*—all muscles loose and limp, baby's weight resting on bed, no pressure on breasts, mind on quiet, regular breathing.

*Back view*—showing how hand can be used to indicate where back aches as it often does during some first-stage contractions.

(Reproduced from the *Reminder Sheets for Exercises, Rest Positions, Breathing and Relaxing Techniques,* published by Maternity Center Association, New York City, with their permission.)

*Sternal* breathing, letting the chest or sternum rise and fall, is used toward the end of the second stage of labor, especially when panting is necessary. *Panting* is done by taking quick shallow breaths with the mouth open; it may be necessary during the actual delivery of the head and shoulders to prevent the birth from taking place too rapidly at this stage.

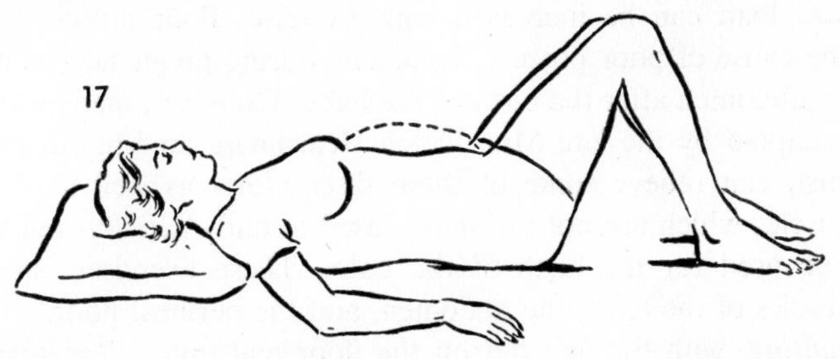


**Fig. 46.** The diaphragmatic or abdominal breath—dotted line shows relaxed abdominal wall raised during slow inhalation when expansion of chest cavity is limited to descent of diaphragm. (Reproduced from the *Reminder Sheets for Exercises, Rest Positions, Breathing and Relaxing Techniques,* published by Maternity Center Association, New York City, with their permission.)

A *combination of intercostal and sternal breathing* consists of rapid breathing with the ribs expanding and coming together at the same time that the sternum is rising and falling. This type of breathing, with the mouth open, is probably necessary toward the end of the first stage of labor when abdominal breathing may become impossible and the time has not yet arrived to bear down with contractions.

*Breath holding* is practiced by drawing in a deep breath with the mouth open, expanding the ribs as far as possible, raising the chest to its maximum, and then holding the breath with the mouth closed, for as long as possible, and finally letting it out quickly. This type of breathing is used for bearing down with contractions during the second stage of labor. The purpose of practice is to prolong the time during which a breath can be held. This exercise and the *pushing* exercise can be practiced later in pregnancy while having a bowel movement. With the lungs inflated the abdominal muscles are contracted and pressure is exerted toward the rectum. This expulsive effort is very similar to pushing the baby through the birth canal after the cervix is fully dilated.

The husband, or nurse, who understands these exercises, and when to use them, is able to give encouragement to the woman in labor and coach her in the proper use of them at a time when she is under stress and may need reminders in spite of long hours of practice.

Muscles not used regularly have poor tone and when given an extra load they are not able to function efficiently and become stiff. The efficiency of the muscles upon which pregnancy and labor place an extra load can be increased with exercise. Poor muscle tone is also the cause of poor posture, backache during pregnancy, and protruding abdomen after the birth of the baby. Exercises, many of which were adapted by the late Mrs. Helen Heardman, an English physiotherapist, can relieve some of these discomforts as well as prepare the muscles which are not ordinarily used in daily activity, but which must be used for the birth of the baby. These exercises condition the muscles of the back, the abdomen, and the perineal floor.

*Squatting,* with the feet flat on the floor and quite close together, is an exercise for strengthening the thigh muscles and for making the perineal muscles more elastic (Fig. 53). It is quite a strain at first, but becomes easier with practice and can finally become a habit in performing many small duties in the home. The squatting position is a common one for delivering the baby in less civilized countries; a modification of this position is assumed on the delivery table. Muscle soreness after delivery due to position is prevented by this exercise.

Assuming the *tailor position* (Fig. 47) and practicing putting the knees as far as possible to the floor strengthens the thigh muscles and limbers up the hip joints. This position can be used while sewing, playing with children, or sitting down to read or rest.

An exercise to make the *perineal muscles* more elastic is to *alternately contract* and *relax* these muscles. This can be practiced in the standing postion, but is usually first learned by lying on the back with the legs extended and the ankles crossed. The buttocks are tightened first, then the insides of the thighs are pressed together, and finally the perineum is drawn in as if to prevent emptying of the bowels or bladder. Relaxation of these muscles is done in reverse order. All of these steps should be performed slowly.

When the muscles of the abdomen and back are strong it is possible for the pregnant woman to stand erect with less strain on the back muscles than when these muscles are weak. Pelvic rocking is an exercise designed to strengthen the back and the abdominal muscles and thereby improve posture and prevent backache.

*Pelvic rocking* can be done in one of three positions; lying flat on the floor, getting on the floor on the hands and knees, or in the standing position. In the lying-down position the back is alternately flattened down to the floor and then arched to increase the hollow in the back. While doing this the shoulders and buttocks must not be

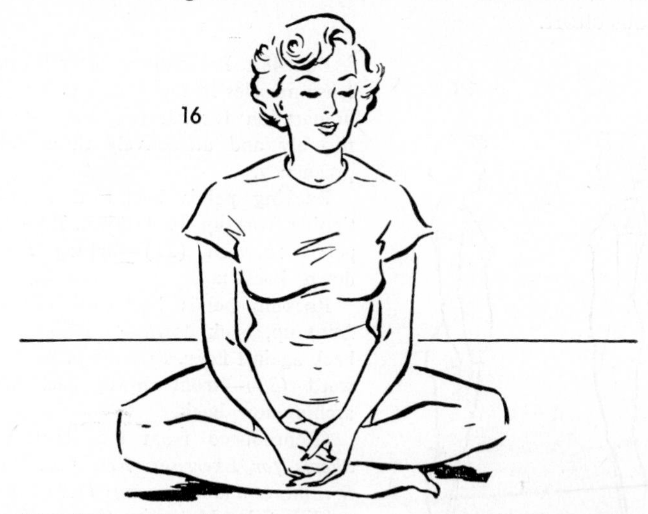


**Fig. 47.** Sitting tailor-fashion, relaxed and comfortable for work or play whenever practical. (Reproduced from the *Reminder Sheets for Exercises, Rest Positions, Breathing and Relaxing Techniques,* published by Maternity Center Association, New York City, with their permission.)

raised from the floor (Fig. 48). When done on all fours, the hands and knees are kept at right angles to the floor and the back is alternately arched and lowered. While the back is arched the head should be dropped and when the abdomen is lowered the head should be raised. The pelvis can also be rocked in the standing position. When this is done while standing up, the feet must be kept together and the feet and shoulders must remain in the same vertical plane (Fig. 48).

All of these exercises should be practiced daily at home, at a special time set aside for them or in the performance of regular household activities. They must be done slowly and calmly and never be carried to the point of fatigue. As with all other muscular activity these exercises should be done for only a few minutes at first; the time can be increased as they require less effort. Sometimes it seems best for the woman to set aside a certain time of day for these exercises. In other cases this seems like a chore and one for which there may not even be time. Many of them can be used while doing the daily housework and while resting. Good body mechanics can certainly be practiced consciously all day while working, standing, sitting, or resting, until they become such a habit that it is no longer necessary to make a conscious effort.

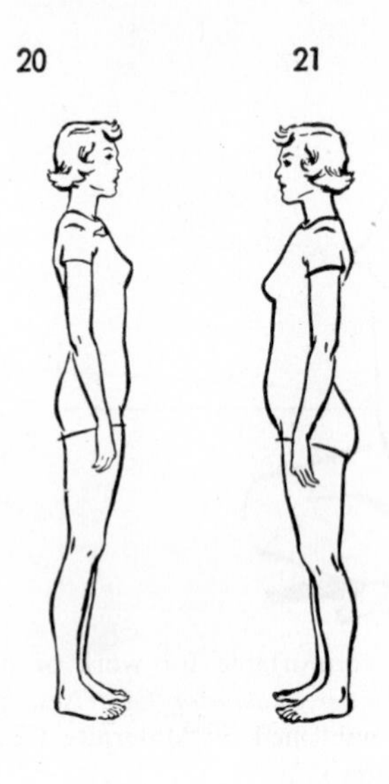


**Fig. 48.** Preventing, or relaxing, tense muscles in low back and hips in preparation for carrying baby comfortably and attractively throughout pregnancy.

Rocking pelvis backward (20)—tipping front up, back down. Rocking pelvis forward (21)—tipping front down, back up.

Rocking pelvis backward (22)—front up, back down—flattening low back against floor. Rocking pelvis forward (23)—front down, back up, arching low back.

(Reproduced from the *Reminder Sheets for Exercises, Rest Positions, Breathing and Relaxing Techniques,* published by Maternity Center Association, New York City, with their permission.)

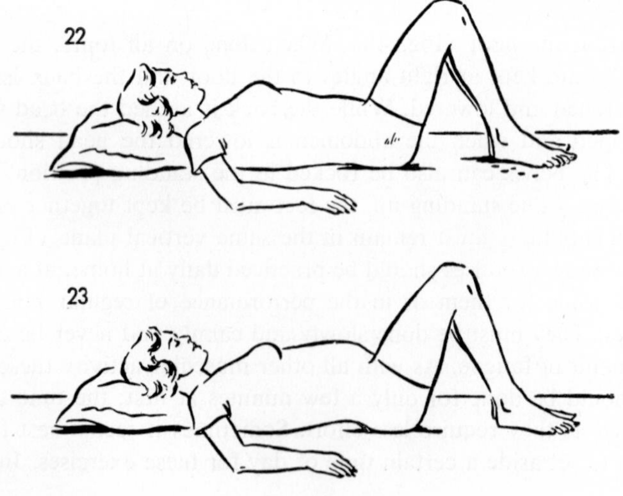

### MATERNAL IMPRESSIONS

In connection with the patient's mental attitude and her anxieties, the nurse may be of great comfort in helping to dispel superstitions and the widely credited and depressing beliefs concerning maternal impressions. After one has traced the development of the human body in the uterus, and even faintly understood its growth and method of nourishment, it is impossible to believe that the mother's thoughts or experiences could in any way deform or mark her child or alter its sex. That the mother's "reaching up," for example, could slip the cord around the unborn baby's neck is manifestly absurd, as well as the previously mentioned superstition about the eighth-month baby's slender chances for survival.

Superstitions, however, are always fondly cherished, for, as Gibbon tells us, "the practice of superstition is so congenial to the multitude, that if they are forcibly awakened, they still regret the loss of their pleasing vision." We can scarcely wonder, however, that even intelligent and educated people hold utterly improbable beliefs about pregnancy, since the most fantastic of them are quite as easy to believe as the thing that we know actually occurs—the development of a human body from a single cell.

These inaccurate beliefs are sometimes serious matters to the young woman, and they should not be laughed at or treated lightly, but explained away seriously. She may be told quite simply that after conception she gives her baby only nourishment; that the baby's connection with her body is through the cord and placenta, in neither of which are there nerves; and that even if the blood could carry mental and nervous impulses, which it cannot, the maternal and fetal blood never come in actual contact with each other. A tale which she has heard about a woman who saw something distressing and later gave birth to a marked child may cease to worry her if she is reminded of the innumerable babies, beautiful and unmarked, who are born to women who have had equally shocking experiences. It is scarcely probable that any woman lives through the 10 months of pregnancy without seeing, hearing, or thinking things that would disfigure a baby if maternal impressions could produce such results, and yet newborn babies are very rarely blemished. Although the ultimate causes of marks and deformities of the fetus are not definitely known, they are probably to be found in faulty development very early in the embryonic life, and, therefore, are not preventable.

## HYGIENE OF PREGNANCY

In coming to the expectant mother's personal hygiene, we find that an understanding of the physiology of pregnancy indicates what this hygiene should include. We shall take it up in detail, however, and describe what is at present considered a reasonable outline of the regimen desired for the average pregnant woman, who is found by careful examination to be normal and free from complications, and needs now to keep well. As has been said, and must be often repeated, the ideal regimen cannot be planned *en bloc* for all expectant mothers. It must be adjusted to the individual and to her circumstances.

### EXCRETIONS

Although the pregnant woman does not have to eat for two, she does have to eliminate the waste and broken-down products from two bodies, through her own excretory organs: the kidneys, skin, lungs, and bowels. True, the amount of the baby's waste is not great, but its elimination is important and increases the strain upon the maternal excretory apparatus.

**Kidneys.** One of the most important factors in prenatal care is promoting the function of the kidneys and watching their output. It is probably more true of the kidneys than of any other organ that a slight abnormality which would not give trouble at any other time may, if neglected during pregnancy, produce very grave results. The patient should be advised to drink the equivalent of at least 7 or 8 glasses of water per day, in addition to other fluids. Milk, tea, coffee, soup, etc., being fluids may constitute about 1 qt of the total 3 qt of fluid taken in the course of 24 hours. It is important for the nurse to explain to the patient, simply and convincingly, that she will greatly help to prevent illness by drinking adequate fluids in one form or another. The patient must understand and thus be convinced of the importance of periodically bringing urine specimens to the doctor for examination. It is essential that a complete urinalysis be done at least once a month during the first seven lunar months, then every two to three weeks, and finally every week in the last month of pregnancy.

If the nurse is called upon to test for albumin, either of the following procedures will serve, unless the doctor specifies a test which he prefers:

*Heat and Acetic Acid Test.* Fill a test tube about half full of urine and gently boil the upper part in a flame; add 5 drops of 2 per cent to 5 per cent acetic acid and again boil gently. The presence of albumin is shown by a white cloud in the upper part of the urine.

*Esbach's Test.* Fill a test tube half full of urine; add 8 to 10 drops of Esbach's solution. The presence of albumin is shown by a white, flocculent precipitate in the upper part of the urine.

**Skin.** Under ordinary conditions the skin serves as a protective covering for the body, helps to regulate the body temperature, and acts constantly as an excretory organ. This last function is performed by the sweat glands which open upon the surface of the body, and there are about 2,000,000 of these minute, tube-like structures in the skin. These glands should be constantly active. Sebaceous and sweat glands daily pour upon the surface of the body an oily substance that lubricates the skin, and something over a pint of water containing waste. Evaporation of this fluid is important in loss of body heat. We are not aware of the constant excretion of fluids, which, therefore, is termed "insensible perspiration," but is continued even in cold weather and must not be interrupted if health is to be preserved. If the oil, dust, particles of dead skin, and the waste material left by dried perspiration are allowed to remain upon the surface of the body they may clog the pores and will develop a distasteful odor. The removal of this material is important esthetically rather than essential to health, however, because it is removed automatically. The fluid evaporates and much of the solid matter is rubbed off on the clothing. The most important aids to the skin's activity are the drinking of plenty of water, deep breathing, exercise, and warm baths; baths serving the double purpose of removing waste matter already on the surface and stimulating the circulation.

This explains to the expectant mother the importance of thorough and regular bathing and of keeping her body evenly warm, especially since there is a marked tendency toward excessive perspiration during pregnancy. Most doctors advise a warm, not hot, shower or tub bath every day. The best time for this warm, cleansing bath, as a rule, is just before retiring, as it is soothing and restful and tends to induce sleep. Very hot baths are fatiguing, particularly during pregnancy. Cold baths usually may be continued throughout pregnancy if the patient is accustomed to them and reacts well afterward. Under these conditions the morning cold plunge, shower, or sponge is beneficial, as it stimulates the circulation and thus promotes activity of the skin. Some doctors permit tub baths throughout pregnancy, up to the onset of labor, while others forbid tub bathing after the seventh month, on the ground that as the patient sits in the tub her vagina is filled with water which may contain infective material. Should labor occur shortly afterward, an infection might result. Shower baths are not attended by this danger of infection. Another argument against tub baths is that as the patient is heavy and somewhat uncertain on her feet there is danger of her slipping and falling while getting in and out of the tub. A rubber mat in the bottom of the tub will help to prevent slipping in those cases where tub baths are taken.

**Bowels.** The bowels, also, eliminate a certain amount of waste material, and every effort should be made to have a daily bowel movement. Unhappily, a large proportion of pregnant women suffer from constipation, particularly during the later weeks, although women who have always had a tendency of this kind may have trouble from the very beginning of pregnancy. Sluggish peristalsis, due to pressure by the enlarged uterus upon the intestines, is probably one large factor, although impaired tone of the stretched abdominal muscles may also be a cause. A decrease in the gastrointestinal tract motility during pregnancy frequently adds to the problem of constipation.

Exercise, the intake of abundant fluids, eating fresh fruit, coarse vegetables, and whole-grain cereals to stimulate peristalsis, and drinking a glass of hot or cold water upon retiring and/or arising are all laxative in their effect. Cathartics and daily enemas should not be taken without the doctor's order. If constipation continues to be a problem it should be brought to the doctor's attention. He may advise the regular use of agar-agar or milk of magnesia.

## DIET

It is advisable for both nurse and patient to understand, and keep constantly in mind, the purposes which are served by the food intake of the expectant mother, and which foods and practices will defeat and which will accomplish these purposes. Although pregnancy is a normal physiologic process it makes a great demand upon the mother's body and her nutrition, and giving special consideration to the mother's food becomes a very important part of prenatal care. The diet should be such that it will promote the health and well-being of the mother and furnish the proper nutritive material for the growth and development of the fetus. Good nutrition adds much toward the maintenance of good health during and after pregnancy and reduces the likelihood of complications during pregnancy and labor. Women with adequate diets are more likely to have healthy full-term babies that are able to survive the neonatal period in good condition than women with poor nutrition; also, the chances of premature and still-born babies are reduced. Proper food during pregnancy is also an essential factor in preparing the mother to nurse her baby successfully.

It was formerly believed that the baby was a parasite taking from the mother's body any nutritive material it needed which was not supplied in her food. Evidence has now been accumulated showing that the fetus, although parasitic to a degree, is not a true parasite, and that the baby as well as the mother suffers from deficiencies. There are many ways in which the fetus may be affected by the mother's food, but one example, which can be cited, is that the structure of the baby's teeth is largely determined by the prenatal diet.

The diet during pregnancy is special in that as pregnancy advances the requirements for protein, minerals, and vitamins are greatly increased whereas the caloric requirement increases at a slower rate; therefore, the food that the mother eats must be selected very carefully to fulfill the needs without appreciably increasing the caloric intake. The dietary habits of the individual should be thoroughly investigated at the first prenatal visit, and necessary changes should be discussed in great detail at this time. If the woman enters pregnancy in a state of good nutrition and is accustomed to eating a well-balanced diet, these changes will not seem great; if her dietary habits have been poor, every effort will need to be made to make sure that she eats the proper food.

The nurse can be very helpful in motivating the pregnant woman to improve her food habits by explaining to her the value of good nutrition for herself and her baby, and by helping her with suggestions and plans for supplementing or changing her usual diet so that it will be adequate. Poor food habits are frequently of long standing and hard to change, and considerable influence may have to be used to change them; therefore, every possible effort must be made to ensure good nutrition during pregnancy and lactation.

To keep the pregnant woman in a state of good nutrition and to supply the needs of the fetus the food requirements are as follows (Chart II).

| | Normal Woman * | Pregnant Woman (third trimester) | Lactating Woman (850 ml milk daily) |
|---|---|---|---|
| Calories | 2300 | 2700 | 3300 |
| Protein, gm | 55 | 80 | 100 |
| Calcium, gm | 0.8 | 1.5 | 2.0 |
| Iron, mg | 12 | 15 | 15 |
| Vitamin A, I.U. | 5000 | 6000 | 8000 |
| Thiamine, mg | 1.2 | 1.5 | 1.5 |
| Riboflavin, mg | 1.4 | 2.0 | 2.5 |
| Niacin, mg | 12 | 15 | 15 |
| Ascorbic acid, mg | 70 | 100 | 150 |
| Vitamin D, I.U. | | 400 | 400 |

* Reference woman: 25 years old; 55 kg [121 lb]; 157 cm [5.2 ft]; normally vigorous.

Chart II. A comparison of the nutritional requirements, as recommended by the Food and Nutrition Board, for the normal, pregnant, and lactating woman. (Proudfit, Fairfax, and Robinson, Corinne: *Nutrition and Diet Therapy,* 11th ed. The Macmillan Company, New York, 1955, p. 229.)

**Protein.** This is a very important part of the pregnant woman's diet and must be supplied in increased amounts in order to meet the needs of both mother and fetus. The Food and Nutrition Board of the National Research Council has recommended 80 gm as the daily requirement for the latter half of pregnancy, an increase of 25 gm above the daily needs of the normal nonpregnant woman. The amount needed by the pregnant woman depends somewhat on her body size; she should have approximately 1.5 gm per kilogram of body weight. These recommended requirements are assuming that the woman is in a good state of nutrition at the beginning of pregnancy.

The mother must have a protein intake which is adequate to maintain her daily needs, sufficient to furnish the 900 gm that are the total net requirements of the fetus and accessory structures for growth and development, and enough to supply that which she needs for the large amount that she physiologically stores in her body during her pregnancy. Studies have shown that pregnant women normally store from 1250 to 2500 gm of protein in their body if circumstances are favorable, apparently as a reserve to provide for a loss which will occur during labor and the puerperium and the large amount required for successful lactation.

Protein foods that are needed daily during pregnancy are 1 qt milk, 1 egg, and ¼ lb of lean meat, liver, fish, or poultry. This will furnish from 60 to 65 gm of protein or approximately three-fourths of the total requirement. Since these proteins are of animal source they are complete proteins and furnish the best building material available, but less expensive sources of protein, such as dried beans and peas and cheese, may sometimes be used as substitutes. Bread, potato, cereals, and other foods that are a part of a well-balanced diet will fulfill the rest of the protein requirement. When the protein needs are properly furnished, many other requirements for good nutrition are quite adequately met.

Many patients may have the false notion that they should restrict proteins during pregnancy and will voluntarily do so unless advice is given to the contrary.

**Carbohydrates and Fats.** These are the energy-giving foods which are necessary to enable the individual to carry on her daily activities. Fat in large amounts will retard digestion because it passes through the digestive system slowly, but a moderate amount is essential and if taken in the form of dairy products, meat, fish, poultry, and eggs will supply other important substances at the same time it is supplying energy. Carbohydrate in the form of milk, fruits, vegetables, and whole-grain cereals and breads will supply protective substances and bulk as well as energy.

If the caloric intake during the course of pregnancy needs to be increased or decreased, it can best be done by altering the carbohydrate and fat intake.

**Minerals.** *Calcium and phosphorus* are essential in the diet as tissue-building material. The requirement is increased during pregnancy to meet the needs of the fetus and allow the mother to store some in preparation for lactation. If protein and minerals are not furnished in sufficient quantity by the diet to supply the baby's needs, his tooth and bone structure will be impaired. The daily requirement of calcium is 1.5 gm. One quart of milk will supply 1.2 gm, and the rest can then easily be obtained from other foods in the daily diet. The phosphorus requirement is probably even higher than the calcium needs, but when the protein and calcium requirements are met the phosphorus will be adequately supplied because foods that are high in these nutrients are usually high in phosphorus also.

Milk is by far the best source of calcium and phosphorus. In fact, it is impossible to ingest an adequate amount of these minerals without sufficient milk in the daily diet. Since milk is an inexpensive source of many other dietary essentials—protein, carbohydrate, fat, vitamins, and fluid—it is really the basis of an adequate diet. It may be used in any form, but because it would be difficult to use a whole quart in cooking some will probably have to be used as a beverage, either as whole milk, skimmed milk, buttermilk, or cocoa. The use of skimmed milk in the place of whole milk is a means of reducing the caloric intake should this be necessary due to an excess weight gain. When used in this form, however, it cannot be considered as a source of vitamin A, although this accessory can be supplied by other foods if necessary. It may be better, however, to reduce caloric intake by eliminating less desirable foods.

The diet during pregnancy does not need to be supplemented by calcium salts if 1 qt of milk is used daily, nor should they be considered an adequate substitute for milk. Besides being a poor substitute they are constipating and must be taken in large quantities to yield an adequate amount of the mineral. There is no substitute for milk, which must also be depended upon for so many of the other required nutrients.

The *iron* requirements also are increased during pregnancy, especially during the latter half, to enable the fetus to build up its hemoglobin and to build a reserve supply of iron for the first three months after birth during which the baby's iron intake is low. If the woman has no anemia to begin with, a diet which daily includes an egg, lean meat or liver, whole-grain products, green leafy vegetables, and fruits, especially dried, will furnish enough iron to supply the needs of the fetus and allow her to store some in her own tissues. If anemia is present iron in the form of medication may be necessary.

*Iodine.* In certain geographic regions, where the soil and water are low in iodine content, the diet is likely to be deficient in this mineral.

Pregnancy requires an increased amount, but this can usually be supplied by the use of iodized salt. Sea foods also are a rich source of iodine.

**Vitamin A.** The need for vitamin A is probably increased to 6000 I.U. daily during pregnancy. This vitamin is essential to the fetus and also helps to furnish the mother with good resistance to infection. Whole milk, eggs, and butter daily, green leafy and yellow vegetables several times each week, and liver once a week are the best sources of vitamin A; but it may be necessary to supplement the diet with vitamin concentrates to furnish the optimum amount during pregnancy. Skimmed milk contains little of the vitamin; whole milk should therefore be used whenever possible. This vitamin is fat soluble and readily stored in the body. Mineral oil used in foods or as a laxative, especially if taken near to a meal, will absorb vitamin A and thus make it unavailable.

**Vitamin B Complex.** *Thiamine* is necessary for the maintenance of a good appetite and the proper functioning of the digestive tract; it is also important for the proper oxidation of foods, by which energy is released for the body needs. Consequently, thiamine needs are increased as caloric intake is increased. It is now thought that the requirements of thiamine are greatly increased during pregnancy and lactation, and unless from four to six large portions of foods rich in thiamine are eaten daily these requirements are probably not met. Milk, eggs, lean meat, legumes, potatoes, and whole-grain or enriched bread and cereals furnish the major amount of this vitamin. Since the appearance of enriched flour and bread on the market it has become easier to obtain the proper amount. When the protein and iron needs are met with food, the thiamine requirement is satisfied. *Niacin* needs are raised with an increased carbohydrate intake. The *riboflavin* requirement of 2.0 mg is easily met if 1 qt of milk, which contains 1.6 mg, is consumed daily. Liver once a week, or more often, will help to ensure an adequate intake.

Adequate amounts of the entire B complex group can probably be supplied by diet alone—a diet which includes milk, eggs, whole-grain products, enriched bread, pork, glandular meats, legumes, green leafy vegetables, and fruit. This group is water soluble, quickly excreted, and poorly stored and must therefore be continually replaced.

**Vitamin C.** This water-soluble vitamin is poorly stored in the body and must be present in the diet in the amount of 100 mg daily for good nutrition. It is present in liberal quantity in fresh fruits (especially citrus), tomatoes, and raw green leafy vegetables. There is seldom a deficiency of ascorbic acid in the summer when fresh fruits and vegetables are readily available and used freely. With proper planning it is possible to maintain an adequate diet during the winter months also.

**Vitamin D.** This vitamin is necessary for the proper utilization and retention of calcium and phosphorus and therefore is very important during pregnancy. It is present in significant amounts in only a few foods—fish, liver, whole milk, cream, butter, and eggs—and even then varies with the seasons. Some foods, especially milk, are now being enriched with vitamin D either by irradiation or addition of a concentrate.

Exposure to sunlight will aid considerably in supplementing the diet, but when this exposure is not adequate, and especially in the winter months, supplements in the form of vitamin concentrates may be necessary to furnish the recommended 400 I.U. daily.

**Water** is very important for the proper regulation of body functions. It is necessary for adequate digestion and absorption of foods and for the proper elimination of body wastes through the kidneys, skin, and bowels. In pregnancy, where the mother eliminates wastes for herself and her baby, a fluid intake of 3 qt daily is particularly important. Most of this fluid intake should be water, with the remainder consisting of milk, soup, and other liquids.

Alcohol should be taken very sparingly or only with the doctor's permission, while tea and coffee should be used with moderation.

**Residue.** The expectant mother should make sure that her food contains a good deal of residue such as is provided by fruit, especially raw; coarse vegetables, particularly uncooked; and whole-grain cereals and bread. This residue increases the bulk of the intestinal contents, which stimulates peristaltic action and thus helps to overcome the tendency toward constipation.

**Caloric Intake.** This is an individual problem and must be determined by the activities of the individual, by the weight at the beginning of pregnancy, and by the weight gain during pregnancy. The caloric requirement is only approximately 15 to 20 per cent above the normal energy needs, this increase being due to an increase in basal metabolic rate. The elevation in metabolic rate is due to the fetal tissues and the hormonal changes in the mother.

Depending upon the weight and activity of the expectant mother the caloric intake should range from 2000 to 2500 calories per day. Since it takes about 2000 calories to supply the pregnant woman with an adequate amount of protein, vitamins, and minerals, there is limited selection of foods outside of those necessary to supply these nutritive requirements.

The pregnant woman should ordinarily be allowed to gain from 9 to 11.4 kg (20 to 25 lb) above the desirable weight for her age and height. The woman who enters pregnancy with a weight below normal for her build may be allowed to gain more by increasing her caloric intake, whereas the overweight woman should restrict her calories as much as possible, making certain, however, that she eats an adequate amount of the necessary foods.

The average pregnant woman will be able to supply her own and her baby's needs if her daily diet includes the following:

Milk: 1 qt
Meat: 4 oz; more if desired
liver at least once a week
Egg: 1
Vegetables: three servings, including one yellow or green leafy, two or three times a week; may be used as fresh, canned, or frozen
Fruits: three servings; including two citrus fruits or one citrus fruit and one glassful of tomato juice
Whole-grain cereal or bread, or enriched bread
Butter: 3 tsp
Water: at least six glassfuls
Iodized salt: used in moderation
Vitamin D: 400 I.U.
Desserts: these are important because they add to the attractiveness of most people's meals, but an excess amount of rich heavy foods and pastries should be omitted; they increase the caloric intake without supplying a sufficient amount of the essential nutritive materials

The expectant mother's meals should be taken with regularity, eaten slowly, and masticated thoroughly. Three average, balanced meals a day will usually suffice, but if the patient has a tendency to nausea early in pregnancy she will often be able to control it by taking a little food regularly five or six times daily, instead of the usual three meals, or if her appetite is small she may wish to eat four to six meals a day.

The mother must not only eat food which will supply the necessary nutritive material for the developing fetus and keep her adequately supplied without a storage of fat, but she must digest and assimilate it. This requires that she guard against overeating, constipation, and indigestion of any kind. Indigestion may be avoided during pregnancy exactly as it is at other times: by eating proper food, by cultivating a happy frame of mind, by exercise, fresh air, adequate rest, and sleep.

As fat is less easily digested and more likely to cause nausea during pregnancy than carbohydrates, it is better for the patient to eat no more fat than usual but to supply any additional energy needed with carbohydrates.

The patient should be advised to avoid fried food, pastry, rich desserts, rich salad dressings, and any food which would ordinarily disagree with her. On the other hand, it sometimes happens that an article of food which is likely to disagree with other people will be easily digested by the pregnant woman, and if it adds to the pleasure of her meals it should not be taboo, since the enjoyment of one's meals promotes digestion. So-called "cravings" are not as common in fact as they are in rumor, but the expectant mother may have a capricious appetite and display strange likes and dislikes for certain foods, possibly because of her tendency to be nauseated.

It is very unwise for the mother, on her own responsibility, to arrange her diet with the idea of keeping her child small or its skull soft and thus make labor easy. In general it is the size of the fetal skull and not the amount of fat distributed over the child's body that makes passage of the baby through the birth canal easy or difficult.

## CLOTHES

The expectant mother's clothes should be light and porous, and fairly loose, so as not to interfere with the circulation or other body functions. They should be so made that their weight will hang from the shoulders instead of from the waist. There must be no pressure on chest or abdomen; no tight garters, belts, or shoes.

Bearing in mind the importance of diversion and amusements, it becomes apparent that in addition to the hygienic qualities mentioned, the expectant mother's clothes should be as pretty and becoming as is consistent with her circumstances (Fig. 49). She is much more likely to go about and mingle with her friends if she is fortified with the consciousness that she is becomingly and well dressed.

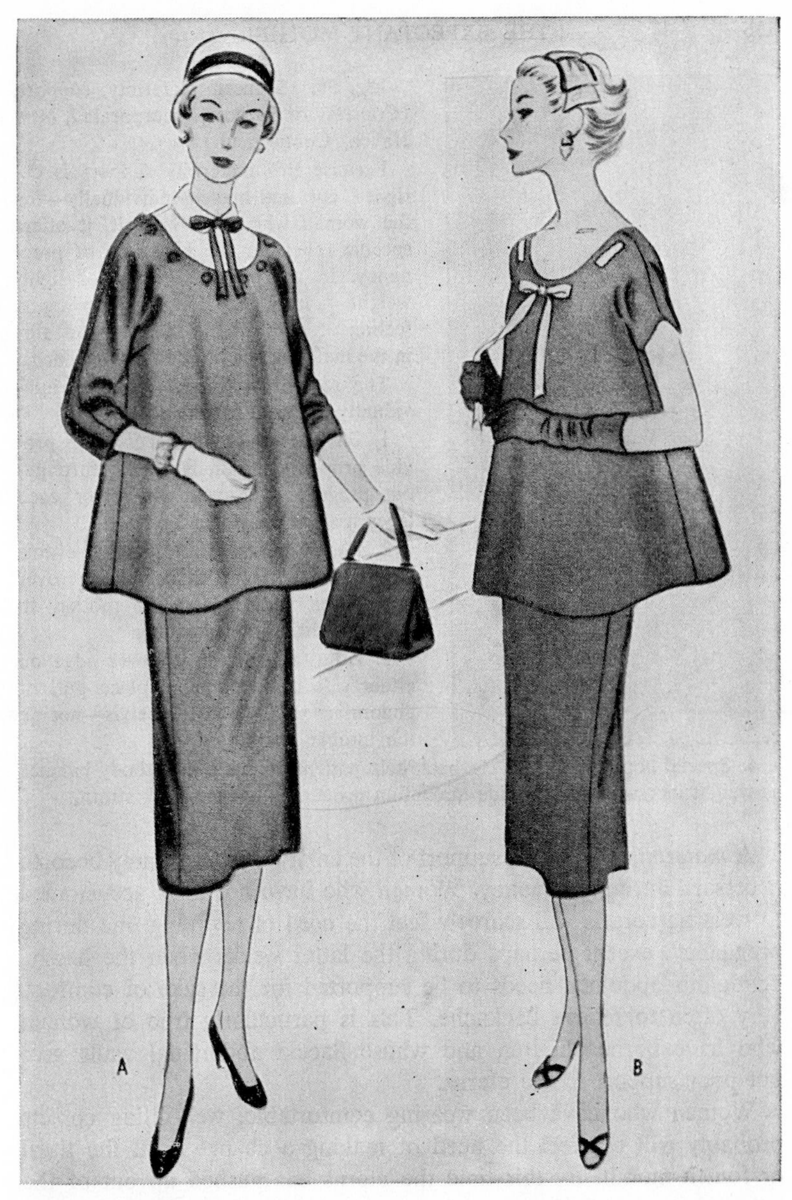


**Fig. 49.** Maternity two-piece dress and detachable dickey—Pattern No. 9938, "McCall's."

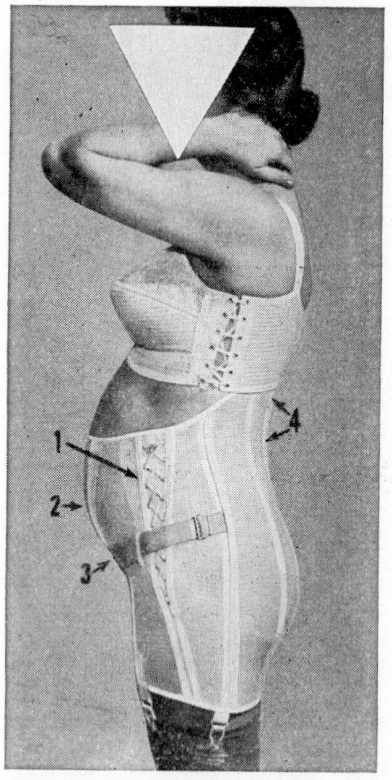


**Fig. 50.** Spencer maternity support. (Courtesy of Spencer, Incorporated, New Haven, Connecticut.)

Because this maternity support is designed, cut, and made—individually—for the woman who is to wear it, it offers specific relief for the backache of pregnancy. In the patient's choice of lightweight fabrics, the support provides a feeling of comfortable security and aids in the maintenance of good body balance.

The maternity brassiere, too, is individually designed for the patient.

1. Easy-to-adjust side lacers help provide proper abdominal support throughout pregnancy. A wide fly under each lacer assures comfort.

2. Elastic center-front panel prevents constriction. Support is curved out over groin area for freedom of motion in walking, sitting, and bending.

3. Adjustable tapes at lower edge on either side of front panel place pull of abdominal support on the pelvis—not on the lumbar back.

4. Special boning and high-cut back help patient maintain good body balance as weight increases and provide maximum protection against back strain.

A *maternity corset,* for support of the enlarging uterus, may become necessary during pregnancy. Women who have not been accustomed to wearing corsets will scarcely feel the need of adopting one during pregnancy, except perhaps during the latter weeks when the heavy, pendulous abdomen needs to be supported for the sake of comfort, very often to relieve backache. This is particularly true of women who have borne children and whose flaccid abdominal walls give but poor support to the uterus.

Women who have been wearing comfortable, well-fitting corsets probably will not feel the need of making a change until the third or fourth month. By this time the uterus has pushed up out of the pelvis, into the abdomen, and accordingly the corset must be constructed so that it will accommodate itself to an abdomen which is steadily increasing in size and also changing in shape, and thus provide support for the abdomen and still not disguise the figure (Fig. 50).

A satisfactory abdominal support should be easily adjustable so that its size and shape can be changed as required by the enlarging uterus. It should give support to the abdomen from below, to hold it up in its normal position, but must give this support without constriction of the upper abdomen. It should always be carefully fitted so that it will be comfortable and never tight. To be entirely satisfactory for adjustability, the maternity corset must be made of soft material and have elastic inserts and side, as well as front or back, lacings. It should extend well down in front and fit snugly over the hips. A maternity corset is not necessarily large and heavy; there are light comfortable ones designed for young women having their first baby, who do not need much support.

If the nurse clearly understands the purpose of a maternity corset, she will be able to explain to the patient why the same style as she ordinarily wears, no matter how large, will not be satisfactory during pregnancy, and may even be harmful. Also, it soon becomes uncomfortable because it tends to push the uterus down into the pelvis and thereby causes backache and cramps in the legs.

Very often the use of an abdominal support during the latter weeks will help prevent, as well as relieve, various discomforts of pregnancy discussed later in this chapter (pp. 152 ff.) under the heading, "Pressure Symptoms." It accomplishes this by lifting some of the weight of the heavy uterus from the blood vessels and ligaments. Backache is also relieved by the use of a maternity corset because it removes the strain of the increased weight of the abdomen from the ligaments and muscles and places it on the pelvic girdle. The corset also gives support to the pelvic girdle which is somewhat loosened during pregnancy.

A *brassiere* which will give good support to the breasts without pressure is important. The modern uplift brassiere, if well fitted, will accomplish this purpose. A brassiere which is adjustable to allow for an increase in the size of the breasts may eliminate the necessity of purchasing a new one frequently (Figs. 50 and 51). Some of these adjustable brassieres are also designed to serve as a nursing brassiere (Fig. 51). They are, therefore, more economical and are available for use immediately after delivery of the baby if desired.

Round garters or rolled stockings should not be worn because they retard circulation in the veins, favor the development of varicosities, and cause muscle cramps. Socks, which so many young mothers wear, eliminate this problem, but when stockings are worn they can be supported by a garter belt which hangs from the shoulders or one that fits at the waist in the back, but below the abdomen in the front (Fig. 52).

The expectant mother's *shoes* also merit attention. The added weight during pregnancy places increased demands upon the feet,

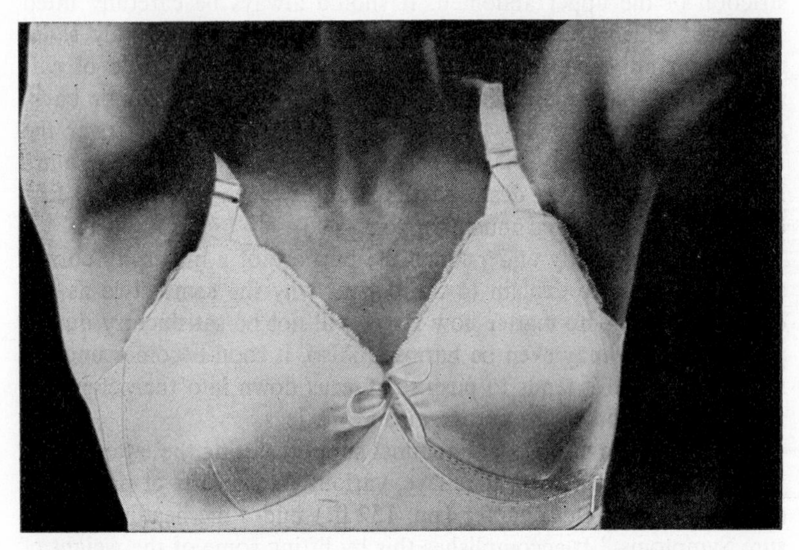

**Fig. 51.** Combination prenatal supportive and nursing brassiere. (Courtesy of Fancee Free Manufacturing Company, St. Louis, Missouri.)

and this weight should be balanced so that it will permit only the least amount of strain and fatigue. The feet may also be larger than usual because they are likely to be somewhat swollen during the latter part of pregnancy, and the increased weight of the body tends to spread them. Another reason for the need of proper shoes is that as pregnancy advances the enlarging uterus falls against the abdominal wall for support, the body's center of gravity changes, and the reaction is to throw back the shoulders which increases the curve of the spine. High heels, by causing a forward inclination of the pelvis, throw the uterus still farther forward. Considerable contraction of the back muscles then becomes necessary to shift the weight farther back for balance. The pregnant woman becomes unstable on her feet and needs broad, firm heels, not necessarily flat if she has been accustomed to wearing moderately high ones. High heels, of course, should be avoided because they not only produce backache by adding to the pull already caused by the abdomen, but also increase the difficulty of walking and the risk of turning the ankles, tripping, and falling.

The shoes then should have a wide heel base, not necessarily low, a good arch for support, and should fit well over the instep. Moccasin type shoes or bedroom slippers do not give good support. A well-fitted Oxford type shoe with a fairly low heel gives a broad base of support, prevents excessive forward tilt of the pelvis, and minimizes the pull on the back muscles. If the woman has always worn high heels the transition to low ones must be made gradually since the calf muscles have become shortened with long use of high-heeled shoes and a sudden stretching will cause muscle aching and pain. The expectant mother will tire more easily and tend to take less exercise than she needs if her shoes are not comfortable.

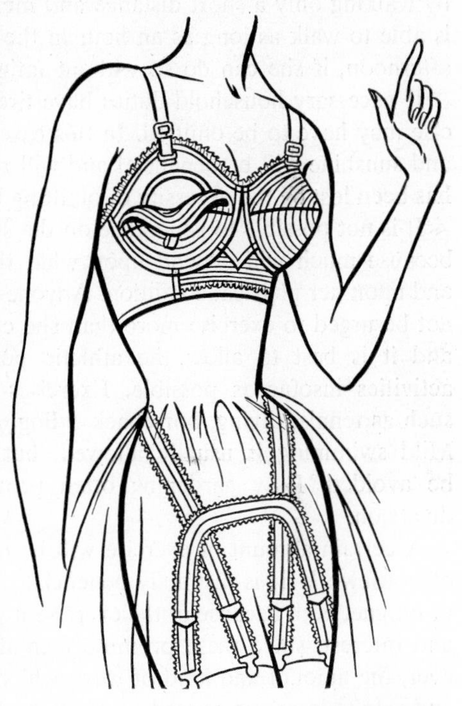

**Fig. 52.** Drop cup nursing brassiere. Garter belt. (Courtesy of Fancee Free Manufacturing Company, St. Louis, Missouri.)

FRESH AIR AND EXERCISE

If the nurse has become aware of the value of promoting all of the normal physiologic processes of the pregnant woman, she already has realized how important are fresh air and exercise to the patient and her expected baby.

Regular outdoor exercise is very important, since it gives exposure to sunshine which is so necessary to general health, promotes digestion, stimulates circulatory and respiratory systems, steadies the nerves, quiets the mind, and promotes sleep. Walking is probably the most satisfactory form of exercise unless the woman has been on her feet all day. It also strengthens some of the muscles that are used during labor. Exercise, however, is injurious if continued to the point of fatigue, no matter how little has been taken. Each woman must be a law unto herself in this matter, therefore, and must be impressed with the importance of stopping before she is tired. She should start by walking only a short distance and increase this gradually until she is able to walk as long as an hour in the morning and an hour in the afternoon, if she can do so without fatigue.

If necessary household duties have tired the woman, outdoor exercise may have to be omitted. In this case rest periods in the fresh air and sunshine will be beneficial and will replace, at least in part, what has been lost by the necessity of omitting the outdoor form of exercise.

It is not possible to generalize on the subject of exercise and sports because much will depend upon what the woman is accustomed to and upon her physical condition. Anyone with sedentary habits should not be urged to exercise more than she can easily do without fatigue, and it is best to allow the athletic person to pursue her normal activities insofar as possible. Exercises that involve violent action such as tennis, diving, horseback riding, or skiing should be omitted. Mild swimming is usually allowed, but rough surf bathing should be avoided. Easy gardening often provides pleasant exercise and diversion.

A certain amount of exercise will be obtained indoors in the form of housework. It is distinctly beneficial, if not continued to the point of fatigue, both because of the exercise it provides and of the diversion and interest, since these promote mental and physical health. However, the amount and kind of work which a woman may comfortably and safely do are so related to what she has been accustomed to that it is not possible to offer more than general suggestions, which will help in the planning for each individual. Heavy lifting should always be omitted.

If the expectant mother is attending training-for-childbirth classes she can practice some of the exercises she is learning while she pursues her household activities; even if she is not attending a regular class, certain suggestions from the nurse will improve her posture and will make her work easier. When stooping or bending is necessary, as they so often are, the bending should take place at the hips or knees while the back is kept straight. Squatting, with the feet in broad stance and turned slightly outward, is easier and more comfortable than stooping. This position can be used many times a day, especially when it is necessary to open low drawers (Fig. 53), pick articles up from the floor (Fig. 54), or care for a child. Picking up the toddler is much easier from a squatting than a stooping position (Fig. 55). By squatting, the mother not only avoids back strain, but actually practices an exercise which, as has been explained previously, prepares her muscles for the position she will assume on the delivery table.

Pelvic rocking is another exercise which can be fitted into the daily routine of work as the woman stands at a sink washing dishes (Fig. 56) or at a table performing other duties. If she dusts or washes the floor on her hands and knees she has an excellent opportunity to practice this exercise, which strengthens the muscles of the abdomen and the back and thus improves posture and prevents backache.

48

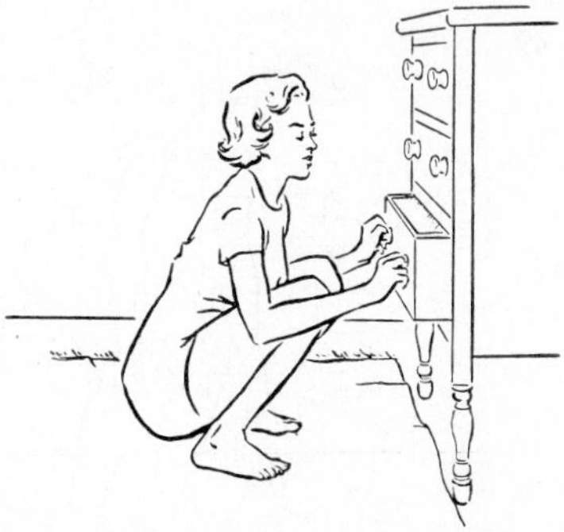

**Fig. 53.** Squatting instead of stooping to reach low drawer or shelf. (Reproduced from the *Reminder Sheets for Exercises, Rest Positions, Breathing and Relaxing Techniques,* published by Maternity Center Association, New York City, with their permission.)

Restriction of work and exercise is frequently imposed between the eighth and fourteenth week of pregnancy, since most abortions seem to occur during this period. Women who have previously had abortions may be particularly urged to moderate their activities in the early months of pregnancy.

## REST AND SLEEP

When we studied the structures of the female body we found that as the abdominal tumor of pregnancy increased in size and weight, the body's center of gravity changed and the pregnant woman was required to make a constant though unconscious effort to stand upright. This is probably one reason for the fatigue which expectant mothers so often feel without apparent cause, and for the fact that they are likely to tire rather more easily than usual. Frequent rest periods are needed by all pregnant women, but are even more necessary for those with poor body alignment than for those who have good posture. Accordingly, the patient may have to rest frequently during the day, at 10- to 15-minute intervals, in order to avoid the ill effects of fatigue (Fig. 57). She should work and exercise in short periods, always lying down when tired and for an hour or two after the noon meal. Many times some rest can be obtained by doing all work that can possibly be done in the sitting rather than the standing position.

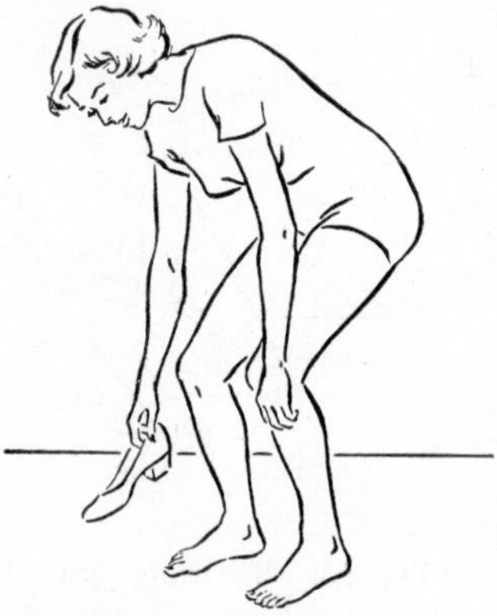

**Fig. 54.** Rising after squatting to pick up shoe or other small object. (Reproduced from the *Reminder Sheets for Exercises, Rest Positions, Breathing and Relaxing Techniques,* published by Maternity Center Association, New York City, with their permission.)

Sitting can be fatiguing unless the hips are well back in the seat of a chair that gives adequate support to the back. The seat must not be so deep, however, that there is pressure under the knees and thus on the veins. The feet should rest on the floor or on a stool of suitable height. Sitting with the legs elevated on a stool, will ensure rest as well as relieve a strain on varicosities and decrease swelling of the feet and legs. To be restful the knees must be in slight flexion and the footstool must be slightly lower than the chair to avoid pressure in the groins. It is often found that a rocking chair, or a straight chair, with armrests and good back support, and a height which allows the feet to rest easily on the floor, or a stool, is a very comfortable place for a rest.

Since eight-hours' sleep is usually considered necessary to keep the average person in good condition, the pregnant woman cannot expect to progress satisfactorily with less. In fact, adequate sleep is so important to her general well-being that she should be persuaded to do everything in her power to secure it.

For good rest a comfortable position must be assumed, preferably on a bed which has a firm mattress, or a bed board, to prevent back strain. In early pregnancy lying flat on the back with a pillow under the head and under the knees may be very comfortable (Fig. 44).

Clothing should be loose, and muscles should be allowed to become loose and limp. Abdominal breathing done at this time will not only add to the practice needed, but will be conducive to relaxation.

Later in pregnancy when the abdomen enlarges it becomes necessary for the woman to lie on her side (Fig. 45). The position should be such that the hips are partially rotated to allow the abdomen to rest on the bed. It may be necessary to use a pillow to support the upper leg. All joints should be bent slightly to prevent muscle tenseness. With conscious effort all of the skeletal muscles can be relaxed in this position. Abdominal breathing should be done for needed practice and for relaxation to induce sleep quickly.

Fresh air during the day, proper ventilation at night, prudent eating, a comfortable bed furnished with warm but light bedding,

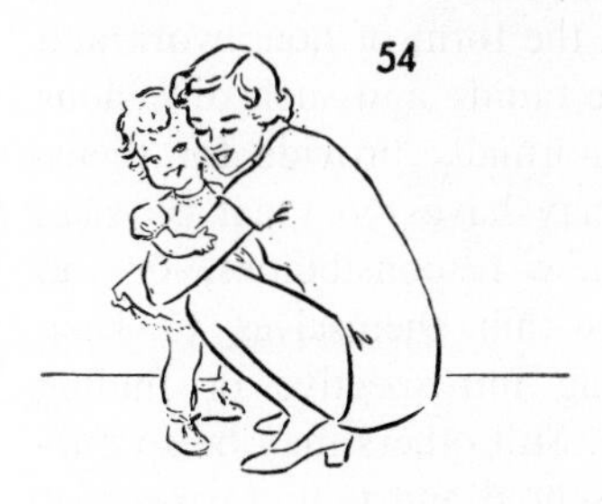


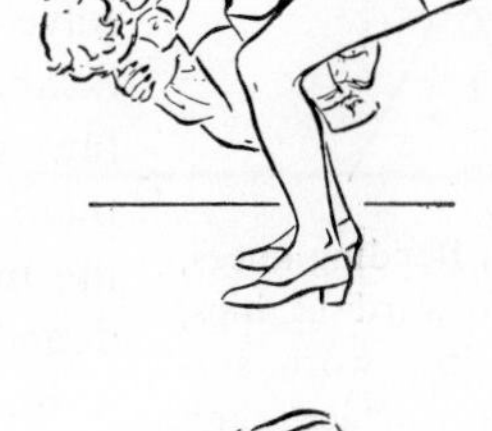


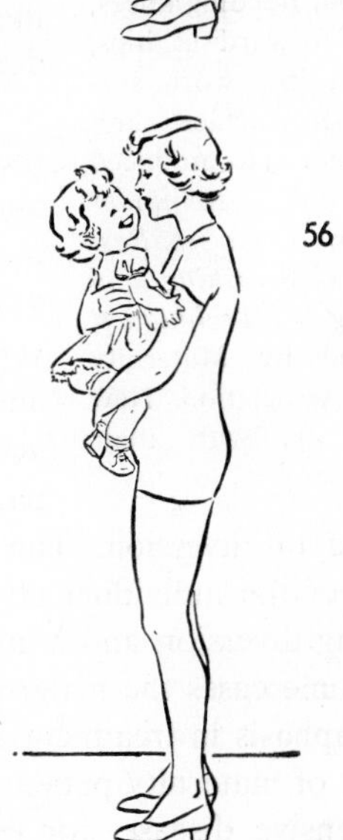


**Fig. 55.** Preventing or reducing strains on back muscles by squatting instead of stooping when picking up toddler:

Gathering toddler in arms (54), hugging her close while rising, tail first (55), ready to carry her without strain (56).

(Reproduced from the *Reminder Sheets for Exercises, Rest Positions, Breathing and Relaxing Techniques,* published by Maternity Center Association, New York City, with their permission.)

warm baths, a hot-water bag to the feet, and a hot drink upon retiring are all conducive to sleep. In addition to these, and perhaps of even more importance, are cheerfulness and a tranquil, untroubled state of mind. It is well for the nurse to make a mental note of that intangible but influential fact, since she can usually exert a great deal of influence in shaping the patient's mood.

31

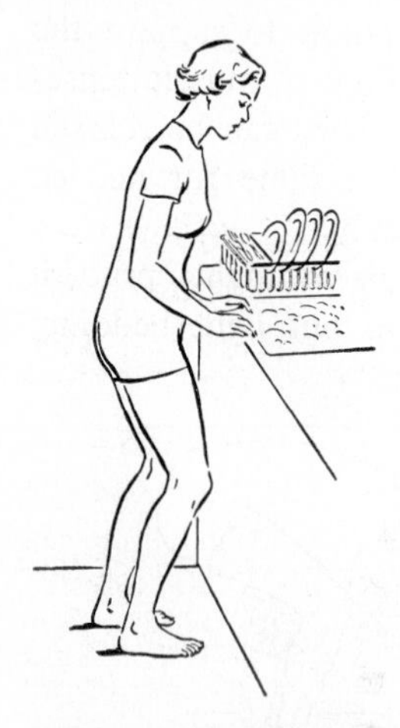

**Fig. 56.** Bending knees, leaning forward at hips, to reach low work surface when surface can't be raised. (Reproduced from the *Reminder Sheets for Exercises, Rest Positions, Breathing and Relaxing Techniques,* published by Maternity Center Association, New York City, with their permission.)

DIVERSION

The matter of diversion and occupation during pregnancy is so important that the nurse is scarcely giving complete care if she overlooks this aspect. Some patients have enough to do in the form of housework and looking after the family and such diversions as they would normally provide for themselves. Others may have too great physical disability, too few responsibilities, or too few resources within themselves to keep them from being introspective or finding life monotonous. Still others may be so burdened with household and family cares that it may be necessary for some member of the family to take over a few of their duties and thereby give them the time and energy needed for entertainment and relief from the monotony of their daily work. Sometimes a very simple suggestion, with a little interest and encouragement from the nurse, will accomplish much toward promoting the patient's mental health. This, of course, is the purpose of diversion. The intelligence, education, and normal interests of the individual obviously must be taken into account when planning diversion and amusement.

In some cases the maternity patient is primarily a medical patient, and emphasis in treatment is inevitably upon medical care. This may be true of maternity patients who have heart disease, tuberculosis, or hypertensive disease, for example. Such patients frequently need a great deal of rest in bed. Other maternity patients who sometimes need prolonged rest are those suffering from toxemia or those threatened with abortion.

It is apparent, therefore, that the nurse will in some instances find herself caring for a maternity patient for whom physical rest is imperative throughout several weeks or even months. The rest that is ordered in such instances is often one important therapeutic measure that prevents the loss or premature birth of the baby or saves the mother from permanent effects of an illness. Accordingly it becomes a matter of utmost necessity for the patient actually to rest as ordered. Merely staying in bed is not enough to ensure physical rest. Mental peace and quietude are necessary no matter what may be the patient's status, location, or intellectual attainments.

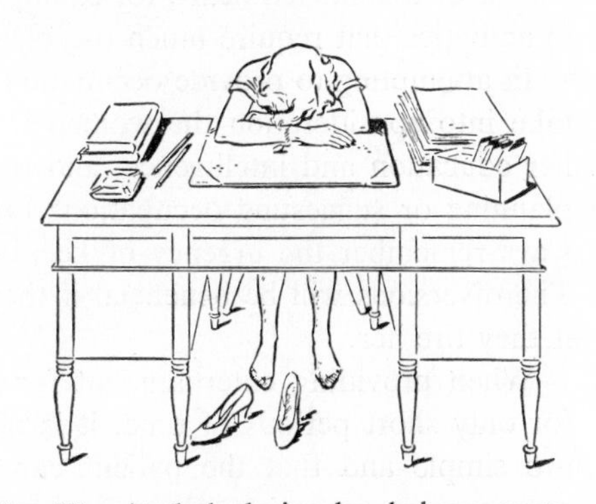


**Fig. 57.** At desk during lunch hour or recess period—all muscles loose and limp, mind on quiet natural breathing. (Reproduced from the *Reminder Sheets for Exercises, Rest Positions, Breathing and Relaxing Techniques,* published by Maternity Center Association, New York City, with their permission.)

It is common knowledge that the unoccupied person is likely to become restless, discontented, and introspective. When one is obliged to be inactive because of physical disability it is almost inevitable that fears and anxieties should present themselves, and as the hours and days go by the disturbing effects of these thoughts roll up like a snowball.

The expectant mother or young mother who is obliged to stay in bed has the same need as any other patient for mental and emotional quiet. With this in mind the nurse will easily appreciate the importance of suggesting or providing diversion for her patient. This is true whether the patient is at home or in a hospital and whether the nurse is solely devoted to one patient or is concerned with the welfare of several in a hospital or through a nursing organization in a community.

It cannot be expected that the busy nurse will be able to give close supervision to a patient's diversion or occupation or that a nurse without special training can suddenly become an occupational therapist. But if the nurse appreciates the fact that diversion is as necessary to certain patients as some of the other medical and nursing care, she will find a way to provide it. Obviously the form of diversion must be approved by the doctor in order that it may not defeat the very ends for which he is striving. The expectant mother suffering from tuberculosis or a damaged heart, for example, might not be able to engage in activities that require much use of arm or shoulder muscles.

In attempting to provide occupation for her patient the nurse must take into consideration the woman's normal activities and interests, her education and intelligence, and the circumstances of her life. In planning or suggesting occupations both nurse and patient must always remember the urgency of keeping within the limits of fatigue. The diversions will be beneficial if they rest the patient, but harmful if they tire her.

When providing entertainment for patients whom the nurse sees for only short periods of time, it is necessary to select projects that are simple and that the patient can work out for herself without assistance or supervision.

Some women may find enough distraction in reading of one kind or another. Very often there is greater satisfaction in working at tangible things. Some women will enjoy a fairly ambitious piece of work that progresses slowly, while others will be more interested in an item that may be completed in a short time.

There is an endless variety of occupations from which to choose. The layette is the first thing that comes to mind in connection with the expectant mother. The small garments are light, easy to handle, and are almost inevitably interesting to the maker.

Knitting, crocheting, and various kinds of needlework are old standbys. They are usually soothing in their effect and have the added value of being creative. Most people like to feel that they are accomplishing something. Knitting bed jackets for one's self or sweaters for children in the family gives one a pleasant sense of achievement. The patient who tires easily, or whose interest is held for only a short time, may enjoy making simple toys for children.

Happily there are many channels through which one may secure suggestions and instructions for all such occupations. An increasing number of hospitals throughout the country have occupational therapy departments where enthusiastic and resourceful workers are glad to respond to requests for help. Even in small towns one finds in the shops the materials and full directions for knitting and crocheting and many kinds of needlework. The women's magazines are inexpensive, and all offer ingenious suggestions and explicit instructions for a great variety of handiwork—garments, fancywork, and household articles. All of the manufacturers of yarn issue excellent booklets of instruction for knitting and crocheting. Patients in hospitals are usually delighted with the opportunity to help make dressings and some of the simpler articles used in connection with the hospital work.

In both cities and towns it is often the friends and neighbors who save the day by teaching and helping a shut-in to do things with her fingers. When the family and friends understand that diversion is not alone pleasant for the patient but also important to her welfare, they are usually very helpful.

The nurse must comprehend the fact that the patient will get more physical rest if her mind and hands have some occupation that is not contraindicated by her physical condition. Although the nurse may have neither time nor resources for providing occupation, she may attain the desired end by enlisting the aids of certain individuals and organizations.

### TRAVELING

In this day, when people travel so much and so easily, it is common to hear discussions as to its advisability for the prospective mother. Like many other details of prenatal care, this question cannot be settled once for all, nor for all stages of pregnancy. Each patient's general condition must be considered, her tendency to nausea, the length of the journey, the ease with which it may be made, and whether or not she has ever had, or been threatened with, an abortion. In general, traveling is less hazardous for the expectant mother today than it was formerly, to just the extent that it causes less strain, discomfort, and fatigue. By many doctors it is considered wise for her to avoid traveling during the first 14 weeks of pregnancy, especially if there is a tendency to abortion, and during the last 4 weeks because labor may begin prematurely. There seems to be no more objection to motoring and flying than to other modes of travel, when the patient's physical condition warrants and when circumstances are such that she can travel smoothly, comfortably, and without fatigue. Obviously, to prevent any impending complications, no journey of any kind should be undertaken at any time during pregnancy without a physician's approval.

### CARE OF THE TEETH

It is important that the pregnant woman give her teeth excellent daily care. It is also advisable for her to place herself under the care of a dentist, as soon as she knows of her pregnancy, telling him of her condition, and having any necessary work done at that time. Additional care consists of assuring that the mineral and vitamin intake is adequate for her own needs and those of the fetus. To supply this need, as has been explained before, it is necessary for her to drink a quart of milk daily and to receive vitamin D in food or in vitamin concentrates.

### BREASTS

The mother may be very anxious to do all that she can in preparation for successful breast feeding. Everything that promotes the expectant mother's general health helps to prepare her to nurse the baby. There is need also for care of the breasts and nipples themselves, to make the nursing satisfactory, and to prevent sore nipples and possibly even breast abscesses.

Briefly, this local care consists of supporting heavy breasts without pressure, attempting to bring out small or flattened nipples, and treating the skin which covers the nipples.

If the patient's nipples are very flattened, she is sometimes taught to begin about the fifth month to try to make them more prominent in order that the baby may grasp them easily. Several methods are advised, all of them in the nature of massage. One simple method is to grasp the nipple between the thumb and forefinger, draw it out, hold it for a moment, then release it and allow it to retract. This should be done over and over, two or three times daily. Another method is to pull the nipple out with a rough towel several times daily. With either method great care must be taken to avoid injury to the nipple. There is no assurance, however, that these procedures will make the nipples more prominent.

Rubbing c towel after 3rd mo. (stim uterine contrac.) toughens nipples.



Toughening of the nipples for nursing has been given much consideration in the prenatal period, and various measures have been advised. For many years it has been customary to recommend that the nipples be carefully washed with soap and warm water each day. This procedure is then followed by the application of lanolin, cocoa butter, cold cream, or petroleum jelly to prevent the nipples from becoming too dry or cracked. There is now a growing tendency to believe that it is advisable to avoid the use of soap and ointments. Elimination of the use of soap is recommended because soap: (1) removes the dead horny cells which serve as a protective covering of the nipple skin, (2) removes the copious secretion of the sebaceous glands, which serves as a protective covering and keeps the skin pliable, and (3) removes the secretion of the sweat glands, which also aids in keeping the skin pliable and in a normal acid condition. Ointments may inhibit evaporation of perspiration and thus may cause the skin to become soft. According to Niles Newton:

> It is usual for women to use particularly generous quantities of soap on their nipples during pregnancy and lactation. This effectively counteracts the effort of the body to prepare the nipple for the abrasive and stretching action of sucking. . . .
>
> One step in the prevention of nipple pain and nipple damage would seem to be to instruct the pregnant and lactating woman to avoid the use of soap on her nipples. . . . She might be told that the skin on her nipples may alter in appearance, but that this is not dirt but merely her body's way of preparing the nipple to withstand the force of the sucking infant.*

## THE MARITAL RELATION

Nurses are not infrequently asked about the wisdom of continuing the marital relation during pregnancy. There is no uniform answer except that abstinence is usually advised during approximately the last four weeks of pregnancy because of the danger of puerperal infection should the patient go into labor soon afterward. When there is a tendency to abortion, intercourse should be omitted either entirely up to the fourth month or at least during the time the woman would ordinarily have her menstrual period. Some doctors advise against intercourse at the time the menstrual period would ordinarily occur

* Newton, Niles: "Nipple Pain and Nipple Damage," *J. Pediat.*, **41**:416–17, (Oct.) 1952.

during the first three months even when there is no history of previous abortion. The patient should always be told to discuss this matter with her doctor and follow his advice.

## COMMON DISCOMFORTS DURING PREGNANCY

There are many minor disturbances which overtake the pregnant woman, and though not serious in themselves, her comfort is greatly increased by having them relieved; her general welfare is thus promoted. The relief of these discomforts, when they are slight or only temporary, sometimes resolves itself into little more than a question of nursing. When long continued or severe, however, they constitute complications which the doctor treats according to indications.

### GASTROINTESTINAL SYMPTOMS

**Nausea and vomiting** are probably the most common disturbances of pregnancy, occurring in about 50 per cent of all cases. The symptoms vary from the slightest feeling of nausea when the patient first raises her head in the morning to persistent and frequent vomiting which then assumes grave proportions and is termed "pernicious vomiting." Although it is possible that even the slightest nausea is due to certain changes in the chemical processes of the body to which an adjustment must be made, there can be no doubt that in many instances the patient's mental attitude is an important factor.

Dr. J. Morris Slemons has made the interesting observation that women who are unaware of their pregnancy for several months are seldom troubled with nausea, while those who erroneously believe themselves to be pregnant sometimes suffer from these well-known symptoms of pregnancy until convinced of their mistake. In other words, although nausea occurs frequently it is not an inevitable accompaniment of pregnancy and may very likely be due to a state of tension. Some emotional tension may well be expected, even when a pregnancy is greatly desired, since certain adjustments must always be made—changes in living arrangements, in budget, or in many other areas. Anxiety, grief, fright, shock, introspection, worry, or any emotional stress may cause nausea when the diet is entirely satisfactory, but indiscretions in diet, rapid or overeating, also may cause nausea and vomiting in the expectant mother.

Although this nausea and vomiting will usually disappear at the end of the first trimester, probably at a time that an adjustment, both physical and emotional, has been made, it can be eased earlier by certain preventive measures.

It must be remembered that the principles of personal hygiene are preventives of nausea during pregnancy, since rest and relaxation, cultivation of a happy frame of mind, and exercise and fresh air all tend to avert this condition. Adequate rest should be stressed as a preventive measure, especially when one realizes that many women experience marked fatigue and lassitude early in pregnancy and that sufficient rest relieves emotional tension to some extent. In addition to easing of tension, certain dietary suggestions, if carefully followed, give relief.

Nausea and/or vomiting of pregnancy may occur at any time during the day but since it appears most frequently in the early morning, as soon as the woman gets up, it is commonly called "morning sickness." This early morning nausea may be relieved in many cases by eating two or three crackers or a piece of toast, with nothing to drink, immediately upon awakening and then lying quietly in bed for 20 to 30 minutes. The patient should then dress slowly and in due course eat her regular breakfast. If nausea occurs at other times during the day the best treatment is for her to eat six small meals a day rather than three large ones in an attempt to keep some food in the stomach at all times. The nausea seems to be worse when the stomach is empty than when it contains some food. Foods that are largely carbohydrate, that do not have a strong odor, and that are of extremes of temperature, either very hot or very cold, give the most relief. It may also be well to take liquids and solids separately instead of taking both at the same meal. Fried or greasy foods should be avoided.

If it is known that nausea occurs at a certain time of day, food should be taken 30 minutes earlier. The patient may be given specific directions as to the times she should eat and the kinds of food she should take and be made to feel that she will get relief from her discomfort if she follows directions carefully. Lying flat and keeping very quiet for a little while after meals, or whenever feeling the slightest premonitory symptom, will frequently prevent and also relieve nausea. Sedatives are sometimes used to relieve the patient suffering from nausea and vomiting. Several of the new tranquillizing agents have been used recently and have shown promise in the management of nausea of pregnancy. Obviously, drugs are given only upon the doctor's order.

**Heartburn,** so called, which is experienced by many pregnant women has nothing to do with the heart. It is caused by a bubbling back of stomach contents into the esophagus and is usually described as a burning sensation first in the stomach and then rising into the throat. It may be prevented, as a rule, by substituting frequent small meals for the usual three larger ones. If frequent small meals do not give enough relief, the doctor may recommend an antacid preparation to be taken at the time of the burning. Many people are accustomed to taking baking soda in a glass of water to relieve heartburn, but this is contraindicated during pregnancy because of its sodium content.

**Distress.** There is another form of discomfort, often vague and ill-defined, commonly called "distress," and occurring after eating. It may be neither heartburn nor pain, but resembles both and makes the patient very uncomfortable. It is usually seen in women who eat rapidly, do not chew their food thoroughly, or eat more at one time than the stomach can hold comfortably. The prevention, naturally, lies in taking small amounts of food slowly and masticating it thoroughly.

**Flatulence** may or may not be associated with heartburn but it is fairly common and rather uncomfortable. It is usually due to bacterial action in the intestines, which results in the formation of gas. As has been explained previously, the pressure of the enlarging uterus upon the intestines and the decreased gastrointestinal tract motility retard normal peristalsis with the result that gas sometimes accumulates to a very uncomfortable extent. It is clear, therefore, that a daily bowel movement is of prime importance in preventing and relieving flatulence and also that foods which form gas should be carefully excluded from the diet. The chief offenders are parsnips, beans, the cabbage family, corn, fried foods, sweets of all kinds, pastry, and very sweet desserts.

## PRESSURE SYMPTOMS

Under the general heading of pressure symptoms are several forms of discomfort resulting from pressure of the enlarging uterus on the veins returning from the lower part of the body, thus interfering with the return flow of blood. This pressure is apt to be greatly increased if lumbar lordosis and tilting forward of the pelvis are marked. As both the cause and relief of these symptoms are associated with the force of gravity, the nurse will usually know what to do in mild cases without further explanation. In general, the heavy abdomen should be supported by a properly fitting corset in case the abdominal muscles are not strong enough to give good support, and the patient should keep off her feet as much as possible and elevate the swollen part. Support of the heavy abdomen not only gives relief but will often prevent the occurrence of pressure symptoms.

The most common pressure symptoms are swollen feet, varicose veins, hemorrhoids, cramps in the legs, and shortness of breath, and although they may appear at any time during the latter half of pregnancy, they grow progressively worse as it advances. If the patient seems to be alarmed over the appearance of these symptoms, her fears may be allayed by the explanation that such conditions are neither unusual nor serious.

**Swelling of the feet** is very common, and sometimes also of the hands; when very slight it may not be serious or particularly uncomfortable. Fluid tends to collect in dependent areas. The edema may be confined to the back of the ankles, or it may extend all the way up the legs to the thighs and include the vulva. Sitting down, with the feet resting on a chair, or lying down with the legs elevated on a pillow will naturally give a certain amount of relief because it redistributes the fluid. It may be easier to keep the legs elevated when a pillow is placed under the mattress than when the effort must be made to keep them on the pillow. If the swelling and discomfort are extreme, the patient may have to go to bed until they subside, but very often she will secure adequate relief by elevating her feet for even a little while several times a day. Since salt increases the retention of fluid, it should be restricted or eliminated from the food as much as possible when edema is present. While employing these harmless and clearly indicated measures to make her patient comfortable, the nurse must be keenly aware of the fact that although edema of the feet, legs, and vulva may be of solely mechanical origin, it is also a sign of toxemia, about the most dreaded complication of pregnancy. As recognition of the earliest signs of toxemia is among the triumphs of prenatal nursing, even the slightest swelling must be reported to the doctor, and immediate steps taken to have the urine examined and the blood pressure checked.

**Varicose veins** are not peculiar to pregnancy, but are among the pressure symptoms which frequently accompany this condition during the later months, particularly among women who have borne children. The superficial veins in the legs will often be equal to the tension put upon them the first time, but will give way as the strain is repeated during subsequent pregnancies. The distention of the veins is not serious as a rule but may be very uncomfortable; aching of the legs is a common symptom even when the veins are not visible. Pain coupled with the unsightly appearance of enlarged veins sometimes has an adverse mental effect. Varicose veins may occur in the vulva although they are usually confined to the legs.

Varicose veins are most apt to develop when it is necessary to stand for long periods of time or to sit with the legs dependent. One preventive measure then is to sit down with the feet elevated. If the patient will constantly keep in mind that she should sit with her feet elevated whenever possible, she will find many instances in which she can do this while doing the daily work that she might ordinarily do standing up. If it is necessary to remain on the feet for the major part of the day, moving about, which improves circulation in the veins of the leg, is better than standing still. When the legs are moved, as in walking, circulation is improved by the massaging action of the muscles close to the veins. Tight bands or round garters interfere with return circulation and should never be worn.

Relief from the discomfort caused by varicose veins is obtained as a rule by keeping off the feet, and particularly by elevating them, and also by the use of elastic bandages. When a woman finds it difficult or nearly impossible to sit or lie down for any length of time, she may accomplish a great deal in a short time by lying flat on the bed with her legs extending straight into the air, at right angles to her body, resting them against the wall or headboard (Fig. 58). This right-angled position, held for 5 to 10 minutes, three or four times a day, by promoting drainage of the veins, will usually help to reduce varicose veins and decrease aching of the legs.

In addition to posture, elastic stockings or spiral elastic bandages will give relief and help to prevent the veins from growing larger. They should be put on before getting up in the morning or after the legs have been elevated for a few minutes so that the veins are relatively empty at the time they are applied.

Elastic stockings offer an advantage over the bandages in ease of application and in appearance, but they are expensive; elastic band-

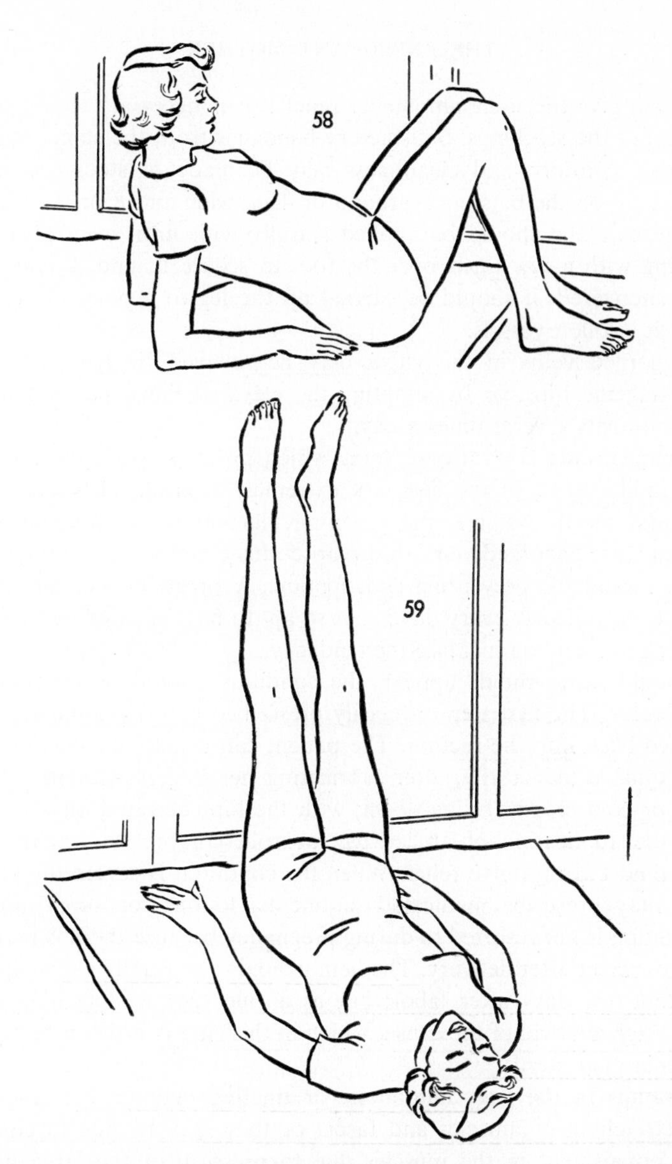


**Fig. 58.** Resting with feet elevated to stimulate return circulation in feet and legs, prevent or reduce enlarged veins and fatigue.

Ready to swing around with buttocks close to wall, and raise feet and legs so heels rest against wall (58).

Right-angle position (59).

(Reproduced from the *Reminder Sheets for Exercises, Rest Positions, Breathing and Relaxing Techniques,* published by Maternity Center Association, New York City, with their permission.)

ages will give the same amount of relief if it is necessary to use them instead of the stockings. Satisfactory bandages from the standpoint of expense, comfort, and cleanliness may be made of stockinet or of flannel cut on the bias, measuring 3 or 4 in. wide and 8 or 9 yd long.

The bandage should be applied spirally with firm, even pressure, starting with a few turns over the foot to secure it, and, leaving the heel uncovered, it should be carried up the leg to a point above the highest swollen vessels.

Engorged veins in the vulva may be relieved by lying flat and elevating the hips, or by adopting the elevated Sims' position for a few moments several times a day.

**Hemorrhoids** are varicose veins which protrude from the rectum, but, unlike those in the legs, are extremely painful. They may also itch and bleed. As it is the straining incident to constipation that causes these engorged veins to prolapse, this condition constitutes one more reason for preventing constipation. A pregnant woman whose bowels move freely every day is not so apt to have hemorrhoids. Hard stools and straining increase the tendency.

Should hemorrhoids appear, the condition should be reported to the doctor. The first step ordinarily prescribed is to have them gently pushed back into the rectum. The patient can usually do this for herself, quite satisfactorily, after lubricating her fingers with petroleum jelly or cold cream. Lying down, with the hips elevated on a pillow, and the application of an ice bag or cold compresses to the anus will almost always give relief. When the condition is severe the physician may prescribe medicated ointments, lotions, or suppositories. Operation is not resorted to during pregnancy because there is marked improvement after delivery. The hemorrhoids are usually worse during the first few days after labor, but as a rule they disappear a short time after removal of the cause, which in this case is pressure made by the enlarging uterus.

**Cramps in the legs**, numbness, or tingling may be the result of overstretching of muscles and fascia or they may be due to circulatory impairment in the muscles due to pressure of the large heavy uterus on the pelvic veins. Less frequently the cramps are caused by a calcium deficiency, this ordinarily being true only when an effort is not made to meet the calcium requirements. The cramps may be very severe. They are most apt to occur while at rest.

Relief is usually obtained by standing on the feet. The cramps may also be relieved by extending the cramped leg, flexing the ankle, and forceably pushing the forefoot upward, with the toes pointing toward the knee (Fig. 59). If cramps occur during labor, or any other time

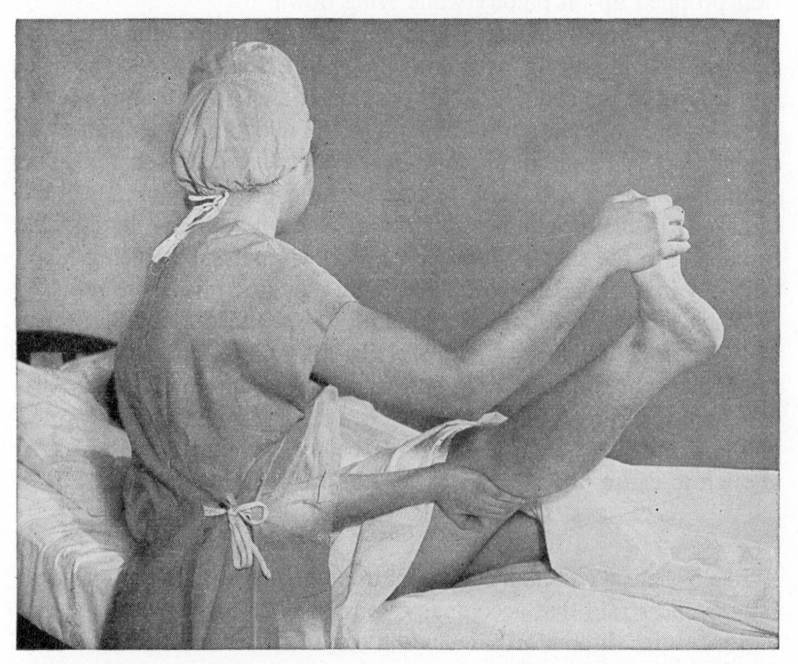

**Fig. 59.** Relieving muscle cramp in the leg by extending the cramped leg, flexing the ankle, and forceably pushing the forefoot upward, with the toes pointing toward the knee.

that the patient cannot get onto her feet readily, this latter method is one the nurse can employ to give her relief. Sometimes the patient will be able to feel the cramped muscle and will automatically begin to massage it to relieve the cramping. Application of a hot-water bottle often gives comfort.

As the baby's head descends into the pelvis the expectant mother may experience **pain in the thighs** and **aching of the perineum.** There is also **increased urinary frequency** and **constipation** due to pressure on the bladder and bowels.

**Shortness of breath,** due to crowding of the diaphragm, is sometimes very troublesome toward the end of pregnancy, and, as may be easily seen, is due to the upward and not downward pressure of the uterus. For this reason it is aggravated by the patient's lying down and relieved by her sitting up, preferably in a straight chair, or being well propped up on pillows while lying down.

Whenever breathlessness seems particularly troublesome it can be relieved by lying on the back with the arms extended above the head and resting on the bed. Since this position stretches the thoracic cavity to its maximum, even normal breathing will allow for expansion of all available lung tissue and breathlessness is relieved. When relief has been obtained by remaining in this position for a few minutes, and especially if this is done before sleep at night, it will soon be possible to change to the side position and relax, without experiencing much difficulty in resting. Intercostal breathing may also give some relief.

When lightening occurs, the breathlessness and the constant sense of pressure of the uterus under the ribs are relieved. The nurse must remember that shortness of breath may be a symptom of cardiac disease and, accordingly, should be watched for and immediately reported to the doctor, especially if it occurs before the uterus has enlarged enough to cause pressure.

### BACKACHE

Backache is a common complaint in pregnancy due to the muscular fatigue and strain that accompany poor body balance. Backache and various other discomforts, including varicosities and swelling of the feet and ankles, may be due to faulty body alignment.

During pregnancy the normal amount of lordosis is increased in an effort to balance the body. It becomes severe if the abdominal muscles are relaxed and in poor tone before pregnancy, which allows for marked protrusion of the abdomen as the uterus enlarges. This causes a great increase in the forward tilt of the pelvis and an increased strain at the sacroiliac joints. With this increased lordosis there is an increase in kyphosis of the dorsal spine and a forward protrusion of the head and neck. This is followed by more stretching and thinning of the abdominal muscles and shortening of the long muscles of the back. Backache is a common result of all of these changes. Since each pregnancy causes further stretching and loss of muscle tone, disturbances are more numerous in women who have borne several children.

A woman who has achieved good body alignment as a young girl will not experience much discomfort from the added strain of pregnancy. The acquisition of good body mechanics should begin in childhood, but if it has not been started then it should begin early in pregnancy, and every effort must be made to improve the posture

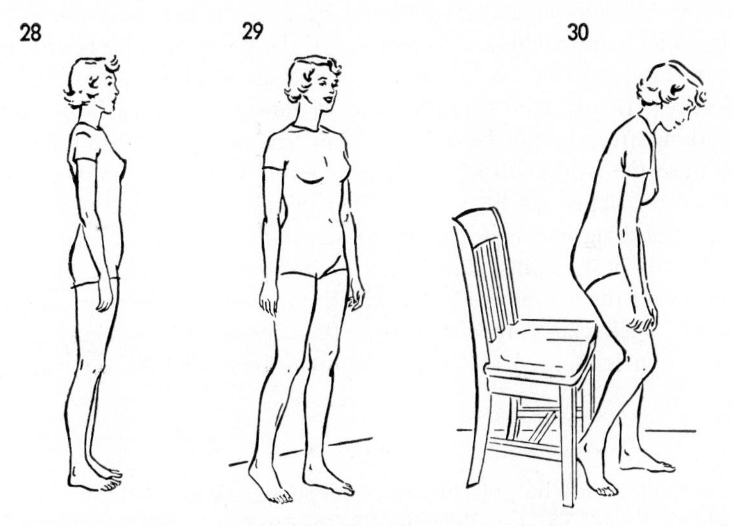


**Fig. 60.** Using good body mechanics in everyday activities to preserve figure, increase efficiency, and reduce fatigue.

Ready for action—head, chest, spine, pelvis, and feet aligned for balanced weight bearing; costal breathing; easy movement (28).

Shifting weight to forward foot to rest while waiting in line (29).

Using leg muscles to lower body weight to chair (30).

(Reproduced from the *Reminder Sheets for Exercises, Rest Positions, Breathing and Relaxing Techniques,* published by Maternity Center Association, New York City, with their permission.)

(Fig. 60). Methods of improving posture have been discussed on pages 120–22 of this chapter.

Good alignment means that the body does not slump, that there are no marked spinal curvatures, and that the forward tilt of the pelvis is minimal. The feet are not unduly flattened or spread at the forefoot. The uterine enlargement is upward rather than forward; the abdomen does not protrude forward to a marked degree, but rather is full nearest the xyphoid.

Exercises, improvement of posture, and abdominal supports which aid in the prevention of backache have previously been mentioned.

Discomfort can also be prevented or relieved by proper arrangement of household appliances. They should be at a working level which makes it possible to keep the arms in a comfortable position and the back straight, with all bending taking place from the hips alone. All working material should be near enough to avoid undue stretching and reaching, and twisting of the body. Ironing boards and work tables should be raised or lowered as necessary and whenever possible. Blocks can often be used to raise working surfaces; when working areas cannot be lowered it may be possible to use footstools to raise the worker to a comfortable level. There are many ways in which the home can be arranged to minimize fatigue and strain.

A waddling gait is apt to be present late in pregnancy due to an instability of the joints. This is the result of relaxation of the sacroiliac joints and the symphysis pubis which normally occurs in pregnancy. Severe backache may accompany this condition, especially if the relaxation is marked and if considerable lumbar lordosis is present.

## INSOMNIA

Insomnia may be present late in pregnancy. It is sometimes a little difficult to get to sleep because the upward pressure of the uterus causes shortness of breath, especially in the recumbent position, and because the activity of the baby may be disturbing. Sleep will be promoted if the side position is assumed and abdominal breathing is instituted, after a few deep breaths have been taken with the arms raised above the head.

## VAGINAL DISCHARGE

The normal vaginal discharge is greatly increased during the latter months of pregnancy, as was pointed out in Chapter 5, so that ordinarily the moderately profuse yellowish or white discharge at this time has no particular significance. As the normal vaginal discharge has antiseptic properties, it should not be removed by douches, which many patients may think they need, unless they are explicitly ordered by the doctor.

Some patients have an abnormally profuse discharge and may suffer from persistent itching and burning. Such symptoms may be due to *Trichomonas vaginalis* vaginitis, to a yeast infection, or to a gonorrheal infection, and should be reported to the doctor.

*Trichomonas vaginalis,* an actively motile, flagellate parasite, may produce a profuse, irritating, foamy secretion, yellowish green in color, and having an unpleasant odor. This discharge is very irritating to the vagina and external genitalia and causes intense itching. It may cause symptoms anytime, but they frequently flare up during pregnancy. There is no specific cure for this condition, but many medications have been used with some relief.

*Yeast infection,* caused by *Candida (Monilia) albicans,* also often flares up during pregnancy because of conditions present in the vagina which are conducive to its growth. It produces a profuse white, watery, curdy discharge which is very irritating to the vagina and external genitalia. This infection is quite easily treated by the application of 2 per cent aqueous solution of methylrosaniline chloride (gentian violet). Nystatin (Mycostatin) (an antibiotic against fungi) has recently been effectively used in the therapy of vaginal moniliasis. It is usually administered in the form of vaginal tablets, but may also be used orally in conjunction with the vaginal treatment.

Whether or not the above conditions need treatment will frequently depend upon the presence or absence of symptoms. The decision rests with the doctor.

A *gonorrheal infection,* of course, should always be treated, regardless of symptoms, both to protect the baby's eyes in its passage through the birth canal and to protect the mother from an infection of the uterine cavity following delivery. This infection can successfully be treated by the use of penicillin.

Smears of the vaginal discharge, to be examined for the gonococcus especially, and also for the presence of yeast or trichomonas, often are taken routinely at the first or an early prenatal visit. If there is reason to suspect a gonorrheal infection a culture may be of more diagnostic value, since the organism cannot always be demonstrated on a smear when the infection has reached a chronic stage. If the appearance of the discharge suggests a trichomonas infection a diagnosis can easily be made by the hanging drop method.

## ITCHING

Itching is a fairly common discomfort, and is possibly a result of irritating material being excreted by the skin glands and deposited upon the surface of the body. The local irritation, if not very severe, usually may be allayed by bathing the uncomfortable areas with a solution of sodium bicarbonate or by taking a starch bath. It is a good plan, also, for the patient to increase the amount of fluids which she is taking, in order to promote the activity of the skin, kidneys, and bowels, and thus dilute the material that may be responsible for the itching and increase its elimination through all channels. Since the excessive use of soap may be irritating, the use of a very bland soap or elimination of the use of soap almost entirely and oiling of the skin following bathing may also help to relieve itching.

Some women complain of discomfort caused by the stretching of the skin over the enlarged abdomen, which becomes so tense it feels as though it might tear apart. There is a very old and widely current belief that this sensation may be relieved by rubbing the abdomen with some kind of an oil or ointment, and that such oiling will not only increase the elasticity of the superficial layers of the skin but the deeper layers as well and that by this means striae may be prevented. There seems to be little foundation for the fear that the skin will tear or belief in the efficacy of the oiling, but if a woman thinks that she is safer and more comfortable after oiling her abdomen, there is certainly no reason why she should not do so.

## EARLY SIGNS OF COMPLICATIONS OF PREGNANCY

It is evident that by teaching the principles of personal hygiene to the expectant mother so convincingly that she will adopt them and, sometimes, by employing simple nursing procedures to relieve the various discomforts of pregnancy, much will be accomplished toward promoting the welfare of both the patient and the expected baby. But this is not enough. The nurse must also be on the alert to detect and report the early signs and symptoms of complications, since there may be times when she will be the first one to see the patient after a symptom has developed.

The principal complications of pregnancy which are amenable to preventive or early treatment are the toxemias, premature terminations of pregnancy, and hemorrhage.

The causes of these conditions and details of treatment and nursing care are discussed together and at some length in Chapter 9, but their most conspicuous, early signs are briefly noted here, since watching for them constitutes a part of prenatal care.

## THE TOXEMIAS

The toxemias apparently result from disturbed metabolism and impaired or inadequate excretory processes. Preventive measures consist largely of teaching the principles of personal hygiene previously described and in promptly instituting treatment upon the appearance of early signs or symptoms. One of the most common symptoms is headache, sometimes persistent and very severe. Others are disturbed vision, dizziness, and more persistent or severe vomiting than could reasonably be called "morning sickness." A rapid gain in weight; puffiness under the eyes or elsewhere about the face, or of the hands; anything more than very slight swelling of the feet and ankles; high or increasing blood pressure; albumin in the urine, amounting to more than a trace; mental depression and epigastric pain—all are possible signs or symptoms of toxemia. A patient in whom even one of these manifestations appears is usually placed under close observation, frequently put to bed and restricted to a salt-poor diet, and efforts are made to promote diuresis.

## PREMATURE TERMINATION OF PREGNANCY

The common symptoms of premature termination of pregnancy (an abortion or premature labor) are bleeding or pain in the small of the back, followed by cramp-like pains in the abdomen, or both. Bleeding or a bloody discharge, irrespective of pain, should be regarded as a symptom of pending labor, and the doctor should be notified at once. The patient should be put to bed promptly and kept quiet until the doctor's arrival. Preventive treatment consists largely of rest, particularly at even the slightest evidence of bleeding or pain, and avoidance of physical shocks and of overwork. Prolonged failure on the part of the patient to feel fetal movements or of the nurse or doctor to hear the fetal heartbeat, after they have once been manifest, usually indicates the death of the child and precedes its expulsion.

## HEMORRHAGE

Bleeding, or a sudden increase in the size of the uterus, with a rapid pulse or general symptoms of shock may be signs of hemorrhage caused by placenta previa or premature separation of a normally implanted placenta. Upon the appearance of any one of these signs the patient should be put to bed and kept absolutely quiet.

### DANGER SIGNALS

To sum up, we find that the following signs and symptoms may be forerunners of serious complications. They should be watched for and reported to the doctor immediately upon their discovery:

1. Bleeding
2. Rapid gain in weight
3. Edema, either general or localized in any part of body
4. Persistent or severe headache
5. High or increasing blood pressure
6. Albumin in the urine
7. Dizziness
8. Visual disturbances
9. Persistent or severe vomiting
10. Fever
11. Pain in the lumbar region followed by cramp-like pains in the abdomen before the expected date of confinement or a steady abdominal pain
12. Marked shortness of breath
13. Sleeplessness or drowsiness
14. Prolonged failure to feel fetal movements
15. Persistent constipation
16. Any new or unusual symptom

When all is said and done, the daily regimen for the expectant mother should be such that she can live a normal, wholesome life; that she is willing, and also able, to weave into her everyday life the principles of personal hygiene which everyone should adopt; that she is carefully watched for complications throughout the entire period of pregnancy, and that these complications be speedily treated.

### BIBLIOGRAPHY AND STUDENT REFERENCES

Blake, Florence G.: *The Child, His Parents and the Nurse.* J. B. Lippincott Co., Philadelphia, 1954.

Bookmiller, Mae M., and Bowen, George L.: *Textbook of Obstetrics and Obstetric Nursing,* 2nd ed. W. B. Saunders Co., Philadelphia, 1954.

Burke, Bertha S.: "Diet and Nutrition during Pregnancy," *Am. J. Nursing,* **52**:1378–80, (Nov.) 1952.

Burke, Bertha S., and Stuart, Harold C.: "Nutritional Requirements during Pregnancy and Lactation," *J.A.M.A.,* **137**:119–28, (May 8) 1948.

Davis, M. Edward, and Sheckler, Catherine E.: *DeLee's Obstetrics for Nurses,* 15th ed. W. B. Saunders Co., Philadelphia, 1951.

Eastman, Nicholson J.: *Expectant Motherhood,* 2nd ed. Little, Brown, and Co., Boston, 1948.

———: *Williams Obstetrics,* 11th ed. Appleton-Century-Crofts, Inc., New York, 1956.

Etherington, Judy: "Old Wives on New Lives. A Study of Prenatal Superstitions," *Pub. Health Nursing,* **44**:537–41, (Oct.) 1952.

Goodrich, Frederick W.: *Natural Childbirth.* Prentice-Hall, Inc., New York, 1950.

Greenhill, J. P. (ed.): *Obstetrics,* 11th ed. W. B. Saunders Co., Philadelphia, 1955.

Heardman, Helen: *A Way to Natural Childbirth.* E. & S. Livingstone, Ltd., Edinburgh, 1950.

Jacobson, Edmund: *You Must Relax,* 3rd ed. Whittlesey House, McGraw-Hill Book Co., New York, 1948.

Krejci, Sylvia: *Teaching Outlines for Mothercraft Classes.* Clara Elizabeth Fund for Maternal Health, Flint, Michigan, 1955.

Kuhns, John G.: "Disturbances in Body Mechanics during Pregnancy," *Pub. Health Nursing,* **42**:536–43, (Oct.) 1950.

Lesser, Marion S., and Keane, Vera R.: *Nurse–Patient Relationships in a Hospital Maternity Service.* C. V. Mosby Co., St. Louis, 1956.

McKinnon, Ann S.: "Body Mechanics in Pregnancy: Nursing Responsibilities," *Pub. Health Nursing,* **42**:595–601, (Nov.) 1950.

Maternity Center Association: "Flint's Prepared Parents," *Briefs,* **16**:4–7, (Dec.) 1952.

———: "Reminder Sheets for Exercises in Preparation for Childbearing." The Association, New York, 1953.

———: "Pert and Pretty," *Briefs,* **18**:15–16, (Nov.) 1954.

———: "Protective Proteins," *Briefs,* **19**:14–16, (Apr.) 1955.

———: "Hemoglobin—A Key to Healthful Childbearing," *Briefs,* **19**:11–12, (Nov.) 1955.

Newton, Niles: *Maternal Emotions.* Paul B. Hoeber, Inc., New York, 1955.

*Prenatal Care,* Children's Bureau Publication No. 4. U.S. Government Printing Office, Washington, D.C., 1949.

Prenatal Education Committee: *A Guide for Teachers of Prenatal Classes.* Welfare Council, Toronto, Canada, 1948.

Proudfit, Fairfax T., and Robinson, Corinne H.: *Nutrition and Diet Therapy,* 11th ed. The Macmillan Company, New York, 1955.

Read, Grantly D.: *Childbirth without Fear,* 2nd ed. Harper & Brothers, New York, 1953.

Stevenson, Jessie L.: *Posture and Nursing,* 2nd ed. Joint Orthopedic Nursing Advisory Service, New York, 1948.

Thoms, Herbert: *Training for Childbirth.* McGraw-Hill Book Co., New York, 1950.

Thoms, Herbert; Roth, Laurence G.; and Linton, David: *Understanding Natural Childbirth.* McGraw-Hill Book Co., New York, 1950.

Wiedenbach, Ernestine: "Childbirth As Mothers Say They Like It," *Pub. Health Nursing,* **41**:417–21, (Aug.) 1949.

Wisconsin State Board of Health: *Nurses' Teaching Outline for Parents' Classes.* Bureau of Maternal and Child Health, State Board of Health, Madison, Wisconsin, 1950.

———: *Booklist for Expectant Parents.* Bureau of Maternal and Child Health, State Board of Health, Madison, Wisconsin, 1952.

———: *Exercises for Natural Childbirth.* Bureau of Maternal and Child Health, State Board of Health, Madison, Wisconsin, 1955.

Woodward, H. L.; Gardner, B.; Bryant, R. D.; and Overland, Anna E.: *Obstetric Management and Nursing,* 5th ed. F. A. Davis Co., Philadelphia, 1955.

Zabriskie, Louise, and Eastman, Nicholson J.: *Nurses Handbook of Obstetrics,* 9th ed. J. B. Lippincott Co., Philadelphia, 1952.

*Chapter 7*

# Mental Hygiene of the Expectant Mother

It may be only once in a long time that the obstetric nurse has a patient who is suffering from such a marked mental disturbance that her condition is diagnosed and treated as a psychosis. But not infrequently the nurse may find she has a patient who is secretly suffering a good deal of mental stress, which also needs to be recognized and treated. In fact, by virtue of the deep significance of the states of pregnancy and motherhood, and the long period of time through which they continue, it is scarcely possible for these experiences not to produce an emotional effect of some sort upon the average woman.

The effect of expectant and actual motherhood upon the individual patient will be dependent upon her character or temperament, her previous mental or emotional habits in meeting good or ill fortune, and the circumstances or conditions of her life that may be affected by the presence of a baby. Sometimes the effect produced by expectant motherhood is a very happy one and sometimes it is quite the reverse. But whether the patient is simply unhappy or is mentally very ill, the nurse's helpfulness will be greater if she has at least some understanding of the cause and character of these mental sufferings.

In the ordinary course of events from birth to death, we are all called upon to adjust ourselves to many different experiences. There are the situations and emotional strains peculiar, first, to early childhood, then to school days; to the period of emancipation from home; for some the responsibility of a life work and, finally, for others there is the adjustment to marriage and childbearing. As we progress through life we develop habits of meeting success, achievement, sorrow, or the disappointments that come; the anxiety or criticism, failure, illness, or poverty. Some individuals habitually face the issues of life, whether large or small, and habitually overcome difficulties for themselves and for other people. Many influences have combined to develop this fortunate type of person; a good inheritance, intelligence, wise training, early implantation of a sense of responsibility and obligation to society. Such persons are described by the psychiatrists as being grown up or psychologically mature.

Others follow the course of least resistance—never face their problems; are thoughtless and inconsiderate in their demands; live from day to day, instead of consciously working out a plan of life; are unable to make decisions and accordingly rely upon the mental and moral strength of others. Such people are referred to as being infantile, or psychologically immature. They are not unlike the baby who gains his end by the unreasoning method of screaming and pounding upon his high chair with a spoon. He is scarcely more irresponsible than the hysterical adult who gains her point by developing a headache, who faints or flies into a rage. Such people make little or poor adjustment to unsatisfactory conditions and have small capacity for endurance or sacrifice.

With not a few women this poor capacity is a result of lifelong indulgence or protection by unwise parents. They never reason out the question of obligation or responsibility because they have never been required to do so.

In the ordinary walks of life such people, instead of squarely facing their problems in an attempt to reach a solution, try to run from them. They try to forget the existence of complications through diversion or change of scene; they may deny the existence of them to protect their own pride or ego from injury. Some persons habitually meet each problem with a hopeless attitude, feel swamped or inadequate or, from the start, are so convinced of failure that effort does not seem worth while. Many others have the familiar reaction of feeling sorry for themselves and show resentment toward fate, or the other fellow, whom they blame for their own lack of achievement. By such means they justify their own failure in meeting the demands made by life.

There are others who cherish trouble in order to win sympathy, make difficulty where there need be none, and steadfastly refuse to acknowledge good fortune or see the silver lining.

Between these extreme types of very mature and immature individuals are ranged people who display innumerable shadings and degrees of psychologic development. Some cope satisfactorily with their life situation because they are so protected that the demands upon them are not great or because the problems are not beyond their capacity for adjustment. Others need a little bolstering up now and then to bridge over the gap between the demands made upon them and their ability to meet these demands. Still others have to be literally carried when disaster overtakes them or they break under the strain.

As might be expected, our ability to stand the big tests or strains that may come to us, our manner of meeting them and their effect upon us, depends very largely upon how we have ordinarily met the lesser trials that have previously come to us. That is, how we have habitually adjusted ourselves to the experiences of life. For, after all, the test of life is a measure of one's capacity for adaptation to these experiences and surroundings.

The test that measures our ability to adapt ourselves may be one big stroke or it may be a long-drawn-out trial which would be of small consequence were it of short duration. It is the persistency and the monotony of a lesser care that so often wears away the rock of our endurance.

If an adjustment required to meet one of life's situations proves to be too much for our adaptive capacity, and we break down under it, our manner of breaking will be characteristic of us or an accentuation of what might have been called our bendings under lesser difficulties in the past.

The expectant mother is no exception to these general principles, since maternity patients are women from every walk of life and have the same joys and sorrows, problems and difficulties, that all women may have. Added to the ordinary conditions of their lives is the experience of preparing for the expected baby and later of fitting that baby into their everyday existence.

Every influence or circumstance that affects the patient's life in the ordinary march of events, whether it is favorable or unfavorable, will have an effect upon her pregnancy and motherhood. Sometimes the anticipated motherhood will increase her happiness and sense of security; on the other hand, it may accentuate already existing problems or even create new difficulties.

The maternity patient, then, is just an average individual already coping with the usual demands of life, who is now confronted with a new and very real situation; a situation that will affect or be affected by, in one way or another, every aspect of her existence—mental, physical, and social. She does not develop nervous breakdowns either more or less frequently than the nonpregnant woman who is under an equal strain. She is merely a human being whose adaptive capacity is being tested. But the test is severe, because there is, perhaps, no greater demand upon the adaptive capacity of a human being than that to which a woman is subjected during pregnancy, delivery, and the months directly following the birth of a child.

It is entirely reasonable that the expectant mother should do much thinking about the effect the baby may have upon the various aspects of her life. She may expect it to create a stronger bond between her husband and herself and thus give her a greater sense of security. Or she may fear that the baby may come between them and excite jealousy. She may resent the idea of being burdened by caring for the baby and having her freedom curtailed. There may be justifiable fear that the baby will have a bad inheritance or an utterly unjustifiable one that the baby will be "marked." There may be anxiety over the added financial strain to be imposed by the baby, and, if there are other children, the mother may be worried by their attitude toward the coming of the baby.

Pregnancy of itself does not affect the brain or mind any more than, for example, it affects the kidneys. The individual has various kinds of mental symptoms or a mental illness if the burden of pregnancy is greater than she can cope with just as the function of the kidneys may be impaired in pregnancy.

It is now generally believed that there is no mental illness which is typical of pregnancy, but that during pregnancy one may see mental disturbances of varying types or severity. The mental symptoms are indications of burdens or conflicts which the patient has been unable to handle satisfactorily. The outward manifestations or evidences of difficulties may appear as restlessness, nervousness, irritability, suspiciousness, or as neurotic vomiting with or without queer food fads; as preoccupations or as undue concern about personal health with various fears and anxiety states; as depression, when the patient weeps, eats little, and has disturbed sleep. Or she may show just the opposite to depression—feel overstimulated, talk too much, and become excited and difficult to manage. She may get to the point of refusing to eat or speak; she may grimace, take queer postures, or show other odd behavior—such signs are indications of an illness of a profound and serious nature.

Aside from the delirium-like experiences sometimes associated with the toxemias of pregnancy, none of the above-mentioned conditions are referable to any disturbance of the physiologic or metabolic functioning of the patient so far as science has yet been able to demonstrate. They are merely accentuations of poor habits of adjustment to difficulties which the patient has shown all her life or evidences of some conflict of which the patient herself may not be aware. Mental disturbances of such severity require skillful handling, but in these cases the nurse will be under the direction of a physician.

Not infrequently the nurse may meet the intangible, undiagnosed conditions which manifest themselves only in fears, worry, or conflicting desires, and she must realize that they may exert an important influence upon the general well-being of the patient during the months of pregnancy and early motherhood. The indications of conflicts or worry may first appear in the attitude of the expectant mother toward the coming of the baby. Its coming is the origin of the patient's happiness or unhappiness. Her attitude in turn is dependent upon what effect she believes the baby will have upon the aspects of her life which are most important to her.

Here it may be helpful to discuss briefly the meaning of "conflict" and the "mechanism" which produces it. As a starting point there must be a recognition of the fact that the deepest and most influential feminine instinct is maternal—the desire to have and care for a child. It is primal. It has been in women since the dawn of Creation and, although in many women it is put down, stifled, or complicated by other desires, it cannot be destroyed. Not a few women deny this instinct, but back of their denial is some reason, conscious or unconscious, which is not harmonious with the idea of motherhood. The woman may be selfish, for example; she may be vain and not want to lose her grace and charm through pregnancy for fear of losing her husband if she becomes less attractive. She may not see the way financially clear to rearing a child or she may set such a standard for motherhood that she is sincerely afraid of being unable to give the child all she believes it should have.

When some such feeling is strong it conflicts with the deeper one of maternalism, and there is a lack of harmony or a "conflict." It is just that—a conflict or struggle between two emotions, and the result is a state of mental unrest. A homely comparison might be found in the digestive disturbance which may follow an effort to cope with food which the patient ordinarily finds difficult to digest. She may have nausea, vomiting, pain, or even more severe symptoms. The severity of the symptoms and their effect upon the patient depend somewhat upon the average vigor or stability ordinarily displayed by the digestive tract under a lesser strain. People with so-called delicate digestions may be greatly upset by certain kinds of food which others are able to digest and so suffer little or no inconvenience.

When a mature individual has a desire which results from our culture or civilization (a wish to preserve her grace or her luxuries, for example) that is in conflict with a deeper primal instinct, she will often be able to reason out the situation, and in the case of approaching motherhood, decide that the baby is worth any sacrifice, any inconvenience, and go joyfully through her period of expectancy. She will glory in the consciousness of her ability to realize the supreme purpose of a woman's creation. In other words, she adjusts herself to the situation, harmonizes the discordant desires, and is mentally undisturbed.

A less mature woman, like a person with a delicate, easily upset digestive tract, will have difficulty in making an adjustment—in harmonizing her instinctive desire for motherhood and her acquired desire for comfort, attention, and the things demanded by convention.

Belief in the overwhelming strength of maternal instinct is so general that society at large takes it for granted every expectant mother wants her baby. This attitude often makes it difficult for a woman to acknowledge, even to herself, a lack of eagerness which may come from anxiety over poor inheritance or from worry over finances which makes her feel unequal to meeting the strain of a first or another pregnancy. This conflict between what she knows is expected of her and her own misgivings may be violent enough to upset her greatly and produce some of the nervous and mental disturbances previously mentioned. This is particularly true if the demands of our cultural state make it necessary for the patient to keep this turmoil below the surface, with no safety valve to relieve the pressure.

This problem of the expectant mother's attitude toward the coming of the baby is very general and varied as well. The mothers of families already large and poverty-stricken are often quite frank in expressing their dismay over the expected birth and lament the prospect of this extra burden. They do not feel the necessity for concealing their feelings or do not "repress" them and sometimes derive relief from being candid. But this is not always the case, since some women grow increasingly anxious over the prospect of stretching an already inadequate income to meet the needs of a family soon to be enlarged. Another real anxiety that gnaws steadily and deeply is uncertainty as to who will keep the home together, look after the husband and perhaps other children while the patient enters the hospital for the birth of the baby. The effect of such anxieties may be seen in sleeplessness, crying spells, depression, and the like.

The mothers of the middle and upper classes are often surrounded by an atmosphere of conventional codes that are stifling to mental honesty. Accordingly, they are less genuine in expressing their true attitude toward the coming child. To some of them—the selfish, self-centered type—the new baby will bring inconvenience rather than hardship, or to the overly conscientious or timid it will mean worry. The importance of their ego may be dimmed. There may be a cutting down of luxuries and of freedom for social activities and increased responsibility with closer confinement to the home. While they give utterance to joy and pleasure over the prospect of having a baby, this does not quite reflect their inmost feelings.

Not a few women find an outlet for the tension caused by their conflict by being fretful and irritable or through conduct which they would have displayed if annoyed or chagrined about something other than the approaching birth of a child. Because of this outlet they are not so likely to break down.

It is by no means the role of the nurse to pry into the affairs of her patients, but she can often become a source of help to a patient suffering from emotional conflict. For one of the most helpful things that such a person can do is to talk and little by little bring out and put into words the buried thoughts, fears, or shame that may be causing the conflict. Very often the listener will say surprisingly little and will express no definite opinions, but by a sympathetic, responsive attitude, free from any tendency to judge or criticize, will encourage the worried person to share her anxieties.

Here it is of grave importance to stress that the nurse observe the strictest ethical attitude toward her patient's confidences. Nothing that the patient discloses or suggests should be repeated to any one but the physician. Reports upon the patient's fears and anxieties should be made to the doctor in the same spirit as reports upon temperature or blood pressure. They are to aid the doctor in forming a clear picture of the patient's condition in order that he may treat her effectively.

It is of the utmost importance not only that the nurse cultivate toward her patient a manner that is sympathetic and understanding but actually to feel these things in her heart. While we may not admire the spoiled, selfish, uncontrolled person we must in fairness remember that she is usually the product of her training, environment, and inheritance. Accordingly, she merits help and understanding rather than condemnation. On no account should the nurse discuss either her patient's mental or physical symptoms, or those of other women, in her patient's hearing. Such discussions are very likely to be misunderstood and give the patient ample food for worry.

Another source of unrest in the mind of the expectant mother, especially during her first pregnancy, is the fear of complications, and even death, in labor. She is reluctant to speak of these things to her husband, family, or friends, lest she appear to lack courage or seem a coward at the prospect of pain. Or she may be unwilling to distress those who love her by admitting her fear. It does no good to say to a frightened woman, "Don't worry." But it may help to ask, "What is it that worries you?" and explain frankly that it is normal and natural for one to have some anxiety about any important change to take place in one's life and that such anxiety is not an evidence of cowardice.

Fear of death and disease are very common traits among people in general, and equally common is the hesitance we all have in acknowledging them. And so the patient keeps these things to herself and turns them over and over in her mind; buries them and tries to put them out of her thoughts. But they stick. Her fear and her dread color everything that she hears, and very often and unwittingly her friends and relatives make matters worse by recounting the unhappy experiences of other mothers that they have known. At the same time these communicative friends do not tell of the immeasurably greater number of women who have come through labor safely, nor does the patient dwell upon these in her mind. She remembers the women who had convulsions, or fever, or a hemorrhage, or the one who died.

Such fears may account for the behavior of some patients during labor who show excitability and distress that amount to little less than frenzy.

The nurse who sees the human being beyond the obstetric case will appreciate the pain which such a conflict causes and by being sympathetic and responsive will try to make it easy for her patient to talk it over. The patient should invariably find her nurse ready to listen and to give assurances of the proved value of the precautions that are being taken to safeguard her and her baby. For not a few women are harassed, not alone by fear that things will go wrong with themselves, but with fear that harm may come to the baby.

Other women are upset because of a habitual inability to make decisions that will bring marked changes in their lives. They find it difficult to accept pregnancy because its consummation will definitely alter their state. Life may prove to be more satisfactory because of the baby, or it may be less so. But in any event it cannot be the same, and they dread making the irrevocable change.

Still another cause of distress is a concern over the possibility of hereditary influence. There may be a family member who is physically deformed, feeble-minded, epileptic, or who has died in a sanitarium or hospital for the mentally ill. The fear that the child may "strike back" to one of these individuals, and be disfigured or suffer mental retardation, may amount to little less than an obsession.

The nurse may often dispel such an anxiety by drawing upon even her slender knowledge of embryology and reassure the patient by explaining erroneous ideas about heredity and pointing out that environment and early training are such important determining factors that a child is more likely to be affected by the example and guidance of his parents during his first few years than by transmission of characteristics.

Attempted abortions during the early months of pregnancy will cause a great deal of mental anguish. Of their effect upon the offspring we know very little. We do know, however, that an unsuccessful attempt to produce an abortion often gives rise to a good deal of secret worry on the part of the expectant mother. It may then be the nucleus of a vague depression during pregnancy, not only because of remorse over wrongdoing, but also because of fear that the child who is coming, in spite of the attempt to destroy him, may pay for the offense by bearing physical marks or mental deficiency. This is another of the anxieties which the patient can seldom bring herself to discuss with her family or even with her physician. But it so occupies her mind that she may allude to it, in a roundabout way, to the nurse whom she sees frequently, as though describing the act of a friend. The nurse who reads between the lines may often relieve a serious tension caused in this way by discussing the matter impersonally. She must give the patient an opportunity to talk and needs to reassure and encourage her to the best of her ability.

Another real cause of worry during pregnancy is the patient's fear that she may not have normal maternal instinct or ability to satisfactorily care for and rear a child. The idea of assuming the physical care and the moral guidance of another human being is often little less than terrifying to a young woman whose responsibilities in the past have been shared or carried by someone else; or to the one who has gone through life hunting for and exaggerating the difficulties in a situation before attempting to meet it; and perhaps to the one who is habitually conscientious in all her relations with other people.

Still another type, and one which presents a much simpler situation, is the expectant or young mother who is scarcely suffering from a mental illness but has a little letdown in her customary poise and self-control, such as we so often see in convalescents and chronic invalids.

Pregnancy, labor, and the puerperium are normal physiologic processes, it is true, but they impose a physical tax. The patient is likely to be very tired during and after labor and may show the same sensitiveness or irritability that any of us show when tired and exhausted. Accordingly, she will merit considerable forbearance on the part of those who surround her.

But when we understand, even faintly, the conflicts which are possible in the mental life of the expectant mother—the incompatibility of her basic maternal instinct and the desires and demands born of our culture and civilization—it is not difficult to see that her adaptive capacity may be sorely tested.

It is well to remember that as individuals we all have different endowments with which to meet the stress and strain of life. The factors which enter into this endowment are constitutional (those we are born with), intellectual, and emotional. It is the caliber of these qualities that determines our adaptive capacity to face our problems and live our lives successfully. It is quite as illogical to expect a man with a weak back to carry a heavy load as it is to expect an individual with poor personality equipment to carry taxing mental burdens without bending or breaking. However, adjustments may be made between the man's heavy load and his inadequate back, perhaps by lightening the load or giving support where he is weak. The same reasoning applies to those unhappy individuals who are coping with difficulties beyond their capacity for adjustment.

It is hoped the nurse may understand from this discussion that the conflicting thoughts which her patient does not express, but buries and keeps below the surface of her mind, are the factors that work harm in her mental or emotional life. If the nurse can persuade her patient to share these thoughts, they will be robbed of much of their power to injure. But this patient, like anyone else, will talk freely only when she talks spontaneously and she will do this only when she senses in her nurse a sympathetic understanding and a sincere desire to be of service. Accordingly, the nurse should always be sensitive to the mood changes of her patient and be alert to recognize, from chance remarks, evidence of secret worries which may be working harm. The nurse will be successful only insofar as she is aware that in each patient the situation and problems are different and that all patients will not respond to the same method of approach.

The foregoing discussion is not meant to suggest that the relief of a patient by means of mental catharsis is necessarily a nurse's function. It is simply that a patient suffering from a conflict is likely to derive a certain amount of relief from talking with someone who understands why she is troubled and above all will not ridicule or criticize her. By virtue of the many hours sometimes spent together by the nurse and patient, the nurse very often happens to be that some one. More than this, the nurse may in such a case be able to give the doctor very valuable information about her patient's mental or emotional state which otherwise might not be revealed. People do not ordinarily find it easy to lay bare their inmost thoughts before the members of their family, and the patient may not discuss her conflict with her physician, which of course is the ideal, since her visits with him are relatively short and do not favor the ambling, desultory conversation into which the nurse and patient may so easily drift. On the other hand, the nurse must not look for trouble in order to be useful or suggest to her patient that it is a common practice among expectant mothers to worry, be fearful, or alarmed, but if the patient displays these emotions the nurse must be ready with tact and common sense to talk over the problems in a normal unprejudiced manner.

The positive course which the nurse may take is to be unfailingly hopeful. Normal, wholesome enthusiasm is extremely infectious. The nurse's genuine pleasure in the coming baby will often lessen in the expectant mother the fatigue and boredom of her pregnancy as well as dread of the delivery and make her more aware of her own real feelings about the child who is soon to be born.

All of the pleas for a tolerant, understanding attitude toward the rank and file of worried or upset expectant mothers are made with particular force in connection with the unmarried patient. Her problem, both to herself and to society, is too complicated to be dealt with adequately as a part of one short chapter. We must bear in mind, however, that reasons for the conflict which may be suffered by any expectant mother are inevitably more pressing in the case of an unmarried woman, and, in addition, she confronts other almost insurmountable difficulties. The nurse's province in all circumstances is to work for the emotional and physical welfare of her patient. It is not within her province to judge, criticize, or condemn. To be helpful the nurse's attitude must spring from an honest desire to see the situation from the patient's standpoint and be sympathetic, understanding, and unfailingly courteous.

To sum it all up: The expectant mother who habitually has not made satisfactory adjustments during her life may be bending under a mental or emotional burden that is heavier than her slender, emotionally immature powers can bear. The nurse's part is to recognize this possibility and realize that, while she cannot attempt to correct the difficulty, she may give the patient hope and courage simply by being optimistic and reassuring.

She may greatly aid the doctor, and thus serve the patient, by appreciating the importance of recognizing and reporting evidences of mental stress. As a result of this awareness it may be that some patient struggling with an emotional conflict will be saved much suffering and even illness because of her nurse's sympathetic insight and understanding.

## BIBLIOGRAPHY AND STUDENT REFERENCES

Blake, Florence G.: *The Child, His Parents and the Nurse.* J. B. Lippincott Co., Philadelphia, 1954.

Bookmiller, Mae M., and Bowen, George L.: *Textbook of Obstetrics and Obstetric Nursing,* 2nd ed. W. B. Saunders Co., Philadelphia, 1954.

Caplan, Gerald: "The Mental Hygiene Role of the Nurse in Maternal and Child Health," *Nursing Outlook,* **2**:14–19, (Jan.) 1954.

———: "Preparation for Healthy Parenthood," *Children,* **1**:171–75, (Sept.–Oct.) 1954.

Chisholm, Rita: "Parents' Classes: A Fertile Field for Mental Health Concepts," *Pub. Health Nursing,* **44**:273–75, (May) 1952.

Cooley, Carol H.: *Social Aspects of Illness.* W. B. Saunders Co., Philadelphia, 1951, pp. 255–73.

Corbin, Hazel: "Emotional Aspects of Maternity Care," *Am. J. Nursing,* **48**:20–22, (Jan.) 1948.

Davis, M. Edward, and Sheckler, Catherine E.: *DeLee's Obstetrics for Nurses,* 15th ed. W. B. Saunders Co., Philadelphia, 1951.

Deutsch, Helen: *The Psychology of Women,* Vol. II. Grune & Stratton, New York, 1945.

Lesser, Marion S., and Keane, Vera R.: *Nurse–Patient Relationships in a Hospital Maternity Service.* C. V. Mosby Co., St. Louis, 1956.

Newton, Niles: *Maternal Emotions.* Paul B. Hoeber, Inc., New York, 1955.

Straus, Barbara: "Mental Hygiene in Pregnancy," *Am. J. Nursing,* **56**:314–16, (Mar.) 1956.

Thompson, Lloyd J.; Barber, Marion; and Woestendiek, Josephine: "Mothers' Classes for Physical and Emotional Health," *Pub. Health Nursing,* **41**:427–31, (Aug.) 1949.

Thompson, Lloyd J., and Lowe, Marie: "Mental Health and Mothers' Classes," *Pub. Health Nursing,* **43**:151–53, (Mar.) 1951.

Walser, Howard: "Education for Parenthood," *Am. J. Nursing,* **52**:566–68, (May) 1952.

Woodward, H. L.; Gardner, B.; Bryant, R. D.; and Overland, Anna E.: *Obstetric Management and Nursing,* 5th ed. F. A. Davis Co., Philadelphia, 1955.

Wooten, Betsy G.: "A Psychosomatic Approach to Maternity Care," *Pub. Health Nursing,* **44**:493–99, (Sept.) 1952.

Zabriskie, Louise, and Eastman, Nicholson J.: *Nurses Handbook of Obstetrics,* 9th ed. J. B. Lippincott Co., Philadelphia, 1952.

Zimmerman, Kent A.: "The Public Health Nurse and the Emotions of Pregnancy," *Pub. Health Nursing,* **39**:63–67, (Feb.) 1947.

## *Chapter 8*

# Some Special Problems of the Maternity Patient

One delightful aspect of maternity nursing is the breadth and richness of its scope. Everything that the nurse knows about people, about life in general, as well as her knowledge of obstetric nursing, comes into use.

One realizes very early that a large part of maternity care involves problems that arise from the simple, homely, human needs that form a part of everyone's life. For expectant mothers do not constitute a class apart—that is, they are not all alike and as a group essentially different from other people, sick or well.

Although pregnancy is not regarded as an illness, it brings with it many of the same practical and financial problems that illness entails. It is recognized, nowadays, that in any illness the patient's mental and emotional life, as well as the financial and domestic aspects, has a definite bearing upon her physical condition. Accordingly, an important profession, medical social service, has developed as an indispensable adjunct to all branches of medical practice.

Social service was inaugurated in the United States in 1905 by Dr. Richard Cabot, who stated the patient's "real trouble is understandable and helpable only when you know:

"1. his bodily state (medical diagnosis and especially prognosis);

"2. his mental state;

"3. his bodily environment (work, wages, food, clothing, housing, etc.);

"4. his mental environment—the influence (good or bad) of his family, friends, enemies, neutral companions." *

This attitude opens up broad vistas in maternity nursing indicating as it does that care is complete and efficacious only when it is related to the patient's physical condition, her mental state, and her environment. Her environment includes the home she lives in, her financial status, and the attitude of the people who make up her household or in any way touch her life.

The patient's problems may be varied and complex. Obviously the nurse cannot solve problems alone, but requires the assistance of others. Needs are discussed here because the nurse can often contribute to the discovery of problems and can assist in directing them to the individuals best able to aid in their solution. As the nurse has undoubtedly seen for herself, effective care of the patient may be made impossible by the existence of certain very homely practical difficulties. If the patient's physical condition demands rest, for example, it is pointless to advise her to stay in bed if her anxieties are too great to make rest possible or if she is the only one to do the marketing, cooking, housework, and washing for the family or if her living conditions are such that she has no place in which to rest satisfactorily.

The nurse's part, primarily, is to be aware always of the fact that each patient may be affected by many influential factors in addition to those of an obstetric nature. Having this awareness of possible complicating conditions, she should try to sense or discover their existence in the life of each of her patients. Here the nurse will have to be very careful. Her success in this respect will be dependent upon her own sensitiveness and insight, her love of people, her sympathy and ability to project herself into the lives of other people because she cares. Her experience with life, her capacity for inspiring trust and confidence, and perhaps above all her innate courtesy in all human contacts—these, more than technical training—will help her to discover her patient's problems. At the same time they will deter her from wounding or affronting her patient by asking tactless or unintentionally impertinent questions. If the nurse is consistently kind and courteous she will by degrees, with little or no questioning, learn the important things to be known about the patient.

Following is a brief discussion of some nonmedical factors that may

* Ninth Annual Report, Social Service Department, Massachusetts General Hospital, 1914; quoted in *On the Social Frontier of Medicine* by Ida Maud Cannon (Harvard University Press, Cambridge, 1952, p. 96).

have a bearing upon the patient's welfare and other family members.

**The Patient's Attitude.** First, perhaps, is the patient's own attitude. Is she obviously happy over the pregnancy or does she resent it for any one of many reasons? Possibly she fears that pregnancy and subsequent motherhood may interfere with her usual pleasures and activities. She may be afraid of losing her husband's affection because of physical unattractiveness and also because of the demands the baby later will make upon her attention. She may feel bitterly toward her husband, and as a result develop hatred or jealousy toward the expected baby. The patient may suffer a sense of guilt because of having wished for or attempted an abortion. She may be afraid of financial inability to give her baby proper care. She may fear a poor inheritance or may dread and fear childbearing because of difficulties she herself has suffered during previous pregnancies or those she has heard of in connection with other women. If the patient experiences fear or resentment because of her condition and is not given relief or guidance, she may not only be unhappy but may become emotionally or mentally ill.

**The Influence of Family Relationship.** Many patients are so happy and satisfied in their married life that there is little or no mental stress or strain. If the husband is happy over the pregnancy, he is likely to be helpful and understanding in his attitude. In some cases the situation is very different, and the patient's unhappy frame of mind is a reflection of the husband's attitude toward her and her pregnancy and serious difficulties that present themselves. Little disagreements, friction, misunderstandings, ordinarily unimportant, may assume serious proportions during pregnancy because of dissatisfaction on the part of either wife or husband. The more worried or irritable either one becomes, the more tense the entire situation. If relations between husband and wife are a little unstable, sometimes he grows less interested and cooperative because she had grown careless about her personal appearance or, through discouragement or fatigue, neglects the home or the meals. If the nurse senses this and encourages the patient to take more pains with her appearance or is able to secure even a little help with the homemaking, it may greatly improve the husband's attitude.

In studying the causes of desertion it is found that in a certain proportion of cases the men desert their wives before delivery and return after the baby is born. The fear of this may give the patient a destructive sense of insecurity. Sometimes the husband is so dependent upon his own mother, as a result of lifelong habit, that he is not a strong support to his wife throughout the pregnancy. Sometimes the patient's dependence upon her own mother gives rise to strain and tension. On the other hand, both these mothers may be very helpful by their attitude toward the coming grandchild. The presence of a congenial woman relative or friend in the house before and after the baby's birth may literally be a lifesaver as will be explained presently. If the patient already has children they should be prepared for the new baby's arrival so that there will be little jealousy on their part. If changes in sleeping arrangements are necessary they should be made a few weeks before delivery. This is particularly important if a child is sleeping in his mother's room and has to give up his bed for the new baby. Other children should be prepared before the baby's birth and with great care, because if it is brought home unexpectedly, an older sibling may be deeply wounded and feel that he is being crowded out of his mother's affections. Complete harmony in the family group is important to each of its members.

**Living Conditions.** It may be that even if the patient lives in very small quarters she will have matters so arranged that she is able to rest and sleep as she should. But the nurse will sometimes find such crowding of family, relatives, or boarders that it is impossible for a patient requiring only normal care to get adequate rest.

If the patient and her husband live in a furnished room, live with relatives, or eat in a restaurant the question of obtaining adequate meals may be quite as difficult as adequate rest.

Lack of conveniences in the home, too many stairs to climb, the necessity to wash, iron, scrub, clean, and market may make everyday living very difficult for the patient to endure. Moreover, if the patient shares a home with other people, relatives, friends or otherwise, there may be enough friction or conflict of personalities to make even a moderately peaceful existence impossible.

**The Patient's Sense of Security.** Every human being carries throughout life a sense of being alone and of fearing it. There is, too, a universal longing for peace and security, and in the maternity patient this is likely to be accentuated since she now has not alone her own needs but those of another human being to consider. Probably the most influential, far-reaching factors affecting the patient's sense of security are her relations with her husband and her financial status. Reference has been made to some of the things which may disturb the husband. Another strain that may be as hard on him as upon the patient is financial anxiety. If the husband has work and there is enough money to provide satisfactory living quarters, domestic service if needed, food and clothes, and to meet the added expense of the coming confinement and the baby's needs, many mental and physical problems will be averted. A lack of money, on the other hand, may create tension, friction, and difficulties that otherwise might not exist. Inability to pay for care may keep the mother from seeking it or from being able to follow instructions that are given.

An increasing number of families now have hospital and medical care insurance, such as that offered by Blue Cross and Blue Shield and many life insurance companies. Industries usually arrange for group-plan health insurance for employees, and the families of employees may usually be included in the insurance benefits for an additional fee. However, in spite of the increasing number of families that have provision for health insurance there are still many others that do not have this plan to aid in the payment of hospital and medical care costs. Not infrequently these families are in the low-income bracket and thus find it impossible to meet the cost of illness.

There are two general groups of financial resources, personal and community. The patient and her husband may be able to raise the needed money through their relatives, church, insurance companies, lodges, or employers. Or assistance may be secured, for families without funds, by the discriminating use of community resources such as family agencies and city relief agencies. Relieving financial anxieties is almost a panacea because a formidable array of difficulties may arise from this one cause.

**Illegitimate Pregnancy.** This is one of the saddest and most difficult situations the nurse will meet. She may take it for granted at the outset that both she and the patient will need assistance, not alone in meeting the immediate situation but also in making the wisest plans for the future of mother and baby. All the mental, physical, and social problems that may confront married women are equally present in the life of an unmarried patient. These are accentuated by the anomaly and insecurity of her position and, added to them, are often the overwhelming problems of a long uncertain future. The patient's attitude toward the situation, and her desire, her ability, or her unwillingness and inability to face her responsibilities are likely to indicate the best course to follow in the interest of both mother and baby.

Sometimes the child's father is willing to marry the patient, and thus many questions are solved. He may be willing to provide part or complete financial support though unwilling to marry. The patient's parents or other relatives or friends may give her financial and moral support. Sometimes they cannot offer either. And so it often happens that the unmarried expectant mother stands alone both as to the present and future problems. Whether the mother shall face society openly and keep and rear her own child, whether she and the father shall singly or jointly support the child in a foster home, or whether the mother shall give up the child permanently and completely—all are questions freighted with importance.

The entire future of two human beings is likely to be shaped by the wisdom and soundness of guidance given at this time. The nurse must not look backward and pronounce judgment; she must consider the future only, and seek aid to make plans to serve the best interests of both mother and baby throughout their lives.

The nurse must, therefore, be familiar with the agencies that are set up to give help and guidance to the unmarried mother, or at least know where to obtain this information, and either she or the doctor must make early referral to them. Thus the doctor, the nurse, and the social worker can cooperate in helping the patient.

In the best interests of mother and baby these problems must never be settled hastily. These agencies, however, all have social workers who are prepared to give excellent advice and assistance to the girl and her family in making a decision as to the best care for both mother and baby, plans that will be most desirable for all concerned.

Decisions may have to be made quite early in regards to whether the girl will continue to live in her home and community or move to another, whether or not she shall continue to work, and who will carry the financial burden. Sometimes a maternity home, where the girl can stay during the prenatal period and until after delivery and until plans have been made for the baby, may be the best solution.

Placing the baby for adoption seems to be the wisest course in most instances for both the baby and his mother, since the mother will have difficulty in assuming the responsibilities of parenthood and in facing the community's usual disapproval. The decision must, however, rest with the mother and this must be made without pressure. If the baby is placed for adoption it can usually be cared for in a foster home, or at least a temporary home, as soon as it is ready to leave the hospital, and the girl can be helped to re-establish herself in her community, in school, or at work.

If the baby is born in a hospital the mother can be spared from any contact with her baby which would make it more difficult for her to give him up, and the nurse should do all she can to protect the mother from questions that other mothers, who do not know the circumstances, will normally ask as they have contact with her—questions about the size and sex of the baby, breast feeding, baby clothes, and many others.

When a licensed agency places a baby in a foster home, both the child and the foster parents will be protected, and the mother is spared any personal contact with the baby and with the home in which her baby is placed. If the mother decides to keep her baby she will need much help and guidance with the physical care of her baby, with financial aid, and with long-term planning for herself and her baby. She may need this assistance over a long period of time.

In an effort to protect the illegitimate child some states have very strict laws regulating the reporting of all cases of illegitimate pregnancy to the state welfare department. This report must be made by the hospital, physician, or nurse having contact with the mother. This department then takes the responsibility for giving guidance through its own social workers or through referral to another agency—public, private, or religious organization.

**Needs Arising from Medical Complications.** A patient may be ordered to stay in bed through entire days, weeks, or even months, because of heart disease, tuberculosis, toxemia, or a threatened abortion. In such a case the rest is quite as urgent as medication, and it is part of nursing care to ascertain whether or not the prescribed rest is mentally and physically possible, since only if complete is it likely to accomplish the desired end.

In some instances the patient may safely be up and about during part of the day and even perform certain light household duties, but be forbidden to go marketing or shopping, climb stairs, walk against the wind, to wash and iron, or do anything that tires her.

There are countless reasons why the doctor's carefully thought-out orders of this nature may be utterly pointless unless the patient is given help of one kind or another. Her frame of mind, her domestic situation, the uncomprehending attitude of her family, the housing situation, inadequate finances, any one or all of these influences may operate to defeat the effort to safeguard her welfare. Sometimes a very simple provision will meet the need: a relative or neighbor to do the marketing; or someone to do the laundry work or to give the home a weekly cleaning. Well-meaning husbands and families may make it very difficult for the expectant mother to give herself proper care solely because they do not appreciate its importance and the patient is given the uncomfortable feeling that she is coddling herself.

The nurse may have to arrange to have a long and serious talk with those who exert the greatest influence upon the patient's everyday life. She may have to talk very simply but seriously in order to make the family see that the fate of two human beings may depend upon their understanding and helpful attitude at this time. The husband or children often can and will do the cooking, dishwashing, and bed-making when they realize how injurious to the patient this work may be.

**What to Do.** By virtue of her relation the nurse is in a particularly favorable position to learn about the patient's mental, physical, and social needs. If she has the wisdom to recognize these needs she has taken the first important step toward relieving them. Having recognized the need, the next step, perhaps, is to decide what changes in the patient's affairs would be most helpful. This gives a goal toward which one can work and suggests the kind of assistance the nurse must seek. To be specific: one expectant mother may be the only one to keep a home together—cook, wash, and iron for her husband and children or other relatives. Obligations at home seem insurmountable when this woman must go to the hospital or even stay in bed at home. The desirable change in such a case would be to supply household assistance so that the patient could stay in bed and not worry about work left undone or would not get up and work as soon as she herself felt able to do so. In another case, the patient might be able to stay in bed but be so harassed over money matters that the mere physical inactivity would be a farce. The ideal here would be to help the husband find a job or perhaps secure temporary financial relief from relatives or a welfare agency. Another woman may be so huddled into tiny quarters with other people that adequate rest and relaxation are impossible, and the only satisfactory solution is removal to another home. And so on throughout the entire, long gamut of possible complications including the subtler, less tangible causes of disquietude previously suggested. Having recognized the need and visualized the condition that might correct it, the next steps may be far from simple or easy. Moreover, the condition that needs to be changed may not be the real problem. For example, the undesirable housing situation is probably due to financial needs. Removal to larger quarters will involve the expense of moving and an increase in rent. During the process of moving, the patient must be taken care of elsewhere, since the effort and discomfort that this entails may result in the complications that it is hoped to avert.

These problems of a social nature usually will have to be handled by workers from social agencies who have the experience and facilities to cope with them effectively, but when the services of social agencies are not available it is the nurse's responsibility to guide the patient to other community resources or to make arrangements for care with other members of the family.

In addition to helping the patient through her immediate pressing need it is very important that the helping hand be so wisely extended that it will not encourage the habit of dependence in the patient or her family. It sometimes happens that ready and adequate relief given in one emergency will deter the patient from attempting to face other subsequent crises without assistance.

Accordingly, the nurse's most valuable service to some expectant mothers may be that of obtaining cooperation with a social agency—always, of course, with the knowledge and approval of the doctor.

The general attitude to take is that if assistance is necessary to resolve the patient's problems there is some channel through which it may be obtained and the nurse must find it. It may require a great deal of thought and experience to accomplish the desired ends in the most effective and economic manner. In large cities there is practically every kind of social and relief agency, and the organization with which the nurse is associated will usually have such definite relations of cooperation that she has only to make a report in order to provide for her patient's social needs. In smaller towns and rural districts where social resources are limited or entirely lacking, the nurse may have to exercise no little ingenuity to secure the necessary support. The first time she confronts social problems that make demands beyond her powers, the obstetric nurse may be discouraged to find that the community has no apparent resources to supply these needs. She may be sure, however, that the resources are there although they may be hidden from view. The nurse may have to start by enlisting the aid of a priest or clergyman, a health department, a woman's club, or some responsible philanthropic individual. There is enormous satisfaction in working out a human problem in this personal, individual way. But the nurse should try to see her patient and her problems in their proper perspective and not involve herself so deeply with the social difficulties of one patient that her service to many others will suffer as a result. It is often more effective and more efficient to delegate certain functions to other people than to attempt to discharge them all one's self. Her quest for assistance on behalf of a troubled, expectant mother may be the starting point for a fine, permanent organization for social or relief work. Many organizations and individuals are ready to help if the need and the way are pointed out to them. More than one nurse has started valuable and sustained work by carrying her local problems to the Parent-Teachers Association, the Grange, the Kiwanis or Rotary Club, the Masons or the Elks, or to a hospital that has not previously had a social service department.

The main theme of this entire chapter is to suggest to the obstetric nurse that she must have a sensitive awareness of the simple, homely, personal needs of her patients, and when occasion arises to seek assistance of such a character that the mother and her baby may derive the greatest and most lasting benefits from the medical and nursing service offered on their behalf.

## BIBLIOGRAPHY AND STUDENT REFERENCES

Block, Babette: "The Unmarried Mother," *Pub. Health Nursing,* **43**:375–81, (July) 1951.

Bookmiller, Mae M., and Bowen, George L.: *Textbook of Obstetrics and Obstetric Nursing,* 2nd ed. W. B. Saunders Co., Philadelphia, 1954.

Brower, Bernice R.: "What Shall I Do with My Baby?" *The Child,* **12**:166–69, (Apr.) 1948.

Byrne, Kathryne: "How a Nurse Can Help an Unmarried Mother," *Am. J. Nursing,* **45**:796–98, (Oct.) 1945.

Cooley, Carol H.: "Don't Let the Social Worker's Services Go to Waste," *Mod. Hosp.,* **70**:77–79, (Mar.) 1948.

———: *Social Aspects of Illness.* W. B. Saunders Co., Philadelphia, 1951, pp. 255–73.

Davis, M. Edward, and Sheckler, Catherine E.: *DeLee's Obstetrics for Nurses,* 15th ed. W. B. Saunders Co., Philadelphia, 1951.

Deutsch, Helen: *The Psychology of Women,* Vol. II. Grune & Stratton, New York, 1945.

Donnell, H. Catherine, and Glick, Selma J.: "The Nurse and the Unwed Mother," *Nursing Outlook,* **2**:249–51, (May) 1954.

Doran, Ruth: "The Unmarried Mother," *Bulletin of Maternal Welfare* (American Committee on Maternal Welfare, Inc.), **1**:11–12, (July–Aug.) 1954.

Newton, Niles: *Maternal Emotions.* Paul B. Hoeber, Inc., New York, 1955.

Smillie, Wilson G.: *Preventive Medicine and Public Health,* 2nd ed. The Macmillan Company, New York, 1952.

Spock, Benjamin: *The Common Sense Book of Baby and Child Care.* Duell, Sloan & Pearce, Inc., New York, 1946.

Woodward, H. L.; Gardner, B.; Bryant, R. D.; and Overland, Anna E.: *Obstetric Management and Nursing,* 5th ed. F. A. Davis Co., Philadelphia, 1955.

Zabriskie, Louise, and Eastman, Nicholson J.: *Nurses Handbook of Obstetrics,* 9th ed. J. B. Lippincott Co., Philadelphia, 1952.

*Chapter 9*

# Complications and Accidents of Pregnancy

The prenatal care which was outlined in Chapter 6 becomes more impressive when one considers the disasters which it is designed to prevent. And the nurse will be more eager and able to watch her patient intelligently and instruct her convincingly if she appreciates and understands something of the conditions which she is helping to avert. She will give more effective nursing care, too, when complications do occur, if she gives it understandingly. In the toxemias, particularly, the importance of the nursing care looms large, since painstaking attention to details may make this care a matter of life or death to the patient.

In considering the complications of pregnancy, the nurse needs to be reminded that pregnancy, labor, and the puerperium are normal, physiologic processes and usually run their course unattended by difficulty. These normal processes, however, may easily become abnormal or complicated, and such complications if untreated may be extremely serious. Watchfulness throughout pregnancy, then, in the interest of early recognition and treatment of abnormal conditions, cannot be too insistently urged.

Some complications that are watched for during pregnancy are peculiar to pregnancy alone, among which are the following:

1. *Premature terminations of pregnancy,* which are designated as abortions, or miscarriages, and premature labors;

2. *Extrauterine or ectopic pregnancy;*

3. *Pernicious vomiting of pregnancy;*

4. *Antepartum hemorrhages,* due to either a placenta previa or a premature separation of a normally implanted placenta;

5. *The toxemias,* including pre-eclampsia, eclampsia, and chronic hypertensive disease. This last condition is not, of course, invariably associated with pregnancy.

There are other conditions not necessarily inherent in the state of pregnancy, but which should be detected and treated early, since their presence coincidently with expectant motherhood may threaten the safety of the patient or the child, or both. Probably the most serious of these possible accompanying disabilities are heart disease, diabetes, tuberculosis, pyelonephritis, syphilis, gonorrhea, and the acute infectious diseases.

Any chronic organic disease is likely to be increased in severity by the strain which pregnancy puts upon the impaired organs, in common with the rest of the maternal body. Acute diseases usually run about the same course in pregnancy, as in nonpregnant women, except when an infection causes an abortion, the stress of which, in turn, reduces the patient's resistance against the complicating disease.

As we consider these various, dreaded complications which may arise during pregnancy, infrequent though they be, we feel that no amount of effort is too much to make, if we can, thereby, save one mother or one baby from their destructive effects. We are stirred by the urgency of preventing a premature ending of pregnancy, for example, when we see it, not so much as simply another obstetric emergency, but in its true, tragic light as the loss of an infant's life and the bereavement of an expectant mother.

## PREMATURE TERMINATIONS OF PREGNANCY

The termination of pregnancy before the fetus is mature is termed an abortion or a premature labor or birth, according to the stage to which the pregnancy has advanced. There have been variations in the accepted meanings of these terms among both lay and medical people.

By the laity the term abortion often is associated with criminal practice and it is seldom used by nonmedical people; miscarriage is a term loosely applied by them to all deliveries occurring before the child is viable or the twenty-eighth week. Medical people, on the other hand, usually use the term abortion, except in their discussions with patients. They designate as abortions all terminations of pregnancy which occur before the period of viability, and designate as premature labor the spontaneous terminations of pregnancy after the child is viable (about the twenty-eighth week) but before it has reached maturity. Some doctors classify a fetus born between 20 to 28 weeks' gestation, weighing from 400 to 1000 gm (14 oz to 2 lb, 3 oz), as an immature fetus rather than an abortus, since such fetuses occasionally survive.

## ABORTIONS

In the nature of things, it is impossible to say how often abortions occur. They sometimes happen so early in pregnancy that the patient is unaware of the accident, or she may mistake the abortion for delayed menstruation. Such information as is available suggests that approximately one out of every ten pregnancies ends in a spontaneous abortion. About 75 per cent of all abortions occur during the second and third month of pregnancy.

### SPONTANEOUS ABORTIONS

**Causes.** There is a variety of causes of abortions; some entirely unavoidable, but some which are believed to be preventable. It is well for the nurse to be familiar with those which occur most frequently, as follows:

*Certain abnormalities of the developing fetus* are inconsistent with life, and are, therefore, a frequent cause of abortion. Dr. F. P. Mall, of Johns Hopkins University, showed after years of investigation that at least one-third of the embryos obtained from abortions were malformed and would have developed into monstrosities had they lived to term. It is often a great comfort to the expectant mother who loses her baby early in pregnancy to realize that had she carried the baby to term it might have been malformed, and that, therefore, she has not lost a normal child. Just why these abnormalities occur is not known, nor is there any known method of preventing or correcting them. The commonest cause is most likely defective germ plasm in either the sperm or the ovum. There also may be such defects in the placental development that the fetus does not derive sufficient nourishment to continue its development and dies very early as a result.

*Certain injuries and abnormalities of the reproductive tract* may cause abortions. A chronic infection may in rare instances be the cause by interfering with proper implantation of the placenta or adequate nourishment of the fetus. Deep lacerations of the cervix, uterine prolapse, fibroid tumors, or developmental anomalies of the uterus may cause abortions either because of their mechanical effect or because of circulatory disturbances of the decidua.

*Endocrine disturbances* may stimulate uterine contractions, especially if there is a deficiency or an imbalance of the hormones necessary to maintain a pregnancy.

*Acute infectious diseases,* particularly pneumonia, tend to cause the death of the fetus and thus cause abortions. Fetal death in these cases is believed to be due to transmission of the exciting agent from mother to child or due to fetal hypoxia.

*Physical shocks,* such as falls, blows upon the abdomen, jumping, tripping over carpets, jars, jolting, or overexertion, may be the exciting cause of an abortion where there is a marked irritability of the uterine muscle. This factor is largely influenced by individual response, however, as a slight jar will cause an abortion in one woman, and a violent experience will have no effect upon another, at the same stage of pregnancy. These shocks are usually contributing factors rather than the basic cause.

It must be borne in mind, however, even in the face of these explanations, that the attitude toward the causes of abortions is undergoing a change. Apparently the most general cause of this accident is inherent in the embryo itself since the majority of those that have aborted are found to be faulty and incapable of complete development. A sound embryo normally attached to the uterine wall is not easily separated while one resulting from faulty germ plasm may be detached and expelled very readily. It is believed that death of the embryo often occurs before separation from the uterus begins.

There are many groundless beliefs concerning the causes of abortions which the nurse may well dispel. For example, it is not possible to separate the embryo from the uterine lining by reaching up or sleeping with the arms over the head. Purgatives and other drugs have much less effect in causing abortions under normal conditions than is generally believed.

**Symptoms.** For the purposes of differentiation in treatment, abortions are usually divided into groups and designated as threatened, imminent, inevitable, incomplete, and complete, but the premonitory symptoms of all the varieties are the same. They are vaginal bleeding and pain that is usually intermittent, beginning in the small of the back and finally felt as cramps in the lower part of the abdomen. Since menstruation is suspended during pregnancy, it is a safe precaution to regard any bleeding during this period, with or without pain, as a symptom of pending delivery. Because it may be possible in some instances to avert an abortion with proper treatment, the nurse should advise any woman who thinks she is pregnant and who has the slightest bleeding to place herself under the care of a physician immediately.

## TYPES OF ABORTIONS

**Threatened.** A threatened abortion is one in which there is some loss of blood associated with pain in the back and lower abdomen, but without expulsion of the products of conception.

**Imminent.** An imminent abortion is one in which the bleeding becomes quite profuse and the uterine contractions become hard enough to cause severe cramps and possibly a bearing-down sensation.

**Inevitable.** An abortion becomes inevitable if the membranes rupture, allowing amniotic fluid to escape, in the presence of cervical dilatation.

**Incomplete.** An incomplete abortion is one in which the fetus is expelled, but the placenta and membranes remain in the uterine cavity. This may go on to completion spontaneously.

**Complete.** A complete abortion, as the term suggests, is one in which all the products of conception are expelled. This is most apt to occur before the tenth week because the anchoring villi may not be very firmly attached to the decidua before this time. Sometimes the entire decidual lining of the uterus, having the appearance of a triangular sac, may be expelled. More often the vesicular ovum surrounded only by decidua capsularis or just the chorionic vesicle with no decidual lining is found. The latter usually has a shaggy appearance or it may be surrounded by a blood clot (Fig. 61).

**Habitual Abortion.** When several succeeding pregnancies terminate in an abortion at approximately the same period of gestation, the woman is said to have habitual abortions.

TREATMENT

**Prevention.** From the many possible causes of abortion given above it can be seen that *good health* in both the husband and wife is an important preventive measure. *Correction of any pelvic disturbance* which might interfere with proper implantation or nourishment of the fetus will also prove valuable.

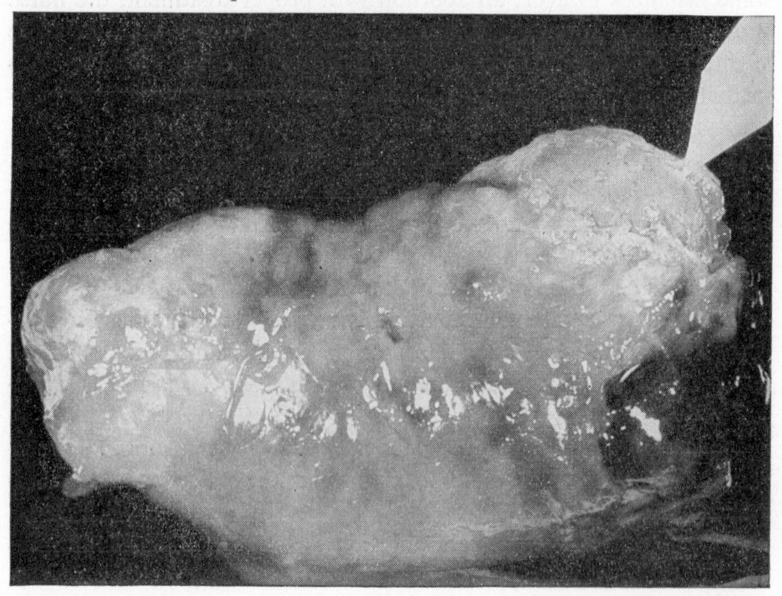

**Fig. 61.** Spontaneous complete abortion at 10 weeks of gestation. The arrow points to a part of the amniotic sac which is not surrounded by decidual tissue. This is the mass of tissue which may have the appearance of a blood clot and which must always be saved for the doctor's examination. (Courtesy of Dr. Madeline J. Thornton.)

Some doctors advise a woman who is pregnant for the first time and who, therefore, does not know whether or not she is likely to abort, to *avoid* such risks as *fatigue,* lifting or moving heavy objects, running, jumping, long trips, or any action which might *jar or jolt* her during the first twelve to fourteen weeks of pregnancy.

In the case of an expectant mother who has had several abortions, greater precautions are advisable, because she is in greater danger of aborting than is a woman who has not had this experience. It is of prime importance that the cause of her previous abortions be discovered and corrected, if possible. In addition to this, she should be particularly careful to observe precautionary measures at the time menstruation would occur were she not pregnant, and as she approaches the stage of her pregnancy at which the previous abortion occurred, she should remain quiet for at least a week before and after the time when an abortion is feared.

*Complete rest and physical relaxation* may be effective preventive measures, and patients with a tendency to have abortions, who have been willing to stay quiet throughout practically the entire period of gestation, have gone through pregnancy without interruption and been delivered of normal babies at term.

*Corpus luteum hormone* is frequently used as a preventive measure, especially where there have been previous abortions, because of the possibility of an endocrine disturbance with a deficiency in this essential substance. A better relationship in the estrogen-progesterone balance is thus obtained. This results in a decrease in the uterine contractions and a better maintenance of the endometrial or decidual lining. More recently estrogen has also been administered. Since estrogen and progesterone are both produced by the corpus luteum and the chorioplacental system, it is believed that where a deficiency in progesterone is present a deficiency in estrogen probably also exists and that the action of one of these hormones depends upon the presence of the other.

Another endocrine disturbance may be a hypothyroidism, and if the thyroid function is found to be depressed administration of *thyroid extract* may be beneficial.

**Remedial.** In the different stages of abortion the treatment employed by most physicians is usually along the following lines:

*Threatened.* If any vaginal bleeding occurs in a pregnant woman she should be put at bed rest immediately and observed closely. It is always important for the nurse caring for these patients to save all perineal pads for the doctor's inspection, in order that he may estimate the amount of bleeding, and to report any increase in bleeding or cramps. She should keep the vulva clean and use sterile perineal pads to prevent infection in case the abortion goes on to completion.

Sedatives, especially the barbiturates, are usually given to keep the patient quiet, and the nurse should restrict the patient's activities to the minimum while there are any symptoms present. Progesterone is administered intramuscularly, and sometimes estrogen is also given.

Symptoms may subside in a few days, stay the same, or become worse so that the abortion becomes imminent. After the symptoms have subsided it is wise to keep the patient in bed for a few more days and then restrict activities for the next few weeks. Progesterone therapy is sometimes continued for several weeks.

If the bleeding continues, the patient is sometimes allowed up rather than kept in bed indefinitely. There is the possibility that a small amount of bleeding may continue for some time even when the pregnancy is progressing normally or perhaps the embryo has died but has not been expelled. Occasionally bleeding is due to causes other than a threatened abortion, such as cervical polyps or areas of cervical erosion. The size of the uterus at subsequent examinations and pregnancy hormone tests will help to determine whether or not the pregnancy is progressing normally or the fetus has died.

*Imminent.* The treatment is the same as for a threatened abortion, in the hope that the symptoms will still subside. If the bleeding does not become so excessive as to greatly exceed the blood loss of a normal menstrual period, it is still possible for the pregnancy to continue, although in many instances it will terminate spontaneously. The moral principles of the Catholic Church permit the emptying of the uterus when the physician is reasonably sure that the fetus is already dead or already detached.*

*Inevitable and Incomplete.* When the bleeding is not profuse in either one of these conditions, it is best to wait and do nothing in the hope that the uterus will expel all of the tissue itself. Blood should be available for transfusion in case the bleeding becomes profuse. Antibiotics may be given to prevent infection. An oxytocic drug may be given to hasten the process of expulsion of tissue.

The nurse caring for these patients should save all perineal pads for the doctor's inspection. Any tissue or blood clots that are expelled must be carefully examined to determine whether or not the abortion has been completed. Since tissue or clots that are expelled from the uterus sometimes remain in the vagina until the patient changes position they are often expelled when she sits up to void. The bedpan must, therefore, always be inspected for clots (Fig. 61).

* See Hayes, Rev. Edward J.; Hayes, Rev. Paul J.; and Kelly, Dorothy E.: *Moral Handbook of Nursing.* The Macmillan Company, New York, 1956, p. 42.

Catholics believe that every fetus should be baptized, regardless of its immaturity or of the circumstances which have brought about its separation from the body of the mother. For details on how to baptize, see pages 340–41.

If at any time bleeding becomes profuse, or if the uterus does not empty itself completely in a few days, operative interference becomes necessary to remove the retained tissues. Because there is always the possibility of infection in any abortion, operative interference is avoided or postponed whenever possible. Since the pregnant uterus is very soft, the retained tissue is more often removed manually than instrumentally, since a curet may very easily be pushed through the uterine wall, and, should this happen, complications are apt to follow. Rigid aseptic technic is always used.

The uterus will usually contract well after it has been emptied and thereby control bleeding, but a uterine pack may be inserted for a period of 12 to 24 hours to further reduce bleeding. An oxytocic drug will stimulate the uterine muscle to remain contracted. Antibiotics are usually administered as a prophylaxis against infection. If the blood loss has been excessive, blood transfusions will hasten recovery.

*Complete.* The treatment and care are exactly the same as are given after a normal delivery. (Chap. 16, pp. 429–41 and 457–62.)

Many doctors follow these various remedial measures with a search for the cause of the abortion just past, in order that it may be corrected if possible and thus attempt to prevent a recurrence.

*Missed.* A missed abortion occurs but rarely, and is one in which the embryo, or fetus, dies and is retained within the uterine cavity for months.

A typical history of such a case is that the uterus grows quite normally until the third or fourth month when signs of a threatened abortion may occur. These soon subside, and it is assumed that the pregnancy is progressing normally, but later examination reveals no further uterine enlargement. Just why the uterus does not expel the dead fetus is not known, but it is known that a dead fetus can remain in the uterus for months and even years without acting as a foreign body and without causing symptoms. If there are no symptoms, nothing is done for a period of time in the hope that a spontaneous abortion will finally occur, since this course seems to be safer than operative interference.

## INDUCED ABORTIONS

In addition to abortions which occur spontaneously there are also induced abortions, and these are designated as therapeutic or criminal, according to the motive for the induction.

**Therapeutic abortions** are resorted to when the patient's condition is so grave that it is believed to be imperative to empty the uterus in order to save her life. Such a condition may exist, for example, when pregnancy is seriously complicated by severe hypertensive renal disease, severe heart disease, and occasionally a condition which is inimical to pregnancy. An abortion induced under these circumstances is countenanced by law, as it is performed to prevent the loss of life from disease. However, it should be noted that the Catholic Church maintains that there is no moral distinction between therapeutic and criminal abortion, and that both are a direct attack on an innocent life. Any Catholic who procures or cooperates in an effective induced abortion is by that fact excommunicated from the Catholic Church.*

Roman Catholic moralists make a distinction between indirect and direct abortion. Indirect abortion is the foreseen but unintended loss of the fetus following upon a medical procedure necessary to preserve the life or health of the mother. The fetus is in no way directly attacked, and the loss of fetal life is a secondary and unintentional consequence. Direct ("induced") abortion is a deliberate termination of pregnancy, the only immediate purpose being the destruction of the fetus. Under this classification would fall criminal and therapeutic abortions. Indirect abortion is allowable for a sufficiently grave reason; direct abortion is never permitted for any reason, because it violates the commandment of God, "Thou shall not kill." Therefore, Catholics who are advised to procure a direct abortion should take counsel with their priest and follow his guidance.†

With advances in medical treatment the indications for therapeutic abortion are becoming less and less, since many complicating conditions can now be more successfully treated during pregnancy than was formerly possible.

As to the legal aspect of the matter, the laws relating to therapeutic abortion vary in the different states, but they are fairly uniform in

* Hayes, Rev. Edward J.; Hayes, Rev. Paul J.; and Kelly, Dorothy E.: *op. cit.*, pp. 43 and 44.

† Hayes, Rev. Edward J.; Hayes, Rev. Paul J.; and Kelly, Dorothy E.: *op. cit.*, p. 43.

their intent and make quite clear the difference between this procedure and the induction of abortion for any reason other than medical necessity.

Whenever a therapeutic abortion seems indicated, one or more doctors are called in consultation and the responsibility for the decision taken by all.

**A criminal abortion** is one induced for other than medical reasons by the use of drugs or instruments, either by the woman herself or someone else willing to induce it, usually known as an abortionist.

Dr. Josiah Morris Slemons wrote of the seriousness of criminal abortion in no uncertain terms, in *The Prospective Mother*. "At Common Law" (an inheritance from England) he tells us, "abortion is punishable as *homicide* when the woman dies or when the operation results fatally to the infant after it has been born alive. If performed for the purpose of killing the child, the crime is *murder;* in the absence of such intent, it is *manslaughter. The woman who commits an abortion upon herself is likewise guilty of the crime.*" *

Since these abortions are often done under unfavorable conditions and with unclean technic, hemorrhage and infection may be frequent complications. Perforation of the uterus during the procedure is also a possibility. If ethical medical aid is sought later, treatment is always conservative. Because of the possibility of infection, immediate operative completion is done only in cases of hemorrhage. The infection is treated with antibiotics, and all efforts are made to build up the patient's resistance with blood transfusions, high-caloric diet, and high-fluid intake. Isolation from other obstetric patients is essential.

## HYDATIDIFORM MOLE AND CHORIOCARCINOMA

A hydatidiform mole is a disease of the chorion in which the chorionic villi become cystic and the chorion assumes a grape-like appearance. These cysts may fill the entire uterine cavity. Usually there is no trace of a fetus. It is dangerous because the growth may invade the uterine muscle, it may be malignant, or a choriocarcinoma may develop later. A choriocarcinoma is a very malignant growth which may develop following a normal full-term pregnancy, an abor-

* Slemons, J. Morris: *The Prospective Mother,* 4th ed. Appleton-Century-Crofts, Inc., New York, 1942, pp. 141–42.

tion, or more likely a hydatidiform mole, making follow-up essential.

In the case of a mole, intermittent uterine bleeding may be present for several weeks. Spontaneous expulsion of the mole often occurs. Since blood loss at the time the vesicles are passed may be severe, the patient must be carefully watched for hemorrhage and blood should be available for transfusion. A curettage of the uterus is usually performed following expulsion of a mole to remove any fragments of tissue which may have remained.

Chorionic gonadotropin tests may be used as aids in the diagnosis if an abnormality is suspected because an increased titer of the chorionic gonadotropic hormone is present in both of the above conditions. The urine will give a positive reaction even when greatly diluted. It is best to collect a 24-hour specimen so that an estimate of the total daily output of the hormone can also be made.

After the expulsion of a mole, the patient should be carefully watched for one year, and frequent hormone pregnancy tests should be made with serum or urine. A positive reaction indicates that some living chorionic tissue is left. This may be benign or malignant but it should be removed after the possibility of a pregnancy is ruled out. If the tissue removed is that of a choriocarcinoma, treatment is directed toward arresting the malignancy.

## PREMATURE LABOR

Premature labor is the termination of pregnancy after the period of viability, but before maturity of the fetus. Premature births are seen with about the same frequency as spontaneous abortions. They usually occur spontaneously.

The premature baby's chances of living are directly proportionate to the length of its uterine life. This has already been stated, but will bear repetition in view of the widely current fallacy that a seventh-month baby is more likely to live than one born in the eighth month of pregnancy. The fact is that, as a rule, the nearer pregnancy approaches term, the more likely is the baby to survive. We ordinarily consider that a premature baby weighing between 1135 and 2500 gm (2½ to 5½ lb) has a favorable outlook if given special care. This care of premature babies is described in Chapter 23.

**Causes.** The toxemias of pregnancy, chronic nephritis, diabetes, pneumonia, typhoid fever, organic heart disease, and in many cases an unexplained or undetermined condition are causes of premature births. Multiple pregnancies, abnormal presentations, premature separation of the placenta, placenta previa, and malformations of the fetus are also frequently found to be causative factors. Hydramnios sometimes brings on a premature labor by so distending the uterus as to stimulate contractions.

Syphilis has in the past been a frequent cause of spontaneous premature birth, but where the serology test is made routinely and adequate treatment given in all cases of positive reaction, there has been an enormous reduction in the number of premature labors and stillbirths.

Labor is sometimes induced prematurely when this procedure may be expected to relieve an abnormality or complications which threaten the life of the mother or baby, or both. The most frequent indication for this course is severe toxemia. The methods employed in inducing labor will be discussed in Chapter 14, "Obstetric Operations and Complications of Labor."

**Treatment.** The care of the patient after a premature labor is the same as that given after a normal delivery. Complications can be avoided if everyone is convinced of the importance of having just as good care after a premature as after a full-term labor. Difficulty in appreciating this is perhaps due to the fact that the small, premature child is expelled more quickly and less painfully than a baby at term.

If the woman is seen at the very beginning of labor, rest in bed, progesterone, and sedation may possibly prevent the uterine contractions from continuing, but sedation should not be given if there is any chance that the baby will be born while the medication is still effective. In premature deliveries, there are more abnormal presentations than at term, and because of the soft bones of the fetus, especially in the cranium, there is more danger of injury to the baby unless it is handled very gently.

## EXTRAUTERINE PREGNANCY

An extrauterine, or ectopic, pregnancy may be defined as a pregnancy which develops outside of the uterus.

Although in the normal course of events the fertilized ovum travels down the fallopian tube and becomes attached to the uterine lining, it may become implanted, and begin its development, at any point along the way between the graafian follicle, from which it has been ejected, and the uterus toward which it is traveling (Fig. 21). If the fetus develops in the ovary, which is extremely rare, it is termed an ovarian pregnancy. If attachment and development of the ovum occur in the tube it is termed a tubal pregnancy, this being the most common type of extrauterine pregnancy.

When the ovum attaches itself to the lining of the tube its history is much the same as when it lodges in the uterus in that it burrows into the mucosa, increases in size, and accordingly stretches the surrounding muscle wall. However, the uterine wall is a thick muscular structure and is capable of preserving its integrity while being distended by the steadily enlarging contents of its cavity. The wall of the tube, on the other hand, is very thin and is not designed to meet the strain of a growing mass such as a fetus. As a result, the pregnancy usually terminates within the first three months in one of several ways. A tubal abortion may occur, and the fetus and membranes are partly or completely extruded from the fimbriated end of the tube into the peritoneal cavity; or the tube may rupture, and the fetus, with or without the membranes, may be expelled into the peritoneal cavity or between the folds of the broad ligament; or death and disintegration of the products of conception may take place within the tube.

The point at which the rupture occurs is mere chance, depending entirely upon where the ovum has attached itself. Rupture occurs either because the chorionic villi, which have the power to invade and destroy tissue, have penetrated the wall or because the weakened wall breaks from pressure. Bleeding will depend upon the point of rupture; a small tear that includes a large blood vessel will result in a severe hemorrhage while a larger rupture that does not injure the large vessels may be less serious. When abortion through the ampullar end of the tube occurs, the bleeding is usually not as profuse or continuous as with rupture of the tube.

The rupture in the wall of the tube may be small and the fetus may not be expelled, or the rupture may be large with expulsion of the entire products of conception. If the placenta is nearly or completely separated the fetus perishes and may be largely absorbed by the maternal organism or it can be mummified. If extrusion occurs before the third month of pregnancy the products of conception are rapidly absorbed. If the greater part of the placenta remains attached to the site of its development, it is possible for the fetus to live and grow and even develop to term. This is called a secondary *abdominal pregnancy.* In this case the placenta may remain surrounded by the tube, but it also grows out and attaches itself to the other pelvic and abdominal organs.

With advances in the field of abdominal surgery, it has become apparent that ectopic pregnancy occurs much more frequently than was formerly believed. It is estimated that this abnormal development takes place in approximately 0.3 per cent of all pregnancies, and, as has been stated, the wall of one of the tubes is the most common site of implantation. Tubal pregnancies have a tendency to recur in the same patient. Little is definitely known as to the causes of this accident, but it is easy to understand they might be found among any conditions that would interfere mechanically with the downward passage of the fertilized ovum and would favor its lodgment in the tube. This might be the case in a diverticulum of the tube or in an infection when the lumen of the tube would be smaller than normal or nearly obliterated as a result of thickening of the lining or adhesions of opposing surfaces. Physical and developmental abnormalities in the reproductive tract which favor decidual formation in the tubes might explain implantation of an ovum before the uterus was reached.

**Symptoms.** It sometimes happens that the patient does not know she is pregnant, and there are apparently no symptoms until the tube ruptures. Frequently, however, there is a history of a missed period and slight vaginal bleeding or "spotting." There may be also slight abdominal pain which the patient attributes to her condition if she knows she is pregnant. Early signs and symptoms of pregnancy may also be present. The uterus enlarges and decidua develops just as in a normal intrauterine pregnancy. When there is some bleeding or the menstrual period is apparently not absent, the blood may be due to bleeding from the large vessels in the decidua; or if the fetus dies the decidua will slough off and cause bleeding. In many cases the first symptom is sudden, excruciating pain in the lower abdomen which may be on either side or diffuse. The patient suddenly feels faint, grows very pale, gives evidence of being in a state of shock, and may sink into a coma. She is suffering from a hemorrhage into the peritoneal cavity, but has no appreciable external bleeding. Upon vaginal examination, the doctor finds the changes normally present in the reproductive tract during pregnancy, and can usually palpate the ruptured tube which he is likely to find much enlarged and exquisitely tender.

Diagnosis before rupture is difficult because the symptoms are vague. It can sometimes be made by the presence of a few symptoms and the palpation of a tumor mass, but any woman who is probably pregnant and has sudden abdominal pain and collapse can most likely be said to have a ruptured ectopic pregnancy.

**Treatment.** The doctor's course usually is immediate operation to excise the affected tube since this condition is very serious. If a diagnosis is made before rupture occurs, it is customary to excise the affected tube as soon as possible in order to prevent rupture of the tube and serious hemorrhage. After rupture has occurred, immediate surgery is necessary to remove the affected tube, and it is usually necessary to give blood transfusions to replace the blood loss.*

The nurse's duty in these cases is to prevent all exertion, to notify the doctor immediately of the symptoms given above, and to give the nursing care for extreme shock. There is little more that she can do pending the doctor's arrival.

If an abdominal pregnancy continues, uterine contractions, termed false labor pains, usually occur. When surgery is not employed until the pregnancy is near term, and if the child is living, the placenta usually has to be left in place because hemorrhage cannot be controlled after its removal. If the fetus has died, the vessels supplying the placenta have probably become obliterated and it can be removed more easily.

## ANTEPARTUM HEMORRHAGE

Antepartum hemorrhage, which is a hemorrhage occurring before or during delivery of the baby, is another serious complication of pregnancy. During the early months bleeding is usually due to abortion, menstruation, or lesions of the cervix and is not severe as a rule, but during the last three months bleeding is almost invariably due to placenta previa or premature separation of a normally implanted placenta, and is often profuse. Sometimes, though rarely, there will be

* Catholic moralists classify this as an indirect abortion, and it therefore carries no moral censure.

vaginal bleeding from a ruptured uterus, but in such cases the external hemorrhage is usually slight.

## PLACENTA PREVIA

Placenta previa is a common cause of late antepartum hemorrhage and is one of the serious conditions arising in obstetrics. With improvement in treatment in the past 10 to 15 years, the mortality rate has been reduced greatly for the mother but continues to remain relatively high for the child. The babies frequently die from asphyxia due to placental separation, or, if born living, the death rate is high due to prematurity.

In order to understand what is happening in this condition, we must go back to the discussion of the implantation of the ovum. We learned that, as a rule, after the ovum entered the uterus it attached itself to a point in the uterine lining high up on the anterior or posterior wall. Unfortunately, the ovum sometimes is implanted so far down toward the cervix that as the placenta develops at that site it partially or completely covers the internal os. It is the extent to which the placenta grows over the cervical opening that determines whether it is of the central, partial, or marginal variety.

*A centrally implanted or complete placenta previa* (Fig. 62) is one which entirely covers the os; *a partial or lateral placenta previa* is one which, as the name suggests, only partially covers the opening, while if it is implanted so high up that only its margin overlaps the os, it is designated as *marginal placenta previa* (Fig. 63) or low implantation of the placenta.

**Causes.** Not much is definitely known about the cause of placenta previa, but it is evident that multiparity is a factor as it is less common among primigravidas and increases in frequency with the number of children a woman has borne. It has been observed also that placenta previa is not only favored by the number of children a woman has borne, but also by the rapidity with which the pregnancies followed each other. When there are frequent pregnancies, there may be more chances of atrophic or inflammatory changes in the endometrium and accordingly a decrease in the blood supply, so that even a placenta attached fairly high may spread out more than normal to get enough blood for its nutritive needs, and in doing this it covers the os.

**Symptoms.** The characteristic symptom is vaginal bleeding which ordinarily occurs some time after the seventh month. The bleeding is frequently intermittent; the first hemorrhage usually stops spontaneously and is very rarely fatal. Frequently, for no apparent reason, the bleeding recurs after the first hemorrhage or there may be slight continuous bleeding from the time of the first attack. After this prelim-

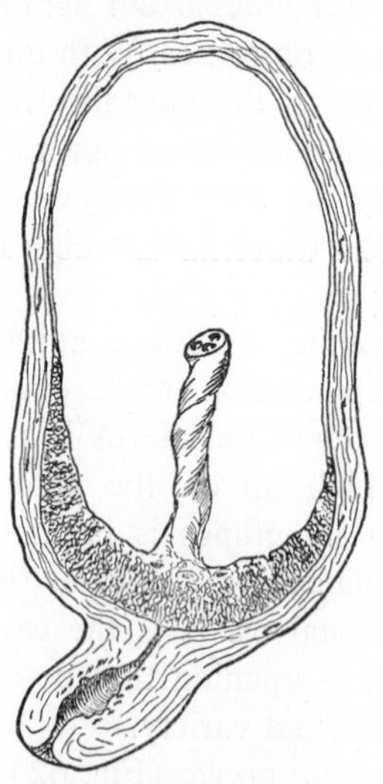

**Fig. 62.** Diagram of centrally implanted placenta previa.

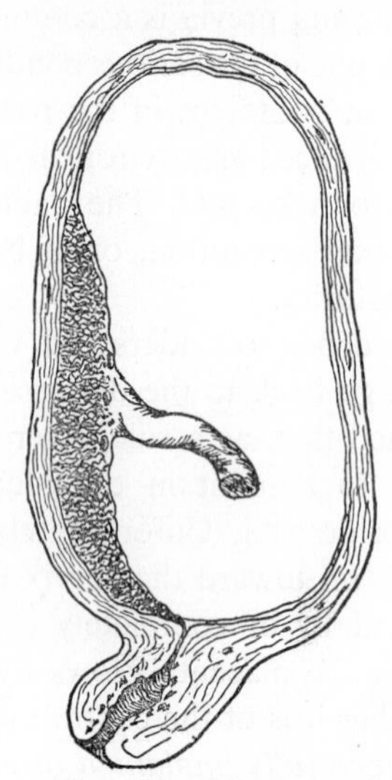

**Fig. 63.** Diagram of marginal placenta previa.

inary bleeding, there may be sudden, profuse hemorrhage with very severe effects. A certain degree of placental separation is inevitable as the cervix thins and dilates during the latter weeks of pregnancy and during labor. This is accompanied by bleeding, since the stretched muscle is unable to contract and thereby compress the open blood vessels.

Outstanding features in the bleeding from placenta previa are that there are no painful or discomforting symptoms due to the bleeding, in contrast to the abdominal pain and tenderness that are frequently associated with the bleeding that occurs in abruptio placentae, and that the uterus remains soft and flaccid, whereas it usually becomes tense when the normally implanted placenta separates prematurely. If bleeding occurs during active labor, there will be the discomfort at intervals that is associated with uterine muscle contractions, but the uterus alternately contracts and relaxes as in normal labor, while complete relaxation of uterine muscle between contractions is usually absent in abruptio placentae.

It has been observed that patients with placenta previa frequently have postpartum hemorrhages, and that they are more susceptible to infection and thrombosis in the sinuses of the lower uterine segment.

**Diagnosis.** A patient with bleeding in the last trimester of pregnancy must always be suspected of having either a placenta previa or an abruptio placentae, but it is sometimes very difficult to make a diagnosis.

A soft-tissue x-ray may be helpful. The placenta as such is not always distinguishable by x-ray, but the placental position can often be located on the basis of being able to visualize on the x-ray an area of thickening of the structures between the fetal parts and the outer uterine wall. The x-ray as a diagnostic method has limitations since it is not always possible to visualize the placental position, and when it does appear to be implanted low on the uterine wall the x-ray may not help to determine how far down it extends. However, if the placenta is seen in a normal position, the x-ray helps to rule out the diagnosis of a placenta previa.

A now frequently used method of diagnosis of placenta previa is to determine by x-ray whether or not the fetal head is displaced from its normal position by a soft tissue mass.

Sometimes air or radiopaque solution is instilled into the bladder before an x-ray is taken, and the relationship between the fetal head and the bladder wall is noted.

Sometimes a diagnosis is made by performing a vaginal examination to palpate for placental tissue. This must always be done under aseptic technic, and very gently to prevent more separation during the procedure. The cervix is usually soft and patulous, and it is fairly easy to feel placental tissue, or at least a spongy mass, between the examining finger and the presenting part. If the cervix is not patulous it is necessary to palpate the lower uterine segment. A boggy mass between the lower uterine wall and the presenting part is most likely placenta. If the head can easily be palpated through the lower uterine segment the placenta is probably not low in the uterine cavity. With placenta previa the head is ordinarily not low in the pelvis, or the presentation is frequently other than vertex.

**Treatment.** It is obviously important for the patient to be taken to the hospital immediately after the bleeding begins, no matter how slight, in order to carry out measures to prevent excessive loss of blood later.

Blood transfusion is a very important part of the treatment whenever bleeding is excessive, since the sudden loss of blood weakens the patient and greatly lessens her chances of recovery. The blood transfusion is of such pressing importance to a patient with placenta previa that crossmatching for transfusion should be done as promptly as possible, and the blood, or donor, kept in readiness to supply the patient's needs. If the patient has lost considerable blood, a 5 per cent glucose solution may be given intravenously to combat shock until the blood is ready for transfusion. Plasma and/or a plasma expander solution may also be used.

When a sterile vaginal examination, or even a rectal examination, is to be done for purposes of diagnosis it should be postponed until blood for transfusion is available, and adequate preparation has been made to do this examination in the operating room and to treat the patient in case of severe bleeding. These examinations should be done gently, in order not to start fresh bleeding, but even with gentle technic there is always the danger that slight manipulation of the cervix may cause severe hemorrhage.

The treatment depends upon the variety of placenta previa, upon the condition of the mother and the fetus, and also upon the parity of the patient.

To understand the treatment the nurse should visualize what is happening. When the internal os begins to dilate, as it does during the latter part of pregnancy, that part of the placenta which overlies it is torn loose, leaving large gaping vessels. These can be closed only by mechanical pressure as long as the uterus is unemptied and accordingly unable to stop the bleeding by contraction of the uterine muscle. This mechanical pressure is best applied by bringing the baby's head down against the placenta. When such a procedure does not seem advisable the baby may be delivered soon to allow the muscle to contract.

Occasionally the cervix is already completely dilated when the woman is examined and the baby can be delivered immediately. If the cervix is not completely dilated it cannot be done manually to hasten delivery without serious results, but rupturing the membranes may bring the presenting part of the fetus down enough to put pressure on the placenta. By allowing the baby's head to drop down, pressure is applied to the placental site and the blood vessels are occluded. Pressure applied to the fundus of the uterus will force the head down lower and exert even greater pressure. This method of treatment is most useful in the multigravidous patient who is already in labor and has only a marginal placenta previa.

If rupture of the membranes does not bring the head down sufficiently to control bleeding, a Willett forceps may be fixed onto the fetal scalp and a pull may be exerted on it to press the head against the placenta. The Willett forceps, which has rounded teeth on the grasping bars, is fixed into the fetal scalp. To exert a pull, a weight of 1 lb is attached to the handle of the forceps by means of a tape hung over the foot of the bed. The forceps is narrow enough to allow for application as soon as the os will admit one finger. Some scalp injury may occur where the forceps is attached, but it is usually not serious. This method is not advised in primigravidas, in cases of partial or total placenta previa, or in cases where hemorrhage has been profuse.

Cesarean section may be the treatment of choice. When the placenta entirely covers the cervical os it is difficult to control the bleeding by other means and the infant cannot be born alive by vaginal delivery. Primigravidas and patients with the placenta partially over the os are often not easily treated satisfactorily with the above-mentioned methods. The cervix and lower uterine segment are very friable because of the vascularity of the placental site; vaginal manipulation may cause severe lacerations and bleeding. Cesarean section forestalls any possibility of cervical lacerations and it also decreases the length of time during which a patient may bleed from placenta previa. Some women, with only slight bleeding from a marginal placenta previa, may not need active treatment, but should remain under close observation until after delivery and where everything is available to control bleeding if necessary. In certain cases of placenta previa, where the baby is still quite small and the bleeding has stopped, delivery is postponed to give the baby the advantage of further development in utero. These patients must, of course, be kept under very close observation. A vaginal examination, done gently, may be indicated, to either confirm or rule out a diagnosis of placenta previa; the bleeding is occasionally due to another, less serious, cause such as cervical polyps.

**Prognosis.** There has been a marked reduction in the maternal mortality in recent years, but the fetal mortality, although showing a decrease, remains high.

## PREMATURE SEPARATION OF A NORMALLY IMPLANTED PLACENTA OR ABRUPTIO PLACENTAE

A placenta previa, as has been explained, is an abnormally situated placenta. It sometimes happens that a placenta which is normally placed will separate prematurely, with hemorrhage as the inevitable result. Premature separation of the normally implanted placenta is the term which best describes this condition, but since this wording is rather long the term *abruptio placentae* is used more frequently.

If the blood escapes from the vagina, the hemorrhage is called *external,* but if it is retained within the uterine cavity it is called a *concealed* hemorrhage. The latter type is much more severe, but also occurs less frequently.

All degrees of separation may take place; the area may be only a few millimeters in diameter or the entire placenta may become detached. Signs and symptoms vary with the amount of separation.

Antepartum bleeding is sometimes due to a very small amount of marginal detachment of the placenta, but this is never enough to definitely demonstrate or diagnose. With abruptio placentae, bleeding first occurs into the decidua basalis, forming a hematoma in it, and splitting the decidua basalis into two portions—one next to the placenta and one next to the uterine wall. As the hematoma becomes larger it separates some of the placenta from the uterus. The amount of bleeding may be small and will then not be recognized until delivery of the placenta, when the region of separation can be seen as a depressed area and containing dark clotted blood. If the bleeding is more profuse the placenta may separate to its margin, and the blood may appear externally by escaping between the membranes and uterine wall. This is then external bleeding.

In the case of a concealed hemorrhage the blood remains behind the placenta, or in some instances it may escape into the amniotic fluid by breaking through the membranes. Usually some bleeding will appear externally later, but if the baby's head is tight in the pelvis or if the membranes are tightly adherent, it does not escape readily. In cases of concealed hemorrhage the detachment of the placenta is usually complete, whereas it is generally incomplete when the bleeding is external. Concealed hemorrhage is frequently associated with toxemia of pregnancy.

In some instances there is extensive intramuscular hemorrhage, possibly throughout the entire uterus, which becomes a bluish or purplish color, and the muscle may lose its power to contract.

The cause of abruptio placentae is unknown. This accident may occur anytime during the latter months of pregnancy or during labor. When the placental separation occurs before labor begins, it is soon followed by the onset of uterine contractions.

**Symptoms.** With external hemorrhage, the chief symptom is an escape of blood from the vagina, frequently accompanied by abdominal pain. The possibility of bleeding due to a placenta previa must be ruled out.

A concealed hemorrhage is an extremely grave complication for both mother and child. The characteristic symptoms are intense cramp-like abdominal pain and uterine tenderness and rigidity. In contrast to the flaccid state of the uterus in placenta previa, in the concealed type of hemorrhage from premature separation the uterus is hard in consistency, being described as "board-like," or "stony," without alternate contraction and relaxation. It is impossible to palpate the fetus because of the tenseness of the uterine muscle. The fetal heart tones will be absent if a considerable amount of the placenta separates.

The nurse caring for a patient in the latter weeks of pregnancy, or for a patient in labor, must know that intense colic-like abdominal pain may be serious. Especially, when caring for the patient in labor, she should not assume that this type of severe abdominal pain is caused by hard uterine contractions. The abdomen should always be palpated to feel the consistency of the uterus and to make certain that the uterine muscle is alternately contracting and relaxing. With external bleeding the uterus may also remain tense between contractions. There is sometimes a gradual, but marked, enlargement of the uterus with concealed hemorrhage.

**Treatment.** Treatment for vaginal bleeding during the latter months of pregnancy should be carried out in a hospital. Therefore, when bleeding begins, immediate arrangements should be made for hospitalization, regardless of amount, for adequate observation and treatment.

The treatment of abruptio placentae depends upon its severity and the extent to which labor has progressed. If contractions have begun and the bleeding is only moderate, labor is ordinarily allowed to proceed normally and unassisted. Rupture of the membranes, so that the uterus can contract around the fetus, may help to control bleeding. Rupture of the membranes also hastens labor and delivery. If labor does not proceed fairly rapidly or if bleeding is profuse, delivery by cesarean section may be necessary to allow the uterine muscle to contract and thus stop the bleeding by closing the uterine blood vessels. Treatment of the accompanying blood loss and shock is very important and is started before surgery is begun.

In cases of premature separation of the normally implanted placenta, as in placenta previa, blood transfusions are indicated, unless the bleeding is very mild. The value of blood transfusions cannot be overemphasized. Crossmatching of the patient's blood for a transfusion should be done immediately upon admission to the hospital, and the blood or a donor should be available at a moment's notice.

In some cases of abruptio placentae there is a failure of the blood-clotting mechanism due to a decrease in the blood fibrinogen level. Frequent tests of the plasma fibrinogen level are often made in order that fibrinogen may be administered intravenously if the patient shows a fibrinogenopenia. It is, therefore, important that fibrinogen be available for treatment if this complication should occur.

If the uterine muscle has lost its ability to contract, due to dissociation of its fibers by intramuscular hemorrhage, removal of the uterus may occasionally become necessary to prevent death from postpartum hemorrhage.

**Nursing Care.** The nurse's duty in the presence of an antepartum hemorrhage, no matter how slight, is to put the patient to bed and to notify the doctor immediately. If the bleeding is slight and the patient is in good condition, it may be enough simply to keep her quiet until the doctor arrives. It may be necessary, however, to give nursing care for shock, which will be evidenced by a rapid pulse, pallor, air hunger, a low blood pressure, cold clammy skin, and faintness.

As nervousness and excitement only tend to increase the bleeding the nurse has an excellent opportunity to try to soothe and quiet a frightened woman, and convince her that she can help herself, in this emergency, by quieting her mind and body.

Pending the doctor's arrival, the nurse should prepare for the administration of intravenous fluids and for examination and delivery of the patient. She can begin preparation of the operative area, for delivery, by shaving it, and have an adequate amount of sterile supplies ready for examination and delivery.

After delivery the woman must be watched *very* carefully for post-partum hemorrhage, and supplies must be available to treat it immediately if indicated. Anuria, or oliguria, may be a complication of abruptio placentae. The urinary output should be carefully watched so that, if it is not sufficient, measures may be taken to attempt to increase it.

**Prognosis.** Prognosis depends upon the type of bleeding, external or internal, and the amount of blood lost. In many cases of external bleeding the loss of blood is only moderate, and the area of placental separation not great enough to interfere with the life of the baby. Bleeding in the external type may, however, become profuse. The concealed hemorrhage is much more dangerous to the mother and the baby than the external variety. The fetus cannot survive, of course, when the placenta is completely separated from the uterine wall, as it usually is in case of concealed hemorrhage. The fetal mortality is also high if the blood loss is large in the external type of bleeding. The maternal mortality depends upon the type and amount of bleeding, the degree of shock, and the promptness with which treatment can be instituted.

## PERNICIOUS VOMITING OF PREGNANCY

Pernicious vomiting of pregnancy, or *hyperemesis gravidarum,* usually occurs during the first three months. We learned in Chapter 5 that a milder form of vomiting, known as "morning sickness," is present in about half of all pregnancies. This mild type consists of a feeling of nausea, possibly accompanied by vomiting, immediately upon arising in the morning, and the patient usually has a capricious appetite. This disturbance appears at about the sixth week and usually disappears spontaneously six to eight weeks later. With some women, however, the vomiting does not disappear during the day, in a satisfactory manner, in which case it is described as "pernicious vomiting."

**Signs and Symptoms.** In pernicious vomiting, the nausea and vomiting in the morning may persist for hours; it may occur later in the day, or even at night; or it may be so persistent that the patient will be unable to retain anything taken by mouth, not even water, at any time of the day or night. There is nausea or vomiting at the sight or smell of food. Vomiting may occur even with a change of position or at the sight of a person entering the room. There may be pain in the stomach, hiccup, and gastric pyrosis (heartburn). Thirst becomes severe. After food is no longer present in the stomach the emesis is composed of mucus and bile. Considerable weight is lost during this period.

Whenever the vomiting seriously interferes with nutrition it is considered pernicious. If it continues long there will be signs of starvation, dehydration, acidosis, and possibly some polyneuritic symptoms. Where there is starvation the carbohydrate supply in the body soon becomes exhausted, and the energy is furnished by fats and proteins. This means an incomplete oxidation of the fatty acids and the presence of ketone bodies in the blood and urine.

A marked weight loss, a dry skin, and signs of emaciation soon appear. The blood chemistry in severe cases may show a decrease in the serum proteins, an increase in the nonprotein nitrogen, and a decrease in the chlorides. Anemia may be present. Acetone is present in the urine.

Occasionally a patient will become extremely ill. The chief signs and symptoms of this very grave condition, in addition to persistent vomiting, may be onset of jaundice; a low-grade fever; a rapid pulse; a reddened, dry, cracked tongue; hemorrhage into the retina; coffee-ground vomitus; a diminished amount of urine containing albumin and casts; irritability, coma, and sometimes delirium. The disease may run its course swiftly with early appearance of coma, or it may persist less acutely for weeks, in which case there is extreme emaciation and prostration. Such a condition is, of course, serious and may terminate fatally.

**Cause.** It is the general opinion that all vomiting of pregnancy is of an organic nature fundamentally. Recalling that some degree of "morning sickness" occurs in about one-half of all pregnant women, it is believed that all forms of vomiting in pregnancy are due to some factor commonly present in normal gestation. This factor is unidentified, but it has been suggested that it may be due to a toxic element, or a maladjustment of maternal metabolism, or a change in gastric motility. Pernicious vomiting may develop when this factor becomes unusually active or when it is present to an extraordinary degree. It is not known why it increases in some cases and not in others. Neuroses or psychologic disturbances due to fear or unwanted pregnancy and all the adjustments that must be made to a pregnancy may, however, play a large part and may be superimposed on the underlying organic cause at any time. An interrelation of the toxic or organic and the neurotic factors is generally acknowledged. The extent to which the patient reacts to the underlying cause is somewhat determined by her emotional stability and her mental reaction to the adjustments it is necessary to make during pregnancy.

**Treatment and Nursing Care.** In many instances pernicious vomiting can be prevented by the proper management of "morning sickness." If the pregnant woman is having early morning vomiting she should be told to eat a cracker or piece of dry toast before arising in the morning, and if there is a tendency to nausea later in the day she can be advised to eat frequent small meals, mostly carbohydrates, every two to three hours, and not to mix liquids and solids. There seems to be less nausea when the stomach is full than when it is empty. Plenty of rest, exercise, and diversion should be encouraged to keep her well occupied.

If the vomiting becomes persistent, hospitalization is advisable. Treatment should be instituted before liver and kidney damage occur. As a rule the best results are obtained by putting the patient to bed and separating her from her family and friends. In the hospital her psychologic conflicts can be helped by rest, sedation, change of environment, and psychotherapy, and the dehydration and starvation can be treated by parenteral fluids and vitamins and a gradual resumption of food.

It must be remembered that since the vomiting may be of emotional origin the patient must be treated with tact and understanding. In the opinion of many psychiatrists the vomiting frequently constitutes a protection, or possibly a protest, which the patient has developed subconsciously because of some reason for fearing or not wanting to become a mother. It is difficult to outline the nursing care of such patients with any degree of precision as no two patients can be cared for in quite the same way. In some cases the patient is a selfish woman who objects to motherhood because of its inconveniences, while in others the prospective mother is tormented by fear of inability to go through her pregnancy successfully, although sincerely wanting to have a child. Or she may be bewildered and overwhelmed by the prospect of the danger of childbirth and the responsibilities of motherhood. Such a patient is a truly pathetic figure, and her distress often may be greatly relieved by a nurse who is endowed with insight and tact. As this subject has been discussed at more length in Chapter 7, "Mental Hygiene of the Expectant Mother," only a word is required here as a reminder that the nurse is likely to need all the resourcefulness and understanding she is capable of offering when caring for patients suffering from pernicious vomiting. The condition never should be made light of, but the patient should be assured that nausea and vomiting are not necessary accompaniments of pregnancy and that with her cooperation the course adopted will end in recovery. In fact, everyone coming in contact with the patient should evince genuine enthusiasm over the successful results that may be expected to follow the painstaking care which has been started early.

If the patient does not show rapid adjustment to the pregnancy, conferences with her spiritual adviser or a psychiatrist may help her with her problem and hasten recovery.

In addition to the necessary mental nursing the patient needs physical care also, since, although her trouble may be of emotional origin, she is, nevertheless, physically ill.

Sedatives are generally given; this may be in the form of sodium phenobarbital hypodermically or some other barbiturate derivative rectally until oral intake is possible. Often one of the new tranquilizing drugs is also used.

For the first 24 to 48 hours after hospitalization the patient will have all food and fluids by mouth, including water and ice chips, restricted in order to rest the gastrointestinal tract. This is usually absolutely the rule even though the patient complains of hunger. As patients with pernicious vomiting usually suffer from a bad taste and dry mouth, a refreshing mouthwash should be used frequently.

Carbohydrates, chlorides, and fluids are given parenterally during the first few days. From 2500 to 3000 ml of fluids are given daily, using partly 5 or 10 per cent glucose solution and partly physiologic saline solution. If the carbon dioxide combining power of the blood is low, ⅙ molar sodium lactate solution is given intravenously. Vitamins are given parenterally; vitamin B is used in large doses if there are any polyneuritic symptoms.

A careful record should be kept of the fluid intake, the urinary output, and all emesis.

After this treatment for two days, small servings of solid food—crackers, dry toast and jelly, dry cereal, baked or mashed potato—are given every two hours, or the solid food is alternated with liquid nourishment in small amounts, not over 100 ml at one time. Hot tea, carbonated fluids, cold fruit juices, and crushed ice are usually easy to retain. Gradually more liquid is allowed so that the patient is taking as much as she desires up to one-half hour before and after the solid food. It is best not to mix the solid and liquid food for another day or two. Some parenteral fluids may still be necessary during these first few days, depending on the oral intake.

All foods should be served in very small amounts, attractively, and either very hot or very cold. The dishes should be removed from the bedside as soon as the patient has finished eating. Anything which appeals to the patient, or for which she has a particular craving, may be given, although generally fats are restricted while carbohydrates are encouraged during the first few days. The diet is increased slowly to six small meals daily, this being followed by a gradual resumption of a regular diet.

If the patient begins vomiting again after having taken food, the treatment of nothing by mouth and parenteral fluids for two days is repeated and feedings are then again gradually resumed.

If vomiting is not controlled after a few days of the above treatment, tube feedings with highly nutritive, vitamin-enriched liquids may be used. The feeding should be administered very slowly, but continuously. A nasal tube is inserted and left in place while the liquid is slowly dripped in from an overhanging bottle which is connected to the nasal tube with a glass connector and rubber tubing. A glass drip bulb in the tubing makes it possible to count the drops per minute; with the use of a screw clamp on the tubing the rate of flow can be adjusted. This rate should not exceed 50 drops per minute and may need to be reduced, or temporarily discontinued, if the patient becomes distressed. These feedings may be continued for two to three days after which solid food is again attempted orally.

The feeding mixture may be prepared in 2- to 3-qt quantities, but only small amounts—200 to 300 ml—may be put into the overhanging bottle at one time; the remainder is stored in the refrigerator. There is danger of large growths of bacteria when the mixture remains at room temperature for long periods of time, especially in very warm weather. The overhanging bottle should be changed two to three times daily, but the nasal tube may be left in place for 24 to 36 hours.

**Prognosis.** The duration and severity of attacks of pernicious vomiting vary greatly. Some patients are ill for a long time, even with careful treatment, and continue to vomit some throughout the pregnancy, while others recover in a few days. There may be a relapse after the patient returns home. Pernicious vomiting may recur in succeeding pregnancies.

Vomiting may end fatally in some cases, especially if liver or kidney damage has occurred, but prognosis is usually excellent with early and persistent treatment. Frequent check on the body weight and for the presence or absence of acetone and acetoacetic acid in the urine is important, since these signs are indicative of whether or not the condition is improving.

## TOXEMIAS OF PREGNANCY

While we grant that childbearing is a normal physiologic process, we know that during the period of gestation there is a narrow margin between health and disease. One is insistently reminded of this when considering the complications grouped under the general head of the toxemias of pregnancy. Since they are an important cause of maternal and fetal deaths they are all serious complications. About 6 to 7 per cent of all pregnant patients have one or the other of these toxemias, and at least one-third of the total maternal mortality rate can be attributed to them. Fetal deaths caused by the toxemias are even considerably greater. It is estimated that many of the stillbirths and neonatal deaths in this country each year are the result of the toxemias of pregnancy.

Although there has been a marked decrease in the maternal death rate in recent years due to the toxemias, they are still a leading cause of death. Many of these deaths are preventable through good prenatal care and early recognition of signs and symptoms of toxemia so that treatment can be instituted before the condition becomes critical.

Nothing definite is known about the cause of the toxemias except that they are due to, or aggravated by, pregnancy. Speculation as to their underlying cause is constantly changing. Some authorities attribute the toxemias to disturbed maternal metabolism. It is known that the general metabolism of the woman changes considerably during pregnancy. Just why all these changes occur is not known, but many of them are believed to be due to a chemical or hormonal stimulation. Many of these changes, especially increase in weight, become more marked during the toxemic disturbances. The toxemias seem to be the result of, or at least are accompanied by, deviations in the usual physiologic changes of pregnancy. However uncertain is knowledge concerning the origin of the toxemias of pregnancy, the entire subject of the treatment is of enormous importance to nurses since the efficacy of both preventive and curative treatment is in a large measure dependent upon skillful and intelligent nursing care.

Although there is not entire agreement as to cause and treatment of the toxemias the general pattern of care is the same. It is generally conceded that all of these patients need to have treatment which will increase diuresis, reduce edema, and reduce blood pressure so that convulsions will not develop. Since the toxemic patient's nervous system is irritated, sometimes slightly and sometimes profoundly, she should be protected from outside irritation and stimulation. This means quiet; a soft light, occasionally darkness in the room, gentle handling, and, with mildly toxic, conscious patients, a pleasant, reassuring, and encouraging manner. Extra care should be taken with unconscious patients that each touch is the lightest and gentlest possible for fear of bringing on a convulsion.

There is not complete agreement as to the classification of the toxemias of pregnancy, but they may be considered as consisting of two main types. The one type is an acute hypertensive disease which occurs only in pregnancy while the other is a chronic hypertensive disease not peculiar to pregnancy, but either first making its appearance in pregnancy or being greatly exaggerated by the added strain of gestation. The onset of the acute disease, which occurs only in pregnancy, is after the twenty-fourth week and usually not until after the thirtieth week, while the chronic hypertensive disease usually, but not always, manifests itself before the twenty-fourth week. They are characterized by edema, hypertension, and/or albuminuria and in severe cases lead to convulsions, coma, and death.

## HYPERTENSIVE DISEASE

Hypertensive disease, also known as essential hypertension or hypertensive vascular disease, is not a true toxemia of pregnancy, but it is frequently first recognized in pregnancy and it presents some of the symptoms of a toxemia. It is due to peripheral resistance produced by involvement of the arterioles which becomes more marked in the severe form of the disease. Although hypertensive disease is not peculiar to pregnancy, it is considered with the toxemias because pregnancy may be an aggravating and possibly a predisposing factor, and because the patient with essential hypertension often develops a superimposed pre-eclampsia or acute toxemia. Hypertensive disease in pregnancy is seen most frequently among pregnant women in the older age group, in multigravidas, and in obese women.

**Signs and Symptoms.** Evidence of this disease is variable. Frequently the only sign of chronic hypertensive disease in pregnancy is the presence of hypertension before the twenty-fourth week of gestation. In many of these women a persistently elevated blood pressure and possibly slight changes in the retinal blood vessels are the only evidences of the disease throughout pregnancy. Signs are typically present from the onset of pregnancy, unlike those of acute toxemia. These women usually feel well with the possible exception of having headaches. A small percentage of patients have a more advanced disease and show varying degrees of cardiac, renal, and/or retinal damage. Blood pressure readings may vary from slight elevation to levels of 300/160 mm Hg. Marked narrowing and tortuosity of the retinal blood vessels and retinal exudates and hemorrhages may be present if the disease is severe, especially if the kidneys are involved. Albuminuria and edema are ordinarily not present, as in an acute toxemia, unless there is severe retinal damage. Some patients have cardiac hypertrophy or electrocardiographic changes.

About 25 per cent of patients with chronic hypertensive disease in pregnancy develop a superimposed pre-eclampsia, and this is apt to occur earlier than pre-eclampsia ordinarily appears. This development may be manifested by a sudden exacerbation of previous signs, sudden weight gain, edema, albumin in the urine, and retinal hemorrhages and exudates.

**Diagnosis.** It may be difficult to differentiate between hypertensive disease and pre-eclampsia unless it is definitely known that the woman had hypertension before her pregnancy. A careful history and physical examination and laboratory studies should always be done. In severe cases cardiac enlargement and functional changes may be present, and kidney function may be decreased. Examination of the eyegrounds may show hemorrhages and exudates which are not present in pre-eclampsia.

The response of the blood pressure, weight, urinary output, and albumin output while the patient is under treatment of bed rest and dietary control may be of value in diagnosis.

Sometimes chronic hypertensive disease cannot be differentiated from pre-eclampsia until some time after delivery. The differential diagnosis can usually be made during the puerperium since in pre-eclampsia the blood pressure usually falls rapidly to normal, the weight decreases rapidly, and the casts and albumin disappear from the urine in from two to four weeks. In chronic hypertension complicating pregnancy, on the other hand, although the blood pressure falls somewhat and albumin, if present, decreases in amount as the patient's condition improves, by the end of the puerperium the blood pressure is still elevated and casts and albumin may still be present in the urine (Chart III).

**Treatment and Nursing Care.** The value of regular urinalyses and observations upon the blood pressure and weight gain, which are included in prenatal care in the interest of prevention, must once more be mentioned. Although hypertensive disease cannot be prevented through prenatal care, evidence of disease can be recognized early and proper treatment instituted if the prenatal care is adequate.

Patients with mild hypertensive disease frequently need only careful evaluation of their cardiovascular status, close observation during pregnancy, and instructions to report untoward symptoms early. Considerable rest and limitation of activity, curtailment of weight gain, and prevention of edema formation are of paramount importance. The more severely ill patient and the one who develops an acute toxemia require hospitalization and intensive treatment.

Hospital treatment and nursing care are about the same as for pre-eclampsia: rest in bed, a high-protein, low-sodium diet, adequate fluids, and close observations upon the general condition of the patient.

Rest in bed and mild sedation may be of value in reducing the

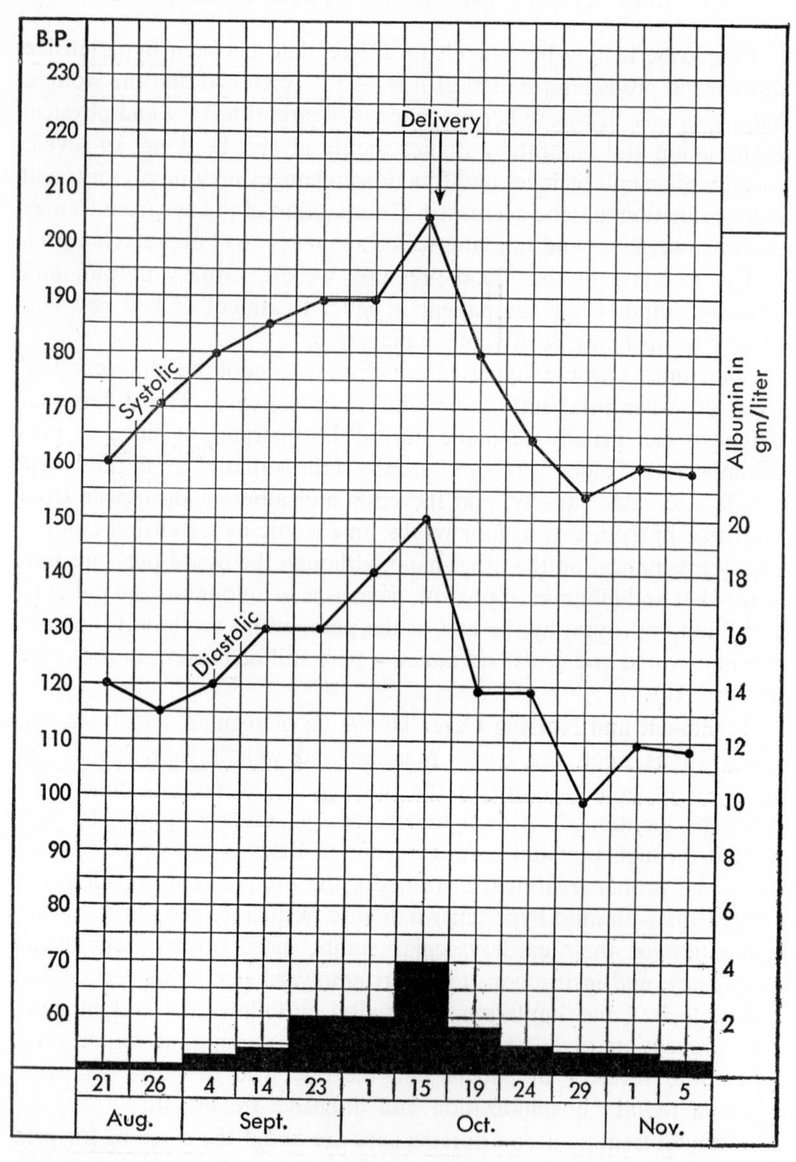


Chart III. Showing persistence of high blood pressure and albumin after delivery of patient with severe chronic hypertensive disease.

hypertension, and some cases will show improvement when placed at bed rest. The nurse should not allow the patient to exert herself any more than is absolutely necessary.

A diet low in sodium and adequate, or sometimes high, in protein content is given. The amount of protein given depends upon the presence of albumin in the urine since an attempt is usually made to supply the basic needs and to replace that which is lost in the urine. Unless the output of albumin is very high, 100 gm of protein per day will frequently supply this need.

Edema is due to an abnormal increase in the amount of fluid that surrounds the cells. To accumulate this additional fluid both water and sodium must be present. The healthy person can consume large amounts of sodium without becoming edematous since she can excrete that which she does not need, but under abnormal conditions sodium accumulates in the body due to poor excretion. This is true in the toxemias of pregnancy. It is on the basis of this knowledge that the low-sodium diet is used in the treatment of patients with edema, to reduce the chances of further accumulation of fluid and to even decrease that present. It is not ordinarily considered necessary to restrict the fluid intake in edematous patients, but the sodium intake must be kept low.

The diet used for patients with edema is often called a low-salt diet because salt is the chief sodium-containing compound used in preparation of food. It is necessary, however, to give thought to restriction of other foods with a high-sodium content when it is necessary to keep the sodium intake quite low.

The average daily diet contains from 4000 to 6000 mg of sodium. If salt is not added at the table and very obviously salted foods, such as ham or salted crackers, are omitted, the sodium intake may be reduced to 2000 mg per day; this salt-poor diet may be sufficient restriction in some cases. On the other hand, in cases of edema, it may be necessary to reduce the sodium intake to 800 mg daily or, in some instances, as low as 200 to 300 mg daily.

It is not only essential for the nurse to know which foods ordinarily have a high-sodium content and therefore need to be restricted, but also to remember that the diet must be so planned that it provides a sufficient amount of the nutritive foods that are essential to the patient. Although sodium is present in all foods, only a few common foods have a natural high-sodium content; these, however, are largely the protein foods of which the patient needs large amounts. Meat, fish, fowl, eggs, and milk are high in sodium. Eggs, which have a high-sodium content, are usually limited to one a day. Cheese is salted and is therefore high in sodium. Meat juices and broths should be restricted because they may have absorbed a considerable amount of sodium from the meat in the cooking process. In general, vegetables contain more sodium than fruits. Beets, celery, and the dark green leafy vegetables have a high-sodium content and should be restricted. Salt brine is used in the preparation of some frozen vegetables; this may add enough salt to the vegetable to be of significance. Frozen peas and lima beans should not be used. Bread and butter must be salt free. Foods that are prepared with salt, baking powder, or baking soda should not be included in the diet. This excludes many commercially processed foods which often contain sodium salts for purposes of preservation, improvement of color or flavor, and as leavening agents. Cooked cereals, prepared without salt, may be used; dry cereals should be omitted with the exception of puffed wheat, puffed rice, and shredded wheat.

Labels should be read on all cooking fats and oils although most are unsalted. It is best to read the labels on all commercially prepared food. Frozen fish are sometimes salted. Most fruits are low in sodium, but occasionally sodium benzoate is used for preservation of fruit juice concentrates. Sometimes salt substitutes contain sodium in another form.

If the prenatal patient is to have sufficient milk, which has a high-sodium content, and all the nutritives that it contains on a diet which greatly restricts sodium, it is necessary to use a low-sodium milk. Some people can drink this milk plain, but many find it unpalatable without additional flavoring, such as chocolate or vanilla and some sugar. Some prefer it served hot with powdered coffee or sugar and powdered cocoa (American process should be used). Low-sodium milk can be used instead of regular milk in the preparation of soups and puddings and in any other cooking.

Unsalted nuts are sometimes used to increase the protein in the diet. One egg and meat or fish, 5 oz, are allowed daily. Canned, unsalted meat and fish can be purchased.

Everything possible must be done to make the low-sodium diet palatable and attractive, and the patient must understand the reason for sodium restriction to obtain her cooperation. Salt substitutes are on the market and can be used, although to some patients they have an unpleasant taste and the patient may prefer to get along without them. These substitutes must not contain sodium in any form. Seasonings help to make the food more palatable; sage, thyme, onion, horseradish, garlic, vinegar, lemon juice, and chili sauce and salad dressings prepared without salt may be used. Jams and jellies are allowed. Desserts will have to consist largely of fruit puddings, cornstarch puddings, fruit pies with unsalted crust, and gelatin mixtures. Low-sodium ice cream and cookies can be purchased or made at home. Fruits serve very well for desserts. Candy, bakery-made desserts, and pudding mixes contain salt.

Tea and coffee are allowed. Most soft drinks and beer contain too much sodium, but Coca Cola is permissible.

Fluids are usually allowed up to 2500 to 3000 ml per day. Water is a good diuretic, and the patient with renal damage may need this fluid to eliminate waste material. Magnesium sulfate, given by mouth daily, may remove some fluid from the tissues.

In order to discover any change in the patient's condition, the weight is checked frequently, sometimes daily, the blood pressure is taken once or twice daily, and an accurate record of the fluid intake and output is kept. Usually all urine is saved for determining the amount of albumin in 24-hour urine specimens. Since any changes in the above may determine further treatment the nurse cannot be impressed too strongly with the importance of accuracy in all of these recordings. Headache, dizziness, and/or disturbance in vision also should be noted and reported to the doctor immediately.

In addition to measuring the output of urine, tests are often made to ascertain as nearly as possible the efficiency of the kidneys' function. The results of such tests as well as the above observations are important in the decision as to the patient's care throughout the remainder of her pregnancy. It should, then, be apparent to the nurse that all these tests must be regarded with great seriousness and carried out with meticulous attention to each detail. Most of them are concerned with the amount of phenolsulfonphthalein or urea that the kidneys are able to excrete in a given time and their ability to dilute and concentrate urine. To ascertain this, specimens of urine are obtained at specified intervals. If there is error in the time of collecting the specimens, misleading impressions may be given to the doctor. For this reason it is of great importance that the nurse carry out all orders and make all reports with absolute accuracy.

Further treatment will depend upon the severity of the symptoms, the findings of the above tests, the results obtained by treatment, and the stage of pregnancy.

**Prognosis.** If hypertensive disease is mild and if pre-eclampsia is not superimposed, the pregnancy usually continues without hazard. Severe hypertension, cardiac or renal involvement, advanced retinal changes, and a superimposed pre-eclampsia may endanger the life of the mother and may result in death of the fetus in utero. Many doctors believe that pregnancy is contraindicated and may recommend that it be terminated in the small number of patients who have a severe form of the disease. If a superimposed acute toxemia develops, there is a high incidence of fetal death in utero and an increased incidence of abruptio placentae. When such a condition does not respond to intensive treatment the doctor may recommend early delivery of the baby. These patients are apt to have a recurrence of an acute toxemia in subsequent pregnancies.

## PRE-ECLAMPSIA—MILD

Mild pre-eclampsia, a hypertensive disease of pregnancy, makes its appearance during the last two months of pregnancy and is the mildest of the toxemias. There is usually some excess weight gain; elevation of blood pressure, systolic usually not above 140 mm Hg and diastolic around 90 mm Hg; and from a fraction of albumin in the urine to 1 to 2 gm per liter. The woman may have no subjective symptoms or she may notice some swelling of the ankles and legs and some headache.

If the signs and symptoms are mild, treatment at home may be sufficient. Extra rest, adequate fluid intake, and a low-salt diet are prescribed. Caloric intake is usually restricted because some of the excessive weight gain may be due to a high-caloric intake, and a large weight gain seems to predispose to toxemia. If improvement is not noticed in a few days, hospitalization with complete bed rest and more intensive treatment ordinarily results in improvement. Return to normal is rapid after delivery.

## PRE-ECLAMPSIA—SEVERE

Severe pre-eclampsia is the term applied to that toxemia of pregnancy which is the immediate forerunner of eclampsia; it is seen more frequently among women who are pregnant for the first time than among those who have borne children.

Pre-eclampsia often responds to treatment if it is prompt and adequate, but if neglected it almost inevitably develops into the most severe aspects of the disease. The imperative need of intelligent supervision and care during pregnancy is once more evident to us, therefore, since this supervision discloses early signs and symptoms which indicate the pressing need for treatment.

Pre-eclampsia seldom appears before the second half of pregnancy, usually not until the sixth or seventh month. At that time edema, hypertension, and albuminuria appear in a patient who has thus far had a normal pregnancy. The disease runs a more acute course than the toxemia associated with chronic hypertensive disease.

**Signs and Symptoms.** Large quantities of water may be stored in the tissues before edema is noticeable, so that an abnormally large weekly gain in weight is sometimes the first evidence of a toxemia. A sudden gain or one of .7 to .9 kg (1.5 to 2 lb), or more, per week should be considered a sign of impending trouble.

Another particularly important sign of pre-eclampsia is a rise in blood pressure. The normal blood pressure for the expectant mother is somewhat dependent upon her age and also upon her previous reading, but a blood pressure of 140/90 mm Hg is usually considered as evidence of impending toxemia. Any increase of 30 mm Hg, or more, in the systolic reading is significant even when this reading is below 140 mm Hg. The diastolic pressure is an even more reliable prognostic sign, and if it rises to and remains at 90 mm Hg, or more, pre-eclampsia must be considered as a possible cause. The blood pressure may rise to 180/110 mm Hg in severe cases; if it rises to 200 or more the toxemia is apt to be due to chronic hypertensive vascular disease.

Following a rapid gain in weight and a rise in blood pressure, changes are noticed in the urine. Albumin is present; at first in only small amounts above the 0.2 gm per 24 hours which the normal pregnant woman may excrete, but it may continue to rise up to 6 to 8 gm per liter. The urinary output may be diminished and in severe cases it becomes very concentrated. In addition to increasing amounts of albumin, the urine also contains casts, red and white blood cells, and epithelial cells.

After the appearance of these three signs the patient begins to notice symptoms; some of these may be due to cerebral hypoxia. Early symptoms which may be observed by the patient are tightness of her rings and shoes because of swelling in her hands and feet. Puffiness of the eyelids and conjunctiva may appear, as well as edema in other parts of the body. The edema may be very marked in the hands, face, abdominal wall, and vulva so that the patient appears quite puffy. She frequently complains of visual disturbances which may vary from a slight blurring, spots before the eyes, and double vision to temporary blindness in severe cases. Visual disturbances are due to retinal edema, spasm of the retinal arterioles, and a detachment of the retina, which reattaches itself in a few weeks post partum. Headache, dizziness, depression, apprehension, and nausea and vomiting are other prominent symptoms, and when the condition is grave there may be epigastric pain, rapid pulse, extreme nervousness, and excitement. Epigastric pain is a late symptom and may indicate that convulsions are imminent. Drowsiness may appear and grow deeper and deeper until the patient sinks into a coma. The child may perish as a result of the toxemia, and a dead, premature baby be born.

**Prevention.** Obviously, prevention is of outstanding importance in any consideration of pre-eclamptic toxemia. The nurse should urge all patients to seek prenatal care early, and report regularly. Since the amount and rate of increase in weight, a rising blood pressure, and the appearance of albumin in the urine are valuable aids in making an early diagnosis of a toxemia of pregnancy, and since these three warning signs are not noticeable to the patient, the need for careful prenatal check is quite obvious. The patient may even feel quite well while these signs are making their appearance. Although swelling of the feet and ankles are frequently present in normal pregnancies they should always be carefully investigated, especially when present on arising in the morning. The nurse should watch closely for the symptoms enumerated above and impress upon the patient the urgent importance of speedily reporting the symptoms that she herself may observe. Both nurse and patient should constantly bear in mind that the best results are obtained by *prompt* treatment of *early* signs.

Restriction of the total weight gain during pregnancy to 9 kg (20 lb) is a prophylactic measure, since patients with an excessive gain in weight are more apt to develop toxemia than those with an average gain. Restriction of the salt intake during pregnancy is also a preventive measure. Restriction of salt is particularly important during the last trimester, and especially for women who are known to be predisposed to toxemia, which includes those with chronic hypertension, obesity, diabetes, and multiple pregnancy.

**Treatment and Nursing Care.** As might be expected, the details of treatment and nursing care of the pre-eclamptic patient vary with the severity of the signs and symptoms. The essentials of treatment, however, may be summed up as rest, increased diuresis, regulated diet, sedatives, and close watching for unfavorable symptoms, and ultimately delivery.

The surest way to have the patient really rest is to put her at complete bed rest, even in rather mild cases, and recovery is usually much hastened by this measure. Sedatives, frequently in the form of sodium phenobarbital, are often given to relieve the patient's nervousness and excitability.

Ammonium chloride may be used to promote diuresis. It does this by inducing acidosis and thus is not used if there is a suspicion of renal insufficiency. It is usually administered in dosages of 4 gm per day for two or three days at a time, with rest periods of two to three days between repetitions of the treatment. Magnesium sulfate or citrate of magnesia, given by mouth every day or two, may help to rid the body of fluid.

Fluids are given up to 2500 to 3000 ml daily, and the high-protein, low-sodium diet, as discussed under the treatment for chronic hypertension complicating pregnancy, is used for similar reasons.

Because pre-eclampsia runs a more acute course than hypertensive disease during pregnancy, the patient must be watched very carefully for any change in her condition. The weight is taken daily, and an accurate record of fluid intake and output is kept to determine whether there is an increase or decrease in the storage of fluid in the tissues. The urine is examined daily for the amount of albumin that is excreted in each 24-hour period and for casts. The blood pressure may need to be recorded every four hours, or even more frequently if the condition seems serious. The retina is examined every day or two for arteriole changes and edema. Any increase in symptoms, such as headache, dizziness, visual disturbances, and nausea and vomiting, should be carefully noted and reported since they may be danger signals. Severe epigastric pain and a feeling of constriction about the chest are regarded as especially grave symptoms, since they frequently are signs of imminent convulsions.

If pre-eclampsia is severe, as indicated by a very high blood pressure, marked edema, low urinary output, large amount of albumin in the urine, and signs of central nervous system irritability, it may be necessary to administer rather heavy sedation to prevent convulsions. Morphine, paraldehyde, or barbiturates may be given to promote drowsiness. Magnesium sulfate may be administered as a central nervous system depressant, hypotensive agents may be used, and hypertonic glucose may be given to promote diuresis. This intensive treatment with drugs is somewhat similar to the treatment of eclampsia and is discussed more completely under that heading.

In the majority of cases of pre-eclampsia, especially when not very severe, the patient improves under treatment. When there is an increase in urinary output, a decrease in the body weight, a decrease in the amount of albumin in the urine, and a fall in the blood pressure, the danger of a serious outcome decreases.

On the other hand, the patient sometimes appears to improve so markedly under treatment that all danger seems to be past, when eclampsia suddenly develops. Convulsions have appeared in patients whose urine was negative and blood pressure normal less than 24 hours before the attack. It must be remembered, therefore, that all patients who have had, or who are suffering from, pre-eclampsia are potential eclamptics until after delivery. Accordingly, although eclampsia is usually considered a preventable disease, it sometimes occurs after the most painstaking and skillful care.

Many pre-eclamptic patients are near term, and labor begins spontaneously. If it does not begin, and if the patient's condition does not improve with the above treatment, delivery of the baby may be considered. From the standpoint of the baby it becomes necessary to weigh the hazards of a premature birth against the possibility of death in utero. Each case must be considered individually, and many factors will influence the course to be followed. Delivery of the baby is postponed until after a day or two of intensive treatment in the hospital, in order to improve the patient's condition to some degree.

If improvement is not apparent after a few days of treatment, and if labor does not begin, the doctor may then consider delivery necessary, in order to prevent convulsions and residual hypertension in the mother and possible intrauterine fetal death. The method of delivery will depend upon the duration of pregnancy and the condition of the cervix. If the patient is near term, and if the uterine muscle is irritable and the cervix is soft and partially effaced, rupture of the membranes, for induction of labor, may be the method of choice. In other cases a cesarean section may be considered.

Treatment and watchfulness are just as important post partum as they were before delivery, since the danger of eclampsia is not past until enough time has elapsed following the birth of the baby to allow for definite improvement.

**Prognosis.** In general, the prognosis for pre-eclamptic patients is good when treatment is prompt. If improvement is not evident with bed rest and medical treatment, delivery of the baby is effective. Recovery is usually quite prompt following delivery, with disappearance of all signs of toxemia in 10 to 14 days (Chart IV). In some cases the hypertension persists, especially if the toxemia was severe or of long duration, or there may be a recurrence of toxemia, at least to a mild degree, in subsequent pregnancies.

Prognosis for the baby is less favorable than for the mother, with stillbirth or premature birth being the greatest hazard.

## ECLAMPSIA

Eclampsia is an acute toxemia occurring before, during, or after labor and constitutes one of the gravest complications that arise in obstetrics. It is characterized by convulsions and coma and sometimes results in the death of mother or infant.

Eclampsia practically always occurs during the latter half of pregnancy and becomes more frequent the nearer term is approached. About two-thirds of all cases occur in primigravidas. It occurs more often in twin than in single pregnancies, and its incidence is greater when pregnancy is complicated by hydramnios. The frequency with which the disease appears has been decreasing each year as more women receive prenatal care, but the incidence is still rather high in areas where economic and social conditions are poor and good prenatal care is not sought or is not readily available.

No one, so far, knows definitely the cause of eclampsia. So much study and investigation have been conducted, however, in search of a clue and so many explanations have been advanced that the condition is sometimes called "the disease of theories." A review of the many theories advanced would probably be more bewildering than illuminating to the nurse and accordingly will not be attempted. Further information may be obtained from an obstetric text.

**Signs and Symptoms.** The signs of eclampsia, as a rule, are those of pre-eclamptic toxemia which have persisted and grown more

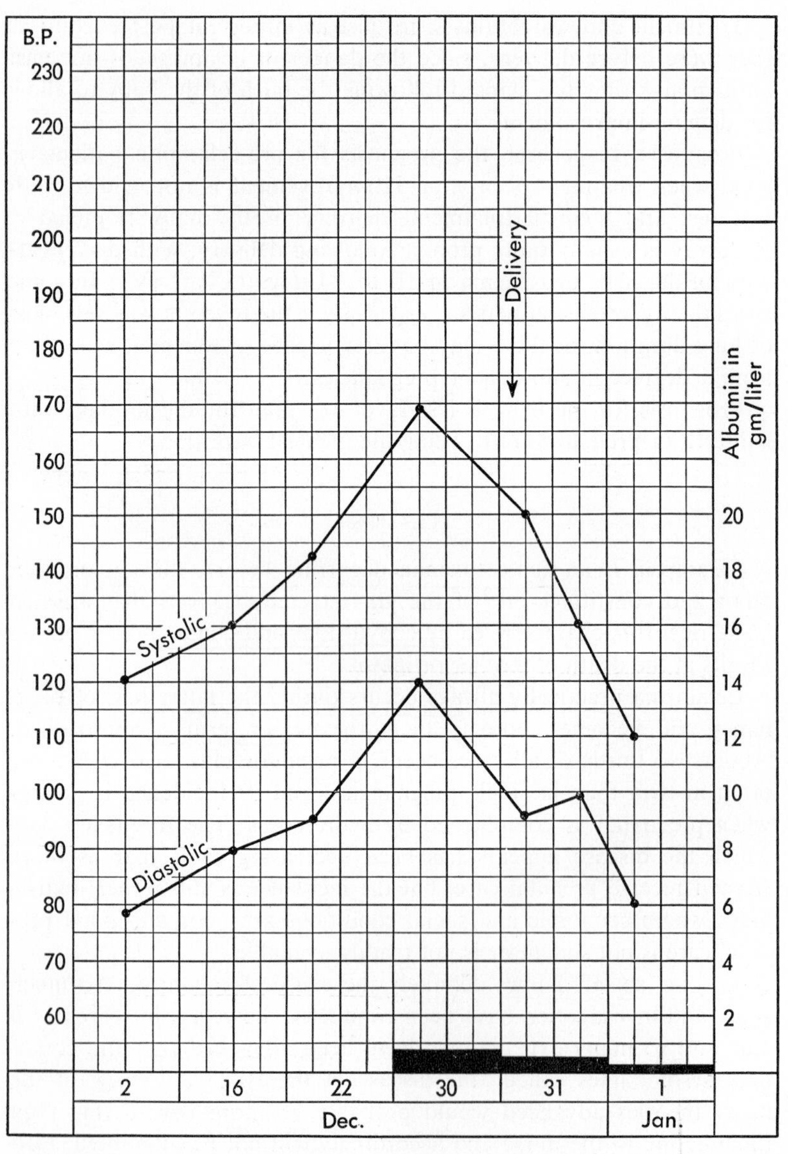


Chart IV. Showing fall in blood pressure and decrease in albumin after delivery of patient with severe pre-eclampsia.

severe, accompanied by convulsions and coma. Edema is present, sometimes to a severe degree; there may have been a tremendous gain in weight. The urine is scanty in amount, frequently less than 600 ml in 24 hours, or anuria may be present. The urine contains many and varied casts, red blood cells, and albumin which varies in amount from a few grams per liter to 10 gm during the acute stage and may even go as high as 30 to 40 gm in severe cases. The average blood pressure is 180/110 mm Hg or it may rise to 200/110. It may, however, be considerably lower in some cases of eclampsia. A rise to 140/90 mm Hg may be serious in an individual who had a very low blood pressure at the beginning of pregnancy.

The symptoms which were enumerated in discussing pre-eclampsia become more severe in the eclamptic patient. There may be visual disturbances such as blurring or even complete blindness usually due to edema of the retina, but sometimes due to brain edema, hemorrhagic retinitis, or retinal detachment. The sightlessness may last for as long as a week after the convulsions have ceased, but there is seldom any permanent damage to vision after eclampsia. Severe epigastric pain and a feeling of tightness around the thorax are signs of an impending convulsion.

Convulsions which are both tonic and clonic in character occur in eclampsia and are very distressing to watch. At first all muscles go into a state of tonic contraction; then they alternately contract and relax. The convulsions are sometimes preceded by an aura, but often are so entirely unheralded that they occur while the patient is asleep. They ordinarily begin with a twitching of the eyelids or facial muscles. The eyes are wide open and staring, and the pupils are usually dilated. Next the whole body becomes rigid, and then alternate contraction and relaxation of all muscles begin. The twitchings proceed from the muscles about the nose and mouth to those of the neck and arms, and so on, until the entire body is in spasm. The patient's face is usually cyanotic and badly distorted with the mouth being drawn to one side. She clenches her fists, rolls her head from side to side, and tosses violently about the bed. She is totally unconscious and insensible to light, and during the seizure respirations cease. Her head is frequently bent backward; her neck forms a continuous curve with her stiffened, arched back. Another distressing feature is the protruding tongue and the frothy saliva, which is bloodstained if the patient is not prevented from biting her tongue by the introduction of some sort of a mouth gag between her teeth. Finally muscular movements become milder, and then the patient lies motionless. After a long deep breath, respiratory movements are resumed. Such is the typical eclamptic convulsion.

The attacks vary greatly in their intensity and duration. There may be only a few twitches, lasting 10 to 15 seconds, or violent convulsions lasting as long as two minutes; their number and severity increase with the seriousness of the patient's condition. In mild cases there may be but one or two convulsions, particularly if the onset is either late in labor or post partum. As a rule, there are several convulsions; 5 to 10 and sometimes more.

The patient goes into a coma after a convulsion, and this also varies in length and profundity; her condition during the intervals being very suggestive of the probable outcome of the disease. If the attacks recur frequently, as they usually do in extreme cases, the patient is likely to remain unconscious during the entire interval. However, she will usually awaken between attacks that are far apart, and this is regarded as a hopeful sign. Some patients have no recollection of the seizures and may even fail to remember anything that happened within several hours, or even days, before the attack. In an occasional case eclampsia is followed by an acute psychosis during which the patient may become very violent. This psychotic disturbance appears about the second or third day after delivery and is usually attributed to the toxemia. Unless the patient has a psychopathic tendency the outlook is good.

During the acute stage the respirations are, as a rule, labored and noisy, and cyanosis may be present. When the pulse is full and bounding, the outlook is considered good. The temperature is often normal or rises to 38.3° C (101° F). It may go as high as 39.4° C (103° F) or 40° C (104° F), in severe cases, and this is a serious prognostic sign.

When eclampsia develops during late pregnancy, labor may begin and the child be born spontaneously, or the fetus may die, after which the condition begins to improve and the infant is born later in a macerated state; or the patient may improve considerably without either the birth or the death of the fetus, but she needs careful watching for return of signs and symptoms.

When eclampsia occurs in labor, contractions usually increase in force and frequency, thus hastening delivery, after which the condition soon begins to improve. Death or expulsion of the fetus is followed by cessation of the symptoms in 12 to 24 hours (coma may continue a few hours or a day), and by ultimate recovery, providing adequate treatment is continued and the condition has not become critical before delivery of the baby or its death in utero has occurred.

In postpartum eclampsia the convulsions occur soon after delivery; almost always within the first 24 hours. They also may occur just once or frequently, and the outcome depends upon whether this is a mild or severe case.

**Treatment and Nursing Care.** Prevention is of first importance. In the vast majority of cases this is accomplished by means of prenatal care and supervision including treatment of pre-eclamptic toxemia. Since there are usually premonitory signs and symptoms—those of pre-eclampsia—before convulsions begin, careful attention to the treatment of pre-eclampsia as soon as any evidence of it appears and delivery of the baby if the condition does not improve with treatment constitute preventive measures.

In the treatment of eclampsia all efforts are directed toward controlling the convulsions, toward promoting vasodilatation to combat vasospasm, and toward promoting diuresis to reduce edema. Convulsions are controlled by the use of sedation and by protection of the patient against any stimulation. A number of drugs may be used for controlling convulsions and for promoting vasodilatation; these may be used either individually or in a combination of several. Since large doses may be necessary for adequate treatment the patient must be carefully watched for untoward reactions. The first essential of nursing care is for the nurse to realize that she is caring for a gravely ill patient and that every detail of the treatment ordered is important and must be executed with skill and understanding.

The intracranial pressure is frequently raised in patients with eclampsia, and they are therefore very irritable, so that any sudden change due to fright or other stimulation may start a convulsion. To this end there are innumerable details to be considered. Every effort is made to keep the patient as quiet and free from stimuli as possible. This is accomplished by keeping her in a quiet, darkened room and by administering morphine or other sedatives as ordered. Every act must be performed as quietly as possible. The nurse should walk lightly. She should consciously guard against kicking or striking the bed. All talking should be in low tones, doors should be opened and closed quietly, and papers should not be rustled or furniture scraped on the floor. The room should be as dark as feasible, with the source of light screened from the patient's eyes. Since any manipulation may excite a convulsion the patient should not be disturbed more than is absolutely necessary. Only the care which is essential for treatment and for observation of the patient's general condition should be given. All manipulation in the form of baths, back rubs, changing of linen, and adjusting of pillows, which is not absolutely essential, should be omitted from the nursing care of the eclamptic patient for fear of starting a convulsion.

Constant nursing care is necessary, however, and the patient must never be left alone for even a second. She must be carefully observed for any change in condition and especially for twitchings, cyanosis, and excessive mucus. Someone must be present to prevent the patient from injuring herself during convulsions and to remove mucus from the respiratory passages as it collects.

Restraint during convulsions should be as mild as possible since resistance only increases the patient's excitement while her need is to be quieted, but she must be protected against falling out of bed and against injuring her tongue. During a convulsion there is a great danger of the patient biting her tongue unless something is placed between her teeth at the very onset to prevent their closing on the tongue. A small roll of bandage, a clean cloth tightly rolled, several tongue depressors wrapped with gauze, or a piece of thick rubber tubing will answer admirably and must always be at the bedside and available for immediate use. Hard wooden mouth gags are not altogether satisfactory because of the danger of bruising or cutting the mucous membranes or even breaking a tooth. If the patient is wearing dentures they should be removed during the acute course of the disease.

Careful watching and proper position are necessary to keep the patient from aspirating excessive pulmonary secretions and vomitus. The comatose patient, or one who is vomiting, is usually turned on one side and the foot of the bed elevated to favor the escape of secretions from the air passages. In addition the nurse may have to swab the unconscious patient's mouth frequently or use suction apparatus to remove mucus. The pulmonary secretions may be so greatly increased that the patient may drown from mucus if it is not removed. Fluids should never be given orally, unless the patient is completely conscious, for fear of aspiration.

Oxygen is of value and is frequently administered, especially if edema of the lungs and cyanosis develop. Often it is administered continuously during the entire period of convulsions and coma.

The blood pressure should be checked every hour or more often, and the urinary output, temperature, pulse, and respirations at least every two hours. A decrease in the urinary output or a rise in any one of the other signs mentioned above is considered unfavorable. An indwelling catheter is usually inserted so that the urinary output can be carefully watched. It should be at least 30 ml per hour. The nurse must check the fetal heart tones at regular intervals and observe the patient carefully for signs of labor. Labor frequently begins after eclampsia develops, and the patient may not be able to report either uterine contractions or vaginal discharge. Examinations, however, should be kept to a minimum.

Morphine is frequently the first drug given when it becomes apparent that the patient needs sedation. It gives the desired action and is readily available. The initial dose may be from 16 mg (¼ gr) to 20 mg (⅓ gr); this will depend upon the size of the patient. Morphine may be continued in subsequent therapy, but many times other drugs are relied upon for sedation. The respirations must be watched and reported if they go below 10 to 12 per minute. In large doses morphine decreases urinary output, increases intracranial pressure, and tends to cause acidosis due to a decrease in elimination of carbon dioxide from the lungs.

Chloral hydrate, which is a powerful depressant, is sometimes used. When given in large doses it may cause a drop in blood pressure.

The barbiturates, or any of their derivatives, produce sleep, relax muscles, and prevent or suppress convulsions. They lower the blood pressure, sometimes to the extent of causing temporary oliguria; when given intravenously the blood pressure must be watched closely for a precipitous fall. The respirations must be watched for depression. When barbiturates are given there is a slight increase in the carbon dioxide content of the blood. Any of the barbiturate derivatives may be used, but amobarbital (sodium Amytal), sodium pentobarbital (Nembutal), and phenobarbital (sodium Luminal) are most commonly administered. The parenteral routes are used for administration; the effect of the drug is most marked when it is given intravenously.

Paraldehyde is another drug which combats convulsions and helps to lower blood pressure. It has no effect on urinary excretion. It is administered rectally with an equal amount of olive oil; there is always the possibility that it may not be retained.

Magnesium sulfate is often used along with some of the other drugs mentioned. It is both a central nervous system depressant and a vasodilator. It therefore controls convulsions and lowers blood pressure, both of which are needed in eclampsia. It is administered intramuscularly, deep into the gluteal muscles, in the upper outer gluteal quadrant, in a 25 to 50 per cent solution about every four hours for 24 hours and then every six hours if the urinary output is fair. The area of administration should be massaged, and a dry warm pack should then be applied. Sometimes the drug is given intravenously, in a 10 per cent solution every hour, until the convulsions are under control; subsequent doses depend on recurrence of convulsions or other signs. With intravenous administration the patient must be observed very closely for sudden respiratory depression.

Magnesium sulfate is eliminated from the body chiefly by the kidneys, and if the urinary output is low it may be retained in the blood until a high, dangerous concentration is reached which may depress respirations and cardiac action and cause coma and death. Rather large doses are necessary, however, to obtain good effect. The patient must be watched for respiratory depression. It is believed that this depression does not occur, however, until after the knee-jerk reflex disappears. The knee-jerk reflex is, therefore, checked before each dose is administered, and the drug is withheld if it is absent. Magnesium sulfate is discontinued if the respirations are below 16 per minute or if the knee jerks are absent, and it is usually not given for longer than 24 hours if the urinary output is only 600 ml or less per day.

An intravenous calcium preparation in the form of 10 per cent calcium gluconate or 10 per cent calcium chloride can be used as an antidote and should always be at hand in case of respiratory depression.

Other hypotensive drugs, such as one of the veratrum aklaloids and hydralazine (Apresoline), have been used to relieve vasospasm; sometimes more than one of these hypotensive drugs is used. The blood pressure must be checked frequently during the administration of any hypotensive drug.

Continuous caudal or spinal anesthesia has been used with some success. It lowers the blood pressure and increases the urinary flow.

Digitalization of the patient is sometimes necessary, especially when pulmonary edema is associated with evidence of circulatory collapse.

Hypertonic glucose is very valuable in the treatment of eclampsia. It is one excellent means of treatment for oliguria, anuria, convulsions, and coma. It promotes diuresis and restores the blood to a more normal state. In the toxemic patient it causes excretion of sodium and chlorides in the urine. The glucose is used to produce a hemodilution and thus establish a normal passage of fluids from the tissues into the circulation and an increase in the urinary output. In this way it decreases brain edema and thus decreases the likelihood of convulsions. It is given in 500- to 1000-ml amounts of a 20 per cent solution over a period of 30 to 60 minutes. Smaller amounts of a 30 to 50 per cent solution may be safer if there is evidence of pulmonary edema or cardiac failure. The optimal amount of glucose at one time is considered to be about 200 gm. Enough should be given to ensure an output of at least 30 ml of urine per hour. Injections are repeated in four to eight hours as indicated by the patient's condition and until normal diuresis begins. Hypertonic glucose has reduced the maternal mortality rate for eclampsia considerably because by its use the urinary output can frequently be increased a great deal and anuria seldom develops.

When the patient cannot take fluids orally a 5 to 10 per cent glucose solution may also be used to provide sufficient fluids and caloric intake and to overcome acidosis. From 2500 to 3000 ml total fluids are usually given in a 24-hour period; larger amounts may cause an increase in the total body fluids. A physiologic saline solution, Ringer's solution, or sodium bicarbonate solution should not be used.

With eclampsia labor may begin any time, but if this does not happen delivery of the baby is postponed until the patient has recovered from the convulsions and the coma. Although the patient's condition improves after either delivery of, or death of, the fetus, the shock that accompanies any delivery procedure when performed while the patient is critically ill outweighs the advantages that follow delivery. As a rule less harm is done by relying on medical treatment to control convulsions and increase urinary output; after improvement in the patient's condition delivery can be accomplished more safely.

Vaginal delivery is preferred, since these patients are not good risks for abdominal surgery, but when the cervix is not ready for easy dilatation a cesarean section may be done. Inhalation anesthesia is avoided in either vaginal or abdominal delivery because of the edema of the lungs.

Induction of labor is usually accomplished by rupture of the membranes; this procedure will either start labor or hasten it if it has already begun. Oxytocin (Pitocin) may also be used, but the blood pressure must be watched carefully because it may rise with the use of this drug. Oxytocin (Pitocin) will probably not produce as much elevation of blood pressure, however, as would the use of posterior pituitary extract.

Since the danger of convulsions is not over for at least 24 hours post partum, the patient must be watched very carefully for convulsions, and the treatment for eclampsia, or at least pre-eclampsia, must be continued post partum until the patient shows definite improvement. It is necessary to watch for shock following delivery by careful checking of pulse and blood pressure. The eclamptic patient's great susceptibility to infection must be kept in mind, and every precaution should be taken during and after delivery to maintain aseptic technic wherever it is necessary.

**Prognosis.** The final outcome depends upon many factors. The prognosis is more favorable after delivery, especially when the urinary output increases. An output of 800 ml or more in a 24-hour period is a good sign. When the coma disappears, the cyanosis disappears, the pulse becomes slow and full, and the temperature becomes normal, recovery can be expected.

When convulsions increase, the coma is prolonged, the urinary output is low, the blood pressure rises to over 200 mm Hg, the temperature rises to above 39.4° C (103° F), and the pulse becomes rapid and weak, the outlook is unfavorable. A lowering of blood pressure when other conditions are improving is a good sign, but a fall in the blood pressure when the pulse is weak and rapid is a sign of cardiac failure. Moist rales in the chest, bloody frothy mucus, and cyanosis are indicative of pulmonary edema and must be considered serious. Hematuria, severe albuminuria, and/or anuria are grave signs. Susceptibility to infection is increased in eclampsia, and it is especially dangerous to the patient since the kidneys and liver may already be damaged.

Death may be caused by pulmonary edema, cardiac failure, or apoplexy fairly early in the disease or when death occurs later it may be due to aspiration pneumonia or marked liver damage. There is considerable danger of pneumonia in eclampsia, due to aspiration of mucus, blood, and fluid which are present in the air passages and can readily be drawn into the lungs by the deep stertorous breathing.

When recovery from eclampsia occurs, it is comparatively rapid. In 24 to 48 hours the urinary output may be as high as 4 to 6 liters per day. An increase in the urinary output is the first sign of improvement. Edema disappears in four to five days, and as the woman loses all this fluid there is a marked difference in her appearance. The patient soon begins to feel well unless she has developed an aspiration pneumonia or other infection. The weight decreases rapidly, the blood pressure drops to normal in about two weeks, the albumin and casts disappear from the urine in about a week (Chart V), and all symptoms subside in from two to four weeks unless the attack is followed by chronic hypertension or permanent kidney damage. This presents a sharp contrast to the recovery from chronic hypertension complicating pregnancy. In the latter complication the elevated blood pressure persists, and casts and albumin may be present in the urine at the end of the puerperium.

All patients who have had either pre-eclampsia or eclampsia should have kidney-function tests done in about six months to determine if any permanent kidney damage has occurred. Some of these patients also have a residual chronic hypertension or they may have a toxemia in another pregnancy; they therefore need very careful watching during all subsequent pregnancies.

The fetal mortality in eclampsia is high due to a decreased amount of oxygen during convulsions, drugs administered to the mother, and prematurity.

## OTHER COMPLICATIONS OF PREGNANCY

Any chronic disease which puts considerable strain on the individual is more serious when present during gestation than in the woman who is not pregnant. The acute diseases are not as seriously affected by pregnancy, as the chronic ones, except that they may cause a spontaneous premature termination of pregnancy which also may lead to complications. In some instances the normal course of pregnancy may be jeopardized by the coincidental disease.

Among the more serious complications of gestation, which are not due to pregnancy, but which it is important to recognize and treat

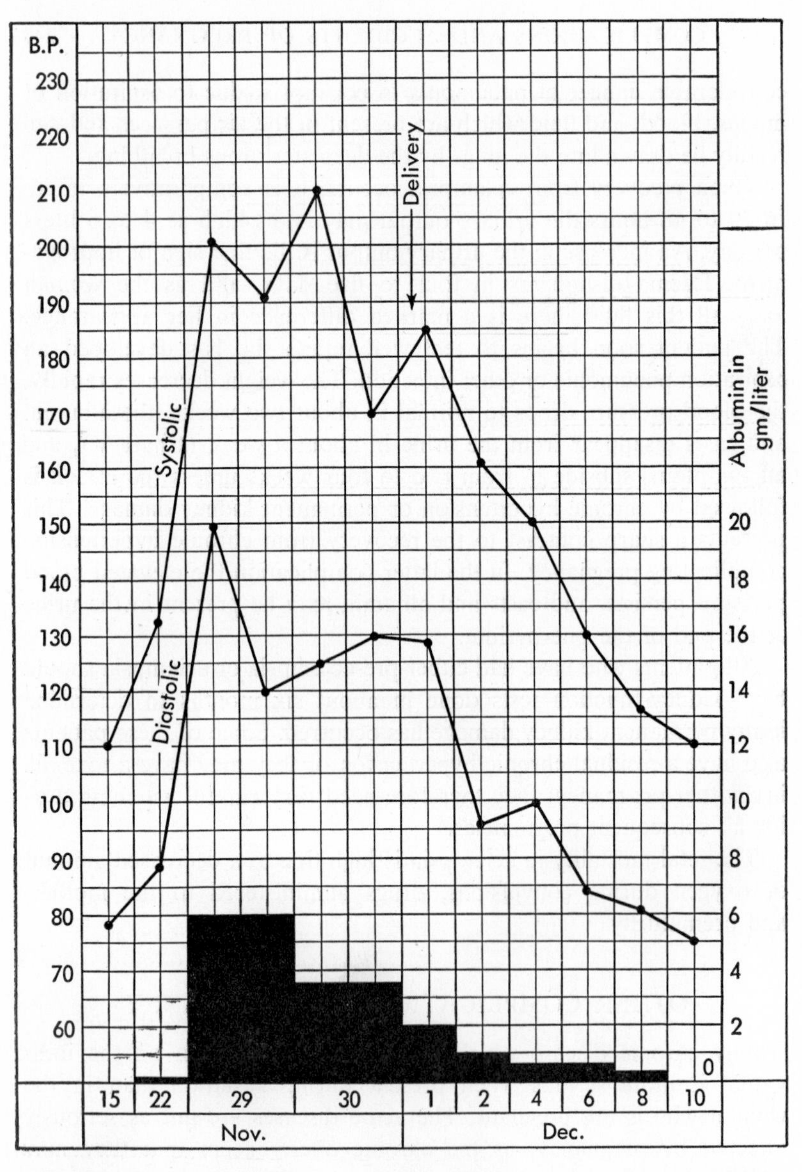


Chart V. Showing fall in blood pressure and decrease in albumin after delivery of patient with eclampsia.

early, may be included the acute infectious diseases, tuberculosis, heart disease, diabetes mellitus, pyelonephritis, syphilis, and gonorrhea.

### ACUTE INFECTIOUS DISEASES

Acute infectious diseases, such as scarlet fever, measles (rubeola), or smallpox, during pregnancy are prone to cause abortion or premature labor either due to transmission of the bacteria or toxins through the placenta to the fetus, due to changes produced in the decidua, or due to a high temperature in the mother. German measles (rubella), in the first three months of pregnancy, may cause congenital anomalies in the infant in the form of cataract, deafness, heart lesions, or mental retardation. Some estimates have placed the incidence of congenital defects up to 25 per cent, or even higher, when the mother has the disease in early pregnancy.

Colds make general anesthesia difficult. In influenza during pregnancy there has, in the past, been a high incidence of premature labor and a rather high mortality rate following delivery. The outlook has become very favorable for both mother and baby since the introduction of the antibiotics. Although these drugs may not be effective against the virus, they may prevent pneumonia as a complication of the disease.

Pneumonia is a serious complication of pregnancy, with premature labor possibly resulting because of a poor oxygen supply to the fetus and because of bacteria which may be transmitted to it. Should labor begin a considerable additional strain is placed on the mother. The treatment of pneumonia has been much more effective in the past few years with the use of the antibiotic drugs, but prevention by the proper treatment of colds is still very important. A cold in the pregnant woman must be considered serious and treated by rest in bed and supportive measures.

There is always danger of puerperal infection with any of the upper respiratory diseases due to the possibility of transmission of organisms, especially the streptococcus, to the genital tract. The incidence of streptococci in the respiratory tract is higher in the individual with an acute upper respiratory infection than in the healthy person.

### TUBERCULOSIS

Since pulmonary tuberculosis is widespread among all classes and is a disease commonly found in young women, it is not surprising to discover it fairly often among expectant mothers. The physiologic relationship between pregnancy and tuberculosis is not yet clearly established and opinions vary, but at present it appears that pregnancy does not exert an adverse effect on tuberculosis.

Since the pregnant patient with a tuberculous infection must receive special care, routine roentgenograms as a part of prenatal care, to detect early lesions, are advisable. If tuberculosis is discovered both the infection and the pregnancy need ideal management. Vomiting of pregnancy and the toxemias may have an unfavorable effect on the disease by interfering with nutrition and metabolism. Since the progress of the disease must be halted and resolution and healing promoted, the patient receives the care she would ordinarily have for a tuberculous infection without a superimposed pregnancy. This treatment remains essentially unchanged during the pregnancy, with possibly some slight modifications in certain cases. Long-term planning is essential for adequate rest and supervision. Suitable arrangements must be made for the care of the baby, since the mother will be unable to care for her baby until her disease is arrested.

As actual rest and relaxation are imperative when bed rest is ordered, the nurse is here reminded that she must make sure that the conditions surrounding her patient will make mental and physical rest possible. If the patient has other children at home, provision for a person to do the housework and care for children or other members of the family becomes necessary.

To reduce the physical strain of labor a low forceps delivery is usually considered advisable for shortening the second stage of labor. Excessive sedation and inhalation anesthesia are avoided, insofar as possible, to prevent suppression of the cough reflex. During delivery and the postpartum period it is important that good drainage of secretions is maintained to prevent accumulation in the bronchi; frequent turning after delivery and encouragement of coughing are important. The mother is not allowed to nurse the baby because of the danger to the baby from exposure to the disease and also because of the added strain this would put upon her. With adequate long-continued care the tuberculous patient may often be carried safely through the obstetric experience and suffer no permanent ill effects.

Tuberculosis is rarely transmitted to the fetus, and there seems to be no predisposition to the disease. The baby may be easily infected by its mother and accordingly is not allowed to nurse at the breast. Nor should the mother care for the baby in any manner because of the danger of contamination by droplet infection. BCG vaccination of the infant born of a tuberculous mother may be considered, but this does not decrease the need for preventive measures against infection of the baby with tubercle bacilli from the mother.

If the patient becomes pregnant after the tuberculosis has responded well to treatment, but while the lesion is still somewhat unstable, the patient must be given all possible safeguards during pregnancy, labor, and the puerperium. Hospitalization during a part of the pregnancy and for a longer than usual period during the puerperium is advisable.

Pregnancy is usually safely attempted, without danger of recurrence of tuberculosis, when a period of two years has elapsed after the lesions have been well controlled. Safety increases with time since this allows for more effective healing.

## HEART DISEASE

In the United States at large approximately 1 to 2 per cent of all pregnant women have some form of heart disease. The danger which this complication imposes upon childbearing women is considerable since, in spite of its rather infrequent occurrence, heart disease is responsible for a relatively large proportion of cases of congestive heart failure and premature labor. The effective work done during the past few years shows that many of these complications may be prevented by early and adequate care. As in many other conditions this fact is of importance to the nurse since it offers her an excellent opportunity to assist the doctor in minimizing the hazards to which heart disease subjects pregnant women.

The first step in the doctor's plan is early diagnosis, the second is detection of early symptoms of heart failure, and the third is prompt and adequate treatment.

The vast majority of cases of heart disease in expectant mothers are the result of rheumatic fever. In the course of rheumatic fever the heart valves are frequently involved or inflamed and suffer permanent injury. Because of the scarring which occurs at their edges, the valves are not able to close tightly and at the same time their orifices become narrowed. It must be recalled, however, that the heart is essentially a pump, the purpose of which is to propel blood through the body. But a pump, even if it has damaged valves, will function adequately if the force behind it is sufficient. Accordingly, women with heart disease usually do very well during pregnancy when the heart muscle is strong enough to pump suitable amounts of blood to the tissues.

The heart must work much harder during pregnancy than it does normally, and the cardiac output increases considerably. When a heart lesion is already present this added strain which usually occurs may lead to serious complications.

Once the doctor has made a diagnosis of heart disease the prognosis and treatment will depend largely upon whether or not the patient is able to carry on her usual activities without undue distress. It may rest with the nurse, in no small measure, to discover if the patient is able to lead a normal life or whether her heart condition so seriously handicaps her that she is forced to rest frequently on account of shortness of breath, for example, palpitation, or pain over the heart.

Heart failure may occur suddenly, without warning, but fortunately, it usually progresses slowly. This is of enormous importance since, if an expectant mother suffering from heart disease is seen frequently and watched carefully, and if evidence of unfavorable signs are immediately reported to the doctor, he will often be able to save the patient from serious disability. With this in mind doctors see many of these patients every two weeks.

Important causes of heart failure in expectant mothers with cardiac disease are overexertion, colds, sore throat, and influenza. If the nurse appreciates the gravity of these precipitating causes she will be able to give the doctor invaluable assistance by impressing their significance upon her patients.

The patient should avoid colds by observing the usual precautions of staying out of crowds and keeping away from people who have colds. Should a cold develop, the patient should stay in bed until entirely recovered. In the presence of even slight heart trouble the doctor will usually guard his patient from the dangers of overexertion by forbidding all heavy work, such as housecleaning, carrying heavy objects, moving furniture, shaking rugs, washing, and the like. He will advise against shopping, marketing, walking against the wind, and climbing hills or many stairs. In addition, the patient will usually be advised to spend 10 hours in bed each night and to lie down at least a half hour after each meal. Excessive weight gain during pregnancy must be avoided. Sodium is often restricted in the diet.

Should the heart condition become more serious, the patient's most imperative need will be mental as well as physical rest. So urgent is this that the nurse must not be content with simply telling the patient to stay in bed several days a week, as the doctor may order, or even to rest continuously throughout whole weeks or months. She must find out whether the patient's living conditions will make complete mental and physical rest possible. If not, it will be necessary to enlist the aid of a friend or relative or paid employee who can stay in the home and relieve the patient of anxiety and the need to attend to her usual household duties. Should such a helper not be available it will be necessary to seek assistance through a welfare agency as is explained in Chapter 8.

Patients with a cardiac disease that normally necessitates little or no limitation of physical activity rarely develop decompensation during pregnancy. Those whose cardiac reserve is limited may have an unfavorable outlook; they must often be greatly restricted during pregnancy and require careful observation for signs of decompensation. For many of these the prognosis is good unless decompensation occurs and does not improve with treatment. In certain very severe cases, particularly if the patient is seen early, the doctor may advise against pregnancy.

The expectant mother who has heart disease must, therefore, be protected in every way possible in order to avert heart failure and also to conserve her forces so that she may meet the inevitable strain to be imposed by the approaching labor. Obviously the patient should be delivered in the hospital. When labor finally occurs the doctor will resort to every known expedient to make it easy. This means relieving the discomforts of labor as much as possible and keeping the patient in bed in a semirecumbent position. Sometimes the patient is delivered while in a semirecumbent position to lessen the strain on the heart. The pulse and respiratory rate must be checked every 30 minutes during the first stage of labor and every 10 minutes during the second stage, and the patient must be watched for evidence of dyspnea. A pulse rate over 115 per minute, a respiratory rate over 28 per minute, and dyspnea are signs of cardiac embarrassment. If the second stage of labor has been reached when these signs appear, immediate delivery is advisable. When they occur earlier in labor, digitalis may be used and a sedative may be administered to provide for rest during labor. The administration of oxygen to the cardiac patient, in labor and for a short time thereafter, is often very beneficial. A low forceps delivery is frequently employed to shorten the second stage of labor unless a spontaneous delivery can be anticipated very soon after complete dilatation of the cervix and with little extra exertion on the part of the patient. The anesthesia must be chosen carefully to avoid cardiac depression or cyanosis.

The patient must be carefully observed for heart failure after delivery even when cardiac distress has not been present during pregnancy. Early ambulation is often not allowed. The cardiac patient is ordinarily kept in bed and in the hospital longer than the average healthy mother even when there have been no signs of decompensation. Having satisfactorily reached this point, the battle is by no means won since the same protection and vigilance that were observed during pregnancy must be continued until the doctor feels it is safe for the patient to undertake the care of her baby and possibly to resume her household duties. Not infrequently the patient may be able to be up and about and yet be unable to meet the added strain imposed by the care of the child.

Throughout pregnancy, labor, and the puerperium it will be absolutely necessary that not only the patient but also her family appreciate the gravity of the situation and give full cooperation in employing what may, to them, seem homely and unscientific precautions. One of the nurse's most important functions will be to support the doctor in impressing upon the patient and her family the urgency of following out every suggestion if the lives of mother and baby are to be protected. It is of equal importance that she assist with making necessary provisions for the mother to receive adequate rest. The patient and her family will usually be very cooperative if they are convinced that the patient does not necessarily face a future of invalidism, but that, on the contrary, she may expect to recover and be able to live a fairly normal life if she does all in her power to prevent heart failure during the periods of strain before and after the baby is born.

## DIABETES MELLITUS

The combination of pregnancy and diabetes mellitus may raise serious problems; the pregnancy may make the diabetes more difficult to control while the diabetes increases the incidence of certain obstetric complications. Fetal and neonatal mortality rates are increased over the general average, and the incidence of congenital anomalies is higher than in infants born to nondiabetic mothers. Present-day treatment has, however, increased the chances of fetal and infant survival, and there is now reason to believe that the average diabetic woman may, under careful supervision, pass through a period of childbearing with a reasonable degree of safety for herself and her babies. The mother with mild diabetes or with a disease of short duration may expect to go through pregnancy without complications, but the one who has severe diabetes, disease of long duration, or vascular or renal damage may have serious difficulty.

Pregnancy in the diabetic patient often results in fluctuating insulin requirement and increased tendency to acidosis. Infections—respiratory, urinary tract, or any other—add to the possibility of acidosis. Toxemias develop more frequently in the woman with diabetes, often early in the second half of pregnancy. If vascular disease existed prior to pregnancy, hypertension may progress, and a true toxemia, with all the previously described signs and symptoms, may be superimposed. The diabetic tends to retain water and become edematous, even without hypertension, and hydramnios often develops. Babies of diabetic women are often large and edematous, and their excessive size may make vaginal delivery difficult. With the above complications, and sometimes even when they are absent, fetal death may occur near the end of pregnancy, or the baby may die soon after birth.

A diabetic patient must have frequent, often weekly, examinations during pregnancy to determine the status of the diabetes and to discover early evidence of complications. Insulin and diet needs must be rigidly supervised. The urine is not necessarily kept entirely sugar free, since there is a normal tendency to a lowered renal threshold for glucose during pregnancy, but the patient's general well-being and blood sugar studies are used as guides in determining her needs. A diet with a restricted sodium intake is recommended, and diuretic drugs may be used whenever edema develops or sometimes even in the absence of signs of toxemia. Some doctors administer estrogen and progesterone because they believe that hormonal abnormalities occur in diabetic pregnancies, and that by the administration of these hormones the chances of fetal survival are improved. The patient is hospitalized whenever this is necessary to stabilize the diabetes; likewise infection, toxemia, and other complications frequently necessitate hospitalization for the diabetic.

A vaginal delivery is often planned if the diabetes is mild and if the pregnancy progresses normally, but a cesarean section may be considered desirable when complications exist or can be anticipated. In a pregnancy complicated by diabetes the baby may develop to an excessive size and thus make delivery through the birth passage difficult, breech presentations are more common, and labor is often prolonged. When a cesarean section is planned it is often performed from two to four weeks before term because the chances of fetal death increase toward the end of pregnancy, and the danger of late complications of pregnancy becomes greater. Development of a toxemia, and/or progression in severity of a pre-existing vascular or renal disease, as shown by an increase in hypertension, edema, and retinal changes, are often determining factors in the decision as to the time and method of delivery.

Whenever food and fluid must be withheld, regardless of the method of delivery that is selected, insulin and intravenous glucose are administered. Since the infant is very susceptible to respiratory distress at the time of birth, analgesic drugs are used sparingly during labor. The patient must be observed during and following labor and delivery for insulin shock, hyperglycemia, or even acidosis. Insulin requirement often changes considerably immediately following delivery, and the nurse must be alert to evidence of either too much or too little insulin. Sometimes severe insulin reactions occur following delivery. The urine must be examined approximately every two to four hours, and blood sugar studies are usually done daily until the insulin and diet needs become stable. Close observation for uterine hemorrhage is important in the immediate postpartum period, because an overdistention of the uterus with a large baby and hydramnios may result in uterine muscle atony. Careful observation and special treatment of the baby, as discussed on pages 800–802, are important at birth, and during the first few days of life.

### PYELONEPHRITIS

Pyelitis, an inflammation of the pelvis of the kidney, is a fairly common and also painful complication of pregnancy. The disease usually occurs during the latter half of pregnancy, and the right kidney is more frequently involved than the left. Although pyelitis means an inflammation of the kidney pelvis, there is also involvement of the ureter. Since the kidney structure is often involved in the inflammatory process the condition is actually a pyelonephritis.

Normally there are peristaltic waves in the kidneys and ureters which drain the kidneys and carry the urine to the bladder. During pregnancy there is atony of the smooth muscle in the ureters, and with this a lessened peristalsis and a stasis of urine. As a result there is some dilatation of the ureters and kidney pelves. Dilatation rarely occurs in the pelvic part of the ureter, but the portion above the pelvic inlet becomes involved. The pregnant uterus may cause pressure on the ureters where they cross the pelvic brim. The enlarged uterus will also displace the ureters to some extent. The right side is apt to become more involved than the left, probably due to inclination of the pregnant uterus to the right. Besides the dilatation and displacement there are also some hypertrophy, which is common in all pelvic organs during pregnancy, and elongation of the ureters. The elongation may lead to curves in the ureters and partial obstruction due to the curves. These changes progress from the fourth to the eighth month of pregnancy and then return to normal in four to six weeks post partum.

Infection occurs rather often because organisms will invade distended tissue more easily than normal tissue. This distention and the decreased drainage of urine will make the urinary tract susceptible to infection. The bacteria may travel upward from the bladder or be conveyed by the lymph and blood streams, possibly from the intestines. The colon bacillus is the most common offender although the streptococcus, staphylococcus, or even the tubercle bacillus may be the infective agent.

**Symptoms.** Frequently the patient will be entirely well, aside from a slight irritability of the bladder causing frequent micturition, and suddenly have paroxysms of acute pain in the region of the kidney, which may be swollen and very painful on palpation. She will have fever and sometimes chills, and a catheterized specimen of urine will contain pus and bacteria. The kidney may suddenly empty itself of pus after which the pain and swelling will subside, only to recur when the pus accumulates again. In severe cases the patient becomes drowsy, toxic, and has a high temperature and pulse. Such signs usually indicate that the infection is spreading from the pelvis of the kidney into the organ itself, this condition being pyelonephritis.

**Treatment.** As soon as the patient shows any signs of a urinary tract infection she should be placed at bed rest and have her fluid intake increased considerably. A urine culture is then made to determine the type of organism causing the infection so that the proper treatment can be instituted. Sulfonamides and antibiotics are very effective in the treatment of urinary tract infections. The drug administered will depend upon the bacteria found in the urine. A patient who has had pyelitis but is symptom free is not considered cured until several urine cultures are negative.

Most infections will respond to treatment quite rapidly, but a reinfection may occur for the same reasons that the first infection developed. There may also be a flare-up in the puerperium. Prompt treatment of all infections is important to prevent fibrosis of tissue which may result from the inflammation. If a chronic pyelonephritis has been present prior to the pregnancy, treatment may be more difficult.

The nursing care consists of the good general nursing that would be given to any patient suffering from an infection, in addition to the specialized treatment ordered by the doctor for each patient.

It has been demonstrated that much may be done toward preventing the development of the disease and also greatly reducing the severity of the cases that do occur. The chief preventive measures are drinking abundant fluids, thus flushing the pelves of the kidneys and the ureters, prevention of constipation, and routine microscopic examinations of the urine at each prenatal visit to discover evidence of infection. The nurse will recall, in this connection, that attention to the intake of fluids and to regular bowel movements, both of which tend to prevent pyelitis, are a part of prenatal care.

### SYPHILIS

The occurrence of syphilis in an expectant mother constitutes a very serious condition meriting prompt and efficient treatment.

Until fairly recent years syphilis was the most frequent cause of fetal death. It was also a very common cause of early infant death, to say nothing of the disastrous effects of congenital syphilis upon those infants who lived. Now, however, in obstetric clinics where Wassermann or other reliable tests are made routinely and adequate treatment is given in all positive cases, syphilis is rated as the least frequent cause of fetal death. Quite as important as the reduced death rate is the absence of syphilis in babies born of syphilitic mothers who have been satisfactorily treated for this disease before or during pregnancy.

The first, and absolutely indispensable, step toward efficient treatment of syphilis in pregnancy is to make one of the reliable diagnostic tests for the disease. One of the important functions of prenatal care is the recognition and treatment of syphilis in pregnant women. Routine serologic examinations are necessary for all patients, since a history of a primary sore or a rash is frequently not elicited and visible signs of the disease are seldom present.

Most states now have laws requiring that a serologic test be done on all prenatal patients at the first visit. Unfortunately all pregnant women do not receive prenatal care, and some of those receiving it do not have a serologic test. Congenital syphilis is a regional problem; there is more in some areas than in others. This is, no doubt, the result of inadequate prenatal care, or none at all. Occasionally, when blood tests have been done and found to be negative, some women are infected after the first prenatal visit. This has led to the proposal that a second serologic test, done in the latter months of pregnancy, may be valuable, at least where there is some suspicion that the disease may recently have been acquired.

One of the purposes of the premarital physical examination laws, enacted in many states, is to discover and treat syphilis before marriage, in order to protect the other partner and the children to be born.

The infection is transmitted from the mother to the fetus by spirochetes, which pass through the placenta, sometime between the fifth month and the time of birth. The father does not transmit the disease except insofar as he infects the mother. The fetus will be infected almost 100 per cent of the time if the pregnant woman acquires syphilis shortly before, at the time of, or shortly after conception, and does not receive treatment. There is some chance that the baby may escape the infection if the mother's disease is of long standing. When the mother acquires her infection late in pregnancy the fetus may escape intrauterine infection, but could acquire the disease by contact with infectious lesions during passage through the birth canal.

Congenital syphilis is one of the serious diseases of infancy that can be completely controlled because its prevention is understood and the method of treatment is excellent. With modern control methods it should be possible to eradicate this disease completely.

Penicillin is used as treatment in all stages of syphilis. It is a safe, effective treatment which quickly eliminates the infectiousness of the disease, prevents later complications, and effectively prevents congenital syphilis. It is easier to administer than the drugs formerly used, rarely has serious toxic effects, and does not require a long period of treatment. Adequate penicillin levels are usually maintained for about two weeks. Even though the mother does not have a negative serology by the time she delivers, a nonsyphilitic baby can be expected if she has shown a favorable response to treatment by monthly quantitative blood tests. Several months may elapse following treatment before a negative maternal blood test is obtained. A rapid drop in titer is expected following treatment of early syphilis, while even a small drop is considered a favorable response in late or latent syphilis; the decline in these cases may be quite delayed and very gradual. Re-treatment is indicated in cases not showing the normally expected response.

If treatment is begun early in pregnancy, infection of the fetus may be prevented. When the treatment is begun so late in pregnancy that the fetus is already infected, effective treatment of the baby in utero can be anticipated as the penicillin, which is administered to the mother, passes through the placenta to the fetus. Re-treatment in succeeding pregnancies is probably not necessary when the mother has once been adequately treated and if she does not become reinfected. For the prevention of congenital syphilis in subsequent pregnancies it is necessary, however, to follow these mothers carefully by monthly examinations and by quantitative serologic tests.

Although the diagnosis and treatment of syphilis are medical questions, the nurse has definite responsibilities and opportunities in advancing the work as a whole. She may aid immeasurably by extending educational work concerning the value of prenatal care and of diagnostic tests for syphilis and subsequent treatment in positive cases.

The nurse in public health work, caring for pregnant women, should make herself responsible for checking that all of these women have had a blood test and that, when indicated, they return to the doctor for proper treatment and regular follow-up care. Upon diagnosis of syphilis in any member of a family, either parent or children, follow-up of all members is necessary in a prevention program. With careful observation of the mother, prevention of congenital syphilis in the future children of this family should be possible.

Since discharges from sores and the blood of syphilitic patients in the early stages of the disease are very infectious, the nurse must observe strict isolation precautions while caring for these patients. She must be particularly careful that body discharges and/or blood from patients in the early stages of the disease do not enter her body through cuts, pin or needle pricks, or her mouth and eyes. Such an accident should be reported at once. Moist dressings and body discharges must be burned; dishes, thermometers, gloves, instruments, and all other equipment used in the care of these patients must be sterilized.

## GONORRHEA

Gonorrhea may be acquired before, during, or after conception and is a serious complication if not adequately treated. Since it may be present in a latent form and not be recognizable by signs and symptoms, patients may need to have vaginal smears taken at their first prenatal visit to discover if the infection is present. Cultures are of even more diagnostic value than smears and should be made whenever indicated.

The vaginal discharge may become profuse and purulent. It may cause great discomfort in the form of irritation and itching of the vulva, or even excoriation of the mucous membrane, and sometimes abscesses of the vulvovaginal glands, but the chief danger to the patient in an untreated gonorrheal infection is that, after delivery, the organisms may travel from the lower genital tract to the uterine cavity and the fallopian tubes, and there set up an inflammation, or possibly cause a general postpartum infection. Sterility may be one of the results of an untreated gonorrheal infection. The greatest danger to the child is infection of the eyes during the passage of the head through the birth canal, and this is the reason for the special care given the eyes of the newborn infant, which is described on pages 334–39.

Gonorrhea does not present the problems today that it did formerly when no specific therapy was available. The infection can be treated very quickly and effectively by the use of penicillin.

The nurse must observe strict isolation technic while caring for these patients until treatment is effective. She should be especially careful not to contaminate her eyes.

## BIBLIOGRAPHY AND STUDENT REFERENCES

Arnold, R. C.; Cutler, J. C.; Wright, R. D.; and Levitan, S.: "Studies in Penicillin Treatment of Syphilis," *Pub. Health Rep.,* **67**:78–89, (Jan.) 1952.

Aycock, W. Lloyd, and Ingalls, Theodore H.: "Maternal Disease as a Principle in the Epidemiology of Congenital Anomalies with a Review of Rubella," *Am. J. M. Sc.,* **212**:366–79, (Sept.) 1946.

Bachman, Carl: "Diabetes Mellitus and Pregnancy with Special Reference to Fetal and Infantile Loss," *Am. J. M. Sc.,* **223**:681–93, (June) 1952.

Ball, Thomas L.: "Management of the Urological Complications of Pregnancy," *M. Clin. North America,* **35**:715–31, (May) 1951.

Blecha, Elmira: "Low Sodium Diets," *Am. J. Nursing,* **51**:464–66, (July) 1951.

Bookmiller, Mae M., and Bowen, George L.: *Textbook of Obstetrics and Obstetric Nursing,* 2nd ed. W. B. Saunders Co., Philadelphia, 1954.

Bunim, Joseph J., and Taube, Harry: "The Management of the Pregnant Woman with Heart Disease," *M. Clin. North America,* **35**:667–76, (May) (1951).

Davis, M. Edward, and Sheckler, Catherine E.: *DeLee's Obstetrics for Nurses,* 15th ed. W. B. Saunders Co., Philadelphia, 1951.

de Alvarez, Russell R.: "Toxemias of Pregnancy," *Am. J. Nursing,* **54**:1486–88, (Dec.) 1954.

Dieckmann, William J.: *The Toxemias of Pregnancy.* C. V. Mosby Co., St. Louis, 1952.

Eastman, Nicholson J.: *Williams Obstetrics,* 11th ed. Appleton-Century-Crofts, Inc., New York, 1956.

Ferguson, James H., and Keaton, Alice G.: "Special Leaflets for Use in Controlling Toxemia and Excessive Weight Gain in Pregnancy," *Am. J. Pub. Health,* **40**:194–200, (Feb.) 1950.

Giblin, Elizabeth, and Osmond, T. W.: "Nursing Care in Toxemias of Pregnancy," *Am. J. Nursing,* **54**:1488–89, (Dec.) 1954.

Gifford, Alice J.; Wright, John J.; Sheps, Cecil G.; and Taylor, Eugene E.: "Congenital Syphilis Can Be Eradicated," *Nursing Outlook,* **1**:28–30, (Jan.) 1953.

Given, William P.; Douglas, R. Gordon; and Tolstoi, Edward: "Pregnancy and Diabetes," *M. Clin. North America,* **35**:659–65, (May) 1951.

Greenhill, J. P. (ed.): *Obstetrics,* 11th ed. W. B. Saunders Co., Philadelphia, 1955.

Jensen, Julius, and Jensen, Deborah: *Nursing in Clinical Medicine,* 4th ed. The Macmillan Company, New York, 1954.

Jones, Julia M.: "Pulmonary Tuberculosis in the Pregnant Woman," *M. Clin. North America,* **35**:647–57, (May) 1951.

Krugman, Saul, and Ward, Robert: "The Rubella Problem," *J. Pediat.,* **44**:489–98, (May) 1954.

Maternity Center Association: "A Word of Caution," *Briefs,* **17**:13–15, (Autumn) 1953.

Moe, Russell J.: "Heart Disease and Pregnancy," *Transactions of the Fifth American Congress of Obstetrics and Gynecology.* C. V. Mosby Co., St. Louis, 1952.

Nelson, Nels A.: "Modern Venereal Disease Control," *Am. J. Nursing,* **50**:75–77, (Feb.) 1950.

Petkauskos, Mary R., and White, Priscilla: "Pregnancy Complicating Diabetes Mellitus," *Am. J. Nursing,* **48**:300–304, (May) 1948.

Proudfit, Fairfax T., and Robinson, Corinne H.: *Nutrition and Diet Therapy,* 11th ed. The Macmillan Company, New York, 1955.

Randall, Lawrence M.: "Pregnancy Associated with Tuberculosis," Transac- *tions of the Fifth American Congress on Obstetrics and Gynecology.* C. V. Mosby Co., St. Louis, 1952.

Reimer, Ann: "Planning the Low Sodium Diet," *Pub. Health Nursing,* **43**:496–98, (Sept.) 1951.

Shafer, J. K.: "Premarital Health Examination Legislation," *Pub. Health. Rep.,* **69**:487–93, (May) 1954.

Shumann, Edward A.: "Obstetric Hemorrhage," *J.A.M.A.* **147**:810–13, (Oct. 27) 1951.

Speiser, Mortimer D.: "Modern Therapy of Syphilis in the Pregnant Woman," *M. Clin. North America,* **35**:631–46, (May) 1951.

Ullery, John C.: "The Management of Pregnancy Complicated by Heart Disease," *Am. J. Obst. & Gynec.,* **67**:834–66, (Apr.) 1954.

Vaux, Norris W., and Rakoff, A. E.: "Estrogen–Progesterone Therapy; A New Approach in the Treatment of Habitual Abortion," *Am. J. Obst. & Gynec.,* **50**:353–66, (Oct.) 1945.

Ware, H. Hudnall, Jr., and Winston, William O.: "Ectopic Pregnancy," *Obst. & Gynec.,* **4**:29–34, (July) 1954.

Woodward, H. L.; Gardner, B.; Bryant, R. D.; and Overland, Anna E.: *Obstetric Management and Nursing,* 5th ed. F. A. Davis Co., Philadelphia, 1955.

Wright, John J.; Sheps, Cecil G.; Taylor, Eugene F.; and Gifford, Alice J.: "Obstacles to Eradicating Congenital Syphilis," *Pub. Health Rep.,* **67**:1179–84, (Dec.) 1952.

Zabriskie, Louise, and Eastman, Nicholson J.: *Nurses Handbook of Obstetrics,* 9th ed. J. B. Lippincott Co., Philadelphia, 1952.

# PART IV. THE BIRTH OF THE BABY

## Chapter 10

## Presentation and Position of the Fetus

Returning for a moment to the pregnant uterus at term, we find it to be a thin-walled, muscular sac containing the mature fetus, attached by means of the umbilical cord to the placenta and floating in the amniotic fluid, which is contained within a sac formed by the amniotic and chorionic membranes.

The average fetus at term is about 50 cm long (20 in.), weighs about 3300 gm (7¼ lb), and is curved and folded upon itself into an ovoid mass, occupying the smallest possible space (Fig. 64). Its most frequent *attitude* is with the back arched, the head bent forward, with the chin resting upon the chest, arms crossed upon the chest below the chin, thighs flexed upon the abdomen, and knees bent. With a few exceptions the long axis of the fetus is parallel to the long axis of the mother, and most frequently the head is downward. It was formerly believed that the child stood upright in the uterus until the end of pregnancy and then somersaulted to the position it occupied immediately before birth (Fig. 65). It is now known that although the fetus may move about and change its position during the early part of pregnancy, it is not likely to greatly alter its relation to the mother's body during the tenth lunar month.

It seems advisable to define here certain terms which are in common use in discussing patients in labor, and which will be employed in the following pages:

*Gravid* refers to a pregnancy regardless of its duration.

*Para* refers to past pregnancies that continued to the period of viability.

A *primigravida* is a woman who is pregnant for the first time.

A *nullipara* (para 0) is a woman who has not had children.

A *primipara* (para I) is a woman who has given birth to one child of viable age. This term is, however, often used interchangeably with primigravida.

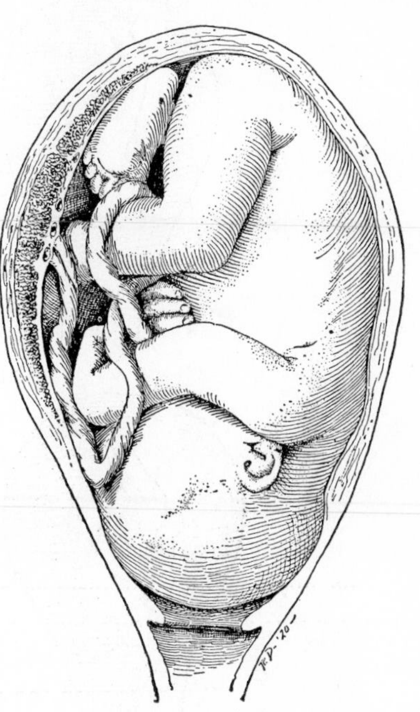

**Fig. 64.** Most common attitude of fetus in uterine cavity at term.

A *multigravida* is a woman who is in her second or any subsequent pregnancy.

A *multipara* (para II, para III, para IV) is a woman who has given birth to two or more children. This term is also often used loosely and applied to the woman who is pregnant for the second time or is in her second labor at which time she is still a para I.

A *parturient* is a woman in labor.

The past obstetric history of a patient is probably more completely described by the use of the terms gravida and para than by the terms primipara and multipara. A primigravida is a gravida I, para 0, during her first pregnancy and labor. If the patient has had an abortion she is a gravida II, para 0. During her next pregnancy she becomes a gravida III, para I. Para refers to pregnancies, not to babies, so that the patient remains a para I even if she delivered twins. She is also a para I if the baby was stillborn or was premature and died, since para refers to a pregnancy which has gone to the period of viability regardless of the condition of the baby.

There is also a terminology, with abbreviations, which is fairly generally used in this country and England to designate the position which the child, about to be born, occupies in relation to its mother's body. A diagnosis of this position is, of course, absolutely necessary to a skillful management of labor, and the nurse should understand the meanings of the terms used, and also their distinctions and subdivisions.

**The presentation of the fetus** is the term which is employed to indi-

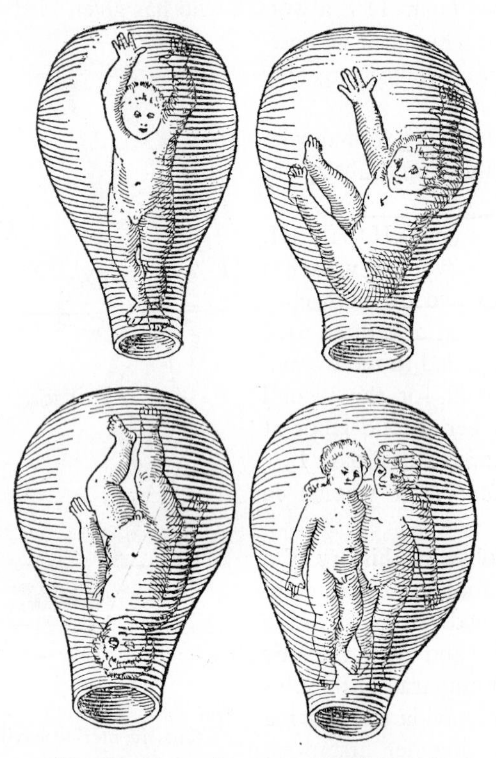

**Fig. 65.** Illustrations from the first textbook on obstetrics, Roesslin's "Rosengarten," 1513, which give an amusing impression of early ideas of the position of the fetus in utero.

cate the relationship of the longitudinal axis of the fetus to the longitudinal axis of the mother. This presentation may be either longitudinal or transverse. In the *longitudinal,* the long axes of the bodies of mother and child are parallel. In *transverse presentations,* however, the child lies across the uterus, with one side or the other at the pelvic brim.

Presentation is frequently confused with presenting part. This latter term is used to designate the part of the baby's body which is over the brim of the mother's pelvis. Thus the part of the fetus which is lowermost is designated as the **presenting part** and gives the presentation its name. In the longitudinal presentation the breech, face, or vertex will be the lowermost part of the fetus. If the buttocks or breech is downward, therefore, it is a *breech* presentation (Fig. 66), and if the head is the lower pole it is termed a *head* or *cephalic* presentation (Fig. 67). The head presentations are divided into two

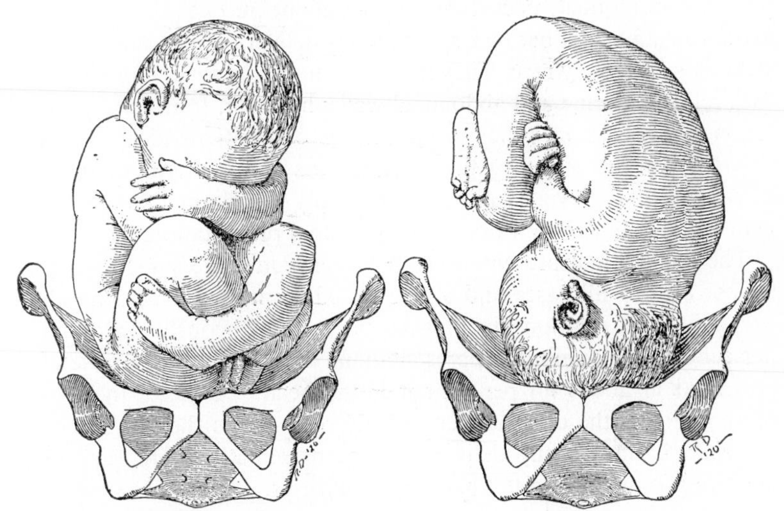

**Fig. 66.** Attitude of fetus in breech presentation.

**Fig. 67.** Attitude of fetus in vertex presentation.

main groups, which are designated, respectively, as *vertex* and *face* presentations. For example, if the baby's neck is so bent that the chin rests upon the chest, the crown of its head, or the vertex, is the part that is lowest in the birth canal and is the part that will be seen first at the vaginal outlet. Therefore, this is called a *vertex,* or *occipital,* presentation. If the neck is bent sharply backward, the face becomes the presenting part and we have a *face* presentation. The large fontanel (sincipital presentation) or the brow (brow presentation) may be the presenting part at the beginning of labor, but these change to vertex or face as labor progresses.

In the breech presentation the thighs may be flexed on the abdomen and the legs flexed on the thighs, and it is then termed a *full breech* presentation; or it may be a *frank breech* presentation in which the thighs are flexed but the legs are extended up on the chest wall. Sometimes one or both feet are lower than the buttocks, thereby becoming the presenting part and making either a single or double *footling* presentation. When only one foot presents, the other leg assumes one of the above positions.

In a transverse presentation the shoulder becomes the presenting part because it is closest to the pelvic brim. The transverse presentations are infrequent, occurring once in about 300 cases, and are regarded as abnormal because spontaneous delivery under such circumstances is extremely rare. They most commonly occur in multigravidas with relaxed uterine and abdominal walls; however, transverse presentation may occur in either primigravidas or multigravidas when the pelvis is contracted, when there are tumors of the uterus or ovaries, when placenta previa is present, or in any condition that interferes with engagement from a normal longitudinal presentation.

The longitudinal presentations, however, constitute something over 99 per cent of all cases and are regarded as normal, since the child occupying this relationship may be born spontaneously. In about 4 per cent of the longitudinal presentations the breech is the presenting part, and in about 96 per cent it is the head. Of these, the vertex presentation is the one most commonly seen and is the one in which the child is most easily delivered. Face presentations are very rare, occurring in only about 0.3 per cent of all cases.

To be able to determine very accurately the relationship of the presenting part to the mother's pelvis the *position* and *variety* also have to be considered.

By **position** is meant the relation of some arbitrarily chosen point on the presenting part of the fetus, to the right or left side of the mother, and **variety** designates whether this point is to the front (anterior), side (transverse), or back (posterior) segment of that side.

Taking these up in the order of their frequency, we find that in vertex presentations the occiput is this arbitrary point on the baby's body which is chosen to describe the position of the child; in breech presentations, the sacrum; in transverse presentations, the acromion process or the scapula; and in face presentations, the chin or mentum.

Presentation, then, describes the relationship of the long axis of the entire fetal body to the mother's body, while position describes the relationship between the baby's occiput, sacrum, shoulder, or chin to the mother's pelvis.

In each longitudinal presentation the presenting part may occupy either the anterior, transverse, or posterior segment of the right or left side of the mother's pelvis, making then six different varieties for each presentation.

If the child is so placed in the uterus that the head is the lowermost part, the neck flexed with the chin on the chest, and the occiput directed toward the mother's left side, and more to the front than to the side, the presentation would be longitudinal with the vertex as the presenting part which would make it a vertex presentation. The arbitrarily chosen point on the child's body (the occiput) would be directed toward the left anterior segment of the mother's pelvis making it a left position of the anterior variety. This is the situation most commonly present, and the description of this presentation and position is left-occipito-anterior which is abbreviated, by taking the first letter of each word, into L.O.A. If the occiput were turned directly toward the mother's left side, neither to the front nor the back, we should have a left-occipito-transverse, or L.O.T.; and if it were directed toward the left posterior segment of the pelvis, the position would be left-occipito-posterior, or L.O.P. As there are three corresponding varieties on the right side, anterior, transverse and posterior, there are six possible positions for the child to occupy in the vertex, or occipital, presentation, as follows:

Left-occipito-anterior, abbreviated to L.O.A.
Left-occipito-transverse, abbreviated to L.O.T.
Left-occipito-posterior, abbreviated to L.O.P.
Right-occipito-anterior, abbreviated to R.O.A.
Right-occipito-transverse, abbreviated to R.O.T.
Right-occipito-posterior, abbreviated to R.O.P. (Fig. 68.)

Similarly, there are six face (Fig. 69) and six breech (Fig. 70) possible positions. If the chin (mentum) is resting in the left anterior segment of the mother's pelvis, the position would be left-mento-anterior, or L.M.A. If the breech presents and the sacrum is in that relation, the position is left-sacro-anterior, or L.S.A. In describing the transverse presentation, four words instead of three may be used; thus, left-acromio-dorso-anterior, or L.A.D.A. There are but four varieties of transverse presentation, since the shoulder is either anterior or posterior: thus left-acromio-dorso-anterior, left-acromio-dorso-posterior, and the two corresponding positions on the right side. Often the entire scapula is chosen to describe the presentation and position instead of the acromion process, and the description can be

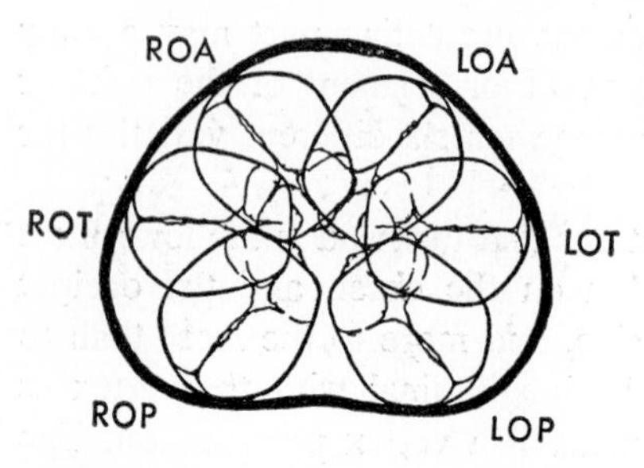


**Fig. 68.** Diagram showing the six possible positions of a vertex presentation as seen when looking at the pelvis from below.

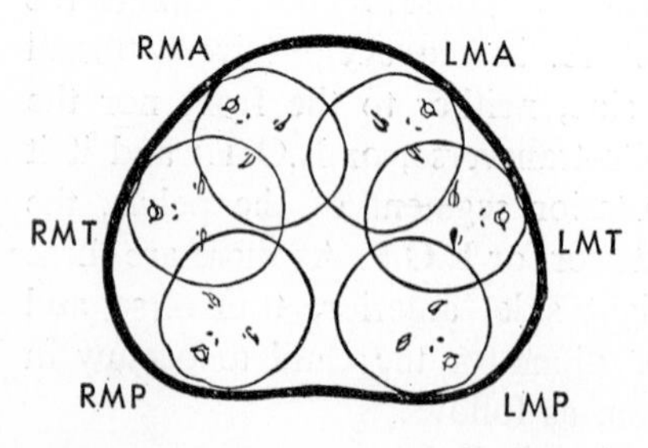


**Fig. 69.** Diagram showing the six possible positions in a face presentation as seen when looking at the pelvis from below.

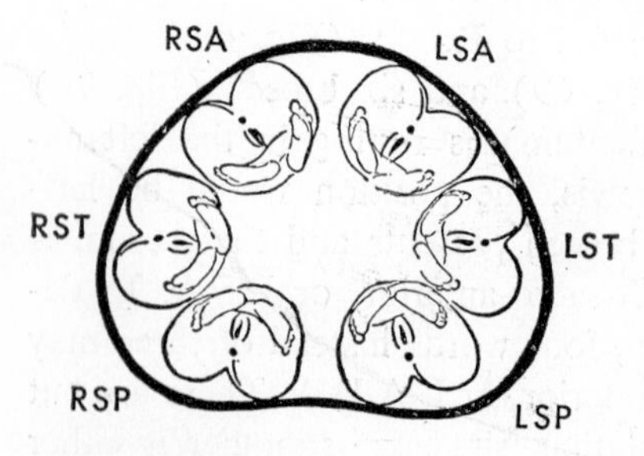


**Fig. 70.** Diagram showing the six possible positions in a breech presentation as seen when looking at the pelvis from below.

given in three words. Therefore, if the baby's head is to the mother's left side and the back lies anteriorly the scapula will rest in the left anterior segment of the mother's pelvis and the position is described as left-scapulo-anterior, or L.Sc.A.

The presentation of the fetus does not become definite until the presenting part enters the superior strait of the pelvis, but it changes less and less frequently as the end of pregnancy approaches.

**Engagement.** During the last weeks of pregnancy, particularly among primigravidas, the top of the fundus settles to the level which it reached at about the eighth month, and the lower part of the abdomen becomes more prominent than formerly. This descent of the uterus is termed "lightening." It may occur gradually or quite suddenly. The patient usually breathes much more comfortably after this change in contour takes place, but, at the same time, she may have cramps in her legs as a result of the increased pressure, more difficulty in walking, frequent micturition and desire to empty her bowels, and the vaginal discharge may be considerably increased. It is at this time that the presenting part enters the superior strait and when the biparietal plane (greatest transverse diameter) of the baby's head has passed through the area of the pelvic inlet it is said to be engaged (Fig. 78).

The time at which engagement takes place depends upon three factors: the parity of the patient, the size and normality of the pelvis, and the size and position of the fetus. It is important for the obstetrician in planning for the delivery to know whether or not the presenting part is engaged, particularly in primigravidas.

Although in primigravidas engagement usually occurs one to four weeks before labor begins, it frequently does not take place in multigravidas until after the onset of labor. This difference is accounted for in the increased tonicity of the uterine and abdominal muscles of women who have not borne other children. In certain abnormalities, or marked disproportion between the diameters of the child's head and the mother's pelvis, engagement may not take place until labor is well advanced, or possibly not at all.

### DIAGNOSIS OF PRESENTATION AND POSITION

The presentation and position of the fetus are ascertained by means of abdominal palpation, vaginal examination, rectal examination, auscultation of the fetal heart, and x-ray.

**Abdominal Palpation.** Palpation of the child's body through the mother's abdominal wall is possible under ordinary conditions during the latter months of pregnancy because the uterine and abdominal muscles are so stretched and thinned that the various parts may be felt through them. Palpation is sometimes difficult in hydramnios and is practically impossible in very obese patients.

By abdominal palpation the size of the baby can also be roughly estimated, and if there is any disproportion between the baby's head and the inlet of the mother's pelvis it can be detected by feeling the baby's head overriding the symphysis pubis.

The employment of abdominal palpation, rectal examination, and x-ray in place of vaginal examination is regarded as an important factor in reducing the frequency of puerperal infections and thus in decreasing maternal morbidity. The explanation is that in general the danger of puerperal infection increases in direct proportion to the number of times a patient is examined vaginally. Since it is known how to diagnose the child's position by these other methods, vaginal examinations are ordinarily used only during labor if information gained by abdominal palpation and rectal examination is doubtful.

Abdominal palpation, as usually practiced, consists of four maneuvers, with the patient lying flat and squarely on her back with the abdomen exposed. The nurse should bear in mind that successful palpation requires even pressure. Cold hands applied to the abdomen or quick, jabbing motions with the fingers will usually stimulate the muscles lying beneath them to contract, thus somewhat obscuring the outline of the child. Such palpation is also very uncomfortable for the patient, whereas firm, even pressure, started gently, with warm hands, causes little discomfort.

*First Maneuver* (Figs. 71 and 75). The purpose of the first maneuver is to ascertain what is in the fundus; this is usually either the head or the breech. The examiner should stand facing the patient and gently apply the entire tactile surface of the fingers of both hands to the upper part of the abdomen, on opposite sides and somewhat curved about the fundus. In this way the outline of the pole of the fetus which occupies the fundus may be made out. If the head is uppermost, it will be felt as a hard, round object which is movable, or *ballottable,* between the two hands, and if the breech, it will be felt as a softer, less movable, less regularly shaped body.

*Second Maneuver* (Figs. 72 and 75). Having determined whether the head or the breech is in the fundus, the next step is to locate the child's back and the small parts in their relation to the right and left sides of the mother. This is accomplished, while still facing the patient, by slipping the hands down to a slightly lower position on the sides of the abdomen than they occupy in the first maneuver, and making firm, even pressure with the entire palmar surface of both hands. The back is felt as a smooth, hard surface under the palm and fingers of one hand; and the small parts, or hands, feet, and knees, as irregular knobs or lumps, under the hand on the opposite side. At the same time the fetal back is palpated it should also be noted whether it is in the anterior, transverse, or posterior part of the right or left side of the abdomen. This information will be valuable in determining the relationship of the presenting part to the anterior, transverse, or posterior part of the mother's pelvis. If the sacrum or occiput is presenting they will be in the same position as the back, and if the face is presenting it will be exactly opposite.

*Third Maneuver* (Figs. 73 and 75). The third maneuver virtually

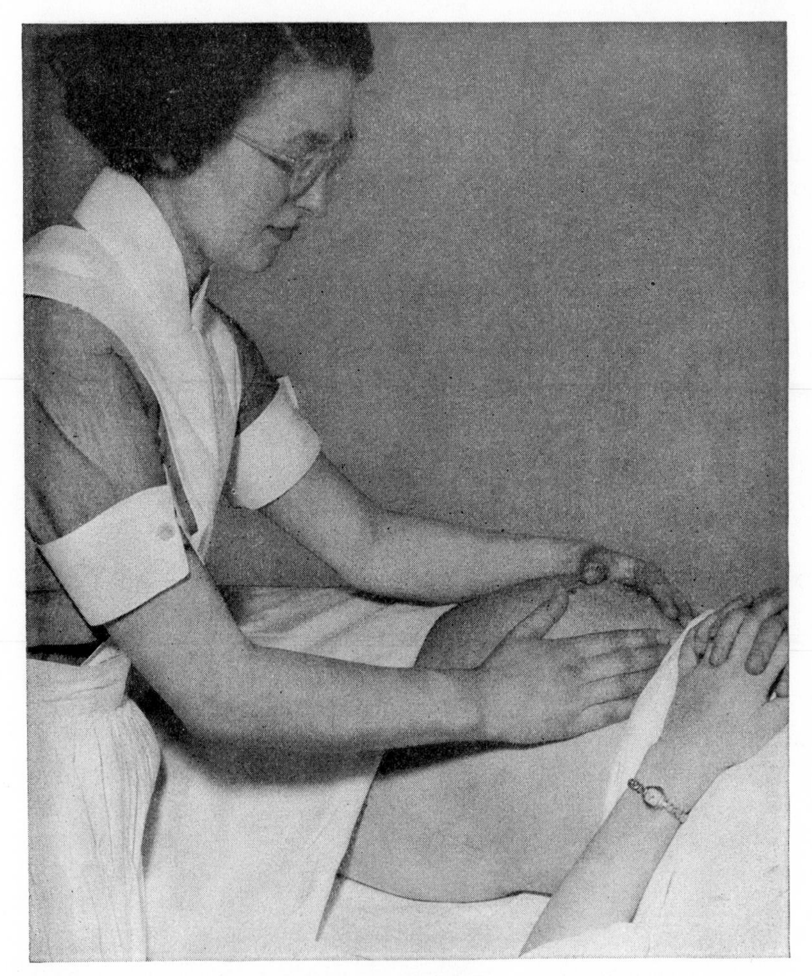

**Fig. 71.** First maneuver in abdominal palpation to discover position of fetus.

amounts to a confirmation of the impression gained by the first maneuver by showing which pole is directed toward the pelvis, but also ascertains whether the presenting part is engaged or floating. The thumb and fingers of one hand are spread as widely apart as possible, applied to the abdomen just above the symphysis pubis, and then brought together to grasp the part of the fetus which lies between them. If the presenting part is engaged it will be fixed in the

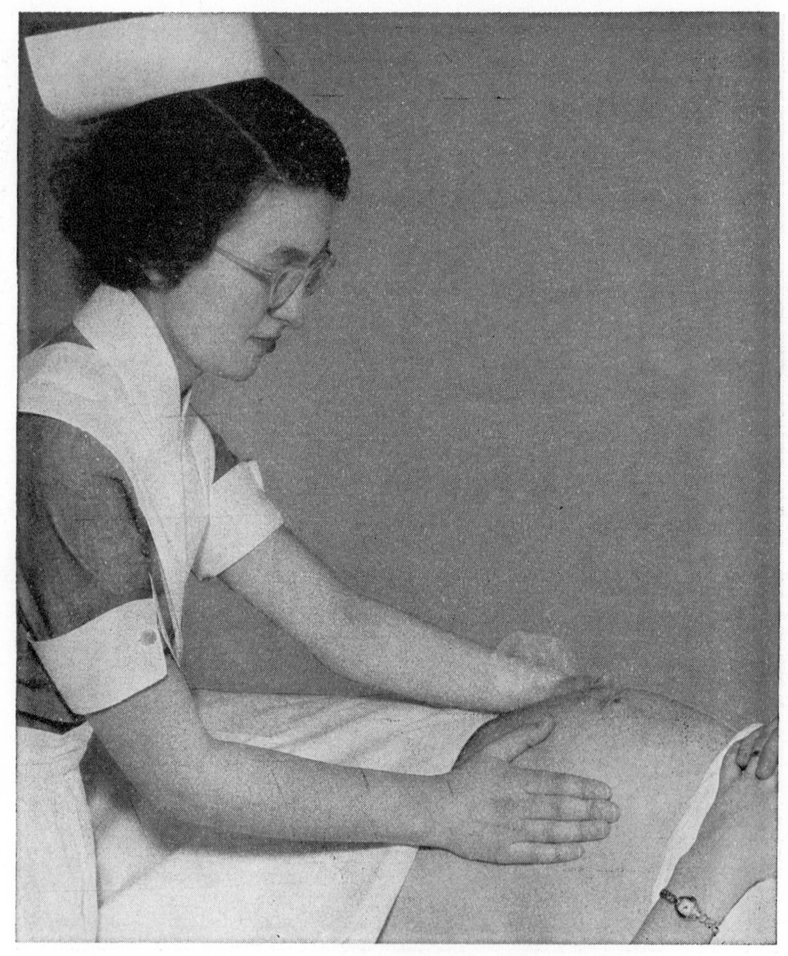

**Fig. 72.** Second maneuver in abdominal palpation.

pelvis, but if not engaged the head will be felt as hard, round, and movable, while the breech will be less clearly defined, but also movable. When the head is deep in the pelvis the anterior shoulder is sometimes felt in this maneuver.

*Fourth Maneuver* (Figs. 74 and 75). The fourth maneuver is of particular value after the presenting part has become engaged. The examiner faces the patient's feet and places the fingers of each hand on

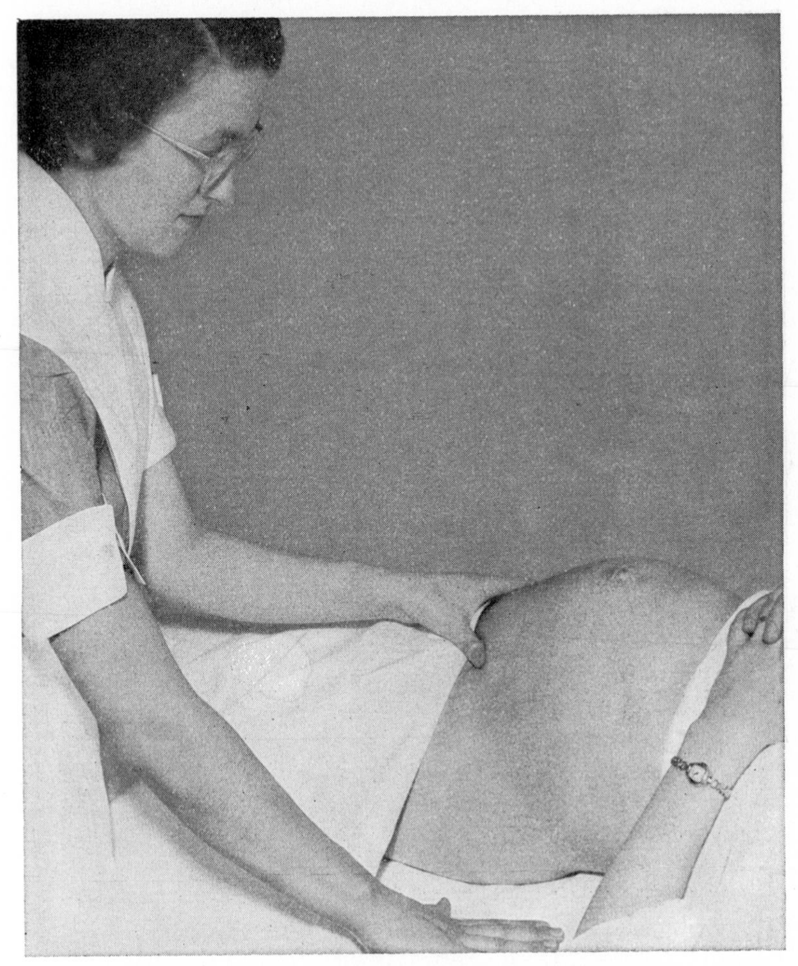

**Fig. 73.** Third maneuver in abdominal palpation.

either side of the midline of the lower abdomen. She points her fingers downward and at the same time slightly inward. The fingers maintain their original position and descend toward the pelvis by displacing downward the movable skin of the abdomen—a sort of gliding movement. If the head is engaged, the fingers on one side or the other will be arrested in their downward progress by the *cephalic prominence,* the most marked protrusion of the baby's head. If this is felt

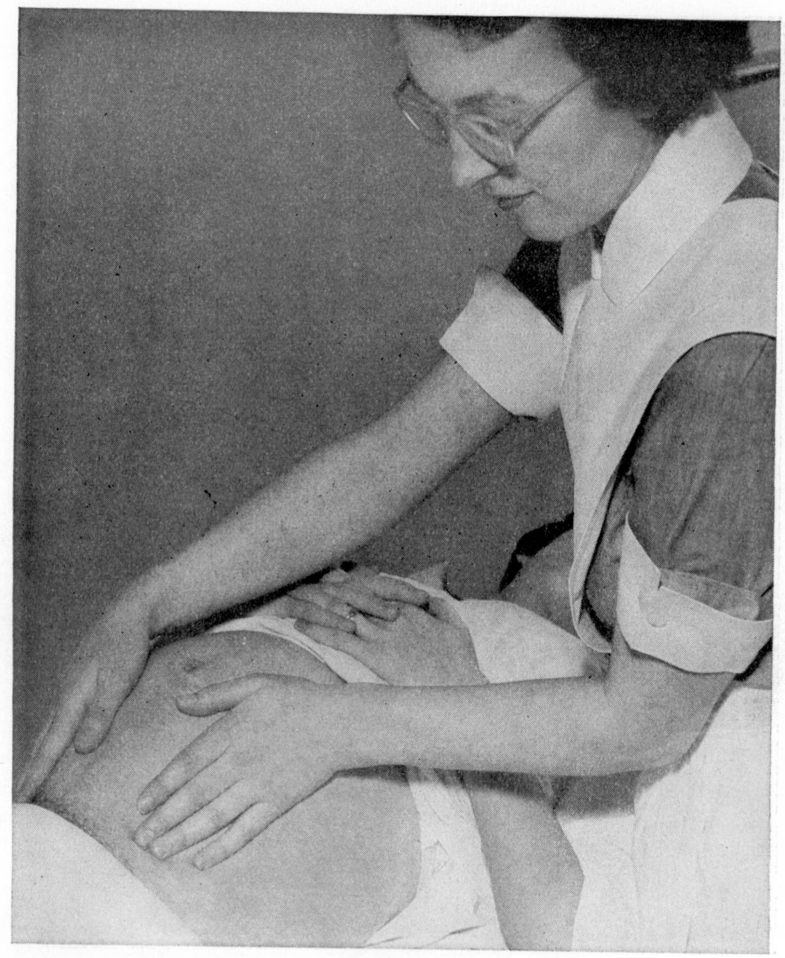

**Fig. 74.** Fourth maneuver in abdominal palpation. (This series of pictures [Figs. 71–74] taken at University Hospitals, Madison, Wisconsin).

on the same side as the small parts of the child, that is, on the side opposite to the back, she then knows that the head is normally flexed and the vertex of the baby is the presenting part. However, if the cephalic prominence is felt on the same side as the back, then she knows that the baby's face is the presenting part. The reason for this is that in a vertex presentation the most prominent point on

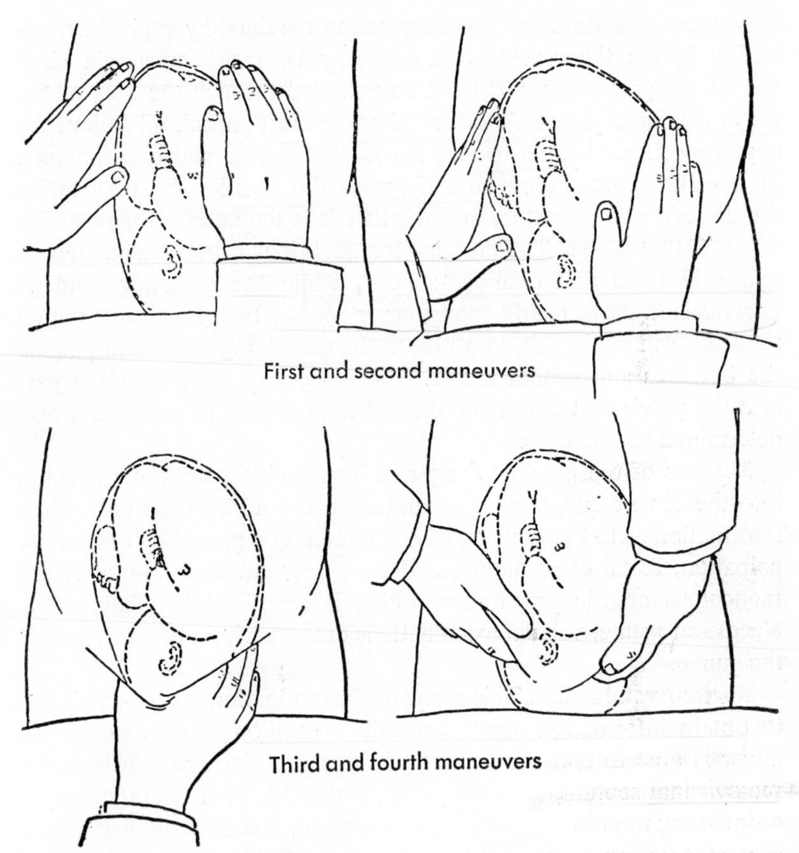


**Fig. 75.** Diagram showing relation of doctor's hands to fetus in the four maneuvers in abdominal palpation.

the baby's head is the relatively sharp projection made by the brow and top of the head, which is so much sharper than the relatively rounded occiput that the fingers slip over the latter and are arrested by the former. On the other hand, in a face presentation, when the head is extended the brow-vertex angle is relatively much less prominent than the very acute angle made by the occiput bent back on the neck. The fourth maneuver tells, also, how far into the pelvis the presenting part has descended. If the cephalic prominence is readily palpable the head has not descended to the level of the ischial spines, and when it cannot be felt at all the head is very deep in the pelvis.

**Vaginal Examination.** The information obtained by vaginal examination before the cervix is dilated may be rather uncertain since the child's presenting part must be palpated through the area of the lower uterine segment. After complete, or even partial, dilatation, the exploring finger is able to feel the sagittal suture and one fontanel, in a vertex presentation, and diagnose the position by discovering the direction of the suture and whether it is the anterior or posterior fontanel that is felt. The anterior fontanel, it will be remembered, is relatively large and diamond-shaped, while the posterior fontanel is small and more nearly triangular in shape. In a face presentation the features may be felt; in a breech the examining finger can palpate the buttocks and genital crease. The descent of the presenting part into the pelvis and the dilatation and thinness of the cervix are also determined at this time.

Because of the possible danger of introducing pathogenic bacteria into the birth canal, vaginal examination should be used only when information as to the progress of labor cannot be gained by abdominal palpation, rectal examination, and the x-ray and then only after the meticulous aseptic preparation which is described in Chapter 12. Needless to state, vaginal examinations are not within the province of the nurse.

**Rectal Examination.** This method of examination is also employed to obtain information about the child's position, as the examining finger is able to feel the surface of the presenting part through the rectovaginal septum, after the cervix is dilated. There is little danger of infecting the birth canal with this method. Rectal examination will also give information as to the amount of effacement (thinning) and dilatation of the cervix, the distance that the head has descended into the pelvis, and whether or not the membranes are ruptured. For these reasons nurses are frequently taught to make rectal examinations, thereby increasing the value of their assistance to the doctor in watching the progress of labor (Fig. 86).

**Auscultation of the Fetal Heart.** This may be helpful in confirming the diagnosis of presentation and position which has been made by palpation (Fig. 76). In the vertex and breech presentations the heartbeat is best heard through the baby's back, and in face presentations it is transmitted through the thorax, which presents a convex surface in this case and fits into the curve of the uterine wall. In anterior vertex presentations the heart is heard within 2.5 to 5 cm (1 to 2 in.) of the midline and below the umbilicus; in transverse, further to the side; and in posterior, well toward the back. Occasionally when the back lies posteriorly the heartbeat is heard best through the anterior chest wall and will then be found near the midline on the opposite side of the abdomen. The information gained from hearing the heartbeat

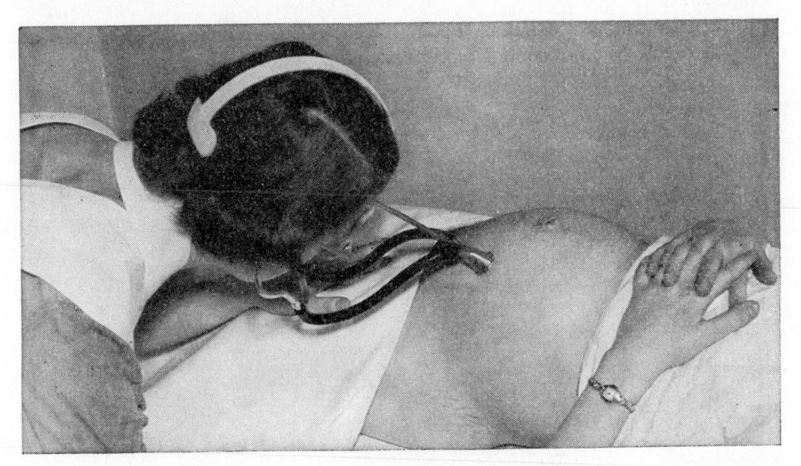

**Fig. 76.** Auscultation of the fetal heart.

can thus be misleading. In breech presentations the heart is heard best at, or near, the level of the umbilicus.

**X-ray.** This is valuable in cases where abdominal palpation is difficult. It can be used to accurately determine position and presentation; to determine the amount of descent, or engagement, of the presenting part; and is a valuable aid in determining the existence of any disproportion between the mother's pelvis and the baby's head (Figs. 10 and 11.) An x-ray is also of value in making an accurate diagnosis when there is a question of multiple pregnancy, it is an aid in estimating the size and age of the fetus, and it may show the existence of fetal abnormalities.

## BIBLIOGRAPHY AND STUDENT REFERENCES

Bookmiller, Mae M., and Bowen, George L.: *Textbook of Obstetrics and Obstetric Nursing,* 2nd ed. W. B. Saunders Co., Philadelphia, 1954.

Davis, M. Edward, and Sheckler, Catherine E.: *DeLee's Obstetrics for Nurses,* 15th ed. W. B. Saunders Co., Philadelphia, 1951.

Eastman, Nicholson J.: *Williams Obstetrics,* 11th ed. Appleton-Century-Crofts, Inc., New York, 1956.

Greenhill, J. P. (ed.): *Obstetrics,* 11th ed. W. B. Saunders Co., Philadelphia, 1955.

Woodward, H. L.; Gardner, B.; Bryant, R. D.; and Overland, Anna E.: *Obstetric Management and Nursing,* 5th ed. F. A. Davis Co., Philadelphia, 1955.

Zabriskie, Louise, and Eastman, Nicholson J.: *Nurses Handbook of Obstetrics,* 9th ed. J. B. Lippincott Co., Philadelphia, 1952.

*Chapter 11*

# Symptoms, Course, and Mechanism of Normal Labor

Labor may be defined as the process by which the products of conception are expelled from the mother's body. It ordinarily occurs about 280 days from the beginning of the last menstrual period. (See Chap. 5.)

The cause of labor is not known. Many theories have been advanced to explain why the uterine contractions, which have occurred painlessly throughout pregnancy, and without expulsive force, finally become painful at about the end of the tenth lunar month and so changed in character as to extrude the uterine contents; but this is apparently caused by a combination of factors. It is not known why some labors occur before and others after the expected date.

The onset of labor is usually marked by a dull low backache and a feeling of tightness in the abdomen. Soon the patient becomes conscious of the uterine contractions through dragging pains which may be felt first in the back and then in the lower part of the abdomen and the thighs, similar to menstrual cramps. Frequently a pinkish mucoid vaginal discharge, "show," is coincident with these early contractions. At first the contractions are weak and infrequent, perhaps 15 minutes apart, but they gradually grow more forceful and occur at shorter intervals. Labor pains are sometimes mistaken for intestinal colic, but when the paroxysms are rhythmical and the uterus is felt, through the abdominal wall, to grow hard as the discomfort increases and soft as it subsides, there can be no doubt but that the patient is in labor. Signs of impending labor may be a gush of amniotic fluid, caused by the rupture of the membranes, or of blood-tinged vaginal discharge.

For purposes of convenience, labor is usually described as consisting of three periods or stages. The first stage begins with the onset of labor and lasts until the cervix is completely dilated; the second stage begins with the complete dilatation of the cervix and lasts until the child is born; the third stage begins immediately after the birth of the child and lasts until the placenta is expelled.

The entire duration of labor may vary from an extremely short time, which is comprised of only a few contractions, to several days of severe and exhausting contractions, but the median length of the first labor in white women is approximately 10½ hours and of subsequent labors about 6¼ hours. The modal duration of labor (greatest frequency of occurrence) is seven hours for a first labor and four hours for subsequent ones. If the median duration of labor is divided into three periods the approximate length of each stage is as follows:

| | *1st stage* | *2nd stage* | *3rd stage* | *total* |
|---|---|---|---|---|
| First labor | 9½ hours | 50 minutes | 10 minutes | 10½ hours |
| Subsequent labors | 5¾ hours | 20 minutes | 10 minutes | 6¼ hours |

The longer labor in primigravidas as compared with multigravidas is due to the greater tone, and thus the greater resistance, offered by the muscles of the cervix and perineum of primigravidous women.

## FIRST STAGE (STAGE OF DILATATION) 0-10 cm

During this period the cervix becomes completely dilated, and it is therefore frequently called the stage of dilatation. The first-stage contractions begin by being mild and occurring at intervals of from 10 to 20 minutes and last from 15 to 30 seconds, but they gradually increase in frequency, length, and intensity until they are forceful and recur every three to four minutes, each contraction lasting about a minute. The discomfort begins in the back, and passes slowly forward to the abdomen and down into the thighs. If the hand is laid upon the abdomen, the uterus is felt to grow very hard at the acme of the contraction, and as it subsides the uterus relaxes. When it is relaxed the uterus rests on the vertebral column, but during a contraction it rises and pushes against the abdominal wall. Its vertical diameter becomes greater during a contraction, its transverse diameter smaller, and the direction of its long axis comes closer to the direction of the superior strait of the pelvis. With the hand on the abdomen the beginning of a contraction can be felt before the patient experiences discomfort and it may be felt to continue a few seconds after the discomfort has subsided.

The patient is entirely comfortable, as a rule, between contractions and, until they become very frequent, will usually feel able, in fact, may prefer, to be up and about, but if she is on her feet when a contraction begins she will usually seek relief by assuming a characteristic leaning position, or by sitting down, until it subsides. The uterine muscle being nonstriated cannot be controlled by the will of the patient but may be influenced for a short period of time by a change in emotion.

The contractions of the uterine muscle dilate and completely obliterate the cervix, which at the beginning of labor is soft, may be from 1 to 2 cm (.4 to .8 in.) long, and have only a very small orifice. The canal is filled with thick mucus which is usually expelled some time early in labor and is known as the mucous plug. In the primigravida the external os of the cervix may be closed or barely admit one finger tip at the onset of labor, but with subsequent pregnancies it is usually open enough to allow one finger tip to pass through easily.

As labor continues the uterus becomes differentiated into two portions, separated by a physiologic retraction ring—an upper contractile portion which becomes thicker as labor advances and a lower portion (the lower uterine segment) which, together with the cervix, becomes thinner and expands as labor progresses. This lower portion and the cervix form the muscular canal through which the baby passes as it is pushed out of the uterus.

With each contraction of the uterine muscle the pressure exerted on the amniotic fluid is distributed equally in all directions. This pressure puts considerable tension on the cervix, which offers the least resistance and is obliterated as a result. Also, with each contraction the uterine muscle pulls on the margins of the cervix and gradually shortens it. This traction from the uterine muscle and the pressure from the amniotic fluid, or the presenting part, brings about a shortening, and finally obliteration, of the canal, known as *effacement*. This effacement begins at the internal os, which becomes widened and gives the cervical canal a funnel-shaped appearance, as the amniotic sac of fluid, or the presenting part if the membranes are ruptured, is gradually forced down into the cervix (Fig. 77).

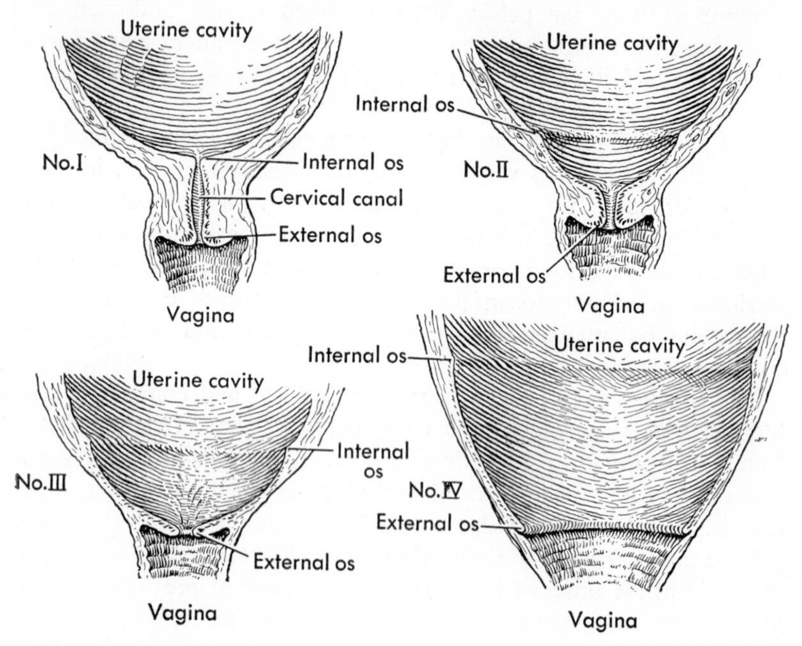


**Fig. 77.** Diagrams showing progress in effacement and dilatation of cervix during labor.

After the cervical canal has become completely obliterated and is continuous with the lower uterine segment, and frequently even before complete obliteration, dilatation of the external os takes place (Fig. 77). This dilatation takes very little time in a woman who has previously delivered a child, since the external os is already partially open at the onset of labor, but a much longer time in the primigravida, where the external os may be closed when labor begins and the resistance of the tissues is much greater. When the external os is dilated sufficiently to permit the baby's head to pass through, or approximately 10 cm (4 in.), the dilatation is said to be complete. Often the cervix has become partially effaced, sometimes completely effaced, and in some instances somewhat dilated, during the last weeks of pregnancy as the result of Braxton-Hicks contractions. Labor ordinarily proceeds more quickly when the cervix is thin and slightly open at the onset of true labor contractions than when it is thick and closed at the beginning of labor.

In the course of this stretching process the cervix sustains many tiny lesions from which blood oozes and tinges the vaginal discharge. This "show," or "bloody show," may appear at the very onset of labor or at any time during the period of dilatation.

As a rule, when the cervix is fully dilated the membranes rupture, and there is a sudden gush of that part of the fluid which was below the fetus in the amniotic sac, but the rupture of the membranes does not necessarily mark the end of the first stage. They may rupture at any time during the first stage, or before the patient goes into labor. Sometimes they retain their integrity until they are artificially ruptured to allow for the birth of the baby. If the membranes rupture before labor starts the contractions usually begin within 24 hours, and the presenting part exerts pressure on the cervix instead of the amniotic sac. The amount of fluid that escapes when the membranes rupture depends upon the position of the presenting part and the point of rupture. Sometimes there is a small dribble of fluid instead of a sudden gush, and the patient may think that she is losing a small amount of urine. After rupture has occurred a little fluid will usually escape with each contraction.

As dilatation advances, the fetus will also descend in the pelvis, and the patient has an increasing, sometimes persistent, desire to empty the bladder and bowels because of pressure upon these two organs by the presenting part. She may vomit, also, when the cervix becomes nearly or completely dilated.

The abdominal muscles should remain completely relaxed during the first stage; the expulsive force in this period should come entirely from the uterine contractions. The patient's utterances at this time may be sharp and complaining in contrast to the groans and grunts which accompany the second stage.

## SECOND STAGE (STAGE OF EXPULSION)

The second stage is sometimes called the stage of descent, or expulsion, of the fetus. The patient should, and is usually quite willing, to be in bed throughout the second stage, during which she should not be left alone. The contractions are regular, occurring at intervals of about two to three minutes from the beginning of one to the beginning of the next contraction. Since the contractions last 50 to 90 seconds and are very forceful, the patient has very little rest. Her face is flushed, and she may perspire freely.

If the membranes have not ruptured earlier they may rupture at this time as manifested by a sudden gush of rather clear fluid from the vagina, or it may become necessary to rupture them artificially. If this is not done they may in some instances not rupture until the baby is born when the child is said to be born with a *caul.*

In the second stage the uterus becomes longer with each contraction, and its transverse and anteroposterior diameters become shorter. This is partly due to a stretching of the lower uterine segment and partly due to a straightening out of the fetus. The fetus straightens out and becomes more rigid and is then extruded due to pressure applied to it from above by the contractions of the uterine and abdominal muscles.

The abdominal and respiratory muscles are brought into active use during the second stage, contracting simultaneously with the uterine muscle and increasing its expulsive force. The abdominal muscles are very important in aiding in expulsion of the fetus. They are apparently controlled by the patient's will at first, and she is able to increase their power by taking a deep breath, closing her lips, bracing her feet, pulling against something with her hands, and straining with all her might and "bearing down." Finally, however, the whole bearing-down process becomes involuntary, especially as more pressure is felt on the rectum, and is accompanied by an intense urge to push and the deep grunting sound which is characteristic of the well-advanced second stage. Under normal conditions, the child descends a little farther into the pelvis with each contraction, and finally the presenting part begins to distend the perineum and to separate the labia (Figs. 95 and 96), advancing at the height of each contraction and slipping back a little as it subsides.

The vagina and perineum are prepared for the great stretching that is necessary to allow for passage of the fetus by a hypertrophy of the muscle fibers and by an increased vascularity. The changes are most marked in the levator ani muscle, which must be stretched considerably, and the perineum, which is changed from a thick wedge-shaped mass of tissue to a very thin structure. As the fetus descends through the vagina the perineum becomes thinner and thinner, and the pressure of the head distends the anus so that the anterior rectal wall can be seen through it. The perineum is frequently torn with the birth of the head unless an episiotomy is performed.

The baby descends into, and through, the mother's pelvis by means of a series of twisting and curving motions, accommodating the long axes of its head to the long diameters of the pelvis (Fig. 78). The

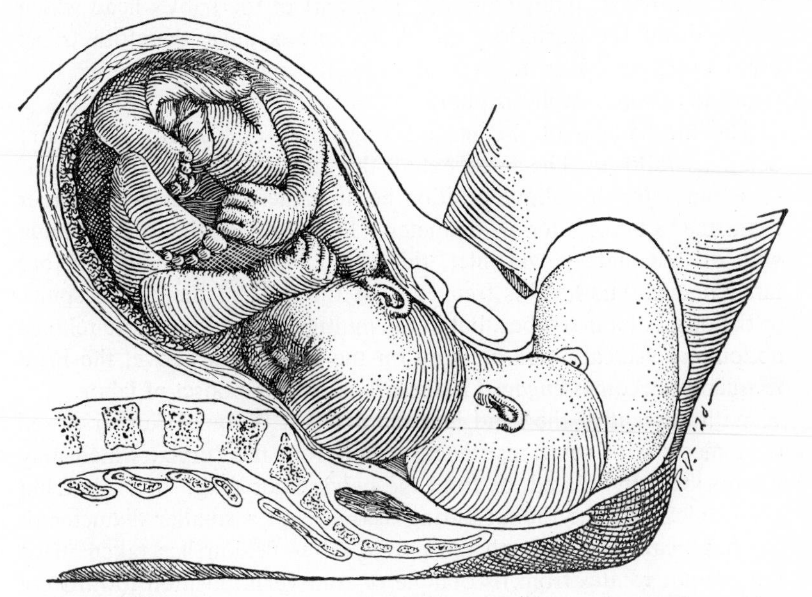

**Fig. 78.** Diagram indicating descent, flexion, internal rotation, and extension of baby's head during birth.

head being somewhat compressible and moldable, because of the open sutures and fontanels, is capable of a good deal of accommodation to the mother's pelvis.

The mechanism of labor, therefore, is virtually a series of adaptations of the size, shape, and moldability of the baby's head to the size and shape of the mother's pelvis. Several movements or adaptations may go on simultaneously. It is an adjustment of the "passenger" to the "passage," and a disproportion between the diameters of the head and the pelvis may interfere with the engagement or descent of the head and constitute a serious complication.

The long diameter of the head must first conform to one of the long diameters of the inlet (Fig. 4), usually transverse, and then turn so that the length of the head is lying anteroposterior in conformity to the long diameter of the outlet (Fig. 5), through which it next passes. As the head descends and rotates it also describes an arc because the posterior wall of the pelvis, consisting of the sacrum and coccyx, is about three times as deep as the anterior wall formed by the symphysis pubis (Fig. 6). That part of the baby's head which passes down the posterior wall of the pelvis must therefore travel three times as far in a given time as the part which simply slips under the short symphysis pubis.

The mechanism of the second stage may be described in more detail as follows: The head enters the superior strait of the pelvis in a transverse or oblique position because these diameters are larger than the anteroposterior diameter (Fig. 4). In the primigravida with an adequate pelvic inlet, this should have taken place before labor began. The head is frequently at the level of the ischial spines at the onset of a first labor, but in the multigravida with a more relaxed abdominal wall and less pressure on the fetus from above, the head frequently becomes *engaged* in the pelvis after the onset of labor.

With *descent* of the head into the pelvis it becomes further flexed as it meets with some resistance, either from the cervix, which may yet not be fully dilated, or from the pelvic floor (Fig. 78). The chin comes closer to the thorax during *flexion,* and a smaller diameter of the head can pass through the pelvis. After flexion has taken place the occiput rotates from its oblique or transverse position toward the symphysis or sacrum so that it is directly anteroposterior and by so doing brings the largest diameter of the baby's head toward the longest diameter of the pelvic outlet (Fig. 5). This *internal rotation* is always necessary for delivery of the head unless it is very small (Fig. 78). The occiput almost always rotates toward the symphysis so that it is directly anterior, but it may in some instances rotate toward the sacrum and be delivered in that position. When the head is delivered with the occiput posterior it distends the perineum more than usual during delivery, and a deep episiotomy is often necessary.

If the occiput enters the superior strait in the posterior or transverse portion of the mother's pelvis it has a longer distance to rotate than when it enters anteriorly. To reach the symphysis it must rotate 135 deg from the posterior or 90 deg from the transverse position while it only rotates 45 deg from the anterior position (Fig. 68). Labor is apt to be more prolonged when the head is in the posterior or transverse position because internal rotation does not take place as readily, or it may occur only partially, or not at all unless aided manually.

After internal rotation, *extension,* another absolutely essential movement, takes place (Fig. 78). The head which is greatly flexed as it reaches the pelvic floor must be extended to be born because the vaginal opening is directed upward and the flexed head would only be forced down against the perineum where it could not be delivered. As the head is pushed down by the contractions, the resistance of the perineum extends the head upward.

In a vertex presentation, left-occipito-anterior position, while the occiput passes under the symphysis and appears at the distending vaginal outlet, the face passes down the posterior wall and along the floor of the pelvis (Fig. 78). As pressure is exerted by the rapidly succeeding contractions, the head pivots about the symphysis pubis, thus extending the neck and pushing the face farther downward and forward. After emergence of the top and back of the head below the symphysis, the forehead appears over the posterior margin of the vagina, then the brow, eyes, nose, mouth, and chin in turn, and the entire head is born (Fig. 78). The baby's head then drops forward, in relation to its own body, with its face toward the mother's rectum and the occiput in front of the symphysis pubis, but soon the occiput rotates toward the mother's left side, resuming the relation that it bore to the inner aspects of her pelvis before expulsion. This is called *external rotation,* or *restitution,* and indicates that the body of the child has rotated. This is caused by the same factors that brought about internal rotation of the head. The undelivered shoulders are now anteroposterior, one under the symphysis pubis and the other resting on the perineum (Fig. 79). Either the lower or upper shoulder may be born first (Fig. 80), followed quickly by the other shoulder, the rest of the body, and the amniotic fluid which was behind the child's body. Thus is the second stage completed.

In face presentation the mechanism of labor is altered from the above description in such a way that it allows the head, which is extended instead of flexed, to rotate and accommodate itself to the pelvis. It is born by flexion instead of extension, and labor is usually prolonged and more difficult.

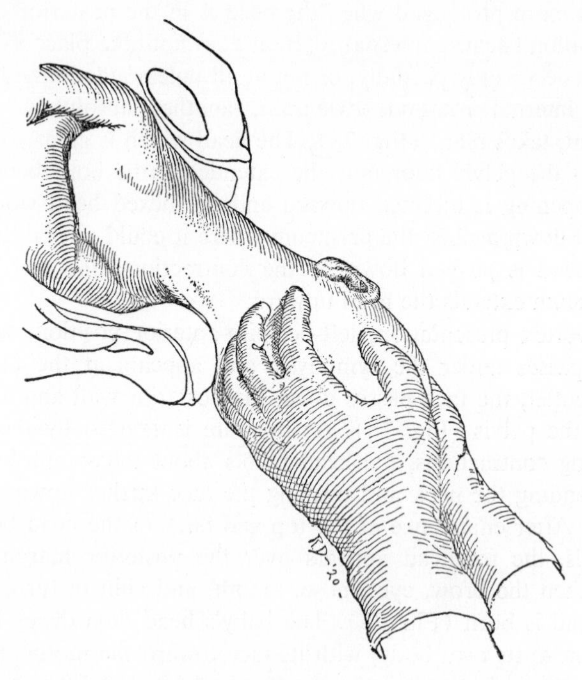


**Fig. 79.** Gentle downward traction is sometimes made to impinge the anterior shoulder under the symphysis pubis.

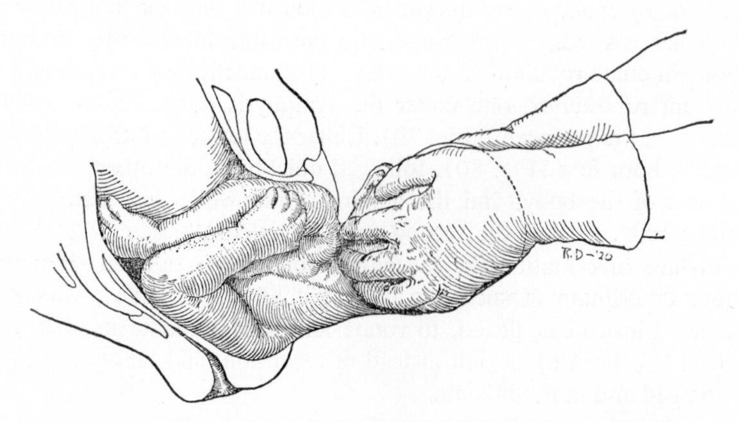


**Fig. 80.** Lifting the head during delivery of posterior shoulder.

## THIRD STAGE (PLACENTAL STAGE)

The third stage, sometimes termed the placental stage, is that period following the birth of the child during which the placenta is delivered. For a few moments after the baby is born the mother lies quietly, and there is a temporary cessation of the uterine contractions; she may sleep as a result of the anesthetic given during the second stage.

The uterus has greatly decreased in size, the fundus now lying just below the umbilicus. It is a firm globular mass above a collapsed lower uterine segment and is freely movable in the abdominal cavity. The uterine contractions are resumed in the course of a few minutes, and as they persist the uterus grows smaller, thereby greatly decreasing the area of placental attachment. As the placenta is noncontractile, it cannot accommodate itself to this decreased area of attachment and so is literally squeezed from its moorings. Separation sometimes occurs as soon as the uterine muscle contracts with expulsion of the child. A change in the shape of the uterus from a discoid to a globular mass during relaxation, and bleeding from the vagina are signs of placental separation.

After the placenta is separated, further contractions push it out of the uterine cavity and into the lower uterine segment. The membranes, which are continuous with the placenta, are peeled from the uterus by the contractions and by traction from the placenta as it falls into the lower segment. As the placenta is pushed into the lower uterine segment it fills this cavity, which has been collapsed, and pushes the fundus up. After expulsion of the placenta the uterine muscle contracts firmly, and the cavity of the fundus becomes very small (Figs. 81 and 82). Signs of expulsion of the placenta into the lower uterine segment or vagina are a rising up of the fundus in the abdominal cavity and a suddenly increasing length of umbilical cord protruding from the vagina. Uterine contractions do not completely expel the placenta, and it must be pushed out of the vagina by contractions of the abdominal muscles or by pressure made upon the fundus by the obstetrician.

It has been generally believed that the placenta is detached from the uterus and expelled from the vagina by means of one of two mechanisms, designated as the Schultze and the Duncan, from the two men who first described them.

In the Schultze mechanism the placenta is described as beginning to separate at the center (Fig. 83), the detached area spreading toward the margin, and the space thus formed filling with blood. The placenta becomes inverted on itself, and the glistening fetal surface

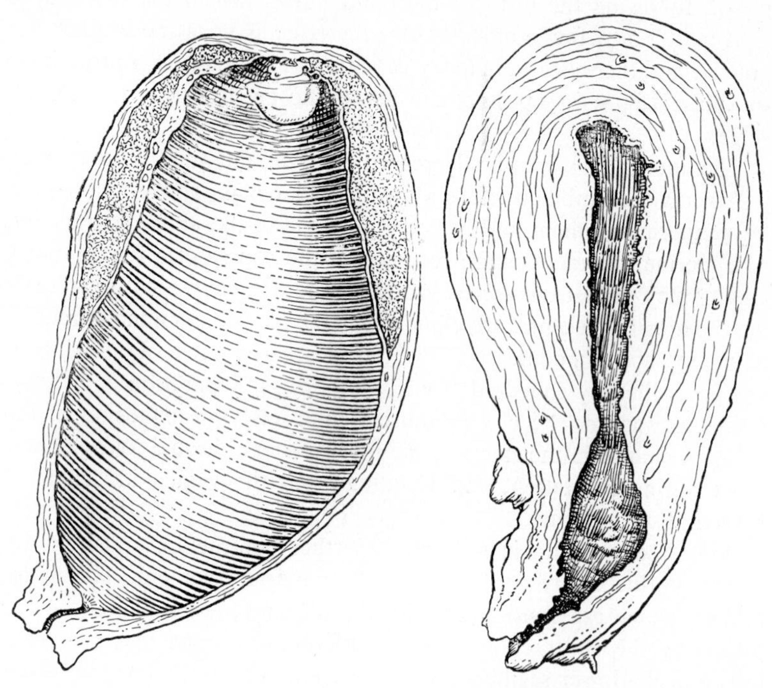

**Fig. 81.** Longitudinal section through uterus showing thinness of uterine wall before expulsion of fetus contrasting sharply with thickened wall in Fig. 82—twin placentas are still adherent in upper segment. (Drawing of photograph of specimen in the obstetrical laboratory, Johns Hopkins Hospital.)

**Fig. 82.** Longitudinal section through uterus, immediately after delivery, showing marked thickening of wall as a result of muscular contraction. (Drawing of photograph of specimen in the obstetrical laboratory, Johns Hopkins Hospital.)

appears at the vaginal outlet. In this case there is practically no bleeding during the third stage, as the inverted placenta blocks the outlet and holds back the blood. In Duncan's mechanism the detachment is described as beginning at the margin (Fig. 83), the placenta rolling on itself in the form of a cylinder whose long axis conforms to that of the uterus. It presents at the outlet by its roughened maternal surface, and there is usually slight but continuous bleeding from the time the separation begins. However, there is some doubt as to whether there are actually two methods of separation and that

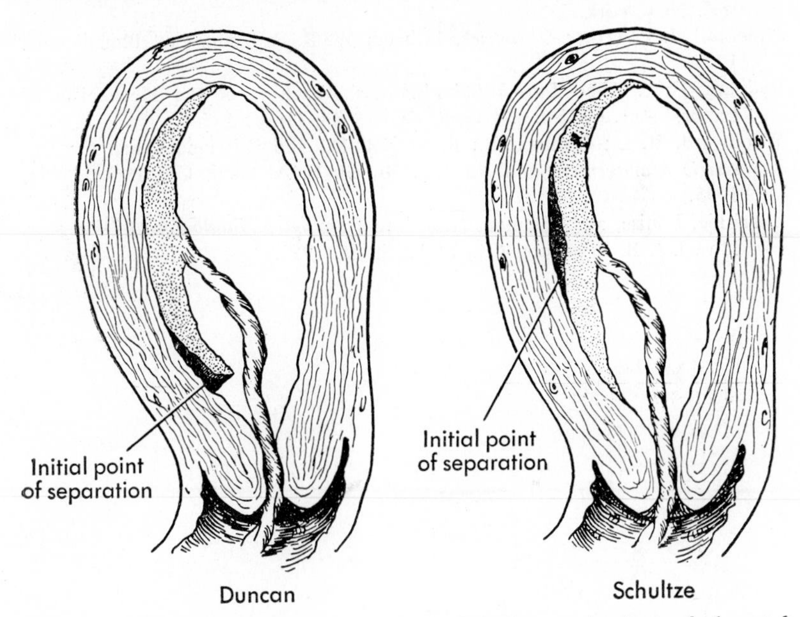


**Fig. 83.** Diagrams showing the Duncan and Shultze mechanisms of placental separation and expulsion.

these may be differences only in the birth of the placenta and not in its separation from the uterus.

A good deal of blood may be lost during the time of placental expulsion and immediately afterward, but this rather profuse bleeding should subside in a few moments. Although the loss of blood may be as much as 400 ml (about 13 oz) without causing serious symptoms, the amount usually lost is from 50 to 200 ml (1.7 to 7 oz). The patient has been through a severe ordeal and at the end of the third stage of labor she is usually tired and cold.

## BIBLIOGRAPHY AND STUDENT REFERENCES

Bookmiller, Mae M., and Bowen, George L.: *Textbook of Obstetrics and Obstetric Nursing,* 2nd ed. W. B. Saunders Co., Philadelphia, 1954.

Busby, Trent: "The Duration of Labor: Mean, Median, and Mode," *Am. J. Obst. & Gynec.*, **55**:846–51, (May) 1948.

Davis, M. Edward, and Sheckler, Catherine E.: *DeLee's Obstetrics for Nurses,* 15th ed. W. B. Saunders Co., Philadelphia, 1951.

Eastman, Nicholson J.: *Williams Obstetrics,* 11th ed. Appleton-Century-Crofts, Inc., New York, 1956.

Greenhill, J. P. (ed.): *Obstetrics,* 11th ed. W. B. Saunders Co., Philadelphia, 1955.

Rydberg, Erik: "The Two Hundred Years' Teaching of the Mechanism of Labor," *Am. J. Obst. & Gynec.*, **68**:236–44, (July) 1954.

Woodward, H. L.; Gardner, B.; Bryant, R. D.; and Overland, Anna E.: *Obstetric Management and Nursing,* 5th ed. F. A. Davis Co., Philadelphia, 1955.

Zabriskie, Louise, and Eastman, Nicholson J.: *Nurses Handbook of Obstetrics,* 9th ed. J. B. Lippincott Co., Philadelphia, 1952.

*Chapter 12*

# The Nurse's Duties during Labor

The extent of the nurse's helpfulness during labor, both to the patient and to the doctor, will depend very largely upon the intelligence with which she grasps that which is taking place and upon her own attitude, as an individual, toward the patient and the miraculous event which approaches. Important as is the preparation of the room, instruments, and linen, this other factor is much more influential. It will be wise, therefore, for the nurse to try to picture the process of labor in each instance and to be guided by a few broad principles that apply to all cases, rather than to try to "memorize" the details of her duties and of the desirable equipment and preparation.

If there is any time in a nurse's career when she should give scrupulous attention to establishing and maintaining asepsis, it is during labor; the patient's progress may, and often does, depend upon it. If there is any time when she should be watchful for developments and for symptoms of complications, it is during labor, because the mother's and/or baby's life may depend upon treatment that follows a prompt report to the doctor. Her powers of adaptability to patient, doctor, and surroundings may be greatly tried, for although they all may be infinitely varied, the nurse must invariably be clear-headed and efficient, and the adequacy of her service must never fail.

The sympathetic insight, which should constantly underlie the work of the obstetric nurse, will be needed at this crucial time of labor in the fullest and finest and completest sense. This is almost her test as a kind and understanding nurse and woman, since she needs to be both. Perhaps she had better imagine for a moment what this occurrence, that we baldly term labor, may mean to the patient, and look at it as nearly as possible from the standpoint of the patient herself. It is one of the most stirring and momentous experiences of her life, particularly if the expected baby is her first child. She is about to realize a long-anticipated dream—that of motherhood. She is also approaching a period of pain, and an event so amazing in its mystery and wonder that to only the most stolid can it fail to be a deeply emotional experience. And so, the young woman, to whom we may refer impersonally as "the patient," is an intensely personal being, at this time experiencing a number of the most poignant of the human emotions: awe, expectancy, doubt, uncertainty, dread, and in some cases fear amounting almost to terror. And through it all she may become exhausted by pain that grows harder and harder to bear.

It is known that the ravaging effects of pain, coupled with great emotional stress, such as fear, worry, doubt, anger, or apprehension, upon the physical well-being of surgical patients are such that recovery may be hindered by fear and worry. Accordingly, many careful surgeons take elaborate precautions to tranquilize a patient who is about to be operated upon, if for no other reason than to increase the patient's chance for recovery. There can be no doubt that nervous and emotional disturbances are detrimental to the physical well-being of the patient in labor, and this fact alone is enough to warrant an effort to avert them. If the nurse appreciates the significance of the emotional influence and shapes her attitude and conduct accordingly, she will thereby help to increase the ease and safety of labor and delivery. Just what that attitude shall be, no one can say, since it must be developed, in each case, in such a way as to win the confidence and meet the needs of the particular patient.

In all cases the nurse should impress her patient with her sincere sympathy and appreciation of the fact that she, the patient, is going through a great emotional and a trying physical experience. Through it all the nurse must give her an opportunity to express her fears and discuss her feelings, and she must be cheerful, encouraging, and optimistic; very gentle, very calm, and reassuring in all that she does in her care for the patient. She must steadily increase the patient's realization of the part which she herself must play in the effort which is being made to carry the event through to a happy conclusion.

The occasion is often a sacred one to the patient, and the nurse should be dignified, even reverential, in her bearing. If the patient feels secure in the belief that her labor is not being taken lightly, that it is being regarded seriously, as it merits, and that every known precaution is being taken, and taken confidently, to safeguard her and her baby's welfare, her actual physical condition will be favorably affected by the mental serenity thus produced.

## FIRST STAGE (STAGE OF DILATATION)

Happily, the onset of labor is usually gradual, as has been described, and there is accordingly ample time during the first stage for deliberate and unhurried preparation for the birth of the baby. The character of the preparation and of the nurse's assistance will vary according to the preferences of the attending doctor, the duration of labor, the circumstances and condition of the patient, and whether she is at home or in a hospital.

**Signs of Beginning Labor.** During the latter part of the prenatal period the patient is instructed to notify the doctor or nurse as soon as she thinks labor has begun. She should notify them when she is conscious of regular contractions occurring about every 10 minutes, if the membranes rupture even though no contractions are felt, or if any vaginal bleeding occurs. Because of their importance these instructions will bear occasional repetition. A multigravida, who has previously had a long hard labor, should especially be urged to call the doctor or nurse early because she may again expect to have a long labor and may postpone notifying someone until there is not sufficient time for adequate preparation.

Since the onset of labor is difficult to define the patient may, in some instances, think she is in labor, and even be quite uncomfortable, only to find that the contractions subside in a few hours. When these perceptible, but nonproductive, contractions cease it is termed a *false labor*. It occurs more often in the multigravida than in the primigravida. As was learned in Chapter 5, the uterus is contracting and relaxing at all times during a woman's life. The painless uterine contractions present throughout pregnancy are called *Braxton-Hicks* contractions. When the patient nears the end of pregnancy these Braxton-Hicks contractions may become painful, similar to true labor pains, but they do not dilate the cervix. These contractions usually occur irregularly, do not increase in intensity, and may continue for days before true labor begins, but when *contractions are regular and increase in strength* true labor has probably started. If the patient has entered the hospital in false labor she must be assured that there is no disgrace in this error and no need to feel apologetic.

It is important that the patient understand the meaning of *rupture of the membranes,* and it may be necessary to use the term "bag of waters" in instructing the patient. It should be explained to her that the bag of waters may break before contractions begin and that while there probably will be a gush of clear fluid from the vagina when this happens, there may be, instead, only a small trickle of fluid at frequent intervals. When a small break in the membranes occurs and there is this occasional trickling of fluid, the patient may believe that she is having urinary incontinence unless she has been properly instructed. It is often important for a patient whose membranes have ruptured to remain in bed, since there is more danger of prolapse of the umbilical cord when she is up and about, particularly if the baby's head is not well down in the pelvis. The doctor will wish to examine the patient after rupture of the membranes and usually wishes to have her admitted to the hospital if she is to be delivered there. Labor usually begins within 24 hours after rupture of the membranes.

A *bloody show* may appear a short time before labor begins, but since it would be difficult for the patient to distinguish between bloody show which is not dangerous, and actual bleeding which is, she should notify the doctor or nurse when this occurs.

**Admission to the Hospital.** If the patient is planning to be delivered in a hospital, she should enter as soon as she is reasonably sure labor has begun. Early admission means less discomfort in traveling, less mental anxiety, and time to prepare for delivery without haste.

Upon admitting the patient to the hospital, which for many is a new and strange experience, the nurse should greet her pleasantly and with a reassuring attitude, and the patient should never be allowed to feel that she is an added burden to the nursing unit. In her conversation with the patient the nurse should obtain the following information: when the contractions began, how frequently they are occurring, approximately how long they last, whether or not the membranes have ruptured, if there has been any bleeding, what the expected date of confinement is, and the number of pregnancies and the number of children the patient has had. All of this information should be recorded accurately and concisely on the record the nurse makes. The number of pregnancies, including miscarriages, and the number of children the patient has delivered may be recorded as gravida and para—gravida referring to the number of pregnancies including the present one, and para referring to the number of pregnancies that have continued to the period of viability including any stillborn infants.

The height and weight of the patient should be measured and recorded upon admission, unless it seems necessary to put her to bed immediately; vaginal bleeding, ruptured membranes, and contractions that are severe enough and close enough to make delivery seem imminent require immediate bed rest. As in the admission of all patients the temperature, pulse rate, and respiratory rate are taken and recorded.

After the patient has been admitted and put to bed she should remain there until the doctor has examined her. This examination will consist of a physical examination, abdominal palpation, auscultation of the fetal heart, and a rectal examination. The nurse should be prepared for this examination by having the necessary equipment in the room. In *preparing for a rectal examination* the nurse should request the patient to lie on her back on the right or left side of the bed, depending upon whether the doctor will examine with his right or left hand, or on her side if the doctor prefers that position. She should be covered with a sheet or blanket and her gown should be well rolled up under her arms. The lower part of the covering sheet or blanket should then be so wrapped about her legs as to protect them and leave the perineal region exposed. To make the rectal examination (Fig. 84) the doctor will need a rubber glove and a lubricating jelly.

After examination of the patient the doctor may order certain laboratory procedures to be done. A urine specimen is usually collected for examination at the time the patient is admitted to the hospital, but the doctor may also wish to have other laboratory studies, such as hemoglobin level and blood count, performed soon after admission.

**Early Preparation for Delivery.** It is a fairly general plan, both in hospitals and in the home, to give the patient a shower or sponge bath at the onset of labor and dress her in a clean gown.

A cleansing *enema* is usually given soon after labor has begun.

This helps to stimulate uterine contractions, especially if a large amount of very warm fluid is used, and it will empty the rectum of material which might be expelled during labor and contaminate the field. If the contractions are already strong a small enema is sufficient, using only enough fluid to empty the lower bowel of fecal

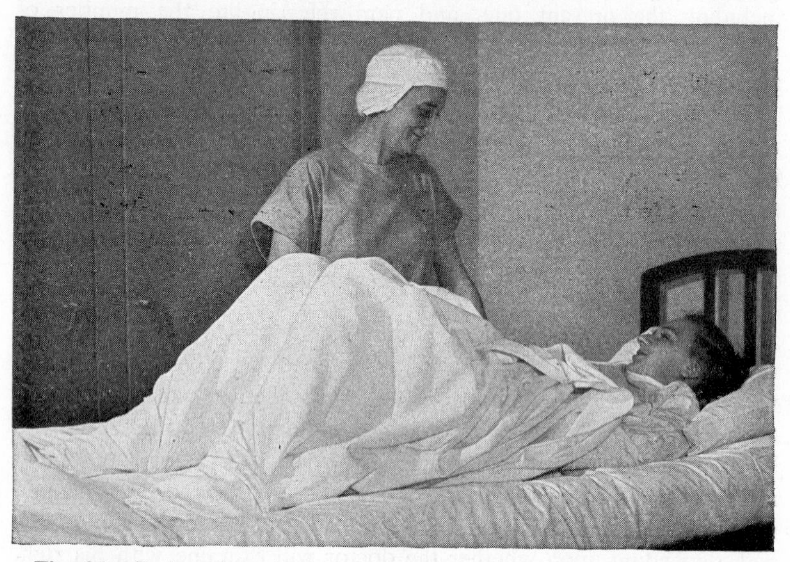

**Fig. 84.** Patient draped with a cotton blanket in preparation for rectal examination. One corner of the blanket is used to cover the right leg; the corner directly opposite covers the left leg; a third corner covers the chest; and the fourth corner may be used to cover the perineal area until the examination is actually performed, at which time it may be pulled up over the abdomen. This drape keeps the patient adequately covered and yet exposes the perineal area sufficiently for the examination.

material. The enema should be given in bed and expelled into a bedpan, as it is not wise for the patient to use the toilet after labor is well in progress. If labor is progressing rapidly it may be necessary to omit the enema entirely because of the possibility of the baby being born while it is being expelled. When the head has descended deep into the pelvis and is making pressure on the rectum, the patient may have considerable difficulty in expelling the enema, and it may then be expelled during the delivery. Those doctors who disapprove of enemas after labor is well in progress believe that solid fecal matter expelled during labor is easier to remove and thus less likely to contaminate the area than the remains of an enema.

The *vulvar and perineal region* is usually *shaved* either before or immediately after the bath and enema, but the time and sequence of the different steps in preparation of the patient are governed by the preference of the doctor and the progress of labor. This procedure will be easier and less uncomfortable for the patient if it is employed as soon as she is definitely known to be in labor. It is not wise, however, to adopt it routinely on admission to the hospital because of the possibility of a false labor. Since the purpose of shaving the area is to remove hair which interferes with adequate skin preparation for the delivery, it is necesary to shave the suprapubic region, the vulva, the inner surface of the thighs, and the anal region. This shaving must be done carefully and completely so that all hair is removed. Before beginning this procedure the nurse must wash her hands carefully to prevent contamination of this area from an outside source. Equipment used must previously have been sterilized. The strokes used in shaving should be from above downward. Sponges used in applying soap should not be returned to the vulvar area after they have touched the anal region. Care must be taken not to allow hair, soap, or water to enter the vaginal opening. All smegma, which may have accumulated in the folds between the labia, should be removed.

After the vulvar area has been completely prepared, the patient, who has up to this time been lying on her back with her thighs separated, is asked to turn onto her side for shaving of the anal region. All other areas should be completely finished before this region is shaved to avoid returning to the cleaner area after preparation of the anal region.

## GENERAL NURSING CARE

**Maintaining Cleanliness.** Precautions must be taken to prevent contamination of the vulva during labor and thereby decrease the danger of introduction of bacteria into the vagina. The nurse must provide clean equipment for the patient's care and must be careful to wash her hands before handling any supplies which come in contact with the patient. Personnel caring for the patient must be free of all signs of infection. To prevent contamination from other patients each must be provided with her own bedpan. The patient must be instructed never to touch the vulva with her hands. A sterile pad of cellucotton or other absorptive material should be kept under the patient to absorb amniotic fluid and bloody discharge draining from the vagina.

To prevent contamination of the vulva a flat pad kept under the patient's buttocks while in bed is preferable to a perineal pad, which may rub from the anal region over the vulva. These pads should be sterilized before use, should be changed frequently, and must be handled in such a way that the side next to the patient is not touched with the hands when it is slipped under her. If the patient has a vaginal discharge while she is up and walking about during early labor, it will be necessary for her to wear a sterile perineal pad, held in place by a T binder or her own belt.

**Activity and Position.** As the contractions are infrequent and mild at first, the patient will usually prefer to be up and about most of the time during the early part of the first stage, when it occurs in the daytime, and many doctors think this important. They feel that patients tend to stay in bed too much during the first stage, since being on their feet would really promote their comfort and this activity has a tendency to make the contractions more regular and efficient. On the other hand, the patient must be cautioned against tiring herself, and should, therefore, lie down often enough and long enough to avoid fatigue. When labor begins at night, it is well to advise the patient to stay in bed and to sleep as much as possible until morning. Even though her sleep is disturbed and broken by the contractions, she will be much less tired in the morning than if she had gotten up and had little or no sleep during the night.

Complete bed rest is indicated if the baby presents in a faulty position, when any complications are present, and when the patient is nearing the second stage of labor. It is also important for the patient to be in bed whenever the membranes have ruptured because of the possibility of prolapse of the umbilical cord. If the patient must be in bed she will probably find the side position (Fig. 45) most comfortable for nearly all of the first stage of labor. As she nears the end of the first stage, when it becomes necessary to change from abdominal to intercostal and sternal breathing, she may have to assume the back position (Fig. 44). While in this position she may wish to have the head of the bed slightly elevated, to relieve strain on her back which is more apt to be experienced when the bed is completely flat.

**Observation of Temperature, Pulse, and Respirations.** These are taken every four hours unless specified to be observed more frequently. An increase in temperature to 37.8° C (100° F) and in the pulse rate to over 100 beats per minute should be reported to the doctor and indicates the need for more frequent observation.

**Observation of Blood Pressure.** The blood pressure should be checked on admission to the hospital and every four to six hours thereafter, unless more frequent observation is indicated by the presence of a toxemia or signs of an impending toxemia. If the patient complains of a *headache* during labor the blood pressure should be checked immediately, since this may be an indication of a developing toxemia. Frequent checking of the blood pressure, even every half hour, may be necessary if it is elevated. The doctor should be notified of an increase to 140 mm Hg systolic and 90 diastolic or even sooner if it was low on admission and appears to be steadily rising. The amount of urinary output should then also be carefully recorded.

**Food and Fluid Intake.** Since it is impossible to estimate the duration of labor it is very difficult to determine whether or not the patient should be urged to eat or drink. She rarely desires food. Some do not retain it because of vomiting throughout labor. Clear liquids are usually offered early in the first stage because labor is an exhausting experience and may continue for many hours. Therefore, the patient should be given aid through nourishment and fluid. Since digestion is slowed by labor and a general anesthetic may be used before labor is ended, solid food is ordinarily withheld, or if given during early labor it should be light and easily digestible. All food and fluid are withheld during the latter part of the first stage, or even during the early part if labor seems to be progressing rapidly, since vomiting during or after anesthesia with the danger of aspiration of stomach contents into the lungs is to be feared. The stomach does not empty well during labor, and food may be retained for 12 hours or longer. The patient may also develop gastric dilatation and may have a large amount of food and fluid in her stomach when she is ready for delivery.

Fluid intake during labor should be recorded. If the patient takes little fluid, or vomits all that has been taken, or if the labor is prolonged it may be necessary to give parenteral fluids. An intravenous infusion of a glucose solution may be desirable every 8 to 12 hours in order to furnish the calories used during labor and to prevent dehydration.

**Output.** The patient should be given a bedpan and encouraged to *void every four hours* or oftener. If she is unable to do so, and the bladder becomes distended, the doctor will usually wish to have her catheterized. Bladder distention is not uncommon, and in extreme cases the bladder may reach to the umbilicus. The nurse should therefore observe the amount of urine which the patient voids and

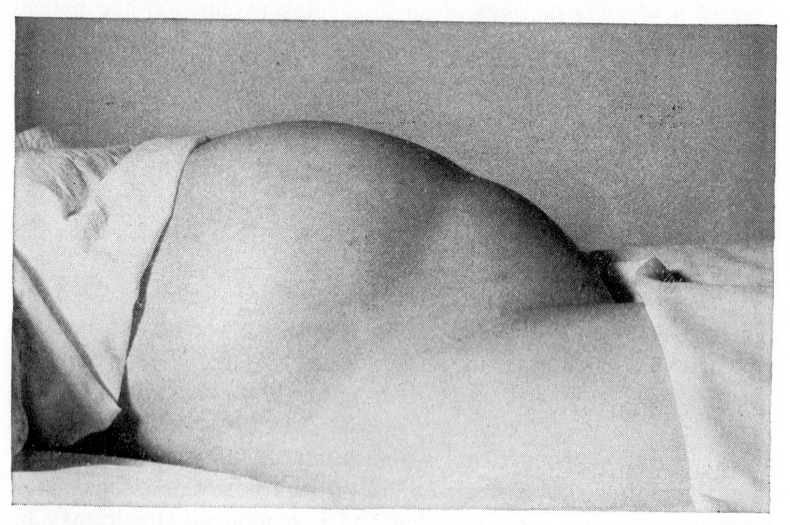

**Fig. 85.** A patient in labor with the lower abdomen showing a distended bladder. The bladder becomes an abdominal organ during pregnancy, and distention is easily visible and palpable.

also watch the lower abdomen for bladder distention. Because the bladder is drawn up in front of the lower uterine segment during pregnancy and thereby becomes an abdominal organ, distention may be observed easily, excepting in very obese patients (Fig. 85).

The seriousness of a distended bladder lies in the fact that it may retard labor (1) by interfering with the descent of the baby's head and (2) through reflex inhibition of the uterine contractions, and the bladder itself may be traumatized, which may predispose to postpartum cystitis. The prevention of a distended bladder during labor is, therefore, of considerable importance.

If a catheterization is necessary, a few special precautions must be observed. To prevent contamination of the vulva the nurse must wash her hands very carefully before beginning this procedure, or preferably wear sterile rubber gloves. Care must be taken that the solutions which are used to clean the area around the urethral orifice, prior to insertion of the catheter, do not enter the vagina. This can be prevented by using sponges moistened just enough to clean, but not soaked with excess solution. To prevent injury, especially if the baby's head is pressing against the urethra, a rubber catheter must always be used. The catheter should be inserted between contractions, since the pressure from the head is less at this time than it is during a contraction, and the patient has less discomfort from the procedure when it is performed between contractions.

The urinary output of the patient in labor should be recorded. This may have special significance if the patient has a toxemia of pregnancy or shows signs of an impending toxemia.

**Support during Labor.** Every patient in labor, regardless of whether or not she has attended mothers' classes and exercise classes, or has read and learned about natural childbirth, will derive much benefit during her labor from the presence of a sympathetic nurse who understands the physical and emotional needs of the individual patient and attempts to satisfy these needs.

The patient who has attended mothers' classes and exercise classes must have much support and encouragement during labor if she is to put into practice that which she has learned. Even the well-prepared patient may become confused and forget while she is under the strain and anxiety of this stressing emotional and physical experience unless she has frequent reminders. Since it is ordinarily not possible for the doctor to attend the patient constantly, the nurse who is with her a considerably longer period of time must have a knowledge of the principles of relaxation and must know how to give support. The care the nurse gives the patient in labor is very important to the patient's success in remaining calm and relaxed.

The nurse must also appreciate that natural childbirth does not mean painless childbirth and that the patient who has attended classes will not be completely relaxed and without anxiety. It does mean that she will make a conscious effort to relax, with help, and that she is willing to tolerate some of the discomfort for the sake of being able to participate actively in the birth of her baby. Natural childbirth does not prohibit the use of analgesia and anesthesia, and it is important that the nurse understand that the patient should be given an opportunity to ask for medication if she needs it. It is, of course, always necessary for the doctor to decide when medication is to be given and what it shall be, but it is important for the nurse to help the patient to realize that she has not failed in her efforts if she needs medication.

The patient who has not been prepared for labor prenatally will need constant support and will respond to the reassurance of a calm, sympathetic, and understanding nurse. Many times a nurse may calm the patient in labor by being with her even at frequent short intervals if it is not possible to stay with her most of the time. The patient's courage will often be strengthened if the nurse will explain, from time to time, the cause of certain conditions that normally arise, and which otherwise might give her alarm, and the reason for certain aspects of physical care. It is the mysterious events, the unexpected and unexplained, that so often terrify. The patient also wishes to have frequent reassurance that she is making progress and that she is cooperating and conducting herself well. In all of this care the nurse must have a good understanding of the psychologic as well as the physical aspects of labor.

It is important to remember that the patient in labor is very alert to her environment. She is acutely aware of the tone of voice, facial expression, disinterest, or false enthusiasm of those around her, but also responds just as easily to a real interest on the part of the nurse. The attitude and conduct of everyone caring for the patient in labor is, therefore, very important. The giving of comfort and strength to the variety of temperaments which the nurse meets among her patients will involve a very sensitive adjustment of manner on her part, but it is an aspect of care which challenges the nurse's ability and one which will give her great satisfaction because of the consciousness of giving a peculiarly needed service.

The husband's presence in the labor room is likewise important in relieving the patient's anxiety and in giving her support, since he does have a vital interest in the birth of the baby. He may already have learned of the support that he can give his wife or he can quickly be given a few instructions. Certainly he can feel helpful by doing the back rubbing that his wife may need, but his mere presence is probably most important.

**Relaxation and Breathing.** It is not recommended that the patient attempt conscious relaxation early in labor, while the contractions produce only a backache, a feeling of tightening in the abdomen, or mild menstrual-like cramps. Conscious effort at relaxation will require close concentration, and because it is tiring the patient should not work at this before it is necessary. During this early stage it is best for her to sit up, walk around, read, or visit with her husband.

When the contractions become hard, conscious effort at relaxation may be started. This will require considerable effort on the part of the patient and careful coaching by the nurse or the husband. As the contractions increase in frequency, intensity, and length, more and more concentration is necessary to achieve relaxation, and every effort must be made to help the patient. The nurse should watch for signs of tenseness, such as tightening of the facial muscles and clenching of the hands, and remind the patient to relax them. If the patient wishes to hold someone's hand this may be comforting, but it must not be a squeezing grip. The nurse can do much to help her get rest between contractions by encouraging her to rest as much as possible during these intervals without making a conscious effort to relax at these times.

Toward the end of the first stage of labor—the transition stage—when dilatation is almost complete, the contractions become very intense, and the patient is apt to become very tired and discouraged. She must increase her efforts to relax and she may have to change from abdominal to intercostal and sternal breathing. It is at this stage that the patient needs much reassurance because there is a great demand on her patience and self-control. Although it may not have been necessary, or possible, to stay with the patient at all times during the early part of labor, especially if she has been relaxing well and if she has felt free to call someone whenever she wished, it does become important for someone to be with her during the period of transition from the first to the second stage. The patient must be given reassurance that this period will not last long. She should be told that as soon as the cervix becomes completely dilated she may push with her contractions and that she will feel better.

**Relief of Pressure Symptoms.** Low *backache,* over the sacral region, may be experienced with each contraction. Massage with the palm of the hand in the form of firm back rubbing, pressure mainly, may give relief. This may be done by the husband or the nurse. A small pillow slipped under the lumbar area may give some comfort.

The patient may complain of *severe cramps in her legs,* especially if the baby's head is low in the pelvis. Relief is frequently obtained by straightening, and slightly elevating the leg, and rubbing it while in that position, and also by flexing the ankle and pushing the forefoot upward toward the knee (Fig. 59). These cramps may return at frequent intervals. As these pains are usually due to pressure they have no serious significance and subside as soon as the child is born.

The patient may also have considerable pressure on her rectum as the baby's head descends low into the pelvis. She should be advised against voluntarily bearing down during first-stage contractions, since the only result at this time will be to waste her strength, which will be needed later, and there is some possibility that this effort may cause small cervical tears. This is one of the points that the nurse will do well to explain: that no voluntary effort on the patient's part, during the first stage, will advance labor, and if she tires herself by making such efforts before the second-stage contractions begin she will not be able to use them as effectively as if she were in a more rested condition. Occasionally, however, there is so much pressure that the patient has a certain amount of involuntary bearing down before dilatation is complete.

This pressure on the rectum may prompt the patient to ask for the bedpan frequently only to find that she cannot use it. With adequate explanation from the nurse as to the reason for this constant feeling of a desire to move her bowels the patient will understand why she does not need the bedpan, the use of which is an effort that tires her. The nurse must, however, not ignore this pressure symptom, since with many patients it is a sign of imminent delivery.

**Observing the Progress of Labor.** The *frequency, duration, and intensity of the contractions* should be carefully noted at frequent intervals. At the beginning of labor the contractions are usually mild, of 15- to 30-seconds' duration and occurring every 5 to 15 minutes, and as labor progresses they become harder and occur more frequently until they are about two to three minutes apart, and last from 50 to 60 seconds or even longer. The patient can be asked to observe the frequency and duration of the contractions in the early stage of labor, but the nurse should time them at regular intervals because the patient's record is usually not entirely accurate. It is only by placing her hand on the patient's abdomen that the nurse can time the contraction and relaxation of the uterine muscle and determine the intensity and duration of the contraction. It is more accurate to determine the strength of the contractions by palpation than to estimate by the patient's reaction since different patients will have different reactions to contractions of approximately the same intensity. Also, in many instances the patient does not feel discomfort at the beginning and end of the contraction so that the actual duration may be longer than the patient's complaint of pain; or she may continue to have discomfort, due to pressure, after the contraction has ended and therefore complain for a longer period of time. The length of the contractions should be recorded from the time the uterus first tightens until it is completely relaxed regardless of the period of time in which the patient feels pain. The frequency with which the contractions occur should be timed from the beginning of one contraction to the beginning of the next and not from the end of one contraction to the beginning of another. If the contractions begin every three minutes and last approximately 60 seconds, there is a rest period of about two minutes, and the frequency of the contractions should then be considered as three-minute rather than two-minute intervals (Chart VI). As labor is entirely a mechanical process

how timing

| Interval | Beginning of Contraction | Duration of Contraction |
|---|---|---|
| | 7 12 | 50 seconds |
| 3 min. | 7 15 | 60 " |
| 4 min. | 7 19 | 60 " |
| 4 min. | 7 23 | 50 " |
| 3 min. | 7 26 | 50 " |
| 3 min. | 7 29 | 50 " |
| 4 min. | 7 33 | 60 " |

Chart VI. A record of the length and interval between uterine contractions. The frequency with which contractions occur is timed from the beginning of one contraction to the beginning of the next. When contractions are timed at various intervals during labor, a chart similar to the above may be kept at the patient's bedside. The frequency and length of the contractions can be recorded for short periods of time. This aids the nurse in accurately recording her observations of the contractions on the patient's record. This chart shows that the patient had contractions of 50 to 60 seconds' duration occurring every three to four minutes.

the more frequently the contractions occur the more progress the patient will make, providing they are of the proper intensity.

A record of both the *fetal and maternal pulse rate* should be made every hour in early labor and every half hour after labor has advanced. To count the fetal heartbeat the abdomen is bared and a stethescope is placed over the area where the heartbeat can be heard best, as described in Chapter 10 (Fig. 76). The fetal heartbeat is a double sound, heard much like the ticking of a watch under a pillow, and is much more rapid than the maternal pulse. The maternal pulse may be mistaken for the fetal, especially when auscultating the lower abdomen, because the pulsations in the aorta may be loud or the sound made by the blood passing through the greatly enlarged uterine vessels may be heard. This is a soft blowing sound and is known as the *uterine souffle*. In counting the fetal pulse it is, therefore, a good plan for the nurse to keep her finger on the mother's pulse to be sure that she does not confuse the sounds of the two heartbeats. The doctor should be notified if the baby's heartbeat is over 160 or below 110 beats per minute.

*Rupture of the membranes,* as manifested by the escape of clear fluid from the vagina, should be reported to the doctor promptly; the cervix may be completely dilated when rupture occurs, the position of the presenting part may change, and there is some possibility of prolapse of the umbilical cord with the gush of fluid, especially if the presenting part is high in the pelvis at the time of rupture. The membranes may break at any time before or during labor, but when rupture occurs after the patient has been in labor for several hours it may be an indication that the cervix is completely dilated. The nurse should instruct the patient to notify her at once if she feels a sudden gush of fluid coming from the vagina. The amount of fluid that escapes will depend upon the point of rupture and the position of the presenting part, and may vary from a small amount which only soaks a portion of the pad under the patient to a quantity which completely saturates the lower bedding. After rupture has occurred some fluid will escape with each contraction.

*Meconium-stained amniotic fluid,* which has a yellowish-green appearance, is an indication of fetal distress, except when the breech is the presenting part, and it should be brought to the doctor's attention. It indicates a relaxation of the sphincter ani muscles of the fetus due to imperfect oxygenation of its blood; this relaxation allows meconium to escape. The fetal heart should then always be checked for rate and rhythm. Meconium in the amniotic fluid does not have significance when the breech is the presenting part because the uterine contractions apply considerable pressure on the baby's abdomen, and meconium is easily forced out of the bowel by this pressure.

As the *transition stage is reached* the patient's entire mien grows more serious. She may also show an increasing amnesia between contractions so that she seems to be unaware of happenings around her. She becomes very warm and may wish to have the room quite cool. Pressure on the rectum increases, abdominal breathing is difficult or impossible, cramps occur or become more marked in the legs and buttocks, and there is tenderness to touch of the back and abdomen. This tenderness may be so marked that the patient requests the nurse not to touch the abdomen to palpate the uterine contractions, and, when necessary, it must then be done very lightly.

An *increase in bloody show,* which is due to tiny lacerations in the cervix, is a good indication that labor is progressing well and the cervix is steadily dilating. There may be considerable increase toward the end of the first stage. Vaginal bleeding, which is a serious complication during labor as explained in Chapter 9, should, however, not be mistaken for an increase in bloody show. The show is a mucoid material containing blood, whereas, bleeding due to placental detachment does not appear to be mixed with mucus.

Toward the end of the first stage of labor, the patient has an *almost continuous desire to empty her bowels* because of pressure made upon the rectum by the descending fetus. If along with this complaint of pressure the patient begins to make *deep grunting sounds* with her contractions and then begins to *involuntarily bear down* with contractions, the second stage of labor has probably begun. Whenever the patient is having bearing-down pains, the perineum should be inspected for bulging at the height of the contractions since *bulging of the perineum* is always a sign that delivery is imminent.

Nurses are frequently instructed to *make rectal examinations* for the sake of increasing the value of their assistance in observing labor. With practice the nurse can learn *to determine the amount of cervical dilatation and effacement, the station of the presenting part in relation to the ischial spines, and the position of the fetus.* A glove, with examining finger well coated with a lubricating jelly, is used for the procedure. The gloves used need not be sterile, but as a preventive measure against infection they should previously have been sterilized by boiling or by steam under pressure. The examining finger should be introduced into the rectum slowly while the patient is instructed to bear down a little in order to relax the sphincters. During the examination the examiner's thumb should be kept back and away from

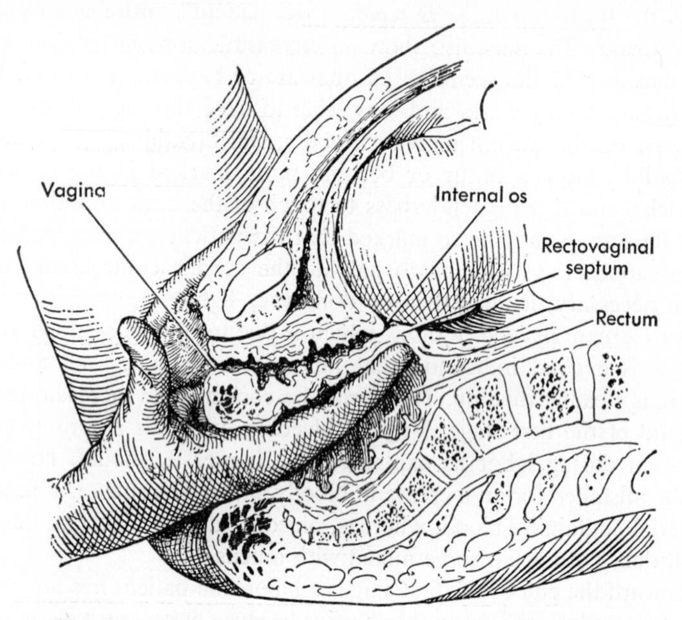


**Fig. 86.** Diagram showing method of ascertaining cervical dilatation and effacement, station of the head, and position of the fetus by means of rectal examination. Examining finger palpates the cervix and head through the rectovaginal septum.

the labia to prevent contamination by rubbing it over the introitus.

The cervix can be palpated through the rectovaginal wall. The opening is felt as a depression with a surrounding circular ridge. By palpation of the diameter of this depression the amount of cervical dilatation can be estimated in centimeters, and by palpation of the thickness of the ridge the amount of effacement is determined (Figs. 77 and 86). The consistency of the cervix should also be noted; one that is soft usually thins and dilates faster than one that is still firm. If the membranes are intact they are sometimes felt bulging through the cervical opening, especially during a contraction. At this examination the degree of engagement of the fetal head should also be ascertained by correlating the level of the head to the level of the ischial spines (Figs. 78 and 86). If the cervix is quite well dilated the cranial sutures and fontanels may be felt for determination of position. Rectal examinations may be made either during or between contractions. An examination done between contractions reveals the amount of cervical dilatation and effacement and the descent of the head while not under pressure of a contraction; one that is performed during a contraction shows the maximum amount of thinning and stretching of the cervix and descent of the head under the influence of the contraction. There may be some recession of the cervical effacement and dilatation after each contraction, but it does not go back to its state before the contraction began since each one makes some change; toward the end of labor this change may be rapid.

There is only slight danger of infection from rectal examinations, and they are practically painless; but since they are disturbing to the patient, especially when performed during a contraction or when the patient is troubled with hemorrhoids, they should therefore not be repeated more often than seems essential. The progress of labor can be followed to a large extent by observation of the symptoms mentioned above. Rectal examinations can be used to confirm the observation that labor is progressing and should be used whenever it is necessary to determine exactly how much progress has been made. These examinations are not always reliable since it is sometimes difficult to feel the cervix, especially if it is very thin.

A *vaginal examination* may become necessary if labor is apparently not progressing satisfactorily and if the findings of the rectal examination are inconclusive. The doctor always performs the examination, seeking the same information that is ordinarily obtained by the rectal examination. The vaginal examination is more accurate than the rectal because the rectovaginal septum does not interfere with palpation of the cervix and the fontanels. The danger of infection demands that every precaution be taken to prevent carrying bacteria from the outside into the vagina. The nurse's duty lies in preparation for the examination by cleaning the skin and draping the patient with sterile towels or draping sheet, and furnishing the doctor with sterile supplies. The doctor wears sterile rubber gloves and is very careful that the examining fingers do not touch anything before they enter the vagina. The fingers are inserted only once, and great care is taken that the labia are well separated before their insertion to prevent touching the inner surfaces of the labia.

*Watchfulness* during labor is of *extreme importance*—watching for symptoms of complications or change in the patient's condition, and watching the progress of labor in order to keep the doctor fully informed about his patient's condition.

Although unexpected symptoms do not, as a rule, develop suddenly during the first stage, the nurse must be nonetheless vigilant for them. The doctor should be notified if the contractions suddenly grow either more or less frequent, or more or less severe; if there is any bulging of the perineum; if the membranes rupture; if there is any bleeding or a prolapsed cord; if there is extreme restlessness or any evidence of unusual distress; if a rising pulse, a temperature of 37.8° C (100° F), an increase in blood pressure to 140 mm Hg systolic or 90 diastolic occur; if the fetal heart rate becomes more than 160 or less than 110 beats per minute; or if there is any marked change in the patient's condition or that of the fetus.

During the early hours of the first stage of labor, if the patient is to be confined at home, the nurse should begin to arrange the room and bed for delivery as described in the Appendix. In a hospital all supplies should always be in readiness for a delivery, but it may be well to check them over carefully to make certain that everything that may be necessary is available.

The end of the first stage is reached when the cervix is fully dilated, at which time the contractions occur about every two to four minutes, are strong and very intense, and the patient begins to feel like bearing down. The membranes frequently rupture at this point, and the vaginal discharge is blood-tinged. The patient should remain in bed and not be left alone from this time on.

To sum up the nurse's duties during the first stage of labor, when the patient may be largely in the nurse's care:

1. She must be a sympathetic, encouraging friend to the patient.
2. She must help the patient conserve her strength by giving her aid and support with relaxation and relieving her discomforts insofar as possible in the best way she knows how.
3. She must observe the progress of labor and watch for symptoms of complications.
4. She must employ technics that will prevent conveying bacteria to the birth canal.
5. She must prepare for the birth of the baby.

## SECOND STAGE (STAGE OF EXPULSION)

The second stage is shorter and harder than the first. The uterine contractions are stronger, more frequent, and more expulsive, and the baby steadily curves and rotates its way down through the birth canal.

With the onset of the second stage the nurse should complete the preparations for the baby's birth, remembering that with a primigravida the baby will probably not be born for about one hour, but may come in half an hour or less if the patient has previously had a baby. The preparation in the delivery room is usually started when the second stage begins in the primigravida, but will need to be made earlier for the multigravida. When the woman has previously delivered a baby it is well to begin preparation as soon as the cervix is approximately 6 cm (2.4 in.) dilated, depending to some extent upon the frequency and strength of the contractions, because in the multigravida the cervix usually dilates very rapidly after it has reached 5 to 6 cm (2 to 2.4 in.), and the baby may be born with as few as one or two pains after complete dilatation. There is frequently not adequate time for complete preparation if it is not begun before the second stage of labor. After the patient has been prepared and draped with sterile sheets and towels, neither they nor the perineal region should be touched with anything unsterile.

**Preparation for Vaginal Examination or Delivery.** Like certain other aspects of obstetric care, the local preparation of the patient for vaginal examination or delivery varies in technic, but the general principles are the same. The desire of all obstetricians is to protect the patient against infection and to accomplish this end with the least possible disturbance to the patient and minimum expenditure of time and effort. The simpler the effective procedure can be made, the more general will be its employment, not alone in hospitals, but also in the patients' homes.

If the doctor wishes to make a vaginal examination it devolves upon the nurse to prepare the patient with strictest adherence to aseptic technic. Vaginal examination made without careful preparation is one of the causes of puerperal infection. As has been previously explained, some obstetricians prefer to make no vaginal examinations during labor when previous examination has indicated that progress is normal, depending rather upon rectal examinations for guiding information. However, we must not lose sight of the fact that vaginal examination is only one of the many ways in which the patient can be infected. Among these are incompletely sterilized or contaminated dressings, instruments, and gloves, and droplet infection

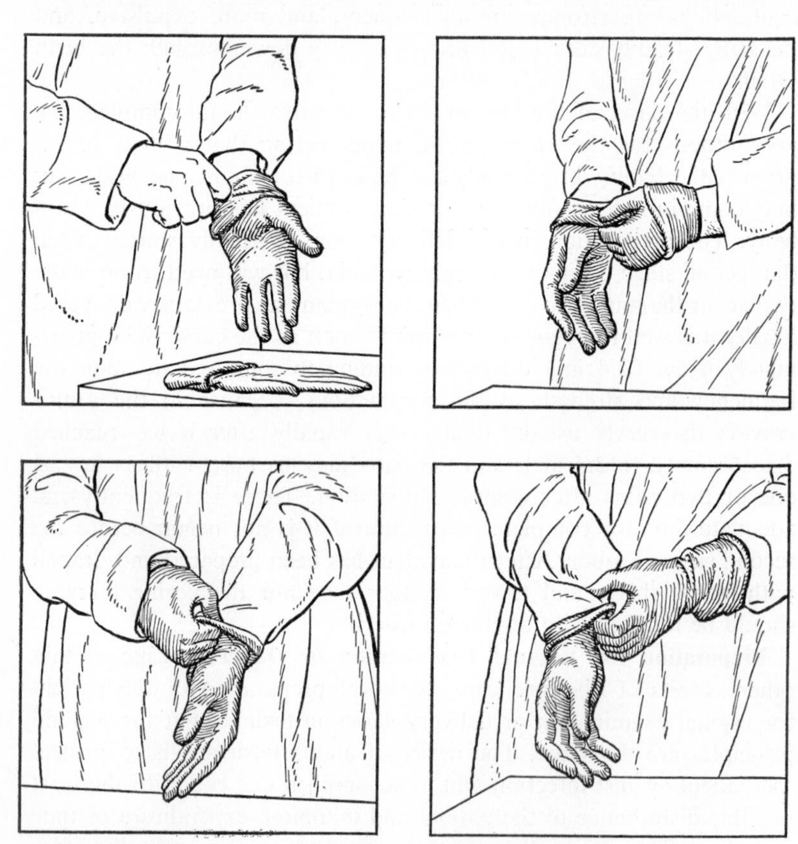

**Fig. 87.** Successive steps in proper method of putting on sterile gloves to avoid contaminating outside of gloves with bare fingers.

Both gloves have been sterilized with the cuffs turned down. The first glove is grasped at the top of the cuff so that only the inside surface of the glove is touched—that part which will come next to the bare hand. The second glove is picked up with the gloved hand placed under the cuff in such a manner that only the outside surface of this second glove is touched; thus the hand already gloved does not touch the hand which is being gloved. The cuffs of both gloves are then pulled up over the sleeves of the gown without touching the bare hands.

(Drawings based on photographs taken at the Long Island Hospital.)

from the nose and mouth of the attendants. This explains the importance of masks on the doctors and nurses as a measure in preventing puerperal infection. Both mouth and nose must be well covered, and the mask must be changed as frequently as possible, but even the mask will not be sufficient protection if any of the attendants has an upper respiratory infection. Therefore, no one with an infection should attend the patient in labor, this being true of infections of other types as well as respiratory. It may be well to mention here that only personnel directly concerned with the delivery should be permitted in the room, and then only when in proper operating room attire.

The perineal region should be regarded as the field of a major surgical operation and be prepared accordingly. Rigid asepsis is important to prevent contamination from without. It is necessary, however, to realize that the area can be made only relatively clean since bacteria from the vulva and anal region are always present. Care must be taken, therefore, to avoid touching the vulva and the surrounding skin insofar as possible during examination and delivery.

A fairly typical method of preparing the patient for vaginal examination or delivery is as follows: The patient should be in bed on a douche pan, or on the delivery table, with knees flexed and well separated, gown tucked up under the arms, and draped with a sheet according to the extent of the area to be prepared. In the hospital this preparation is ordinarily done in the delivery room with the patient on the delivery table and the legs up in stirrups. With the patient in this position the doctor can work more easily than with her feet on the bed, and she will be in a position for any operative procedure that may be necessary (Fig. 88). Care must be taken *to prevent a strain on the ligaments of the pelvis* during the positioning of the legs in the stirrups. They must not be separated too widely and one leg should not be placed higher than the other. To avoid this straining it is therefore also important that both legs be put up and taken out of the stirrups simultaneously; it is likewise necessary that the legs be strapped to the stirrups immediately after being placed there, to avoid the danger of having the patient move a leg out of the stirrup. For a similar reason they must never be unstrapped, after the delivery, until the very moment they are to be put down on the table. The patient may be partially under the influence of an anesthetic and may accidentally move her legs.

Here it is well to remind the nurse of her obligation to protect the patient from the embarrassment of unnecessary exposure at any time during labor. The field which is prepared must be uncovered, and while the patient is being prepared for examination or delivery a certain amount of exposure is unavoidable, but there are many ways in which

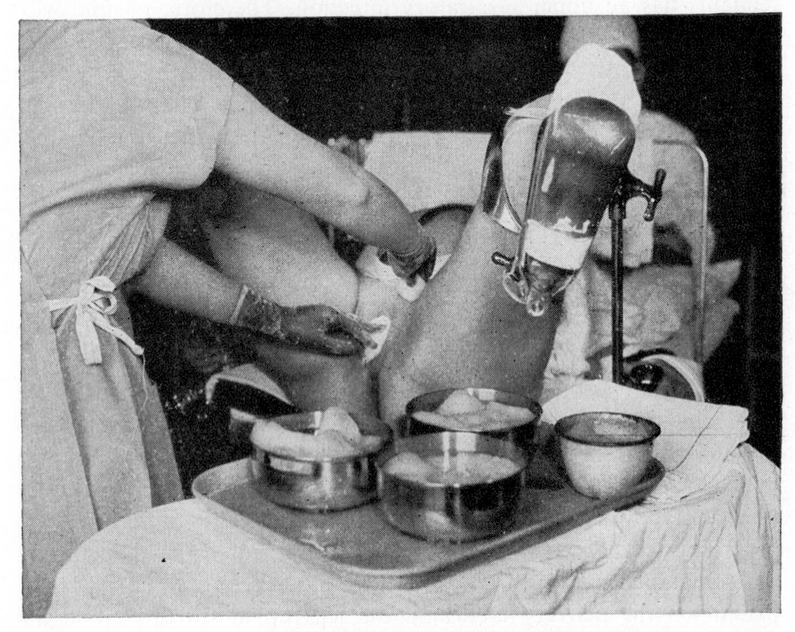

**Fig. 88.** Patient on delivery table with legs in stirrups, and nurse ready to wash the perineal area in preparation for sterile vaginal examination or delivery. (This and succeeding pictures of a normal delivery [Figs. 88, 91, and 94–101] taken at University Hospitals, Madison, Wisconsin.)

the nurse may show her consideration for the patient in this connection and the patient always appreciates this effort.

After the patient has been positioned the materials needed for preparation should be conveniently arranged on a table nearby. The nurse should clean her nails, prepare her hands and arms with soap and warm water, as she would for any surgical operation, put on a pair of sterile rubber gloves, and then prepare the patient (Figs. 88 and 89).

Some obstetricians have the entire area from the umbilicus to the knees prepared while others prepare only the suprapubic region, the

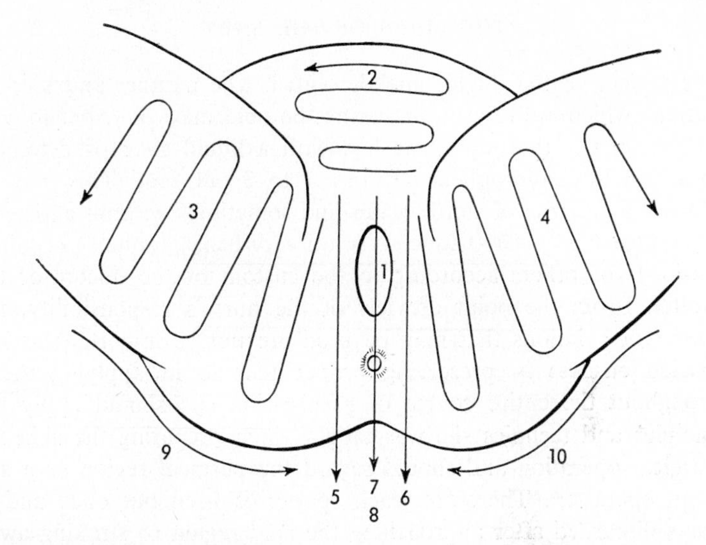


**Fig. 89.** Diagram showing the sequence and direction of the strokes used in washing the perineal region for delivery.

1. A dry cotton ball is held over the introitus to prevent the solution which is used for washing from entering the vagina.
2. One cotton ball is used to wash the mons veneris and the lower abdomen; the washing is begun at the upper aspect of the labia majora and continued upward toward the umbilicus.
3. Another cotton ball is used to wash the inner aspect of the right thigh. Beginning in the crease of the groin and continuing outward toward the knee, these strokes should be made with a back-and-forth motion and must always be carried well underneath the thigh.
4. Another cotton ball is used to wash the inner aspect of the left thigh in the same manner.
5. One cotton ball is used to wash the right labium majus and the area to the right of the anus with one downward stroke. It is discarded when the table is reached.
6. Another cotton ball is used to wash the left labium majus and the area to the left of the anal region with one downward movement.
7. The dry cotton ball, which has been held over the introitus, is now discarded, and a cotton ball is used to wash, with one downward stroke, directly down the middle over the vulva and the anus.
8. The above step is repeated with another cotton ball.
9. Another cotton ball is used to wash that part of the right buttock which is close to the delivery table. The movement is toward the anal region, and the cotton ball is discarded when the anus is reached. This step may be used to complete the washing of the buttock that was not possible in step 3 since washing down too low at that time would have meant touching the table and contaminating the nurse's gloves.
10. The left buttock is washed in the above manner.

inner surface of the thighs, and the vulva. The number and kind of solutions which are used in preparing the field may vary, but in general the area is thoroughly washed with a liquid soap or detergent containing hexachlorophene (G-11) 1 to 3 per cent. This may be followed by a rinse of sterile water and sometimes with an antiseptic solution, such as 1:1000 aqueous solution of benzalkonium (Zephiran chloride), or others according to the custom of the doctor or the hospital. From the point of view of the nurse's responsibility, the number of solutions that may be used are not as important as her conscientiousness in preserving proper technic in applying them. Throughout the entire course of preparation she should apply the principles and technics she was taught when preparing the skin for a surgical operation and should regard the perineal region as a site for an operation. Therefore, each sponge is used but once and is always discarded after approaching the anal region or stroking away from the vaginal opening in any direction. This washing should proceed from the center outward in order not to carry infectious material from an unclean to a clean area, which in this case is the vaginal outlet. The suprapubic region and lower abdomen are washed across, back and forth, working up from the symphysis pubis; the strokes on the thighs are up and down working from the groin out toward the knee; those used to clean the groins and vulva are toward the anal region and away from the vagina, *never toward it,* and the fluids poured upon the vulvar region must never run into the vagina from over surrounding skin. Some obstetricians instruct the nurse to press a sterile cotton ball between the labia against the vaginal opening while she is washing and flushing the adjacent areas, to avoid the introduction of unclean fluids. After the surrounding areas have been prepared the labia are separated and the inner surfaces washed from above downward and flushed by pouring the solution directly between the folds. A dry sterile towel or pad is slipped under the buttocks. It may occasionally be necessary to apply these solutions very hastily or even to omit some of them entirely when the delivery is imminent. If there is time for some preparation, but not for all of the steps, it is best to use the soap and water to remove the blood and mucus, which usually collects on the skin, but there may only be time to pour a solution of one of the antiseptics over the area. Every precaution must still be taken to avoid contamination from the anal region.

Next the patient is draped with sterile linen, but before handling the linen the nurse should remove the gloves she used for the preparation and put on a sterile gown and a fresh pair of sterile gloves. Since it is impossible to sterilize the skin, as much of the prepared area as possible should be covered with sterile drapings. Sterile leggings or towels should be placed over the legs and as deeply into the groins as

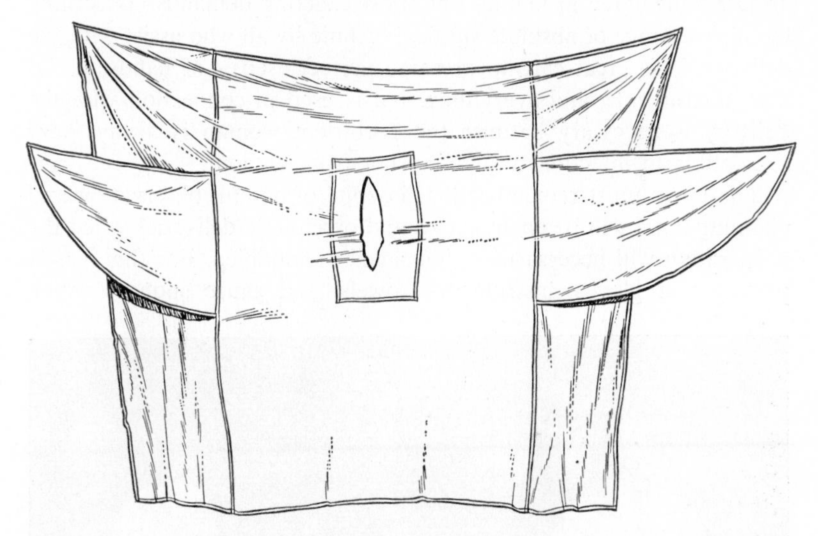

**Fig. 90.** A perineal sheet with leggings attached, thus making it possible to drape the patient with one motion. The oblong opening fits over the perineal region to expose the operative area.

possible and sterile sheets placed over the abdomen and under the buttocks. These can then be held in place with sterile towel clips or sterile safety pins. If the patient is on a delivery table with the legs in stirrups, a sterile perineal sheet with leggings attached and an opening over the perineal region can conveniently be used (Figs. 90 and 91). If the patient is delivered on a bed the area under her will become wet with amniotic fluid and blood; extra thicknesses of sheet or towels should be used under the buttocks and between the patient's legs to prevent contamination from the bed or table underneath.

Other methods of preparation may be used, but regardless of the method that is used the nurse must remember the general principles of asepsis and adjust herself to the preferences of the individual doctor. On one point, and this concerns the nurse, there is absolute agreement; it is that everything brought to the perineal region, or used in any way in connection with the delivery, must be sterilized properly. She may be certain that all doctors will want caps and masks, sterile gowns and gloves, and sterile towels, gauze, and instruments. No matter how simple or elaborate the preparation may be, all obstetricians agree in making the most exacting demands concerning the maintenance of absolute surgical technic by all who assist with the delivery. This great care to preserve perfect asepsis of hands, dressings, instruments, and everything that is used in connection with the delivery is necessary because the parturient woman is always very susceptible to infection brought to her from without.

The nurse must remember that in spite of careful observation and planning there will be emergencies and precipitate deliveries when the preparation will necessarily be curtailed or modified. For this reason packages of gloves, instruments, towels, and gauze sponges which

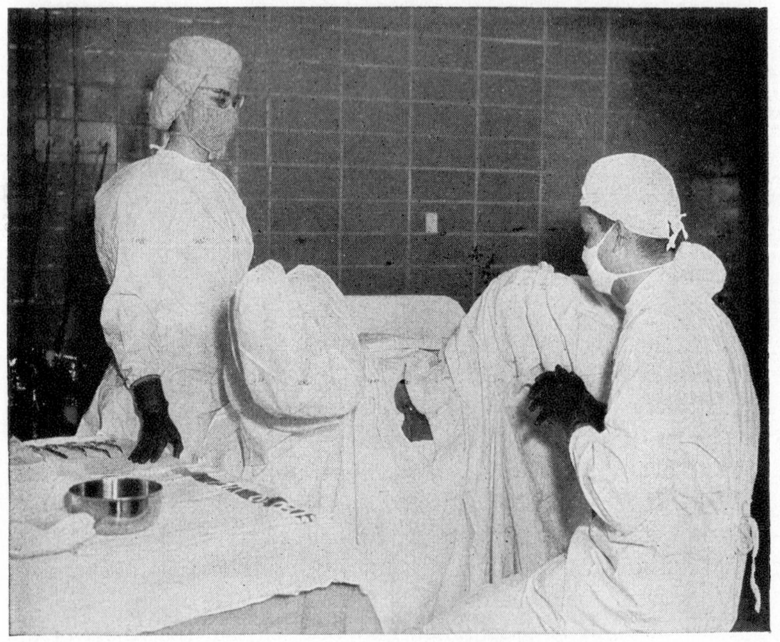

**Fig. 91.** Everything in readiness for the delivery. The patient is on the delivery table with legs in stirrups, and the perineal area prepared and draped with sterile sheets. The doctor and the nurse are dressed in cap and mask and sterile gown and gloves, and the sterile instruments, gauze, and towels are in readiness.

have previously been sterilized should be readily available for immediate use.

In preventing contamination, much depends upon the actual sterilization of the rubber gloves either by boiling or by steam under pressure, and the method of putting on the gloves, in order that once having been sterilized, they may be kept so (Fig. 87). Although the hands are carefully prepared by scrubbing, they cannot be made absolutely sterile, and, therefore, in relation to the gloves which are sterile, the bare hands must always be regarded as unclean. Too much thought and attention cannot be given to the sterilization and handling of gloves, since the postpartum course may depend upon their aseptic condition. The same is true of the instruments used during delivery which also may be sterilized by boiling or by steam under pressure. In the hospital the draping sheets, towels, and instruments are most easily prepared by placing them in heavy linen

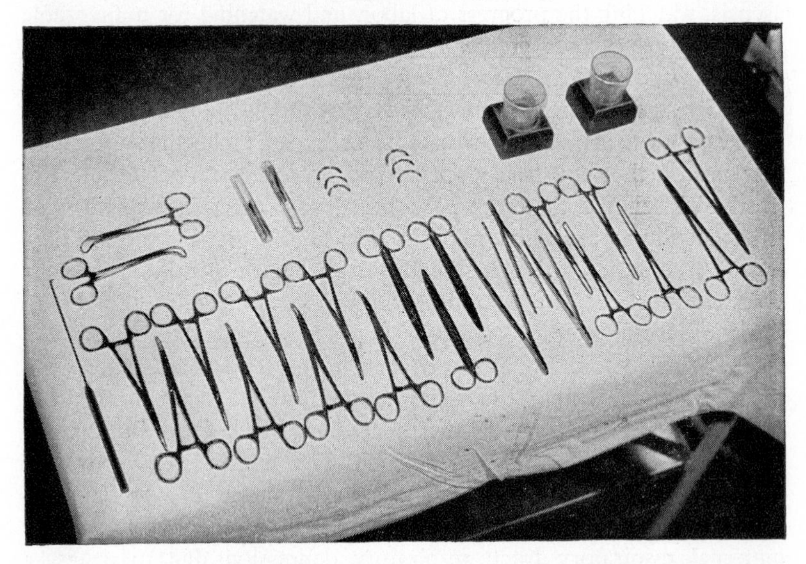

**Fig. 92.** Instruments which may be necessary for a normal delivery and the repair of an episiotomy or a laceration.

*Above:* Two towel clips; catgut, chromic, size No. 00, and/or 000; taper and/or trocar point curved surgical needles; medicine glasses in holders for antiseptic solutions.

*Below:* Membrane hook; eight curved Pean forceps; one Mayo dissecting scissors; two straight operating scissors; one tissue forceps with teeth; one dressing forceps, without teeth; one Russian tissue forceps; four Allis tissue forceps; two needle holders.

wrappers of double thickness and sterilizing them with steam under pressure in a wall autoclave. Modifications will necessarily have to be made for home deliveries as described in Appendix I.

In addition to the sterile instruments (Fig. 92), basins, and a supply of sterile towels and gauze sponges, the nurse must remember that there should be, for the baby, an umbilical cord tie or clamp and dressing, blankets, a heated crib, identification material, silver nitrate solution or penicillin for the eyes, an aspirator, and oxygen and intubation equipment in case the baby needs resuscitation. Also needed are equipment for giving anesthesia to the mother, suture material for repair of the perineum, and supplies for control of bleeding from the uterus after delivery of the placenta, which means that oxytocic drugs, parenteral fluids, and uterine packer and packing must be available.

**Process of Delivery.** During the second stage the preservation of asepsis, watching the progress of labor, and watching for unfavorable symptoms are of even greater importance than during the first stage.

*Watching the Fetal Heart Tones.* Fetal distress may be brought about by an interference with the oxygen supply to the fetus, which may be due to a number of causes, or by an abnormal amount of pressure on the fetal head as it passes through the birth canal. The heart tones should therefore be watched very carefully and checked as frequently as every five minutes. The fetal heart may slow a little during a contraction, but it should quickly return to normal between contractions. Careful observation of the rate and rhythm of the fetal heart is the best method of recognizing an impending fetal asphyxia. There is an almost immediate change in the fetal heart action with the development of hypoxia. Oxygen administered to the mother will in many instances satisfactorily treat hypoxia in the fetus and thereby prevent respiratory depression at birth. This is especially true when the fetus is deprived of an adequate oxygen supply due to low concentration of oxygen in the anesthetic agent, obstruction in the maternal respiratory tract, respiratory depression due to drugs, a failing maternal circulatory system, placental separation, or pressure on the umbilical cord during contractions. High concentrations of oxygen may be administered to the mother between, as well as during, contractions while awaiting spontaneous delivery or while preparation is being made for an operative delivery if this is indicated.

*Artificial Rupture of the Membranes.* If the membranes have not ruptured by the time the patient is prepared for delivery they are

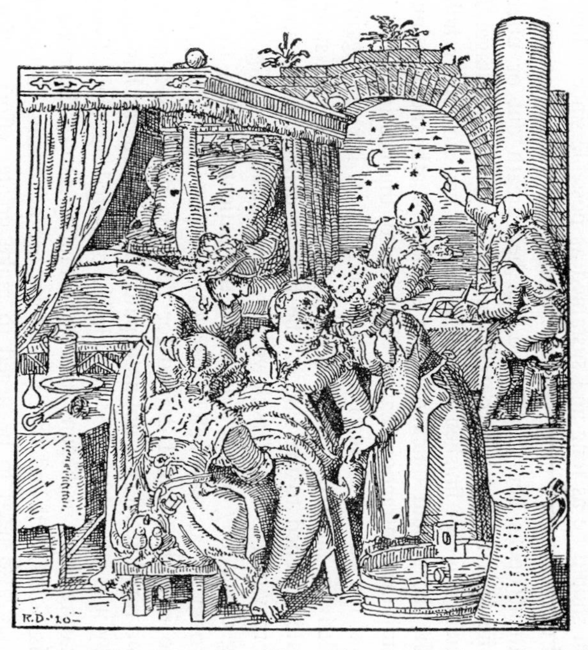

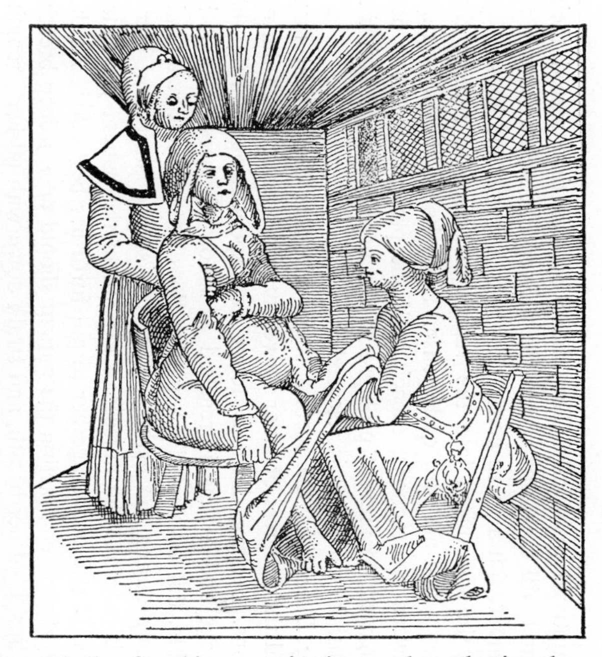

**Fig. 93.** Old prints illustrating early ideas of suitable methods of making examinations and conducting deliveries, furnishing interesting contrast with present-day methods. Concern seems to be divided between the patient and the signs of the zodiac in the picture at the left.

usually ruptured artificially. They have by this time served their purpose and will now only retard the delivery. A sterile forceps or an instrument with a sharp point, known as a membrane hook (Fig. 92), may be introduced into the vagina and used to rupture the membranes which are now quite tense. They should always be ruptured between contractions, especially if the presenting part is not deeply engaged, to prevent prolapse of the umbilical cord with the sudden gush of fluid that is released.

*Bearing Down.* As the second stage advances the patient may greatly aid the progress of labor by voluntarily bearing down during contractions. Bearing down is reflex and spontaneous during the second stage and a time is reached as labor advances when it is unavoidable, but occasionally a patient does not use this reflex advantageously during the early part of the second stage and some coaching is helpful. The nurse can explain to the patient just what she should do and encourage her to put forth her best effort. At the beginning of each contraction the patient should take a deep breath, close her lips, hold her breath, and strain down with all her strength. Each push should be as long and sustained as possible since a long-continued effort is much more effective than short grunting attempts. If the patient opens her mouth and lets her breath out or utters sounds, she fails to use her contractions to the best advantage. If the contraction is not finished when the patient can no longer hold her breath, she should quickly take a second breath and continue pushing until the contraction ceases. The effect of this bearing down is increased if the patient flexes her knees and braces her feet against the bed, delivery table, or stirrups, and if she is provided with straps or a handle attached to the side of the bed or delivery table upon which she may pull as she bears down with the contractions (Fig. 94).

Bearing down may be started before the patient is taken to the delivery room, or at least before her legs are put into stirrups and before she is prepared and draped for delivery, if she is a primigravida and rapid delivery is not anticipated. After a woman has once had a baby it is advisable to be completely prepared for the delivery before bearing down is begun. It is important to assure the patient that she is doing well and that her efforts are advancing the baby, but she may also need to be urged to make greater effort. Before the head can be seen at the outlet or its advance noted by perineal bulging, the stage of its descent is often ascertained by palpating through the perineum, the fingers of a gloved hand pressing upward on one side of the vulva.

*Preventing Rapid Delivery of the Head.* As soon as the perineum bulges, efforts should be made to prevent perineal tears, or if an episiotomy is performed, to prevent extension of the incision. Tears

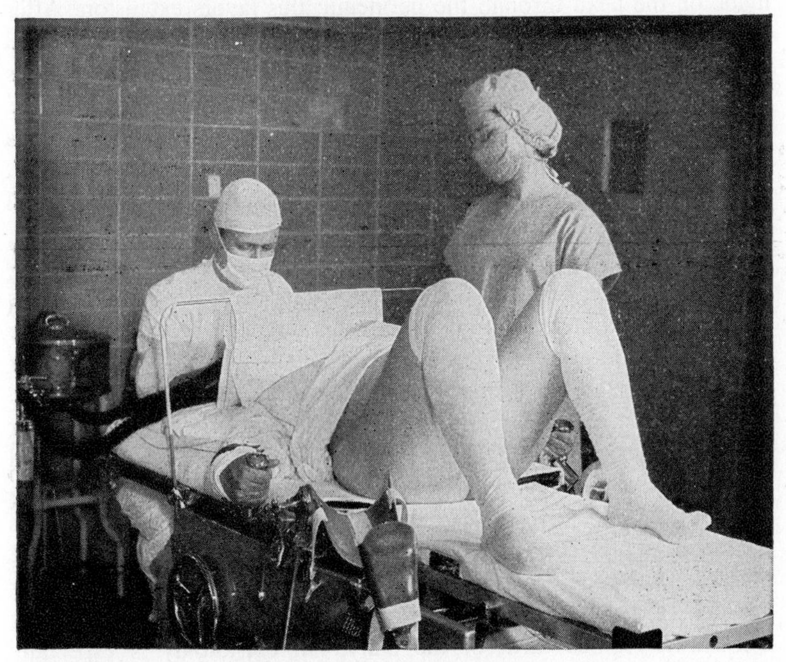

**Fig. 94.** Patient receiving a few breaths of a nitrous oxide and oxygen mixture for analgesia, and pulling on the handles at the sides of the delivery table while bearing down during second-stage contractions. This bearing down may be started before the patient's legs are put up in stirrups and before she is prepared and draped if rapid delivery is not anticipated.

cannot always be prevented, but their frequency can be reduced by not allowing the head to be delivered too rapidly at the acme of a contraction. Sometimes when the perineum has been offering considerable resistance to the head this resistance is suddenly overcome, and one contraction may force the head through with a tear as a result. Imperfect extension of the head is another common reason for perineal tears because it is forced down against the perineal body instead of upward to the vaginal opening. For these reasons it is well to put pressure on the head after it becomes visible, partly to further extend it by bringing it closer to the lower margin of the symphysis pubis and partly to prevent it from being extruded too rapidly. In many instances the doctor will deliver the head between contractions by Ritgen's maneuver. In this method the head is delivered by pressure made on the head through the perineum; this favors extension. After the head has descended far enough to distend the vulva with its parietal areas the doctor covers his gloved fingers with a sterile towel, places them directly before or behind the anal region, and makes pressure upward through the perineum to deliver the head between contractions in a slow and controlled manner. See Figures 95, 96, 97, and 98 for appearance, advance, and birth of the head during normal delivery.

*Episiotomy*. Many obstetricians prefer to facilitate delivery by cutting through the perineal body with a pair of blunt scissors. This operation is termed *episiotomy* and will usually prevent tears. The incision is sutured after labor just as a tear would be repaired. This incision starts at the posterior margin of the vaginal opening and may be made either directly in the midline down to the sphincter ani muscles or at a 45-deg angle to either side, the latter being termed a mediolateral episiotomy. It is ordinarily made during a contraction and with the patient receiving analgesia. It is usually performed when the head is low enough to distend the perineum and apply some pressure to the incision. Generally it is done before undue stretching has occurred, but not so early as to allow for excessive blood loss while awaiting the birth of the baby. An episiotomy is especially useful in cases of breech presentation; in cases of rigid perineum to prevent pounding of the baby's head against the perineum; when rapid delivery is necessary; or where a laceration seems inevitable. It is the belief of those who perform this operation that the muscles of the perineal floor will be spared undue stretching; that the opening will not tear further, or if further tearing does occur that it will continue in the same line; and that the clean-cut incision may be repaired more easily than an irregular tear. The midline incision is easy to repair, heals well, and probably heals with less discomfort to the patient than the mediolateral, but there is danger of extension through the sphincter muscles if further tearing does occur. With the mediolateral episiotomy, extension can be made without damage to the

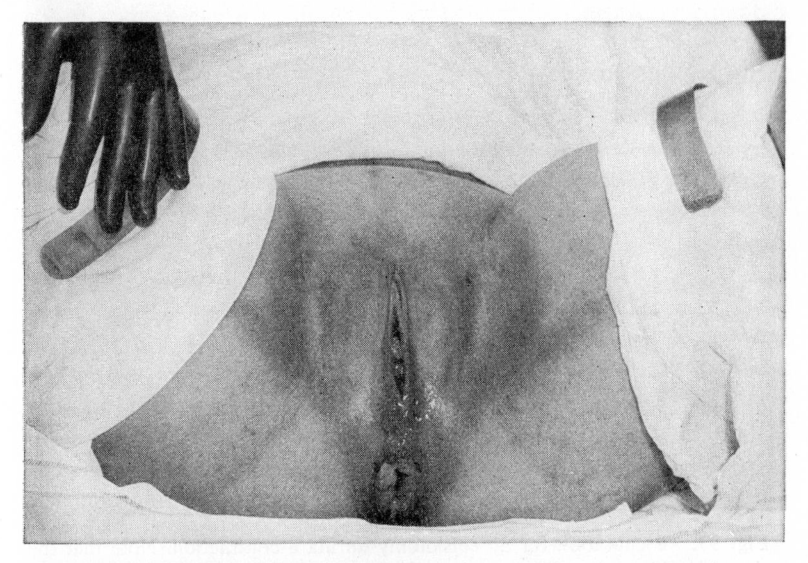

**Fig. 95.** The baby's head is appearing at the vulva at the height of a contraction; separation of the labia is beginning.

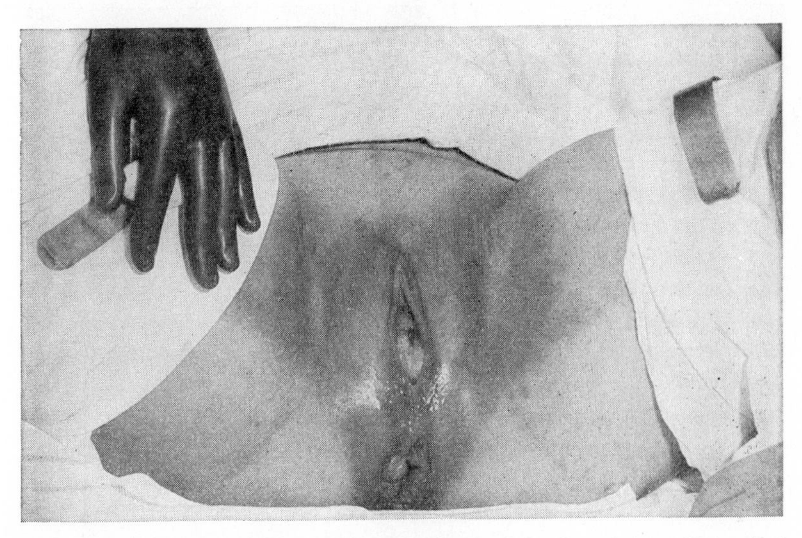

**Fig. 96.** Advance of the head is indicated by distention of the vulva and of the perineum.

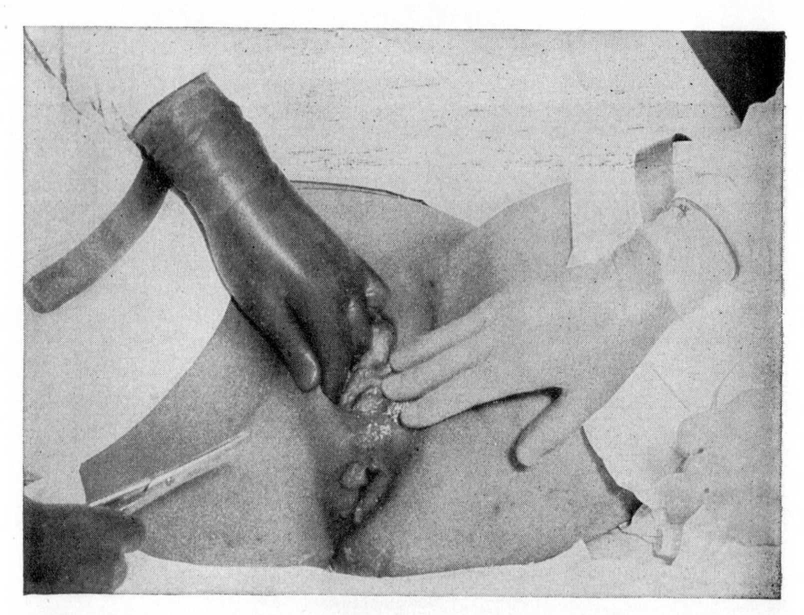

**Fig. 97.** Preparation for an episiotomy during a contraction. Note that the perineum has become quite thin and that the anus has begun to distend.

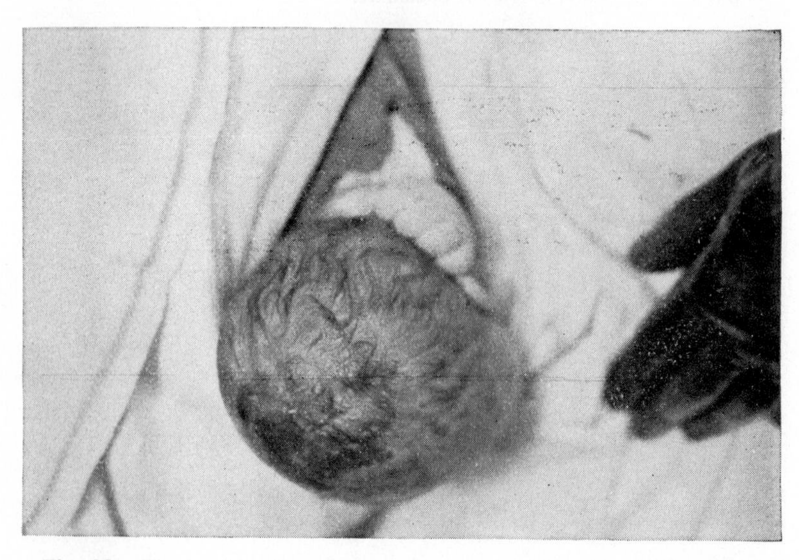

**Fig. 98.** The head has been born, and external rotation toward the right has taken place. In this delivery a hand has prolapsed alongside the head; this is not ordinarily the case.

sphincter muscles, and it is, therefore, ordinarily employed in unusual presentations.

*Palpation for Umbilical Cord around the Neck.* Immediately after the birth of the head the obstetrician palpates the baby's neck to determine whether or not loops of umbilical cord surround it. Quite frequently one or more loops of cord do encircle the baby's neck and they may be so tight that the vessels become constricted. If these coils of cord are fairly loose they may be slipped over the head, but if they are tight the cord should be clamped and cut immediately. When the nurse is acting as the doctor's assistant, she should be prepared to hand him quickly two clamps and a blunt scissors.

*Delivery of the Shoulders and Body.* The shoulders appear at the vulva as soon as external rotation of the head has taken place and they are usually born spontaneously, but it may be necessary to hold the head between the two hands and make downward traction to fix the anterior shoulder under the symphysis pubis and then upward traction to deliver the posterior shoulder (Figs. 79, 80, and 99). After the shoulders are delivered the rest of the body will usually follow quickly, but if traction must be made it should be done gently and only in the direction of the long axis of the baby so as to avoid bending the neck on the body and thus prevent excessive stretching and injury of the brachial plexus. Moreover, the nerves of the arm may be injured when too much pressure is made with the fingers in the axillae. Pressure on the mother's abdomen will help to deliver the shoulders and body. As soon as the body is delivered the baby is grasped by the feet and held with head down for postural drainage (Figs. 100 and 101).

## CARE OF THE BABY IN THE DELIVERY ROOM

At the end of the second stage of labor the newborn baby who, sometimes, is not breathing quite satisfactorily and whose cord is still uncut requires immediate attention.

**Establishing Respirations.** After the baby has been brought safely into the world, it is of greatest possible importance to make sure that it begins its separate existence by crying lustily, in order fully to expand its lungs. This provides for oxygenation of its blood, which has taken place, until now, through the placental circulation. The removal of this placental supply should stimulate active respiratory movements. The mechanism of respiration is established before birth, and respiratory movements have occurred during intrauterine life; therefore, if the baby does not breathe at birth there must be some

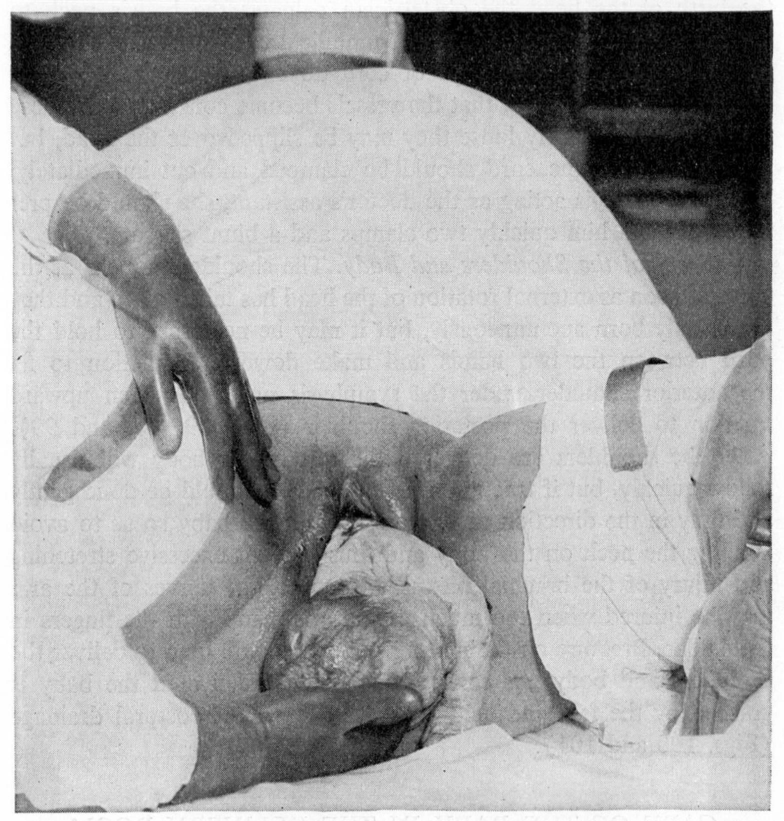

**Fig. 99.** The anterior shoulder has been delivered; birth of the rest of the body follows quickly.

serious cause for failure of this function, and any infant not breathing within 30 seconds is not normal physiologically and must be considered in danger of asphyxia.

In many cases the baby cries satisfactorily without aid, but not infrequently must be stimulated to do so. In all instances the first step is to clear the air passages of the mucus lodged in the mouth and throat, by some one of the many approved methods. The baby should be held up by its feet, with the head hanging down and the neck curved sharply backward, immediately after birth to allow mucus and fluid to drain from its mouth and nose by gravity (Fig. 100). Some doctors disapprove of holding the baby up by its feet, on the

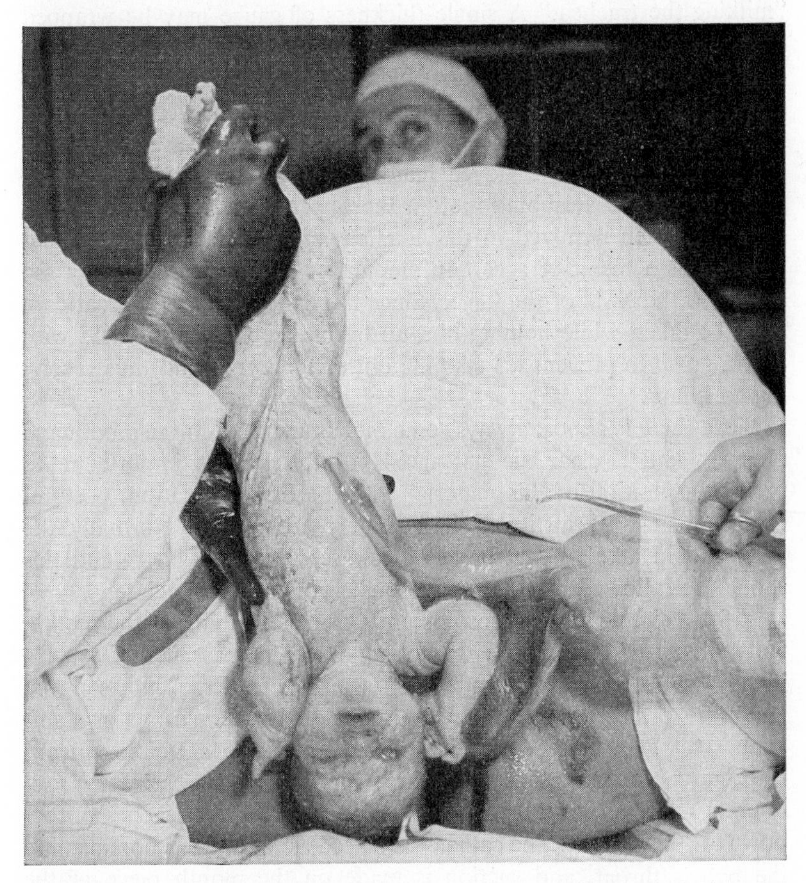

**Fig. 100.** The baby is grasped by his feet and held with head down for postural drainage of secretions from the respiratory tract. The doctor is palpating the umbilical cord for cessation of pulsation before clamping and cutting it.

ground that this procedure may do harm by increasing the intracranial pressure, especially where a difficult operative delivery has been performed and where the possibility of a cerebral hemorrhage or a tendency toward it is present; instead, they lay the baby at once on its right side and swab out its mouth.

While holding the baby by its feet, the removal of mucus may be aided by stroking the neck in the direction of the mouth to facilitate drainage from the pharynx and trachea. This is sometimes called "milking the trachea." A single thickness of gauze may be wrapped around the finger and wiped about in the back part of the baby's mouth, although many doctors object to this procedure for fear of abrading the very delicate mucous membrane, no matter how lightly this is done. Sometimes a soft rubber ear syringe is used. At times the index finger of the gloved hand, without gauze, is used; with a quick but gentle swabbing motion the finger is suddenly withdrawn. Mucus is often removed in this manner and respirations stimulated, possibly as a result of a certain amount of suction produced by the sudden withdrawal of the finger. Since the baby is slippery, great care must be taken while holding him up by his feet that he is held with a firm grasp to prevent his slipping out of the hands and thus receiving an injury.

Since there is almost always some mucus and fluid in the mouth and pharynx and a clear air passage is of the utmost importance to prevent aspiration of this material with the first inspiration, postural drainage must be instituted immediately after birth. Normally the baby should take its first breath a few seconds after birth, and this should be followed by a loud vigorous cry almost immediately.

If these simple methods of postural drainage, wiping of the mouth, and milking of the trachea do not clear the air passages of mucus, it may be necessary to introduce an aspirator into the baby's throat and remove the mucus by suction. A soft rubber ear syringe or a soft rubber catheter, No. 14 or 16 French, attached to a DeLee mucous trap may be used for this procedure (Fig. 102). The catheter is frequently more effective than the ear syringe because it reaches farther down into the throat. The catheter is placed as far back as possible into the baby's throat, and suction is made on the mouth piece of the mucous trap (Fig. 103). The position of the catheter should be changed frequently. Postural drainage may be continued while this procedure is carried out. The catheter should have only one opening, or if it has more these should all be very close to the end, since any efforts at suction may only result in drawing up air through the second opening if it does not reach down to the level of the mucus.

If the baby does not cry well after the mucus is removed, he often may be stimulated to do so by gently rubbing the back, gently spanking the buttocks two or three times, or by spanking the soles of the feet. After the baby has cried well, he may be laid on his mother's abdomen, care being taken not to make traction on the cord, or the cord may be cut and the baby placed on a table or in an incubator

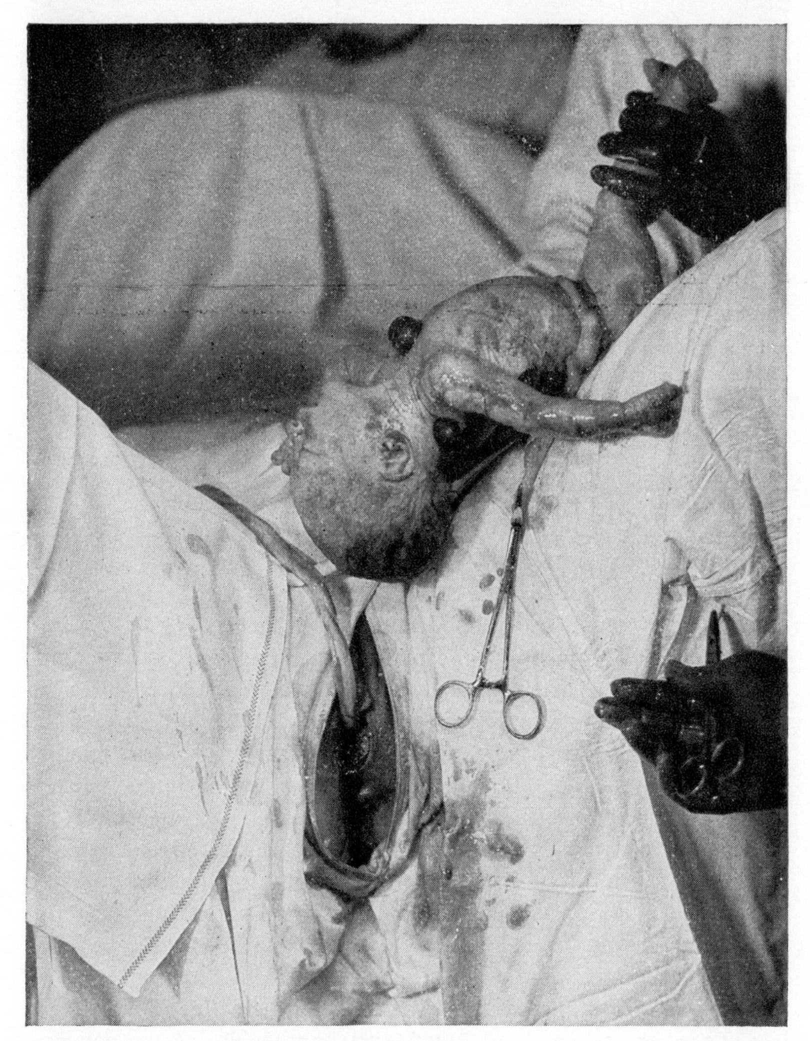

**Fig. 101.** The umbilical cord has been severed, and the baby is moved to another table or an incubator for tying and dressing of the cord and for all other necessary care.

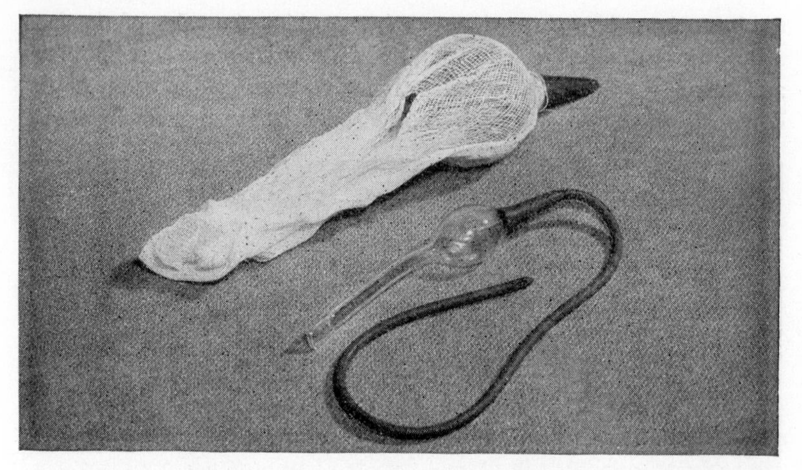

**Fig. 102.** Equipment which may be used to remove secretions from the baby's mouth and throat.

(*Top*) Soft rubber ear syringe. A piece of gauze placed around the syringe prevents slipping when it is handled with rubber gloves.

(*Bottom*) A soft rubber catheter of size No. 14 French with only one opening near the end, attached to a glass mucous trap.

for further care. If he does not cry after slight stimulation, the umbilical cord is clamped and cut and he is moved to a table or an incubator for resuscitation as discussed on pages 763–68.

**Care of the Umbilical Cord.** The cord is compressed by two clamps about 5 cm (2 in.) from the baby's abdominal wall and cut between the clamps. It may be necessary to apply the clamps as soon as the head is born, but whenever possible it is best to wait a few minutes or until the cord stops pulsating. If the cord is not cut until it ceases to pulsate the baby will receive about 100 ml of blood from the placenta of which it is otherwise deprived. This blood is especially valuable because of its iron content, since the amount of iron the baby receives during the early months of life is very small. It is also possible to supply the baby with oxygen through the cord, until the placenta separates, by administering oxygen to the mother; but similarly the baby may receive anesthesia through the cord if it has been necessary to deeply anesthetize the mother during the delivery, and immediate clamping of the cord may then be important to protect the baby (Figs. 100 and 101).

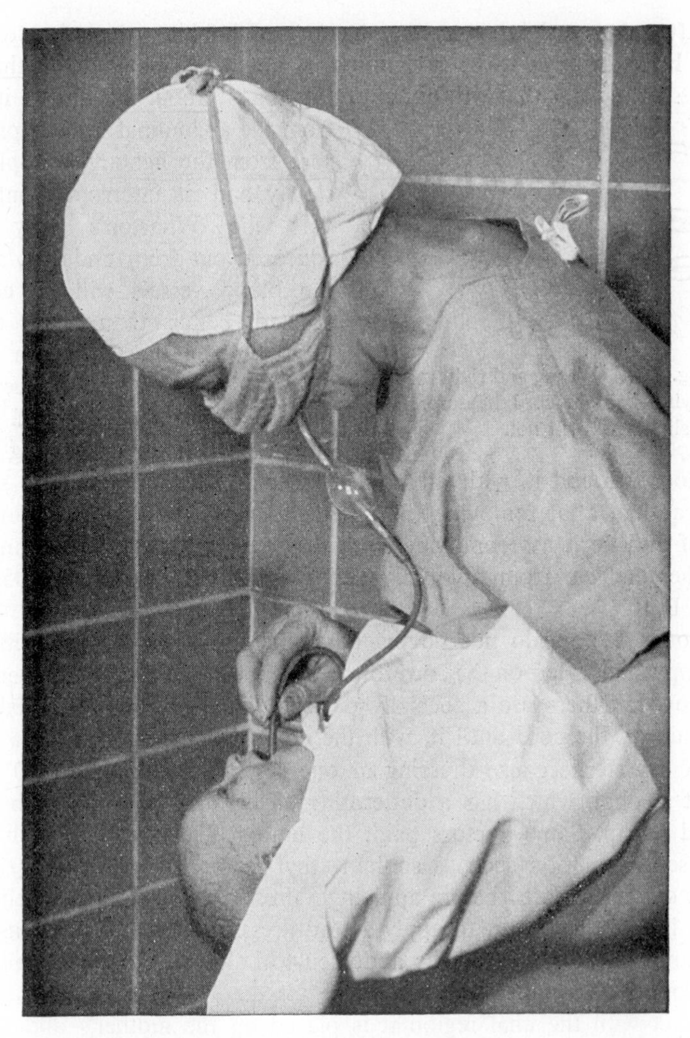

**Fig. 103.** Nurse using a soft rubber catheter to remove secretions from the mouth and oropharynx. The catheter is placed as far back as possible into the baby's throat and is moved about frequently. Suction is being made on the mouthpiece of the glass trap. The mucous trap collects the secretions and thus prevents them from entering the mouth of the operator. The use of postural drainage during this procedure aids in the removal of secretions.

After the cord is clamped a ligature of bobbin, which is strong and heavy enough to be noncutting, is applied. This is tied tightly, in a square knot that will not slip (Fig. 104), about 2.5 cm (1 in.) from the abdominal wall. If pressure from the ligature is applied slowly and at interrupted intervals the Wharton's jelly is squeezed out from under it, and the blood vessels will be constricted better than with one rapid pull on the tie. When the Wharton's jelly is not squeezed out it may escape later and the cord will then retract leaving the tie loose around it, with subsequent bleeding. It is considered a safe precaution, after removing the clamp, to bend the cord back upon itself and tie it a second time with the same ligature, as the danger of hemorrhage from a loosely tied cord is serious. (Figs. 105 A and B.)

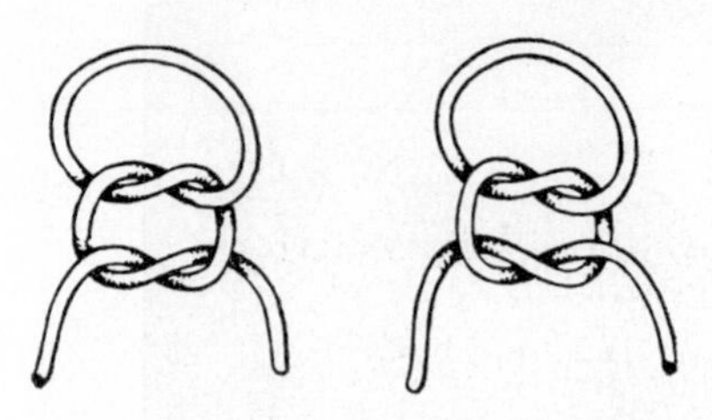

**Fig. 104.** Wrong and right method of tying knot in cord ligature. *Left,* will slip; *right,* will not.

Some doctors do not tie the cord, but crush the vessels with a clamp which is left on the cord for several hours and then permanently removed. Others use a specially devised clamp which is allowed to remain on the cord until it, with the cord, drops off.

A dry sterile gauze dressing or one saturated with 60 to 70 per cent alcohol, which has a desiccating effect, may be applied to the cord stump. Some doctors paint the umbilical cord stump with an antiseptic solution such as sodium ethyl mercurithiosalicylate (tincture of Merthiolate) before applying a dressing. Some doctors believe that it is not necessary to apply a cord dressing. If a dressing is used, a band is placed around the abdomen to hold the dressing in place.

To prevent contamination of the placental end of the cord by contact with the anal region it is placed on the mother's abdomen until the placenta is expressed. It should remain clamped until the placenta is expelled, because of the possibility of another child in the uterus and the danger of its bleeding to death through the open cord (Fig. 101).

**Care of the Eyes.** The infant's eyes may become infected during birth if gonococci are present in the birth canal, but proper care of the eyes at birth will prevent almost all cases of ophthalmia neonatorum. A germicide properly dropped into the eyes as soon as possible following birth will kill any organisms that are present.

The Credé method, made famous by the Viennese obstetrician who

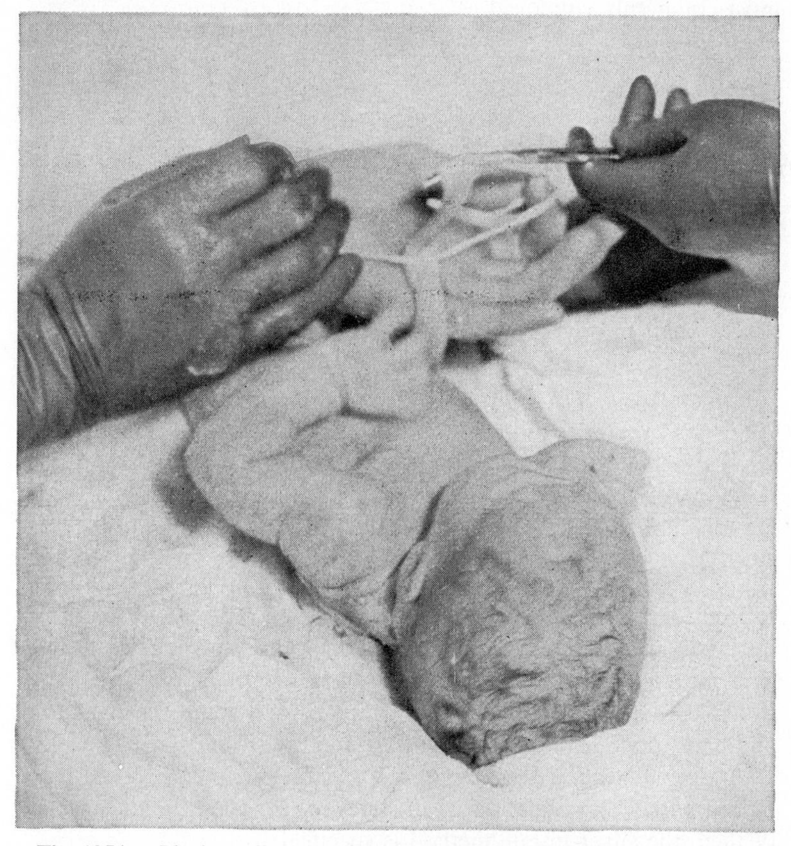

**Fig. 105A.** Placing a ligature of strong heavy bobbin on the umbilical cord. (One type of clamp which is used, instead of a ligature of bobbin, to constrict the umbilical cord can be seen in Fig. 168.)

introduced it in 1881, was to drop from a glass rod, a single drop of nitrate of silver, 2 per cent, into each eye immediately after birth. The routine use of this prophylaxis reduced the occurrence of ophthalmia in Credé's clinics from 10 per cent to 1 per cent among the newborn babies. This treatment has been variously modified, and other and weaker silver solutions, such as silver nitrate 1 per cent, mild protein silver (Argyrol), or strong protein silver (Protargol) are used with satisfactory results. Of these silver solutions, silver nitrate, 1 per cent, is considered the best and is the prophylactic most commonly employed.

Since it has been demonstrated that penicillin is highly gono-

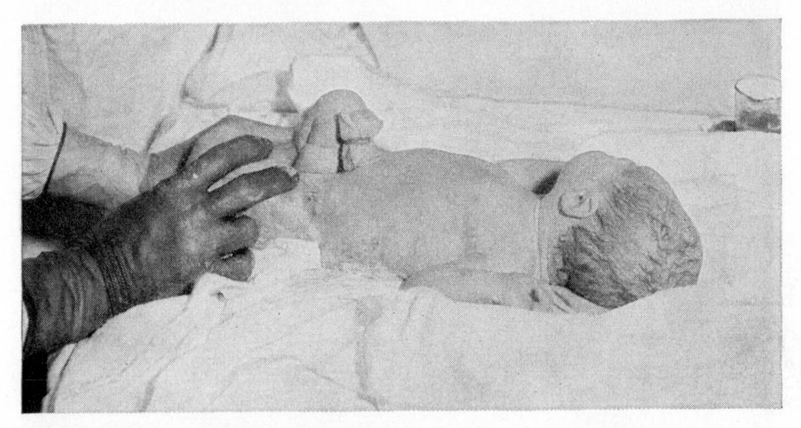

**Fig. 105B.** A sterile gauze dressing applied to the cord stump. A sterile rubber band may be used to secure the dressing; the band may also help to constrict the umbilical cord blood vessels.

coccocidal, its use has often been highly recommended as a prophylactic agent against ophthalmia neonatorum and it is being used as a preventive treatment in some instances. Its efficiency is unquestionable, but it, as well as silver nitrate, has some disadvantages, and many doctors do not wish to abandon the silver nitrate treatment.

A prophylactic treatment against ophthalmia neonatorum is required by law or regulation in all states in this country, and in many of them the silver nitrate method is specified.

The silver nitrate solution may be dropped between the baby's lids, immediately after the birth of the head and before the birth of the entire body; or immediately after the delivery of the baby is completed; or the treatment may be postponed until after the third stage of labor when there is more time to give it. The procedure must always be carried out very carefully to ensure adequate treatment. The outer surface of the eyelids should be carefully wiped from the nose outward with a sterile cotton ball moistened with sterile water to remove mucus, blood, and vernix; the lower lid should then be pulled down as far as possible and 2 drops of a 1 per cent solution of silver nitrate placed into the conjunctival sac (Fig. 106). After the lid is released the solution will spread over the entire conjunctiva. Care must be taken not to drop the medication directly on the cornea where it may cause trauma and injury. Many doctors will leave the

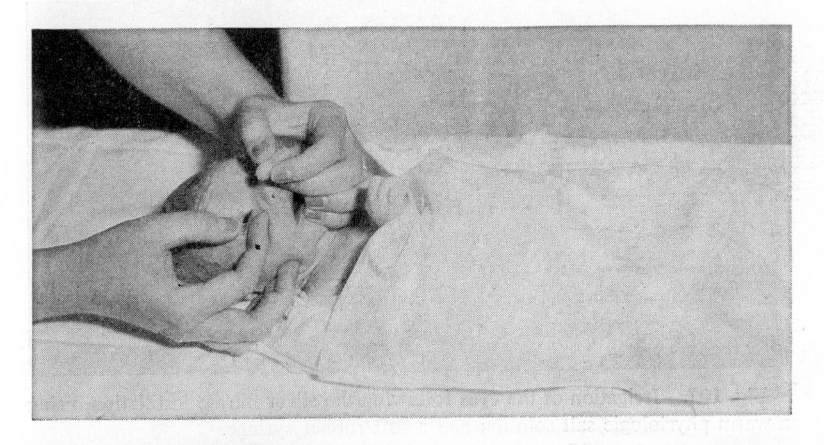

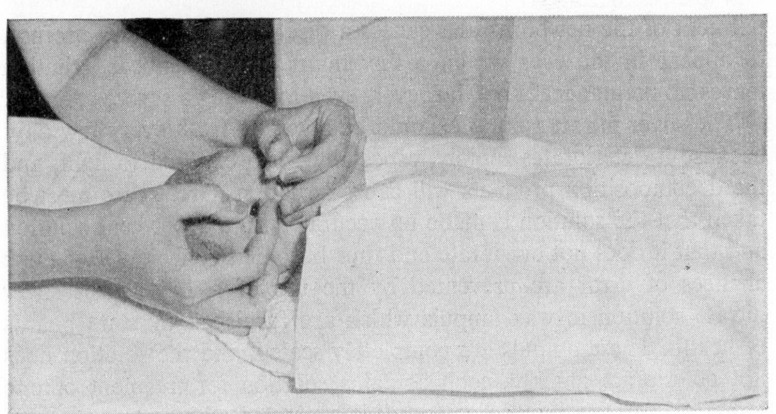

**Fig. 106.** Placing the drops of a 1 per cent silver nitrate solution into the conjunctival sac for the prevention of ophthalmia neonatorum.

(*Top*) The eyelids are not sufficiently separated, and there is danger of dropping the medication directly on the cornea, where it may cause trauma and injury.

(*Bottom*) The eyelids have been separated sufficiently to permit placing the medication on the lower eyelid or into the conjunctival sac.

silver drops in situ for one to two minutes and then irrigate the eyes with a warm physiologic salt solution, using a soft rubber syringe (Fig. 107). This will wash out the excess silver nitrate and form a precipitate with the remainder. This irrigation may prevent chemical irritation from the silver nitrate which occurs in approximately 50

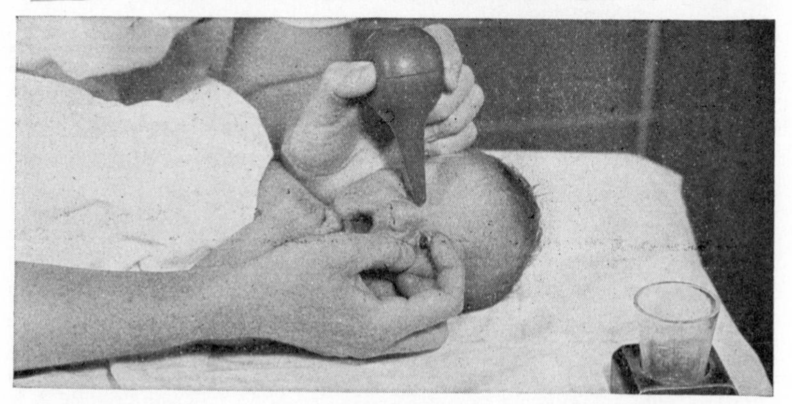

**Fig. 107.** Irrigation of the eyes following the silver nitrate instillation, using a warm physiologic salt solution and a soft rubber syringe.

per cent of the newborns and causes a discharge, sometimes profuse, to appear in the eyes within a few hours. This chemical irritation leaves no permanent effect, however, even following a severe reaction.

The silver nitrate solution should be made up fresh every few days because it deteriorates rapidly, especially when exposed to light, and the decomposition products will cause irritation. Great care must be taken that the solution is made up accurately in a 1 per cent solution and that it does not evaporate and thus become stronger. All of these chances of error are prevented by the use of a 1 per cent silver nitrate solution in wax ampuls which are furnished by state boards of health. These ampuls are completely sealed, and the solution does not deteriorate quickly; each contains solution for treament of one baby. To use the ampul one end of it is pierced with a sterile needle, and the solution squeezed out one drop at a time.

When penicillin is used as a prophylactic agent against ophthalmia neonatorum it may be administered either intramuscularly or as a topical application by placing penicillin ophthalmic ointment into the eyes. To prevent the penicillin solution, which is used for intramuscular injection, or the ointment, from becoming inactive they must be properly preserved by being kept in a refrigerator, and care must be taken that they are not used beyond the expiration date.

**Warmth, Gentle Handling, and Protection from Infection.** At this juncture it seems pertinent to stress three points which must be remembered throughout the entire regimen of the baby's care, namely: the importance of protecting him from infection, chilling, and exhaustion. Cleanliness, warmth, and gentleness are imperative. Immediately after birth the baby finds himself in a room which is many degrees cooler than the very warm habitat from which he has just emerged. Suddenly deprived of his mother's help he is struggling to establish independent functions, chief of which at the moment are respiration and circulation. Body warmth is a valuable aid in helping to establish normal functions, and accordingly the baby should be kept warm from the beginning. For this purpose there should be a small cotton flannel blanket in readiness with which to cover him during the interval that elapses between his birth and the time at which he can be placed into a warmed crib. This blanket should previously have been sterilized to prevent infection, especially of the umbilical cord before it has been dressed. Gentle handling is imperative during the removal of mucus, stimulation of respirations, and treatment of the eyes.

**Inspection for Abnormalities.** Before the baby leaves the delivery room the doctor inspects him for abnormalities, especially any gross deformities such as hydrocephalus, spina bifida, cleft lip and palate, imperforate anus, and birthmarks. He also observes the baby's color, and looks especially for jaundice, which necessitates immediate blood studies, and generalized cyanosis, which may indicate the presence of atelectasis or congenital cardiac defects. He may also examine the child for tongue-tie, since the membrane can easily be cut with a pair of sterile, unused scissors from the delivery table at this time.

**Identification.** If the delivery takes place in a hospital the baby must be marked *before it is taken from the delivery room.* A simple yet absolutely dependable system is necessary. Most commonly used are adhesive labels applied to the back on which the baby's name and other data are written, name necklace or bracelet (Fig. 108, *bottom, left*), and identification tapes with identical numbers for both the mother's and the baby's wrists (Fig. 108, *top*). Foot or palm prints may also be taken (Fig. 108, *bottom, right*). Many hospitals use more than one system as a double check on the baby's identity.

**Baptism.** The Roman Catholic Church teaches that no child can reach Heaven without being baptized. Parents who are Roman Catholics wish to have their baby baptized if it is in danger of death. If time permits, a priest should be called to administer baptism. If there is not sufficient time, the nurse should perform the baptism. Baptism is conferred by pouring ordinary water on the child's forehead while

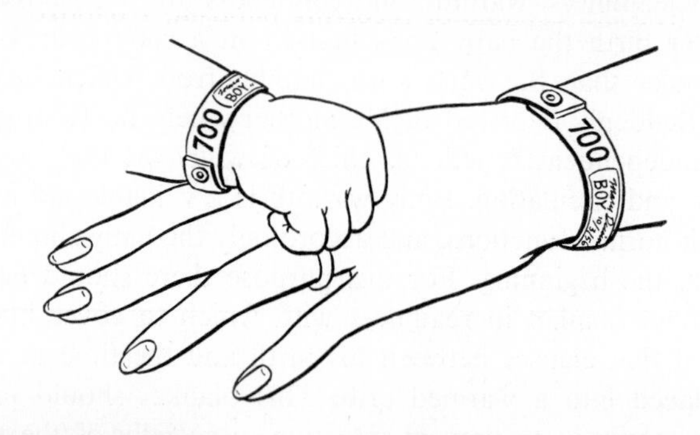


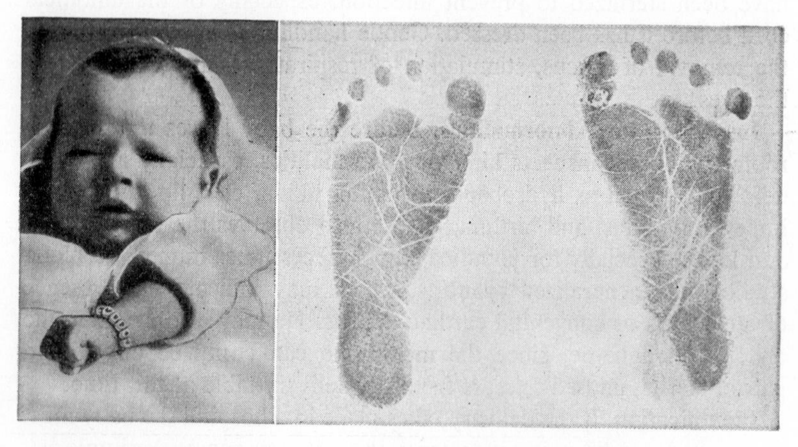

**Fig. 108.** Several methods of identification of the newborn infant.

(*Top*) Two-section OB Ident-A-Band divided into two separate bands bearing identical numbers—one band for the mother, one band for the baby. (IDENT-A-BAND-Made and manufactured by Franklin C. Hollister Co., 833 North Orleans, Chicago, Ill.)

(*Bottom, left*) A bracelet (or necklace) of Name-on-Beads is put on the baby before he is taken from the delivery room. (Courtesy of J. A. Deknatal & Son, Inc., Queens Village, L. I., N. Y.)

(*Bottom, right*) Footprints.

saying the words: "I baptize you in the name of the Father and of the Son and of the Holy Spirit." It is necessary for validity that the nurse have the intention of doing what the Roman Catholic Church wishes. The Church teaches that every fetus and embryo should be baptized if possible. When it is doubtful that the subject is capable of receiving baptism, conditional baptism is administered with the form: "If you are capable of receiving baptism, I baptize you in the name of the Father and of the Son and of the Holy Spirit." *

Most Protestants observe infant baptism. Those who practice this rite usually desire to have their baby baptized if his condition is serious. The doctor or nurse should, therefore, consult with the parents to determine their wishes regarding their baby's baptism, and arrange to call a minister of their faith. If time does not permit calling a minister, an emergency baptism may be performed by anyone else. If time does not permit for consulting with the parents regarding their baby's baptism the doctor or nurse should baptize the child, since many Protestant parents consider this rite very important and desire to have it done. The baptism is administered by pouring water, usually with the palm of the hand, over the child's head, and at the same time saying the words: "I baptize thee (or you) in the name of the Father and of the Son and of the Holy Ghost." If time permits, the Lord's Prayer and/or Apostles' Creed may also be spoken; however, these are not essential to the rite of baptism.

## THIRD STAGE (PLACENTAL STAGE)

The third stage of labor and the hour immediately following delivery of the placenta are very hazardous to the mother and require careful management because of the great danger of hemorrhage.

After the birth of the baby, the doctor may request the nurse to place one hand on the mother's abdomen in order to feel the fundus and to keep him informed concerning its size and consistency. It should be observed only, and not massaged, before the placenta is delivered. With separation of the placenta the fundus will change from a discoid to a globular mass. Bleeding from the vagina may begin or increase, since, as a rule, there is little bleeding until the placenta

* Hayes, Rev. Edward J.; Hayes, Rev. Paul J.; and Kelly, Dorothy E.: *Moral Handbook of Nursing*. The Macmillan Company, New York, 1956, pp. 84 ff.

has separated. After the placenta descends into the lower uterine segment the fundus rises and may be felt as a firm mass at or above the umbilicus. Since the placenta is entirely separated from the uterus at this time its complete expulsion is usually effected by firm, steady, downward pressure on the fundus in the direction of the pelvic inlet.

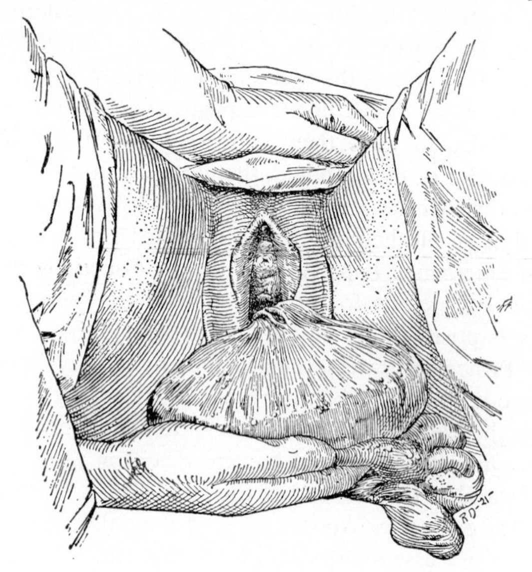

**Fig. 109.** Delivery of the placenta.

In this way pressure is exerted on the placenta with the fundus. The obstetrician holds his hand just below the vaginal outlet, to receive the placenta (Fig. 109), which he turns over and over in his hands, thus twisting the membranes, and gradually draws it away from the mother, the membranes trailing after in the form of a twisted and tapering cord (Fig. 110). Or alternatively they may be grasped with a forceps and removed by gentle traction; this method is especially useful if the membranes have torn away from the placenta. It is important that the placenta and membranes be carefully examined to make sure that they are intact, because, if fragments of either are retained within the uterus, they will prevent its firm contraction and thus may be a cause of postpartum hemorrhage. For this reason, only very gentle pressure and traction are used in expressing the placenta and withdrawing the membranes, since the use of force might

definition of inversion

leave small particles adherent to the uterine lining. Another important reason for exerting only gentle pressure and traction is that if much force is used at this stage it may cause inversion of the uterus. This involves prolapse of the uterine fundus, through the cervix, into the vagina, and is a very grave obstetric accident. Having been inspected,

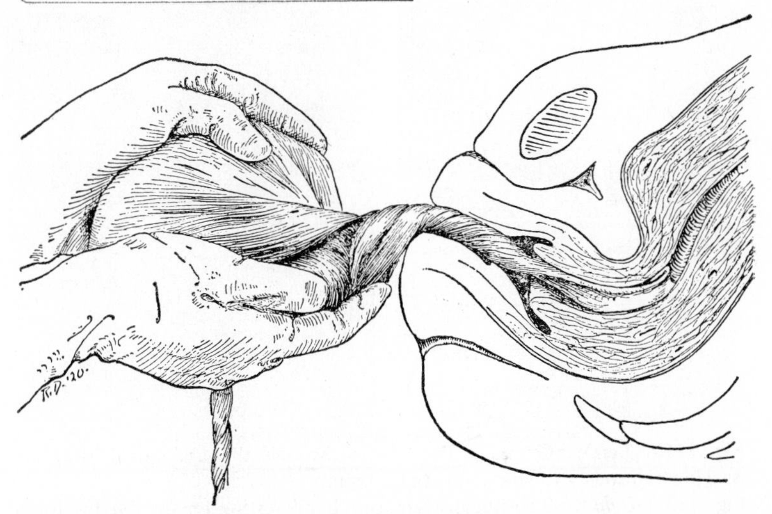

**Fig. 110.** Twisting the membranes while withdrawing them from the uterus.

the placenta should be placed in a covered receptacle to be disposed of as the doctor directs; sometimes the physician wishes a laboratory examination of the placenta, and it must be saved for this purpose.

With the birth of the placenta comes a gush of blood from the uterine vessels, some of which are as large as a lead pencil and are at first widely gaping. The bleeding usually subsides very shortly, however, as the blood vessels are closed by involuntary contraction of the network of uterine muscle fibers in which they are enmeshed, and which are sometimes referred to as "living ligatures." If the bleeding continues, this contraction should be stimulated by massage. After birth of the placenta the uterus should be a firm hard mass. The doctor or nurse must keep a hand on the fundus at all times so that any relaxation may be detected immediately and the uterus massaged until it again contracts. This is done by firmly grasping the uterus through the abdominal wall and kneading it vigorously. Rubbing the top of the fundus with the fingers is usually not enough.

The fundus should be grasped by the entire hand, with the thumb curved across the anterior surface and the fingers, directed deep into the abdomen, behind it, or it may be held between the two hands—one to give support and the other to massage (Fig. 111).

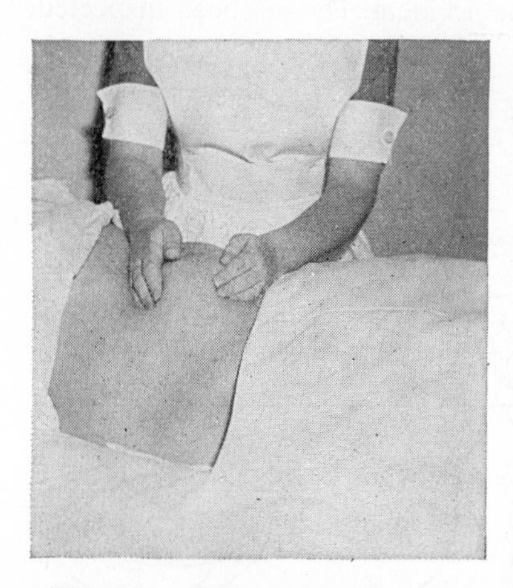
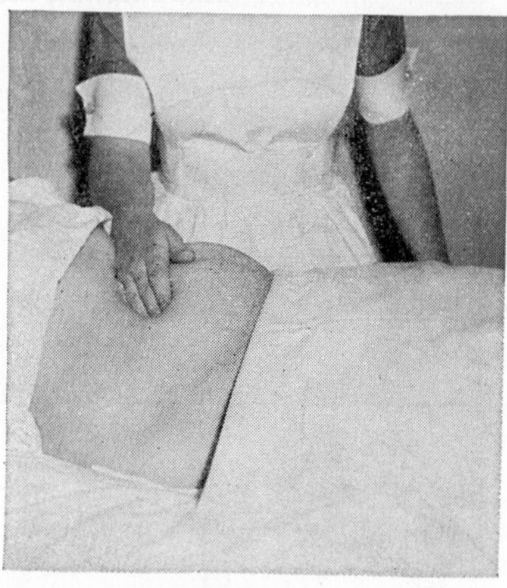

**Fig. 111.** (*Left*). Grasping the uterus through the abdominal wall and massaging vigorously to stimulate contraction.

**Fig. 112** (*Right*). The nurse keeps one hand resting on the fundus for at least one hour following delivery of the placenta to observe the consistency, size, and height of the uterus. This is an essential safeguard against postpartum hemorrhage.

After delivery of the placenta, drugs with an oxytocic action are usually given to further stimulate contraction of uterine muscle fibers. Ergonovine 0.2 mg (1/320 gr) or oxytocin (Pitocin) 10 oxytocic units (international standard) is most frequently used.

Ergonovine is an alkaloid of ergot, a fungus which grows on rye and other grains. It is a powerful stimulant to uterine muscle contractions and exerts an effect which may last for hours. The contraction of the uterine muscle is sustained following administration of the drug and aids greatly in controlling postpartum bleeding. Ergonovine may be administered orally or parenterally. It is prepared in tablet form in doses of 0.2 mg (1/320 gr) for oral administration and in ampuls of 1 ml containing 0.2 mg (1/320 gr) for either the intramuscular or intravenous route. The uterine muscle contracts almost immediately following intravenous injection, within a few minutes following an intramuscular injection, and even within 5 to 10 minutes following oral administration, since the drug is readily absorbed from the gastrointestinal tract. Ergotrate, which is a trade name for ergonovine, is a term frequently used as a synonym. A partially synthetic ergot alkaloid known as methylergonovine (Methergine) is often used in place of ergonovine. It is also prepared in 0.2-mg (1/320-gr) doses and may also be administered by either the oral or parenteral routes.

Posterior pituitary extract, obtained from the posterior lobe of the pituitary gland, also produces marked contractions of the uterine muscle, but unlike the long-sustained contractions produced by ergonovine these contractions are sustained for only 5 to 10 minutes, after which there are intermittent periods of relaxation. The periods of rhythmic contractions are very strong, however. Posterior pituitary extract has two fractions; the one with great oxytocic properties is known by the name oxytocin (Pitocin) and the other with marked vasopressor and antidiuretic properties by the name vasopressin (Pitressin). Since hypertension and water retention are common problems in the complications of pregnancy the pressor and antidiuretic principle may be undesirable; for this reason it seems better to administer the oxytocic fraction alone in preference to giving the entire posterior pituitary extract. This drug has no value administered by the oral route. It is prepared in 1-ml ampuls of 10 oxytocic units (international standard) and is administered intramuscularly.

When these medications are administered intramuscularly they are often most easily given into the deltoid muscle. It is important to use a needle at least 2.5 cm (1 in.) in length in order to reach the muscular tissue of the arm. The area should be thoroughly massaged for quick absorption. If the uterine muscle does not contract well after the administration of either one or both of these drugs, a second dose of ergonovine may usually be administered with safety.

These drugs are sometimes administered immediately after delivery of the baby to hasten separation of the placenta, but there is a possibility that the cervix may clamp down and retain the placenta and thus necessitate manual removal. This is especially dangerous in home deliveries where conditions are very unfavorable for operative procedures.

These drugs are also, in some cases, administered at the time the shoulders of the baby are being delivered. When given at this particular moment the uterus, which is already contracting down rapidly as its contents diminish, contracts very forcefully and separates the placenta. If the placenta is then immediately expressed, before the uterus reaches a tetanic state due to the oxytocic drug, it is usually possible to remove it without difficulty, since the lower uterine segment has just recently been dilated with the birth of the baby. When these drugs are used before delivery of the placenta it is in an effort to reduce the blood loss of the third stage, but the incidence of retained placenta is always higher when oxytocic drugs are administered before its delivery than when they are withheld until the end of the third stage. In many instances it is safer to let nature take its course in separation of the placenta, and some doctors strongly object to the administration of any drugs until the third stage is completed.

Occasionally separation of the placenta is delayed or spontaneous separation does not take place. If there is no excessive bleeding, it is often best to wait and make occasional attempts at simple expression. If, after one-half hour, attempts at expression are still unsuccessful, the doctor will usually decide that manual removal is necessary. He introduces his hand into the uterus and separates the placenta from its wall. Strictest aseptic technic is necessary to prevent infection. The doctor always changes his gloves (preferably putting on gauntlet gloves) before this procedure, and the patient is re-prepared as necessary.

## REPAIR OF EPISIOTOMY OR PERINEAL LACERATION

A large proportion of women require repair of either an episiotomy, a laceration, or both, following the birth of the baby. A laceration may be no larger than a nick in the vaginal mucous membrane, it may extend down into the perineal body to any degree, or it may even extend entirely across the perineal body and tear through the rectal sphincter. The causes of these tears are generally conceded to be rigidity of the perineum, a sudden expulsion of the child's head before the perineum is fully distended, contraction of the outlet of the bony pelvis, certain abnormalities in the mechanism of labor, and excessively large fetal shoulders. Lacerations may be prevented or limited in many cases by skillful delivery of the child, but in spite of the most careful efforts, tears of some degree occur in most primigravidas and probably in many multigravidas unless an episiotomy is done. These injuries are usually described as being of the first, second, or third degree, according to their extent.

*A first-degree tear* is one that extends only through the vaginal mucous membrane and perineal skin, usually at the margin of the perineum, without involving any of the muscles.

*A second-degree tear* is one that extends down into the perineal body and involves fascia and muscle of the levator ani, or even extends down to, but not through, the rectal sphincter. Such a tear usually extends upward into the vagina on one or both sides, making a triangular injury.

*A third-degree tear* extends entirely across the perineal body and through the rectal sphincter and sometimes up the anterior wall of the rectum. This variety is often called a *complete tear,* in contradistinction to those of first and second degree, which are incomplete. A third-degree tear should occur only very infrequently.

These lacerations, or an episiotomy, are repaired either in the interval between the delivery of the baby and expulsion of the placenta or after delivery of the placenta. Equipment is usually available to anesthetize the patient, the field is still clean, and sutures can readily be put into place. The instruments needed will consist of round or trocar point Mayo catgut needles, needle holder, tissue forceps, scissors, and two or three hemostatic forceps. Chromic catgut sutures, No. 00 or No. 000, are used most frequently. (See Fig. 92 for delivery instruments.) As the few instruments necessary for perineal repairs should be sterilized and placed in readiness before delivery, there is no further preparation for the nurse to make.

Sometimes tears occur in the labia or around the urethra. These may be only slight abrasions or they may be deep enough to bleed freely. If it is necessary to repair a tear around the urethra thin nontraumatic needles and fine catgut suture, No. 00 or smaller, are ordinarily used, since the tissue in this area is thin and tears easily. An indwelling catheter may be placed into the bladder for a few days to prevent trauma or tension on the sutured area, which may accompany a catheterization should the patient be unable to void.

## IMMEDIATE AFTERCARE OF THE PATIENT

After delivery the vulva is cleaned of blood by using sterile cotton balls, water, and forceps; the thighs and buttocks are dried; and a sterile perineal pad may be applied. The patient is moved to a clean, freshly made bed, a sterile bed pad is slipped under her hips, and a fresh gown is put on to replace the one that was worn during delivery. The perineal pad is very commonly held in place by a T binder, with which all nurses are familiar, but some doctors prefer an abdominal binder to which a perineal strap is attached. This abdominal support may be a straight swathe or a Scultetus bandage, varying with the preference of the doctor. Other doctors do not use either an abdominal binder or a perineal pad; they prefer that a large, absorbent, sterilized pad is placed under the patient to receive the discharge.

If the patient has had a general anesthetic she may vomit, just as she might after an anesthetic for any other operation. She is usually tired and cold at the conclusion of labor and may even have a nervous chill. Although this chill is not serious, the patient is nonetheless uncomfortable and she should be warmly covered, and a hot-water bottle should be placed at her feet.

Unless the anesthetic has been deep or prolonged the patient will soon awaken and will wish to see her baby. She will be much happier and rest better during these next few hours if the baby is brought to her room as soon as she awakens so that she and her husband may see the baby. After this efforts should be made to provide for rest and quiet. She should be made as comfortable as possible by a change of soiled perineal pads, by the proper amount of covering, and by being allowed to assume a comfortable position. The room should be quiet, somewhat darkened, and well ventilated. Medication for pain relief, such as morphine, may be ordered, especially if there is perineal pain from the repair of a tear or an episiotomy. The patient usually has great thirst due to restriction of fluids in the latter part of labor and the loss of fluid in the effort that is exerted during labor and delivery, and, unless nausea persists, she will wish to have large amounts of cold water to drink. Ordinarily fluids are not contraindicated, and, unless there is some reason for withholding them, the nurse should give the patient cold water, or other liquids, as soon as she wishes and in the quantity she desires.

In addition to observations regarding the patient's condition in general, the majority of doctors require that the nurse shall stay with the patient and keep one hand resting on the fundus for at least an hour after delivery as a safeguard against postpartum hemorrhage (Fig. 112). This period is sometimes referred to as "the placental hour." As long as the fundus is felt through the abdominal wall as a firm, hard mass, its irregularly arranged muscle fibers are contracted upon the blood vessels and will prevent an escape of blood. If the fundus feels soft and boggy its muscle fibers are relaxed; constrictions are accordingly somewhat released from the open vessels, and serious bleeding may occur unless these fibers are stimulated to contract again. The nurse who is entrusted with the care of the patient at this time has a grave responsibility, since the uterine muscle may suddenly relax and a severe hemorrhage may occur very quickly. In order to fulfill this trust properly she must watch the consistency, the size, and the height of the uterus; observe the patient's pulse rate; and watch for the appearance of excessive external bleeding. Not more than one to two pads should be saturated by bleeding during the first hour. There may be, however, concealed bleeding, with all the blood retained in the uterus, and it is for this reason that the size of the fundus must be carefully watched. The desirable state is for the fundus to be hard and round at or below the level of the umbilicus. The doctor should be immediately notified of any departure from the normal. The uterus should not, however, be massaged unless it does relax because massage may cause uterine muscle fatigue; this fatigue then predisposes to relaxation. Unnecessary massage also makes the patient very uncomfortable; the uterus is always very sore and sensitive to any manipulation after delivery.

If there has been no relaxation of the uterine muscle during the first hour after delivery of the placenta there is usually no great danger of hemorrhage. The patient may then be made comfortable in any position she desires and left to rest, but the nurse must still return frequently to check on the consistency of the uterus and the amount of bleeding through the vagina.

## POSSIBLE EMERGENCIES DURING LABOR

**Delivery by the Nurse.** It sometimes happens that labor progresses with unexpected rapidity, or that the doctor is unavoidably delayed, and the nurse is accordingly confronted with the emergency of being alone with the patient during part or all of the delivery.

When the baby is making such rapid descent that the nurse expects it may be born before the doctor's arrival, she may somewhat slow labor by instructing the patient to open her mouth, breathe deeply, and try not to bear down during contractions. Exerting force, however, to delay the birth is very dangerous from the standpoint of injuring the baby and causing it to have marked hypoxia, and the nurse is never justified in forcefully holding back the baby's head.

The nurse should put on a pair of sterile rubber gloves or cover her hand with a sterile towel, whichever is more easily available, and apply moderate pressure to the head as it is advancing with contractions, not with the intent of retarding delivery, but to prevent a rapid, unassisted birth. It is the rapid distention of the perineum that causes lacerations; also the sudden expulsion of the baby's head at the height of a contraction may cause injury to the baby's brain. As the scalp appears at the introitus the nurse should apply pressure to the head during contractions to prevent its sudden expulsion and to keep it well extended by pressing it up toward the symphysis pubis so that the perineum may be stretched slowly. The head should be allowed to come down a little farther with each contraction. After the brow is visible, pressure may gradually be released and the head allowed to emerge, or the patient may be asked to bear down between contractions to deliver the head between, rather than with, the force of a uterine contraction.

The nurse should remember that there need be no haste in the delivery of the head since a slow delivery is less dangerous to both the mother and the baby than rapid expulsion. After the head is born, it drops down toward the mother's rectum, and external rotation, or restitution, takes place.

The shoulders are usually born spontaneously, but if traction is necessary the nurse may grasp the head with both hands, curving the fingers of one hand under the baby's chin, and of the other, under the occiput, and make gentle, downward traction in order to slip the anterior shoulder from under the symphysis pubis; she should then pull gently upward, to deliver the lower or posterior shoulder after which the rest of the body follows easily. The mother may be asked to bear down to assist with the delivery of the shoulders. When traction is used it must be very gentle to prevent injury to the baby's neck or arms.

The baby should immediately be held up by his feet; mucus and fluid should be cleared from his air passages, and he should be made to cry at once. Respirations are usually spontaneous in this type of delivery. The nurse's hand should then be placed on the mother's abdomen to palpate the uterus for size and consistency and to make certain that the patient is not bleeding. If the uterus remains firm there is no necessity of delivering the placenta before the doctor's arrival even though it has apparently dropped into the lower uterine segment.

The nurse should also know that there is never a need for haste to cut and tie the umbilical cord even in case the placenta is separated soon after the baby is born. Bleeding does not occur through the surface of the placenta. An intact umbilical cord prohibits moving the baby any distance or giving him much care, but if he is covered he will be sufficiently warm until there is time to give him further attention. After his breathing is well established he does not immediately need other care. Understanding that there is no haste to care for the umbilical cord gives the nurse an opportunity to attend to other matters that may be more urgent. When there is time the nurse can obtain sterile tie and scissors, clean the umbilical cord with an antiseptic solution, and tie and dress it under conditions that are as clean as possible.

Sometimes delivery has taken place before the doctor or nurse arrive. Immediate attention must be given to the baby to prevent him from aspirating fluid in his attempts to breathe or even drowning in the amniotic fluid which escapes after delivery. As soon as the baby's breathing is established the mother must be observed for any evidence of excessive uterine bleeding, and care of the mother and baby should be continued as outlined above.

Throughout all this the patient will be frightened, and it is very important to give her just as much reassurance as possible. She will be able to cooperate much better during the delivery if she has confidence that she is being cared for adequately than if she is not given support in her fear. The nurse must reassure the patient that everything is going well and must explain to her that the doctor has been notified and will arrive as soon as possible. She must not leave the patient alone—not even for a moment—during this time. The baby may be born very suddenly while she is away, and it is also very frightening to the patient to be left alone, even if the birth is not imminent. There is usually someone else who can summon the doctor—other employees or a relative.

**Prolapsed Cord.** If the umbilical cord should prolapse through the cervix into the vagina, or even protrude from the vagina, at any time during labor, in the absence of the doctor, the nurse should elevate the patient's hips in the hope that gravity may lessen the pressure on the cord as it lies between the presenting part and the pelvic bones and thus lessen the danger from impaired circulation. The elevated Sims' position or the knee-chest position are often helpful or the foot of the bed may be elevated very high on blocks or on a chair.

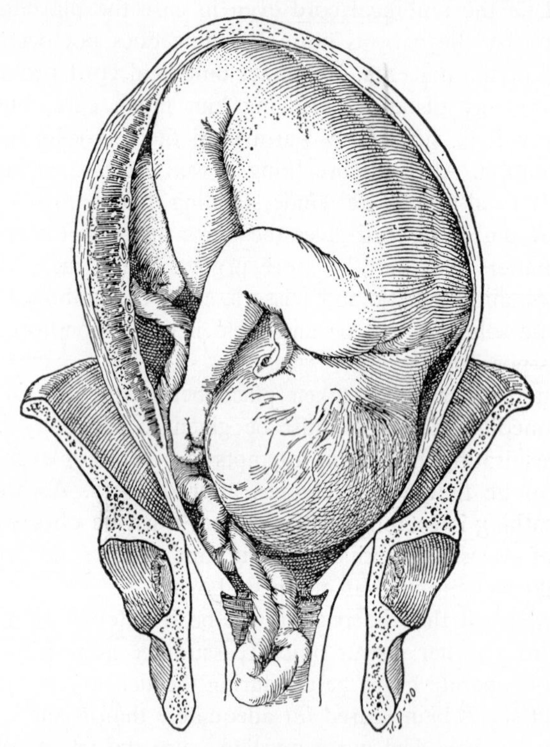

**Fig. 113.** Showing how a prolapsed cord may be pressed between baby's head and pelvic bones, thus cutting off placental circulation.

The nurse should make hasty preparations for the doctor either to apply antiseptics to the cord and replace it, or, if cervical dilatation permits, to deliver the child as quickly as possible by an operative procedure. It may be necessary for the nurse herself to hold the prolapsed cord up in the vagina while awaiting the doctor's arrival. Interference with the placental circulation by pressure on the cord frequently results in asphyxiation of the baby (Fig. 113).

**Postpartum Hemorrhage.** If a postpartum hemorrhage occurs, in the absence of the doctor, the nurse must massage the fundus while someone else elevates the foot of the bed on blocks or the seat of a firm, straight chair and calls the doctor. The nurse must continue massaging the fundus and not leave the patient for even a moment to do anything else. In anticipation of a postpartum hemorrhage, the nurse must have a clear understanding of the doctor's orders, particularly in regard to the administration of ergonovine, which is so widely and efficaciously used to check postpartum bleeding. This subject will be discussed in detail in Chapter 18, "Complications of the Puerperium and Nursing Care."

## BIBLIOGRAPHY AND STUDENT REFERENCES

Blake, Florence G.: *The Child, His Parents and the Nurse.* J. B. Lippincott Co., Philadelphia, 1954, pp. 29–52.

Bookmiller, Mae M., and Bowen, George L.: *Textbook of Obstetrics and Obstetric Nursing,* 2nd ed. W. B. Saunders Co., Philadelphia, 1954.

Corbin, Hazel: "Childbirth without Fear," *Am. J. Nursing,* **47**:392–93, (June) 1947.

Davidson, Harold H.: "Penicillin in the Prophylaxis of Ophthalmia Neonatorum," *Obst. & Gynec. Surv.,* **7**:147–54, (Apr.) 1952.

Davis, M. Edward, and Sheckler, Catherine E.: *DeLee's Obstetrics for Nurses,* 15th ed. W. B. Saunders Co., Philadelphia, 1951.

DeMarsh, Q. B.; Alt, H. L.; Windle, W. F.; and Hillis, David S.: "The Effect of Depriving the Infant of Its Placental Blood," *J.A.M.A.,* **116**:2568–73, (June 7) 1941.

Domino, Edward F.: "The Ergot Alkaloids," *Mod. Hosp.,* **80**:98–106, (May) 1953.

Eastman, Nicholson J.: *Williams Obstetrics,* 11th ed. Appleton-Century-Crofts, Inc., New York, 1956.

Franklin, H. Charles: "Prophylaxis against Ophthalmia Neonatorum," *J.A.M.A.,* **134**:1230–35, (Aug. 9) 1947.

Gill, Meyer J.: "G-11 Takes the Scrub out of Scrub-up Procedures," *Mod. Hosp.,* **75**:67–68, (Oct.) 1950.

Goodrich, Frederick W.: "Experiences with Natural Childbirth," *Pub. Health Nursing,* **41**:122–25, (Mar.) 1949.

———: *Natural Childbirth.* Prentice-Hall, Inc., New York, 1950.

Greenhill, J. P. (ed.): *Obstetrics,* 11th ed. W. B. Saunders Co., Philadelphia, 1955.

Heardman, Helen: *Relaxation and Exercise for Natural Childbirth.* Williams & Wilkins Co., Baltimore, 1950.

Hogan, Aileen: "Bomb Born Babies," *Pub. Health Nursing,* **43**:383–85, (July) 1951.

House, Dorothy E.: "The Patient in Labor," *Am. J. Nursing,* **39**:1328–33, (Dec.) 1939.

Hurlburt, Maretta, and Oscadal, Julia: "The Obstetric Recovery Room," *Am. J. Nursing,* **49**:136–37, (Mar.) 1949.

Javert, Carl T.: "The Immediate Postpartum Period as a Fourth State of Labor," *Am. J. Obst. & Gynec.,* **54**:1028–32, (Dec.) 1947.

Kartchner, Fred D.: "A Study of the Emotional Reactions during Labor," *Am. J. Obst. & Gynec.,* **60**:19–29, (July) 1950.

Lesser, Marion S., and Keane, Vera R.: *Nurse–Patient Relationships in a Hospital Maternity Service.* C. V. Mosby Co., St. Louis, 1956.

Maternity Center Association: "Is It the Baby Who Pays?" *Briefs,* **13**:2–6, (May) 1949.

———: "Labor Is More than Mechanics," *Briefs,* **13**:3–5, (Oct.) 1949. (Digest of an article by Dr. Grantly D. Read published in the *British Journal of Medicine,* April 16, 1949.)

———: "Uterus at Work," *Briefs,* **14**:2–4, (June) 1950.

———: "Watch Your Language," *Briefs,* **19**:3–6, (Jan.) 1955. (Digest of an article by Horace H. Hughes published in *Nursing World.*)

———: "Primitive Labor in Africa," *Briefs,* **19**:8–10, (Oct.) 1955. (From an article by Dr. Grantly D. Read in *Parent's Magazine,* July, 1955.)

———: "Soranus of Ephesus Master Obstetrician," *Briefs,* **19**:2–6, (Nov.) 1955.

Mitchell, Mildred M.: "This Is Positive Identification of the Newborn," *Hosp. Management,* **77**:46–47, (June) 1954.

Newton, Niles: *Maternal Emotions.* Paul B. Hoeber, Inc., New York, 1955.

Read, Grantly D.: "An Outline of the Conduct of Physiological Labor," *Am. J. Obst. & Gynec.,* **54**:702–10, (Oct.) 1947.

———: *Childbirth without Fear,* 2nd ed. Harper & Brothers, New York, 1953.

Stafford, G. T., Jr.: "The Obstetrical Recovery Room," *Mod. Hosp.,* **81**:83–85, (July) 1953.

Thoms, Herbert: *Classical Contributions to Obstetrics and Gynecology.* Charles C Thomas, Publisher, Springfield, Ill., 1935.

———: *Training for Childbirth.* McGraw-Hill Book Co., New York, 1950.

Thoms, Herbert, and Goodrich, Frederick W.: "Training for Childbirth," *J.A.M.A.,* **140**:1256–58, (Aug. 20) 1949.

Thoms, Herbert, and Wiedenbach, Ernestine: "Support during Labor," *J.A.M.A.,* **156**:3–5, (Sept. 4) 1954.

Wiedenbach, Ernestine: "Childbirth As Mothers Say They Like It," *Pub. Health Nursing,* **41**:417–21, (Aug.) 1949.

Woodward, H. L.; Gardner, B.; Bryant, R. D.; and Overland, Anna E.: *Obstetric Management and Nursing,* 5th ed. F. A. Davis Co., Philadelphia, 1955.

Zabriskie, Louise, and Eastman, Nicholson J.: *Nurses Handbook of Obstetrics,* 9th ed. J. B. Lippincott Co., Philadelphia, 1952.

*Chapter 13*

# Analgesia and Anesthesia

Those of us who are accustomed to seeing anesthetics used to relieve patients of some of their pain during labor find it hard to realize that until comparatively recent years women went through labor and delivery without the use of pain-relieving drugs.

The use of anesthesia was introduced into obstetric practice in 1847 by Sir James Y. Simpson of Scotland, who first used ether, but later adopted chloroform when he learned that it also had anesthetic properties. Its use in America was subsequently introduced by Dr. Walter Channing of Boston.

In the early days the idea of using anesthesia during labor was greeted with a storm of protest, both from the clergy and the laity, because of their belief that the relief of women in childbirth was contrary to the teachings of the Bible, as set forth in God's curse on Eve, when He said, "In sorrow thou shalt bring forth children" (Genesis 3:16). Drs. Simpson and Channing, however, pointed out that the Bible said, when Eve was created from Adam's rib, "And the Lord God caused a deep sleep to fall upon Adam, and he slept; and he took one of his ribs, and closed up the flesh instead thereof" (Genesis 2:21).

In the vast majority of cases today some agent is employed to lessen the pain of the woman in labor. The reasons are that not only is it humane, but it also promotes the physical and mental welfare of the patient to make her labor as painless as is consistent with her safety and the safety of her infant. It is well known that severe pain is a very exhausting experience. In addition, the muscular relaxation obtained with anesthesia is sometimes necessary to facilitate the work of the obstetrician. Analgesia in labor also relieves many patients of the terror and fear which they might otherwise suffer. As has been explained in Chapter 7, "Mental Hygiene of the Expectant Mother," such an emotional experience may contribute to subsequent mental difficulties in certain unstable women. The agents used to relieve pain may be described as anesthetics, which produce an inability to appreciate sensation; analgesics, which relieve pain; and amnesics, which produce loss of memory. The widespread and indiscriminate use of these drugs has resulted in injury to both mother and baby. An ideal drug should relieve pain, without producing unconsciousness, should be applicable at all times, should not interfere with uterine contractions, and above all else should be absolutely safe for both mother and baby. No drug has yet been discovered that will give absolute pain relief and still be safe for both mother and child. Many drugs have been used and even considered ideal for a short time, but none has perfectly stood the test of time. Moderate doses of many drugs, if properly administered, will give considerable relief from pain and mental distress without great danger of asphyxia to the baby. Large doses within too short a time of delivery are sure to cause fetal respiratory depression with its subsequent ill effects. The kind of drug and the time of administration are very carefully chosen by the doctor for the individual patient.

In recent years doctors have reduced the use of analgesia in some of their patients by preparing them mentally and physically for natural childbirth, which is uninhibited by the use of large doses of drugs.

## PHYSIOLOGIC LABOR

According to Dr. Grantly Dick Read, a London obstetrician, who first published his work in 1933, women can be prepared for a natural physiologic labor in which there are no fear and tenseness because they learn to regard it as a natural process. The patient knows what to expect because she has been taught the physiology of pregnancy, the development of the baby, and the method of relaxation; she is determined to relax completely with each contraction, thereby making it entirely effective in dilating the cervix. By physiologic labor Dr. Read means labor and delivery without great discomfort and with no shock or injury to the mother or baby, this labor being uninhibited by mechanical, chemical, or psychologic factors. The psychologic factor is largely responsible for interference during labor; therefore, by psychosomatic treatment analgesia, anesthesia, and forceps deliveries can be reduced in many cases, thus lowering the maternal and infant morbidity and mortality rates.

Although physiologic labor is possible in many patients it cannot be satisfactorily conducted in all women. Some are not emotionally fitted because they are not able to exercise the patience and self-control that are essential in natural labor. These women need and should be given as much analgesia as can safely be administered. Other patients need interference during labor and delivery because of complications of pregnancy; it is only the normal patient that is suited for an entirely physiologic labor.

Much of the pain of labor can be overcome by education. As previously mentioned, many women do not know what to expect during labor; they are apprehensive because they do not know the meaning of all that takes place, they keep wondering what will happen next, and they are left alone during labor. They have heard that severe pain accompanies labor and they are afraid. This fear produces a state of tension and tension causes pain. Through the sympathetic nervous system, during a state of tension, the circular muscle fibers of the uterus, which should be relaxed, are contracted and antagonistic to the longitudinal fibers which are trying to dilate the cervix during contractions. The tension that is present also causes involuntary spasm of the abdominal and back muscles which leads to still more pain.

Fear must be overcome by education as early as possible in the prenatal period. The processes of labor must be explained, and the patient must develop confidence in herself so that she will feel that she can have the baby without difficulty. To be unafraid she must also have complete confidence in her obstetrician and feel free to ask any questions that she wishes. During the prenatal period physical efficiency should be improved by teaching exercises, controlled breathing, and relaxation. These can be taught to a group, in a class, and do not necessarily have to be taught by the obstetrician. Physical therapists and nurses have frequently supervised these exercises. The exercises are not long or difficult; they involve the abdominal and leg muscles and are not necessarily the kind that make muscles stronger, but rather more elastic and flexible. An easy posture, which does not overly protrude or draw in the abdomen, is also taught to help in preventing backache and a tired feeling during pregnancy. Proper breathing is utilized in the relaxation of the body and the mind, and, therefore, controlled breathing and relaxation, both of which are important in labor, are taught. When the body is relaxed it is not possible to have physical and mental tension. Exercise, controlled breathing, and relaxation after being taught and supervised in class can be practiced daily at home.

When labor begins, the signs of which the patient now knows, she notifies the doctor and he sees her early. She is in a good emotional state, and everything must be done to keep her that way. The labor room must be quiet and peaceful with no hurry, confusion, or unnecessary conversation, and the doctor or nurse should stay with her for an hour or more to make sure she remembers her teaching of how to relax during a contraction. When she is relaxing well it is not necessary for someone to stay with her at all times, but she should feel that she can call someone whenever she wishes. Her husband should be allowed to stay with her. There should be complete relaxation of the body; no tossing about or facial contortions. If the patient wishes to hold someone's hand this may be comforting, but it must not be a squeezing grip. As labor progresses and the contractions become harder the respirations become faster and deeper, and it will be necessary to give the patient much reassurance because there is now a great demand on her patience and self-control. This is especially true at certain periods; one of these periods being when the cervix is almost completely dilated, since the last few contractions of the first stage are the most uncomfortable. Analgesia may be necessary at this period, and the patient should know that it is available.

After the second stage begins, analgesia is probably not necessary. Where the patient has been relaxing with contractions during the first stage she now must be reminded to relax completely between contractions. She takes deep breaths and pushes during contractions—when the uterus pushes—and when the contraction ceases she takes a few deep breaths and relaxes completely. In this way a state of partial amnesia is produced which allows for complete rest and recovery of the uterine muscle for the next contraction.

With pressure on the perineum and crowning of the head there may be fright and expectation of severe pain. Considerable reassurance is again necessary, and the patient must be reminded not to contract the perineal muscles. Being unafraid prevents involuntary contraction of these muscles. During this stage the patient may grunt and groan as anyone would during hard physical labor, but she should not cry out because with this she may lose her self-control. Analgesia should be available at this time if the patient wants it. The mother is asked to stop bearing down when the head is about to be born so that the uterine contractions alone can advance the baby slowly, thereby allowing time for adequate perineal relaxation to prevent laceration. Episiotomies are frequently made at this stage.

Much of physiologic labor is having complete confidence in herself and her obstetrician, and in having mastered self-control. It gives the mother much satisfaction to have had the baby naturally born and to have been completely aware of his birth. With this type of labor there is less necessity for operative interference, postpartum hemorrhage is rare, and the mother is anxious to breast-feed her baby.

## ANALGESIC AND AMNESIC DRUGS

Drugs which produce a stage in which the patient is drowsy and sleeps between contractions, but does not entirely lose consciousness, are often administered during labor. The patient may complain at the height of the contraction, but sleep between contractions. These drugs are sometimes supplemented by one which produces forgetfulness. The patient may appear to be conscious of considerable pain during the contractions, but be unable to recall it later. Scopolamine is most frequently used to produce this amnesic effect.

**The Opium Derivatives.** The narcotics are quite generally used because they are relatively safe and do not produce the restlessness that may follow the use of many of the other drugs. For this reason they can more easily be used in the home. The opium derivatives give good analgesia and usually have no serious effect on the baby if administered at least four hours before delivery takes place. Sometimes one injection of scopolamine is also given. It produces amnesia and may also counteract any respiratory depression which may follow the administration of an opiate.

Morphine, or other opiate, is usually given when the patient is making some progress in labor, as shown by the presence of from

3- to 4-cm (1.2- to 1.6-in.) dilatation, if the discomfort caused by the contractions is such that the patient warrants receiving a pain-relieving drug. To get the full effect of the drug the patient should be psychically prepared by being told that she is being given something for relief of pain; the room should be darkened and all unnecessary noise should be excluded.

The opiates are usually not repeated except in long labors and usually not given to patients in premature labor because narcotics are very dangerous to the premature baby, sometimes even when as many as eight hours have elapsed between administration of the drug and the birth of the baby. Pantopon and dilaudid are other opiates sometimes used.

Meperidine (Demerol), a synthetic drug resembling morphine as an analgesic and atropine as an antispasmodic, is now used considerably for pain relief in labor. It may be administered orally or intramuscularly in doses of 50 to 100 mg (¾ to 1½ gr) and is sometimes repeated in a few hours. It is frequently given with scopolamine; the resultant effect being analgesia and amnesia. In large doses it produces respiratory depression.

Meperidine (Demerol) or an opiate and scopolamine combination may be used for its analgesic and amnesic effect. The analgesic drug and scopolamine, 0.43 mg (1/150 gr), are usually given at the first injection, and then scopolamine may be repeated in smaller doses one or more times. Sometimes the analgesic is repeated much later. Scopolamine is used mainly to produce amnesia. Scopolamine ordinarily promotes drowsiness, but in patients who have pain it frequently produces excitement and restlessness. These patients sleep between pains, but may become restless during a pain and become very excited and complain bitterly. After the delivery they usually do not have much recollection of discomfort. Because of the extreme restlessness that some of them show they must be watched constantly. The effects of the drugs may accumulate in the baby and cause respiratory depression.

**Barbituric Acid Derivatives.** The barbiturates are employed quite frequently in labor. Those of short to moderate duration, such as amobarbital (sodium Amytal), pentobarbital sodium (Nembutal), or secobarbital (sodium Seconal), are most commonly used. They have a hypnotic effect, produce relaxation, and relieve fear and tension. When used with scopolamine, narcosis and amnesia result. They may be given early in labor, when used either alone or with scopolamine, because these drugs do not affect the uterine contractions. The dosage is usually 0.1 to 0.3 gm (1½ to 4½ gr) by mouth for the first dose with one or two repetitions of 0.1 gm (1½ gr) if necessary. Scopolamine 0.43 mg (1/150 gr) is usually given hypodermically soon after the first dose of barbiturate and may also be repeated. It aids in producing amnesia and it may counteract some of the respiratory depression which follows the administration of a barbiturate. These patients need careful watching to prevent them from injuring themselves by the restlessness and excitement that are caused by the drugs. Due to excitability and poor cooperation the incidence of operative deliveries is increased. The barbiturates depress the respiratory center, and if large doses have been given, the baby may be severely asphyxiated.

**Paraldehyde.** Paraldehyde may also be given to the patient in labor to produce amnesia. It may be used alone or in combination with scopolamine, the barbiturates, or opium derivatives. It may be administered orally or put into olive oil and given rectally. It has a disagreeable taste, an unpleasant odor, and may be vomited when administered by mouth or expelled when given by rectum.

**General Remarks.** Agents given systemically traverse the placenta. There is thus a direct relationship between the dosage of any sedative drug, the time of administration, and fetal asphyxia. It is always difficult to decide the best time for the administration of an analgesic. The complaints of the patient, the amount of cervical dilatation, and the rapidity with which labor is progressing are factors taken into consideration. Sedatives may, in some instances, retard labor, especially if given early. They may affect the baby when not enough time has elapsed between administration of the drug and delivery of the infant to allow for elimination of the drug. If labor is progressing rapidly, especially in the multigravida, it is not wise to give an analgesic drug since there will not be sufficient time for its elimination before delivery. The severe second-stage contractions, and even the latter part of the first stage, can be relieved by inhalation anesthesia.

After administration of any drug the nurse must watch the mother and the unborn baby carefully. The mother must be watched for respiratory depression. Careful observation of the strength and frequency of the contractions is necessary; labor may be slowed or it may progress rapidly. It is frequently difficult to decide from the patient's reactions when the second stage is reached. If a drug which causes excitement is given, the mother must be watched every moment to prevent her from injuring herself. The fetal heart tones should be checked frequently to observe the reactions of the fetus to the drug. Slight degrees of hypoxia, which apparently have no ill effects upon the mother, may have a deleterious effect upon her baby.

## INHALATION ANALGESIA AND ANESTHESIA

The common inhalation anesthetics are nitrous oxide, ethylene, cyclopropane, chloroform, ether, and trichloroethylene. In obstetrics these agents are sometimes used during the latter part of the first stage of labor to produce analgesia and during the second stage for one of two purposes: either to anesthetize the patient for delivery, or for analgesia at the height of contractions. The latter means that the agent is given with each contraction, but consciousness is maintained; this has been called anesthesia *à la reine,* after Queen Victoria, upon whom it was first employed at the birth of her seventh child, in 1853.

It must be remembered that inhalation anesthesia also affects the baby, perhaps mostly by decreasing the oxygen supply, and that many of these patients have already had an analgesic drug. If the mother becomes cyanotic at any time, hypoxia is produced in the fetus.

Many patients vomit because food and fluid have not been withheld as for elective surgery. They may become cyanotic and may aspirate food. A suction apparatus should always be available in the delivery room, and it should be possible to place the patient in a Trendelenburg position very readily. Before beginning inhalation anesthesia, atropine or scopolamine is often given to reduce secretions in the respiratory passages. Since food and fluid leave the stomach slowly during labor, only light, easily digestible food or a liquid diet without milk should be given during labor, and many doctors prefer that the patient have only sips of water or no fluids after the cervix reaches 7- to 8-cm (2.8- to 3.2-in.) dilatation in the primigravida and 3 to 4 cm (1.2 to 1.6 in.) in the multigravida.

Inhalation analgesia may decrease the strength and frequency of the uterine contractions, but by relieving the discomfort of the contraction there is usually more cooperation from the patient in bearing down. Because of the tendency to uterine inertia the blood loss may be greater during the third stage, but the use of drugs with an oxytocic action will usually overcome this inertia.

**Nitrous oxide and oxygen** are often used to produce analgesia with each contraction in the second stage. This mixture is given as soon as the patient begins to have a contraction, and by the time it is at its height she loses sensation of pain, but continues to remain conscious. Some obstetricians do not begin analgesia by this method until the cervix is fully dilated, while others begin its administration late in the first stage. During the second-stage contractions the patient is asked to take two or three deep breaths of the mixture and with her lungs full to hold her breath and bear down as long as possible. If the contraction is long she may take another deep breath and bear down a second or even a third time. As soon as the contraction begins to subside pure oxygen is given to get as much as possible to the baby. Because nitrous oxide is rapidly absorbed and eliminated, it makes a very good analgesic agent up to or even during the actual delivery. During delivery of the head the analgesia may be deepened with the mixture, or may be augmented with ether or one of the other gases. This mixture is not satisfactory for deep anesthesia.

Nitrous oxide should be administered only by an experienced anesthetist because it requires high concentrations of the gas to produce analgesia (60 to 80 per cent) and there is great danger of producing hypoxia in the fetus if it is not carefully administered. An experienced anesthetist can vary the concentration of nitrous oxide and oxygen as indicated by the reactions of the baby and the strength and duration of the contractions. The patient should never become cyanotic. If properly administered it may be used for analgesia over a rather long period of time during the second stage of labor without reducing contractions and without danger to mother or baby. From this standpoint it is a very good analgesic agent in obstetrics. Its disadvantages are that it is used with safety only by an experienced anesthetist and that it requires heavy expensive apparatus for its administration. When these difficulties can be overcome, its use is attended by very satisfactory results.

**Ethylene** is not as generally used as nitrous oxide. Its effect is rapid and higher concentrations of oxygen can be used with it than with nitrous oxide, but it has an unpleasant odor and it is very explosive. A great disadvantage is its inflammability. It must be administered by an experienced anesthetist.

**Cyclopropane** is the newest of general anesthetics. It is a valuable anesthetic agent, but it is highly explosive and it must be administered only by an experienced anesthetist. It is safe for the baby since as high as 80 to 90 per cent oxygen can be given with it. It is therefore valuable as an anesthetic for operative deliveries. It may also be used to augment nitrous oxide, just as the head is being delivered, because a much higher concentration of oxygen can then be given. It is not used for intermittent pain relief because its explosiveness prohibits frequent removal of the mask.

**Chloroform** was at one time the most generally used obstetric anesthetic, but it is now used only occasionally because it may have adverse effects upon the heart and it may damage the liver if the anesthesia is prolonged. The advantages of chloroform, which still commend it at times, are that it is easy to give, is quick in its action, is pleasant to inhale, is followed by little or no nausea, gives excellent muscular relaxation, and is well tolerated by the unborn infant. Its disadvantage is that it has only a very narrow margin of safety. If it is necessary to administer an anesthetic in a patient's home chloroform and ether are most frequently used; of these chloroform is easier to administer and is not explosive, but ether is the safer one to use.

Chloroform is less irritating to the patient and requires less time to produce anesthesia. It is not inflammable and can more safely be used if there is an open flame anywhere near the patient's room. Chloroform may be administered by dropping only a few drops of the liquid on a handkerchief held above the patient's face, this being draped loosely over the hand of the person giving the anesthetic. A tight cylinder is not necessary. To regulate the drops carefully a wedge may be cut into the cork of the bottle and a piece of gauze or cotton may be used as a wick from which to drop the liquid. Whenever chloroform is administered it is necessary to keep a finger on the patient's pulse constantly because of the narrow margin between the anesthetic dose and the toxic dose; the pulse will show changes by becoming weak, irregular, or varying in rate if the patient is receiving too much. The anesthetic must be stopped immediately if any change is noted in cardiac action.

**Ether** is mainly used for continuous anesthesia, as in operative deliveries, and especially when it is important to have good muscle relaxation. It is not very satisfactory for analgesic purposes because it takes effect so slowly that if given for analgesia the patient rarely gets the maximum effect when she needs it the most, unless it is administered by an experienced person. It is unpleasant to the patient because of its irritation to the respiratory passages. In spite of this it

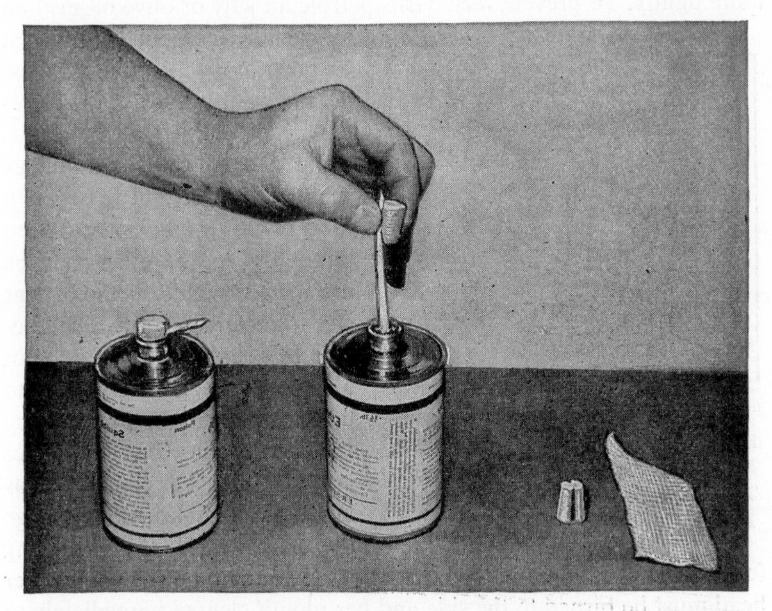

**Fig. 114.** *Right to left:* gauze wick, cork with two grooves, insertion of wick and cork into ether tin, dropper ready for use. (Leigh, M. Digby, and Belton, M. Kathleen: *Pediatric Anesthesia.* The Macmillan Company, New York, 1948.)

is usually a good analgesic to use in the home during the second stage of labor. Its advantages are that it has a wider margin of safety than most of the anesthetic agents, especially in the hands of an inexperienced person; it is also inexpensive and requires no elaborate equipment. A mask may even be made by placing a handkerchief over a newspaper cylinder. Ether may also be given as a rectal instillation, in olive oil or mineral oil, for purposes of analgesia.

Since ether takes effect slowly it must be administered as rapidly as possible when used for analgesia. The anesthetist must be ready to have the patient begin inhaling it as soon as a contraction begins. It is better for the anesthetist to keep a hand on the patient's abdomen and judge, by palpation, when the contractions begin and end than it is to ask the patient to tell when she feels contractions begin and cease.

When ether is used to produce anesthesia the cylinder should fit quite tightly. To prevent face burns petroleum jelly or olive oil may be applied to the skin. Care must be taken not to drop any of the liquid into the eyes; it is, therefore, well to cover them with a towel. If some of the liquid does accidentally get into the eyes, a drop of castor oil may be placed in each eye. The ether may be dropped as rapidly as the patient can tolerate the odor; if she begins to cough, a few breaths of air should be given. It is well to talk to the patient while giving the anesthesia, but all other noise should be eliminated as much as possible. At one stage the patient will get a tingling feeling due to changes in the circulation. If at any time she vomits, her head must be turned to the side and her mouth cleared immediately to prevent aspiration.

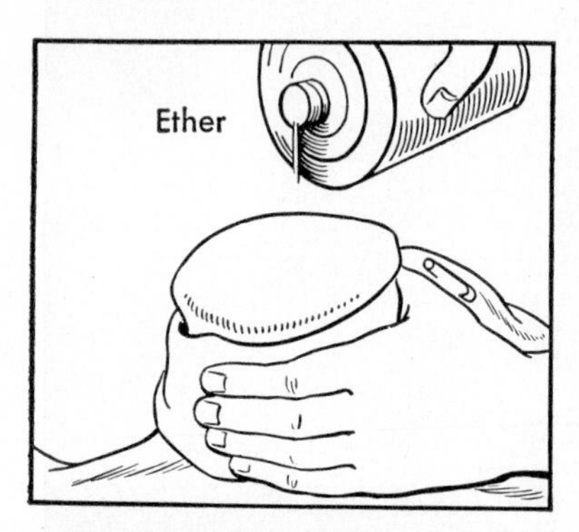


**Fig. 115.** Open drop ether anesthesia. (Leigh, M. Digby, and Belton, M. Kathleen: *Pediatric Anesthesia.* The Macmillan Company, New York, 1948.)

It will take a large amount of ether and from 3 to 15 minutes of administration for the patient to reach an unconscious stage. If she blinks her eyelids when touched she is still awake. After she is unconscious it will take very little more ether to keep her asleep. The patient's breathing, pulse, color, and pupil reaction must be watched closely, and if any danger signs appear such as shallow, irregular breathing, irregular pulse, cyanosis, and failure of the pupils to contract when exposed to light the anesthesia must be discontinued immediately. The airway must be watched carefully, and support must be given to the chin, because relaxation of the jaw and throat muscles may cause obstruction.

**Trichloroethylene, Also Known as "Trilene."** This is a volatile liquid which may be used for analgesia or light anesthesia. As an anesthetic agent it may be sufficiently effective for delivery, but it does not give marked relaxation. By means of an inhaler, which the patient can use and which supplies her with a mixture of trichloroethylene and air, it can be self-administered for analgesic purposes with each contraction during the latter part of the first stage of labor and sometimes during the second stage. It may be used in conjunction with other medications or other anesthetic agents. During the second stage it may be used alone or with other methods, commonly pudendal block or saddle block.

Trichloroethylene is not inflammable when mixed with air, but precautions must be taken when it is used with oxygen. There is no excitement reaction with its use. It has a fairly pleasant odor, is not irritating to the respiratory tract, does not increase salivary secretions, and seldom induces nausea and vomiting. Analgesic concentrations do not affect the blood pressure, respirations, and heart rate, but changes may be noticed when it is used for anesthesia. Trichloroethylene is not recommended for patients with cardiac disease or a toxemia of pregnancy. It does not appear to prolong labor or cause fetal asphyxia. Trichloroethylene may be valuable for purposes of analgesia in the latter part of the first stage of labor when delivery is anticipated so early that medications given orally or hypodermically could not be eliminated before delivery and thus would affect the baby. Because trichloroethylene is inexpensive, the equipment is easy to transport, and it may be self-administered, it can easily be used in the home.

For self-administration the inhaler is prepared by pouring 15 ml (½ oz) trichloroethylene into the cylinder and rotating it in order to saturate the absorbent material lining the walls of the cylinder. For purposes of analgesia the patient is instructed to hold the mask lightly over her mouth and nose and to inhale the vapor at the onset of a contraction (Fig. 116). Two or three breaths usually provide sufficient analgesia. She must be instructed to breathe quite deeply, since trichloroethylene is less volatile than other volatile anesthetic agents. When it is used for the second stage the patient is instructed to take a few quick breaths and then bear down. The inhaler is equipped with a nonrebreathing mechanism, and the expired air is blown into the atmosphere.

The collar on the cylinder of the inhaler is adjustable and can be set to regulate the potency of the vapor that is to be inhaled. When it is set at a minimum concentration very little of the inhaled air comes in contact with trichloroethylene, and the concentration of the vapor that the patient breathes is very low. When it is set at a maximum practically all of the air that the patient breathes comes in contact with the absorbent material in the inhaler, which is saturated with the liquid, and the patient receives a high concentration of

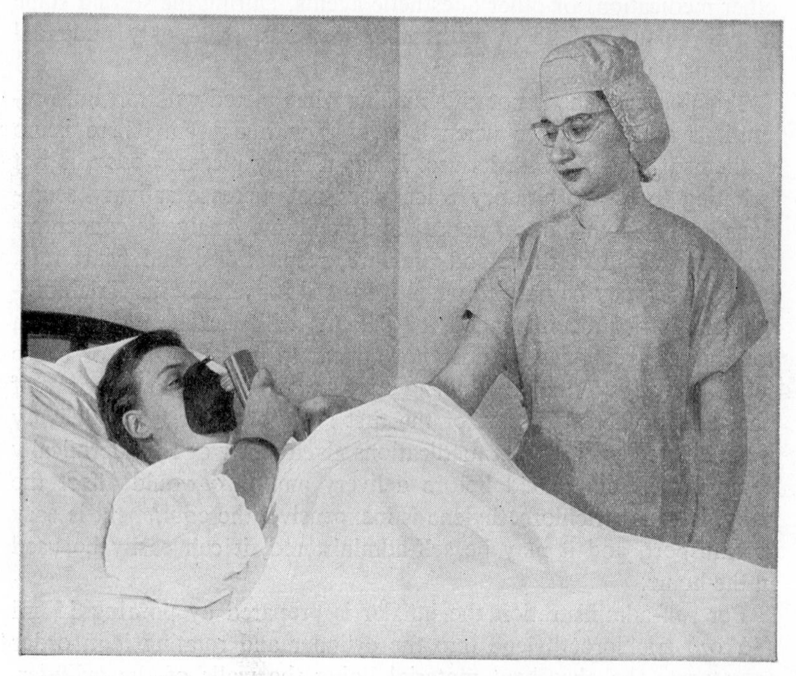

**Fig. 116.** Self-administration of trichloroethylene (Trilene) for purposes of analgesia during contractions in the latter part of the first stage of labor.

trichloroethylene. For obstetric analgesia the setting may be adjusted to supply approximately 0.65 per cent trichloroethylene in air; this may be somewhat increased or decreased as seems necessary by the patient's reaction. With analgesic concentrations there is usually no loss of consciousness, but the patient may experience slight dizziness, tingling, and numbness. If unconsciousness is induced by the inhalation of too much vapor, safety is ordinarily assured, because the patient will drop the mask, inhale only pure air, and recover consciousness rapidly. It is necessary, however, to watch that the patient does not have the hand, which is holding the mask, propped in such a manner that it cannot fall away when consciousness is lost; therefore, the patient must never be left alone. It is important, however, that no other person hold the mask for the patient. A wrist band which straps the inhaler to the patient's wrist prevents it from falling to the floor.

Trichloroethylene should be stored in closed containers and away from light. Any unused amount in the inhaler should be discarded each day to prevent any possibility of danger from the decomposition products which result from oxidation. When used for anesthesia it must never be used in a closed circuit with soda lime, since a chemical reaction between these two substances produces a compound which is toxic to the nervous system.

**General Remarks.** With any general anesthetic the patient's pulse must be watched carefully, the air passages must be kept open to prevent cyanosis which is dangerous to both mother and baby, and the fetal heart tones must be checked every few minutes. It is possible for the anesthetist to auscultate the fetal heart tones if a Leffscope, which has a heavy stethoscope bell, is fixed to the patient's abdomen with adhesive tape, over the area where the fetal heart is best heard (Figs. 117 and 118). With a piece of tubing on the stethoscope bell, long enough to reach from the patient's abdomen to the head of the

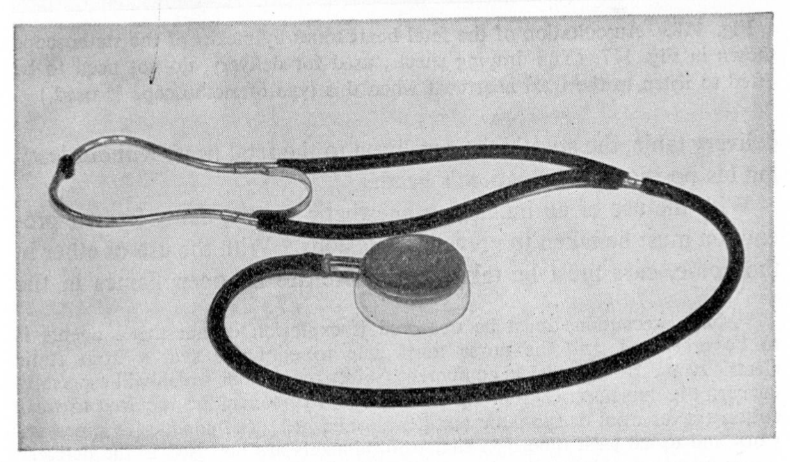

**Fig. 117.** A heavy stethoscope bell which may be placed over the area where the fetal heart is best heard and fixed to the patient's abdomen with adhesive tape. A piece of tubing long enough to reach from the patient's abdomen to the head of the delivery table permits the anesthetist to listen to the fetal heart without leaving his position at the patient's head.

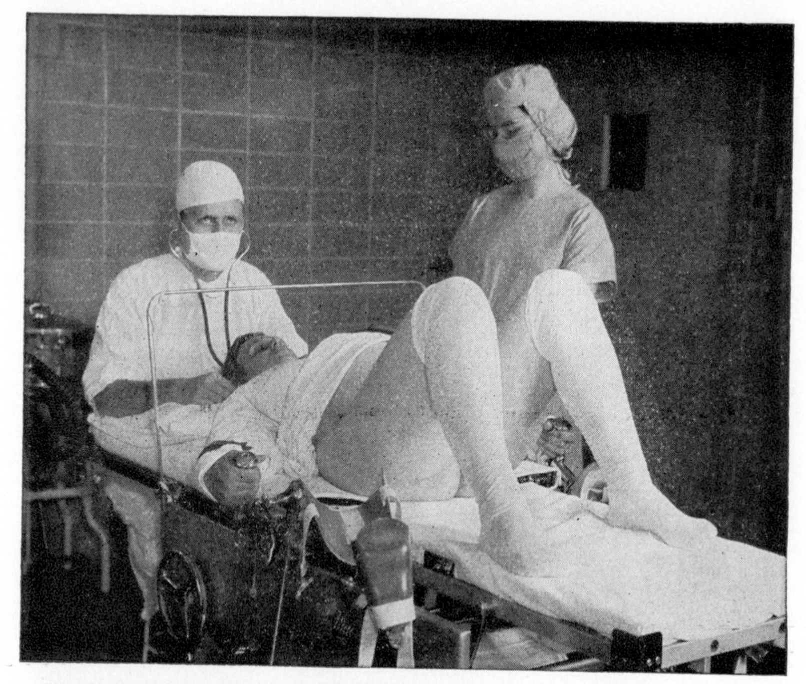

**Fig. 118.** Auscultation of the fetal heart tones by means of the stethoscope shown in Fig. 117. (The draping sheets, used for delivery, do not need to be lifted to listen to the fetal heartbeat when this type of stethoscope is used.)

delivery table, the anesthetist can listen to the fetal heart without leaving his position at the patient's head.

With the use of all inhalation anesthetic agents, every known precaution must be taken to prevent explosions.* With the use of ether in the home, care must be taken that there are no open flames in the

* Many precautions must be observed if explosion of anesthetic agents is to be prevented, and the nurse must help to eliminate sparks from static electricity and from electrical equipment. Safety regulations which will especially concern the nurse are: (1) that all delivery room personnel are required to wear cotton (never wool or synthetic textile) clothing; (2) that conductive shoes are worn and tested each time; (3) that wool blankets are not used in the delivery room; (4) that only conductive rubber material is used on the delivery table and anesthesia equipment; (5) that anesthesia equipment is not touched while anesthesia is in progress; (6) that all appliances are grounded; and (7) that all electrical appliances are kept in good repair. (Further information may be obtained from "Recommended Safe Practice for Hospital Operating Rooms," pamphlet No. 56. National Fire Protection Association, Boston, Mass., 1956.)

room. Under all conditions it is important to remember that no matter what kind of anesthetic or analgesic is given, it is necessary to guard against the very prevalent tendency to talk freely while the patient is losing consciousness. Many patients suffer great mental distress because of hearing, or partly hearing, conversation not intended for their ears, which takes place in their hearing while they are incompletely anesthetized.

*Emergency Administration of Anesthesia by an Unskilled Person.* Unless it is absolutely essential to do otherwise, only an experienced anesthetist should administer an anesthetic, but if an unskilled person must assist it is known that ether is, by far, the safest agent. The doctor must always assume the responsibility for the anesthetic, but there are instances in which it becomes necessary for a nurse, under the guidance of a physician, to administer it. The nurse must always remember that she is using a powerful drug and that she has two patients to consider.

## REGIONAL ANESTHESIA

Procaine (Novocaine), piperocaine (Metycaine), dibucaine (Nupercaine), lidocaine (Xylocaine), and tetracaine (Pontocaine) are some agents used for local anesthesia. They may be administered by local infiltration of tissues in the operative area, by spinal injection, or by injection into the caudal canal.

**Local Infiltration.** Local anesthesia is accomplished by injection of an anesthetic drug directly into the vulvar and perineal tissues. It has no value as an analgesic during labor, but is useful for perineal anesthesia during delivery of the baby and may also be used for local infiltration of tissue for cesarean section. Local anesthesia is simple to administer and it is not dependent upon a second person. It does not interfere with uterine or abdominal muscle contractions. It has no ill effects upon the mother with the exception of an occasional adverse reaction due to the dosage or rapid absorption of the drug. It is particularly valuable when inhalation anesthesia is hazardous. There is no danger of aspiration of fluid by vomiting and thus no danger of pulmonary complications.

The nurse's duties consist of preparing the syringe and needle and solution for injection. A 20-ml syringe and No. 20-gauge needle which is 5 or 6.2 cm (2 or 2.5 in.) long are used for the infiltration. Procaine hydrochloride, 0.5 to 1 per cent solution, is most commonly employed as the anesthetic agent; from 30 to 100 ml of solution may be used. This solution should be fresh, preferably prepared from ampuls of stock solution at the time of use. Dilution should be made with physiologic saline solution. An ampul of epinephrine (Adrenalin) 1:1000 should be available, because the doctor may wish to add a few minims to the procaine solution before it is injected.

The patient is usually prepared and draped as for delivery, and when the head appears at the vulvar opening, the tissues of the vulva and the perineal body are injected with the solution. The tissues must be handled gently. The patient's cooperation is necessary during the injection; she can be aided in her efforts by being encouraged and comforted. The physician should talk to her during the procedure, and unless the nurse must be occupied with other duties in the delivery room she should be at the head of the delivery table where she can easily talk with the patient, give her encouragement, and reduce apprehension.

**Pudendal Block.** This is a regional anesthetic similar to local infiltration of the perineum, but one in which the anesthetic agent is placed deeper into the tissues, and anesthesia of the pudendal nerve is effected. The technic and drug used are similar to perineal infiltration with the exception of a 10- to 12½-cm (4- to 5-in.) needle in order to facilitate the deeper placement of the solution. There is greater relaxation of tissue with this technic.

**Caudal Analgesia and Anesthesia.** By this method analgesia and anesthesia of the pelvic region are obtained through the injection of one of the local anesthetic agents into the caudal space, which is the area within the sacrum at the lowermost part of the bony spinal canal. A dural sac separates this space from the spinal cord. A number of sacral nerves emerge from the dural sac and pass through this space. By filling the canal with an anesthetic solution the pain sense of these nerves can be abolished, and anesthesia is thus produced in the pelvic region supplied by these nerves. The anesthetic solution can be placed into the caudal canal with a spinal needle inserted through a foramen present at the lower end of the sacrum. If the anesthesia is to be of short duration a single injection of anesthetic solution may be made, and the needle immediately removed. When the analgesia is to be of long or indefinite duration, known as continuous caudal anesthesia, frequent injections must be made. These are accomplished by inserting a polyethylene tube or a specially designed malleable needle into the caudal canal; either of these may be left in place to facilitate injections. Anesthesia may be started when the patient is in active labor and cervical dilatation has reached 3 to 4 cm (1.2 to 1.6 in.). To prepare the patient she is placed in the Sims' or knee-chest position and the skin over the sacral and coccygeal region is washed with soap and water and painted with an antiseptic solution. The needle is inserted into the sacral canal and attempts at aspiration are made. If the dura has been pierced, and spinal fluid is obtained, the procedure is discontinued, because a large injection of medication into the spinal canal is dangerous or fatal. Analgesia is usually present in 5 to 15 minutes or at least in 30 minutes following injection. If analgesia is satisfactory sensations are lost in the pelvic region, and the pain of uterine contractions is relieved. The lower extremities become tingly and motor weakness develops. Supplemental injections are given as frequently as indicated by the patient's reactions; these may be necessary approximately every 40 to 60 minutes. Caudal analgesia may be continued indefinitely, at least for six to eight hours, or even longer.

When successfully administered this method gives relief of pain without great inhibition of the uterine contractions and gives good perineal relaxation. Since the anal sphincter also relaxes, the bowel should be empty. The baby is born without the effect of any drug. However, this is a specialized procedure, there are dangers involved, and its usefulness and safety depend upon the experience of the administrator; it is therefore a procedure which must be limited to hospital use. This may be a valuable method of anesthesia when a general anesthetic is contraindicated.

Some of the contraindications to its use are certain obstetric complications, such as bleeding and shock, and spine deformities. Operative deliveries are increased because the patient has no urge to bear down with the contractions although she is able to do so when told. Ill effects sometimes occur due to the circulatory depression and vascular collapse, with a drop in blood pressure, which may follow the injection. The blood pressure must be carefully watched. The administration of a vasopressor may be indicated. In cases of hemorrhage or shock of obstetric origin, caudal analgesia is contraindicated because of its vasodepressor action.

The nurse's duties will consist of sterilizing the equipment necessary for the caudal injection and supplying the doctor with sterile rubber gloves, draping towels, and skin antiseptics. The site at which the needle is placed must be protected and kept clean. Since the patient is unaware of her contractions after analgesia is begun, the progress of labor must be observed by palpation of the abdomen for frequency and strength of contractions and by performing rectal examinations. The bladder must be observed for fullness and catheterization performed as necessary.

**Spinal Anesthesia.** With this method, anesthesia of the operative area is produced by the injection of one of the local anesthetic agents into the subarachnoid space. This is done either by a single injection or by a continuous method. Spinal anesthesia, when used for obstetric patients, is largely used for cesarean sections, since anesthesia can be obtained without affecting the baby and there is not as much need to hurry to deliver the baby as with inhalation anesthesia. When used for vaginal deliveries, a high spinal anesthesia retards labor and operative interference may become necessary.

With the patient on her side, a spinal needle is inserted into the subarachnoid space through the third or fourth lumbar interspace. If one injection is to be used the anesthetic agent is usually dissolved in a few milliliters of spinal fluid, injected, and the needle removed. This anesthesia lasts for approximately one hour. If the continuous method is to be used a small plastic catheter is passed through the needle, taped into place, and injections of the solution are made in small doses until the anesthetic level reaches to approximately the costal margin. After surgery has been started repeated small doses will be necessary. By the continuous method the level of anesthesia, as well as the blood pressure, can be better controlled than with the single injection.

The use of spinal anesthesia requires trained personnel. It is contraindicated in cases of obstetric hemorrhage or shock and in patients who have central nervous system lesions. Drug sensitivity may be a complication. The blood pressure may fall precipitously following injection of the drug, accompanied by vomiting, pallor, weak pulse, and cold sweats. The blood pressure must be watched very closely, and measures must be taken to combat any serious drop. Intravenous fluids begun before, and continued during, the spinal anesthesia help to stabilize the circulatory system and also provide a means of giving intravenous drugs very readily should this become necessary. A postpartum headache, sometimes severe, may be a complication. Spinal anesthesia does not affect the baby, except in cases where there is a precipitous drop in blood pressure. The patient is usually kept in a recumbent position for 12 to 24 hours as ordered by the doctor.

**Saddle Block (Low Spinal).** This is also a spinal anesthetic in which one of the local anesthetic agents is used, but differs from the one described above in that the drug is localized in the conus of the dural sac, this being facilitated by the addition of glucose to the anesthetic agent which makes it heavy. Such anesthesia is of relatively short duration. It is not ordinarily used for relief of labor pains, but for delivery only, and must be planned so that delivery will take place in approximately one hour after injection of the drug.

The patient must be in a sitting position for injection of the agent. This position is very distressing to her at this time in labor, and the nurse must do all she can to provide adequate support for her to lean upon while in the sitting position and also to reassure her during the procedure.

A spinal needle is inserted into the subarachnoid space through a lumbar interspace; when spinal fluid is obtained the anesthetic agent is injected. The patient remains sitting for approximately 30 seconds; the time must be accurate but varies with the drug used. At exactly the proper time, following injection, she is placed on her back with her head on a pillow to keep the neck sharply flexed. Anesthesia occurs in that area of the body which would ordinarily come in contact with a saddle while riding horseback. The leg and thigh muscles and the abdominal muscles are not greatly affected. As with other spinal anesthesia a fall in blood pressure must be watched for and combated, and a postpartum headache may be a complication. A recumbent position may be ordered for 12 to 24 hours following delivery.

## INTRAVENOUS ANESTHESIA

This route is sometimes used for anesthesia in forceps deliveries and cesarean sections with thiopental (sodium Pentothal) being the agent employed. It is not a satisfactory method when good muscle relaxation is necessary. To avoid fetal narcosis the baby must be born within eight minutes after starting the anesthesia. This means that all preliminary preparation, such as the application of skin antiseptics, draping, and check of equipment, must be completed before anesthesia is begun. Laryngospasm in the mother is a complication, but in most instances this can be prevented by the use of atropine or scopolamine as a premedication. The patient should receive oxygen while under the influence of the anesthetic.

## BIBLIOGRAPHY AND STUDENT REFERENCES

Ayerst, McKenna, and Harrison, Limited: "The 'Duke' University Inhaler." The Company, New York, 1952.

———: "Trilene." The Company, New York, 1952.

Bookmiller, Mae M., and Bowen, George L.: *Textbook of Obstetrics and Obstetric Nursing,* 2nd ed. W. B. Saunders Co., Philadelphia, 1954.

Davis, M. Edward, and Sheckler, Catherine E.: *DeLee's Obstetrics for Nurses,* 15th ed. W. B. Saunders Co., Philadelphia, 1951.

Eastman, Nicholson J.: *Williams Obstetrics,* 11th ed. Appleton-Century-Crofts, Inc., New York, 1956.

Falls, F. H., and Falls, John L.: "Obstetric Anesthesia Mortality," *Bulletin of Maternal Welfare,* **1**:9–10, (July–Aug.) 1954.

Flowers, Charles E.: "Increasing the Safety of Obstetrical Anesthesia," *Bulletin of Maternal Welfare,* **2**:9–11, (Jan.–Feb.) 1955.

Freed, Frederick C.: "Administering an Anesthetic to a Maternity Patient," *Pub. Health Nursing,* **30**:697–700, (Dec.) 1938.

Greenhill, J. P.: "Anesthesia in Obstetrics," *Am. J. Obst. & Gynec.,* **54**:74–81, (July) 1947.

——— (ed.): *Obstetrics,* 11th ed. W. B. Saunders Co., Philadelphia, 1955.

Griffin, Noyce L.: "Preventing Fires and Explosions in the Operating Room," *Am. J. Nursing,* **53**:809–12, (July) 1953.

Hershenson, Bert B.: "Modern Trends in Obstetrical Anesthesia," *Am. J. Obst. & Gynec.,* **63**:559–69, (Mar.) 1952.

Hingson, Robert A.: "Continuous Caudal Anesthesia Requires Expert Nursing Care," *Am. J. Nursing,* **46**:747–51, (Nov.) 1946.

National Fire Protection Association: *Recommended Safe Practice for Hospital Operating Rooms,* pamphlet No. 56. The Association, 60 Batterymarch St., Boston 10, Mass.

Pickrell, K. L.; Stephen, C. R.; Broadbent, T. R.; Masters, F. W.; and Georgiade, N. G.: "Self-Induced 'Trilene' Analgesia in Plastic Surgery, with Special Reference to the Burned Patient," *Plast. & Reconstruct. Surg.,* **9**:345–54, 1952.

Read, Grantly D.: "An Outline of the Conduct of Physiological Labor," *Am. J. Obst. & Gynec.,* **54**:702–10, (Oct.) 1947.

———: *Childbirth without Fear,* 2nd ed. Harper & Brothers, New York, 1953.

Thoms, Herbert: *Training for Childbirth.* McGraw-Hill Book Co., New York, 1950.

Thoms, Herbert, and Goodrich, Frederick W.: "Training for Childbirth," *J.A.M.A.,* **140**:1256–58, (Aug. 20) 1949.

Thoms, Herbert, and Wiedenbach, Ernestine: "Support during Labor," *J.A.M.A.*, **156**:3–5, (Sept. 4) 1954.

Watson, B. P.: "Commemoration of the Centennial of the Introduction of Anesthesia in Obstetrics by Sir James Y. Simpson," *Am. J. Obst. & Gynec.*, **56**:205–12, (Aug.) 1948.

Woodward, H. L.; Gardner, B.; Bryant, R. D.; and Overland, Anna E.: *Obstetric Management and Nursing*, 5th ed. F. A. Davis Co., Philadelphia, 1955.

Zabriskie, Louise, and Eastman, Nicholson J.: *Nurses Handbook of Obstetrics*, 9th ed. J. B. Lippincott Co., Philadelphia, 1952.

*Chapter 14*

# Obstetric Operations and Complications of Labor

Unhappily, not all labors run the smooth and uncomplicated course which has thus far been described. Certain abnormalities sometimes arise to complicate delivery; these may necessitate operative interference or relief. In the presence of complicated labor there is little that a nurse can do alone, but her preparation and assistance will be more effective if she understands the purpose of the operations, and she will better appreciate the importance of certain signs which she is required to watch for and report when she realizes the extreme seriousness of the conditions that produce them.

The complications which necessitate operative procedures at the time of delivery are of either maternal or fetal origin. Among those arising in the mother may be contracted pelves that produce marked disproportion between the passage and the passenger, antepartum bleeding, toxemias of pregnancy, certain chronic diseases, uterine inertia, and pelvic tumors. Chief among those due to the fetus are certain presentations which make spontaneous delivery doubtful or impossible and evidence of fetal distress.

Rigid aseptic technic in the use of all equipment is absolutely essential in operative delivery because of the added risk of infection from manipulation of the tissues in the reproductive tract that cannot be made aseptic. It is important that the hands are prepared properly by careful scrubbing before surgery and that sufficient sterile gloves, draping sheets, towels, and instruments are available.

Except for cesarean sections the patient is placed in the lithotomy position for delivery, with the legs held up by stirrups. The buttocks should extend over the edge of the table for 2 to 3 in. to give the operator the maximum amount of room for the necessary manipulative procedures (Fig. 88). In the hospital a delivery table with suitable stirrups is used, whereas in the home a narrow table and improvised leg holders are necessary. Complete anesthesia is usually necessary, and whenever it is possible an anesthesiologist should administer the anesthetic agent so that the obstetrician can devote his full time to the surgery. The patient is prepared as described in Chapter 12 by shaving the pubic hair and by washing the skin of the lower abdomen, the inner surface of the thighs, and the vulva with soap and water and applying antiseptic solutions. She is then draped with sterile leggings and sheets or with a special draping sheet that has the leggings already attached so that it can be slipped on in one motion. This sheet contains a rectangular opening which exposes the perineal area (Fig. 90).

The instruments that are needed will include those ordinarily used for a normal delivery (Fig. 92), and in addition those necessary for the particular operative procedure that is contemplated. The added hazards of an operative delivery, to both mother and child, make it imperative to have available all equipment necessary for the management of postpartum hemorrhage and for overcoming fetal asphyxia.

Before any operative procedure is started the patient is catheterized, since a full bladder interferes with bimanual palpation, with descent of the presenting part, and later with expulsion of the placenta. There is also some danger of injury to the bladder if it is distended during delivery and especially during manipulative procedures.

## OBSTETRIC OPERATIONS

**Forceps.** The forceps is an instrument which is used to extract the child's head in certain conditions in which progress is arrested and which may thus result in dangers, immediate or remote, to the mother and/or child. The value of forceps in obstetrics can scarcely be overestimated; before its invention the only operative method of delivering a live baby was by means of version and extraction, and in these cases the fetal death rate was high. Prior to the advent of forceps, the obstetric instruments in use were designed for the destruction of the child in utero. Use of forceps may be hazardous, however, and this method of delivery should be carried out only when all conditions for proper application are fulfilled.

The forceps was devised and first used in great secrecy, early in the seventeenth century, by a Dr. Chamberlen, in England, who

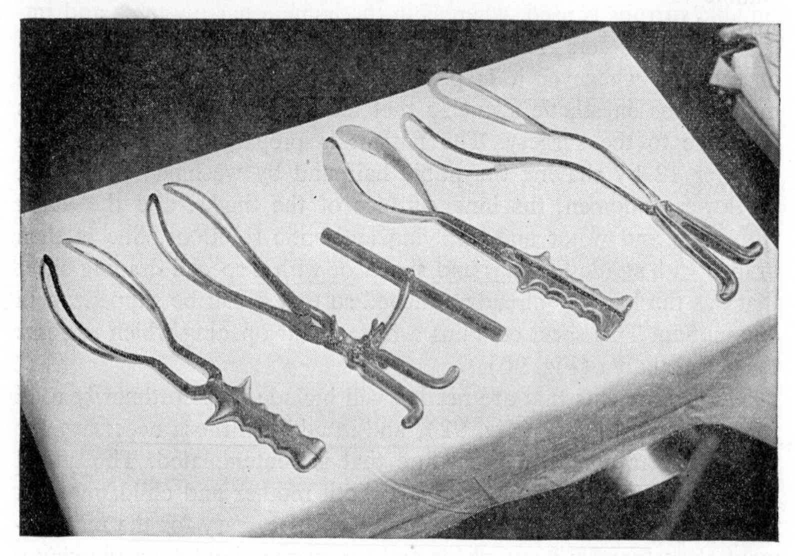

**Fig. 119.** Several kinds of obstetric forceps. *Left to right:* Simpson; Tarnier, with axis traction attachment; McLean-Tucker; Piper, for delivery of the after-coming head in breech extraction.

jealously guarded all information relating to his invention from everyone but members of his own family. There were several doctors in the Chamberlen family who practiced obstetrics and who used the forceps, but knowledge concerning the nature of the instrument and methods of using it were not shared with members of the medical profession outside of that family until the beginning of the eighteenth century. Since that time the use of forceps has been widely extended, and the original Chamberlen instrument has been so modified and improved by different obstetricians that there are now a large number and variety in existence and in use (Fig. 119). Over 600 kinds, varying in size and shape, have been designed. The type of forceps does not make as much difference as its application and use. Each doctor usually becomes accustomed to one kind and uses it almost exclusively.

The forceps consists of two parts, designated as the right and left blade according to the side of the pelvis in which it lies when it is applied to the baby's head. Each blade is curved outward to fit around the baby's head and curved upward to correspond to the axis of the mother's pelvis. These are known as the cephalic and pelvic

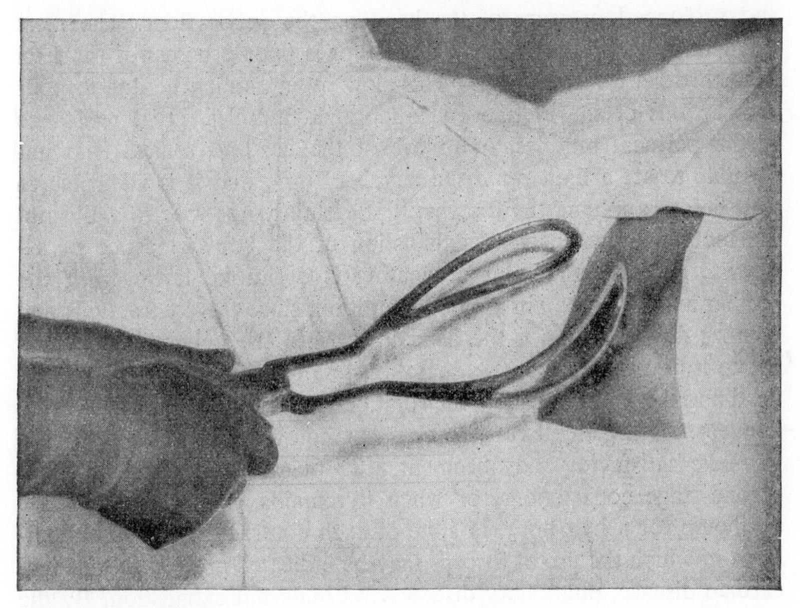

**Fig. 120.** Orientation for L.O.A. position (Simpson forceps). (From Eastman, N. J.: *Williams Obstetrics,* 11th ed. Courtesy of Appleton-Century-Crofts, Inc., New York.)

curves (Fig. 119). A few blades are solid but most are fenestrated. Since the left blade always fits to the left side of the mother's pelvis and the right blade to the right side, the nurse who is assisting the doctor will be able to distinguish the right from the left blade easily and hand him the correct one, when he asks for it, if she articulates the blades and holds them before the vulva to visualize the forceps in position (Fig. 120).

There are two groups of indications for the use of forceps, those relating to the condition of the child and those relating to the mother. Indications for their use in the interests of the child are signs of fetal distress, such as a change in the rate or rhythm of the fetal heartbeat and sometimes the passage of meconium. In head presentations the escape of meconium suggests paralysis of the rectal sphincter muscles, due to imperfect oxygenation, caused by interference with oxygenation and/or circulation of placental blood. Fetal asphyxia may be due to many causes, among which are too much analgesia or anesthesia, premature separation of the placenta, pressure on the umbilical cord, and prolonged pressure of the head on the pelvic floor. The most frequent indication for the use of forceps is poor progress of the fetal head through the birth canal. This slow progress may be due to poor contractions of the uterine and abdominal muscles, great resistance of the perineal muscles, or failure of the head to rotate. It is impossible to set a limit upon the length of time that it is advisable to wait before applying the forceps; it is certainly not wise to wait until the mother shows signs of exhaustion or the baby evidence of asphyxia. A certain amount of waiting is desirable, however, if the mother and baby remain in good condition, since the contractions and bearing down will push the head lower into the pelvis and perhaps rotate it and thus make the operation less dangerous. The lower the head and the more complete the rotation the less the danger of forceps delivery. As a general rule, forceps is employed when the head fails to make satisfactory advancement after one to two hours of good, second-stage contractions, or when it remains in one place on the perineum for a half hour, in spite of such contractions. Other conditions in which the use of forceps may be indicated are severe toxemia, cardiac disease, pulmonary disease, and maternal exhaustion. By the use of low forceps in these conditions the exertion of the second stage of labor, which might menace the life of the mother, is alleviated.

Forceps operations are usually designated as *high, mid,* or *low,* depending upon the level to which the head has descended into the pelvis when the forceps is applied. If the head is at the superior strait and has not become engaged, it is a high forceps operation; mid forceps, if the head is halfway down, the lowermost part of the skull being on a level with or below the ischial spines; and low forceps, when the skull is on the perineal floor. The application of low forceps is a simple operation and attended by little danger to mother or child, mid forceps is more serious, and high forceps is practically never used in the present day. Many forceps operations today are *elective low forceps* deliveries. To be termed an elective low forceps the skull must be on the perineal floor with the head already visible at the vulva and the sagittal suture in an anteroposterior position. Only gentle traction is necessary, and the operation is quite simple. The procedure is elective instead of indicated when it is expected that spontaneous delivery could take place within 15 to 30 minutes. It is performed to relieve the mother of the strain of the last part of the second stage, to prevent overstretching of the perineum since an episiotomy is performed earlier than if delivery were spontaneous, and to relieve the cerebral tissues of the infant from a long period of pressure against the perineum. Sometimes pain-relieving agents interfere to some degree with the mother's bearing-down ability, and this operation hastens the delivery in such cases.

Before applying forceps the operator must satisfy himself that all conditions are favorable. There must be complete dilatation of the cervix; otherwise severe lacerations with hemorrhage may result. There must be no considerable disproportion between the size of the head and the pelvis because extraction would then be very dangerous to both mother and child. The head must be engaged, the position of the child's head must be known in order that the forceps may be properly applied, and the membranes must be ruptured since the forceps may slip or prematurely separate the placenta. It is also necessary that the head must not be so large or so small that the forceps will not grasp it securely.

Before beginning the operation the doctor will usually wish to lubricate his gloves for vaginal examination and lubricate the blades of the forceps so that they will slip into place more easily. Special precautions must be taken to use a lubricant which is absolutely sterile. There is considerable danger of contamination when a lubricant is squeezed from a tube because of the small opening and the inadequate protection from the cover on the tube. A liquid, such as tincture of green soap, sterilized in an autoclave and poured from a bottle which has a sterile cover that fits well over the edge is much safer. Many times the doctor will wish to use an antiseptic solution on his gloves and in the vagina during the vaginal examination. Some operators manually dilate the vaginal outlet and pelvic floor with the hand before applying the forceps in order to decrease the resistance of the muscles and thus decrease the incidence and degree of perineal tears and the amount of traction necessary on the forceps. An episiotomy is ordinarily done for similar reasons.

An accurate diagnosis of the position of the head is important before the blades are applied because they should be placed to the sides of the head and over the ears. A hand in the vagina guides the blades into proper position (Fig. 121 A-D). The blades are

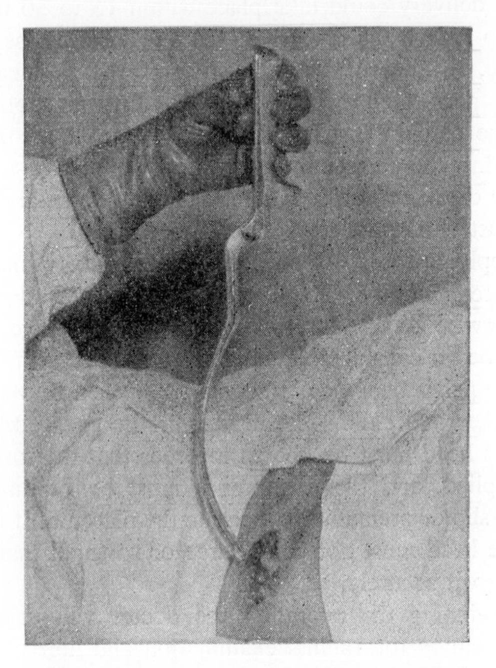

**Fig. 121A.** Low forceps: The left handle held in the left hand. Simpson forceps. (From Eastman, N. J.: *Williams Obstetrics,* 11th ed. Courtesy of Appleton-Century-Crofts, Inc., New York.)

applied separately; the first to be placed is usually the one that fits over the posterior ear. The handles are locked after the blades are in place; if they are on correctly the handles will close easily. Some compression of the head is unavoidable, but should be reduced to a minimum so as to prevent intracranial hemorrhage with injury to the brain.

The forceps is used mainly to make traction to deliver the head, but sometimes must be used to rotate it also. Rotation takes place with traction unless the position is occiput posterior or occiput transverse. In these instances the operator may either rotate the head manually before application of the forceps or perform a forceps rotation of the head. In doing a forceps delivery, nature is imitated as much as possible. Gentle intermittent traction, with as little force as

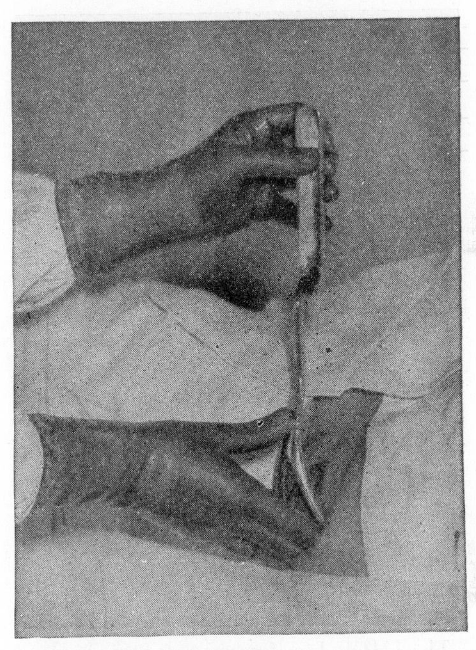

**Fig. 121B.** Low forceps: Introduction of left blade to left side of pelvis. (From Eastman, N. J.: *Williams Obstetrics,* 11th ed. Courtesy of Appleton-Century-Crofts, Inc., New York.)

necessary to advance the head, is made in the direction of the axis of the pelvis (Fig. 122 A-D). The traction is applied with the arms of the operator flexed and the elbows close to the thorax so that body weight is not used in the pull. The head is allowed to recede in the intervals between each application of traction, as it does in a spontaneous delivery. Except in those instances where the condition of the mother or baby indicate that speed is imperative, the head should be delivered slowly enough to allow for adequate dilatation of the perineum. The head may be delivered completely with the forceps, or the blades may be removed after the head is well advanced and the delivery completed by Ritgen's maneuver. The blades must always be removed gently to prevent injury to the ears. During the entire procedure the fetal heartbeat must be observed almost continuously.

All operative deliveries are potentially dangerous, and if the forceps

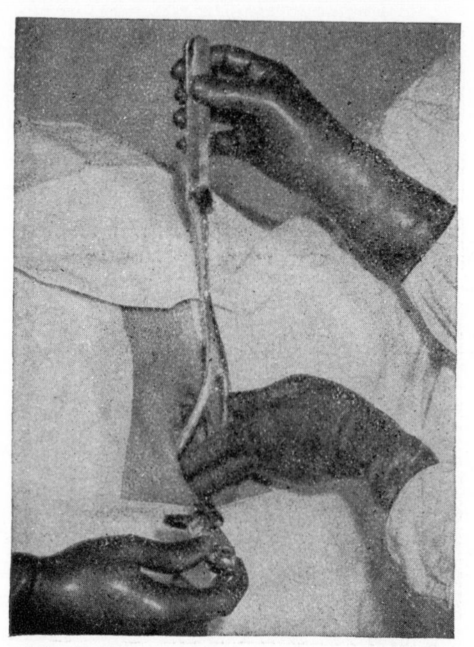

**Fig. 121C.** Low forceps: Left blade in place; introduction of right blade by right hand. (From Eastman, N. J.: *Williams Obstetrics,* 11th ed. Courtesy of Appleton-Century-Crofts, Inc., New York.)

is incorrectly applied or if delivery is attempted through an incompletely dilated cervix or a contracted pelvis, the dangers to mother and baby are very great and may be fatal. The dangers are reduced to a minimum, however, when the forceps is applied with the proper indications and technic.

**Breech Extraction.** In most cases of breech presentation, particularly among primigravidas, it is necessary to assist nature in the delivery of the child. This is known as breech extraction and may be either partial or total depending upon how far the baby has been delivered spontaneously before traction is made to complete the delivery (Fig. 123). This procedure was probably the earliest obstetric operation performed. Complete anesthesia is usually necessary at such times, and a lithotomy position, with the buttocks over the end of the table, is used to facilitate ease of manipulation. Preparation for delivery

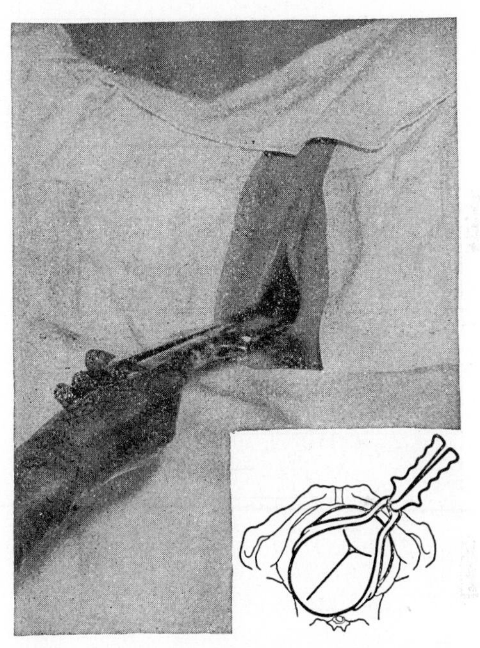

**Fig. 121D.** Low forceps: Forceps has been locked. (From Eastman, N. J.: *Williams Obstetrics,* 11th ed. Courtesy of Appleton-Century-Crofts, Inc., New York.)

must be made early so that extraction is possible as soon as the umbilicus appears, following which the fetal heartbeat may show evidence of interference with circulation in the umbilical cord. The fetal heart tones, therefore, must be watched very closely during the second stage of labor. In the majority of cases, no effort is made toward assistance until the body is born as far as the umbilicus, but as soon as it has been extruded thus far it is considered important to complete the delivery within a reasonable time—approximately five to eight minutes—in order to prevent asphyxia of the infant, which may be due to pressure on the cord between the head and pelvic bones or due to separation of the placenta after the uterus is partially emptied. The umbilical cord may be palpated at this time to determine if pulsation is present or absent. Even when pulsation has been interfered with, complete delivery of the head does not necessarily have to be accomplished rapidly, but it must be delivered far enough

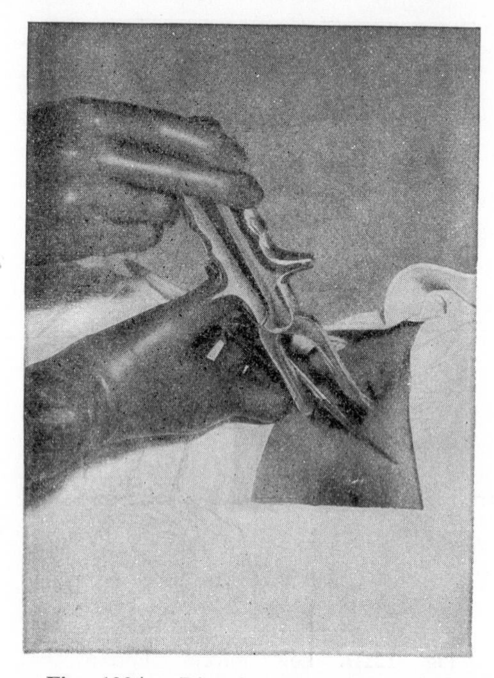

**Fig. 122A.** Direction of traction in low forceps (namely, outward and upward): Left mediolateral episiotomy may be performed. (From Eastman, N. J.: *Williams Obstetrics,* 11th ed. Courtesy of Appleton-Century-Crofts, Inc., New York.)

to allow access of air to the baby's mouth so that pulmonary respiration can be established. The body can usually be held in a position to favor drainage of mucus and amniotic fluid from the respiratory tract, and mucus should be wiped from the mouth.

When the baby's body is born to the umbilicus his feet or legs are grasped by a towel, to prevent the hands from slipping, and downward traction is made on the body until the lower halves of the scapulas are outside the vulva. During this procedure the nurse may be called upon to make pressure on the uterus to keep the baby's head flexed, and to prevent the arms from becoming extended upward above the head; this pressure also helps in expelling the child. The shoulders are delivered after one of the axillae has appeared; when the arms

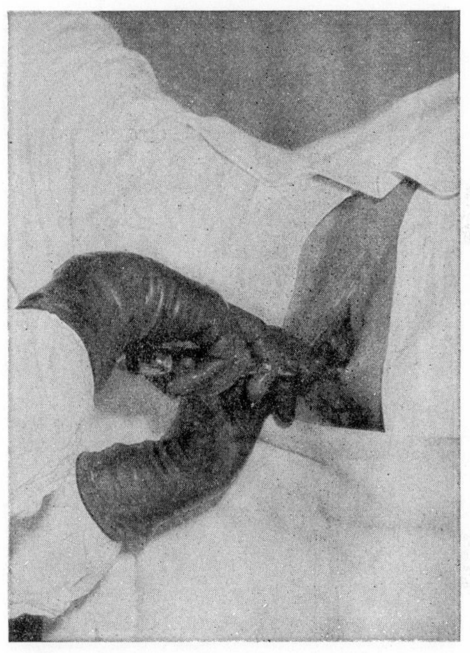

**Fig. 122B.** Direction of traction in low forceps (namely, outward and upward): Horizontal traction, operator seated. (From Eastman, N. J.: *Williams Obstetrics,* 11th ed. Courtesy of Appleton-Century-Crofts, Inc., New York.)

remain flexed this is relatively simple. The body is drawn upward toward the groin of the mother to deliver the posterior shoulder and bent down to deliver the anterior one (Fig. 124). The arms usually follow spontaneously after each shoulder is delivered. However, if the arms are extended above the child's head, they must be swept down across the chest by the operator's hand, introduced into the vagina. Unless the fingers reach the elbow and are used as splints, fractures of the humerus or clavicle may occur during delivery of the extended arms. Occasionally the arm lies around the back of the neck, known as nuchal arm. Delivery then becomes still more difficult.

After delivery of the shoulders and arms the body rotates spontaneously or is rotated manually so that the back is directed upward

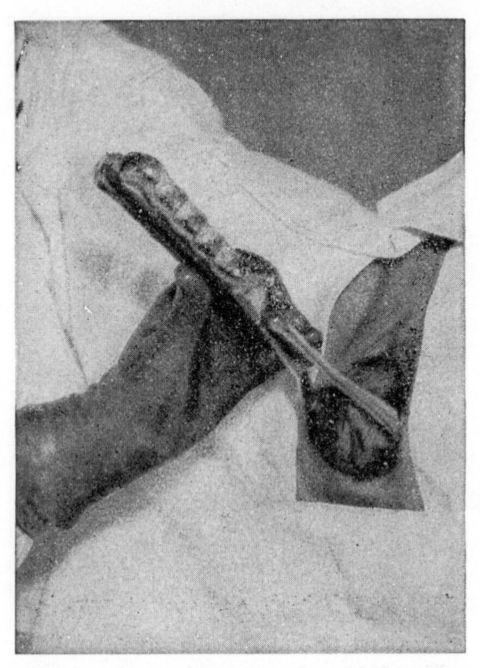

**Fig. 122C.** Direction of traction in low forceps (namely, outward and upward): Upward traction. (From Eastman, N. J.: *Williams Obstetrics,* 11th ed. Courtesy of Appleton-Century-Crofts, New York.)

in line with the mother's abdomen. The head is then in position to be delivered. Delivery is usually completed by what is known as Mauriceau's maneuver, which consists of keeping the head flexed with one hand, while the body of the child is supported on the arm, and making downward traction with the other hand which is placed over the shoulders. At this juncture, delivery is facilitated by an assistant making suprapubic pressure (Fig. 125 A and B). The occiput appears beneath the symphysis pubis, after which the body is lifted upward and the mouth, nose, forehead, and entire head are born. Sometimes the after-coming head is delivered by forceps rather than by means of Mauriceau's maneuver, and the nurse should be prepared for this possibility by having the forceps ready. If rotation of the head is

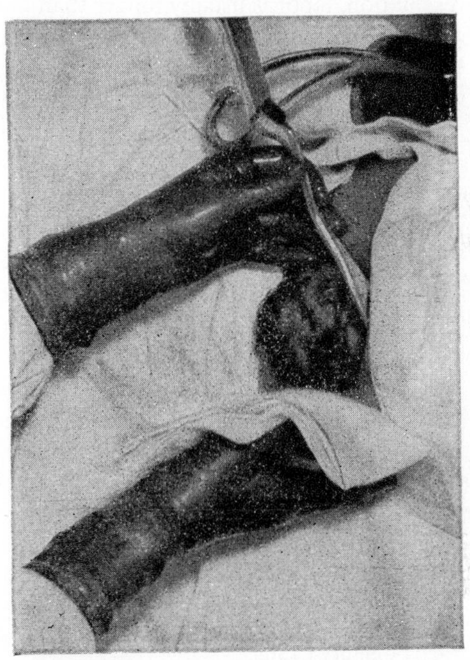

**Fig. 122D.** Direction of traction in low forceps (namely, outward and upward): Disarticulation of blades. Beginning of modified Ritgen's maneuver. (From Eastman, N. J.: *Williams Obstetrics,* 11th ed. Courtesy of Appleton-Century-Crofts, Inc., New York.)

impossible, it becomes necessary to deliver it from the occiput posterior position.

Occasionally, due to some condition which is dangerous to the mother or child, extraction becomes necessary before the breech has been delivered spontaneously. In these cases the hand is introduced into the vagina and the feet are grasped and brought down by traction, or the fingers are hooked into the groins and downward traction is made. Pressure on the mother's abdomen should always supplement traction on the body. Delivery in this manner is difficult and especially so when the breech is high. The cervix must always be completely dilated before any attempts at extraction are made; otherwise deep cervical lacerations result.

In breech presentation, labor is usually longer than in vertex presentation because the membranes frequently rupture early and the breech does not make a good dilating wedge. The incidence of prolapse of the umbilical cord is higher than in a vertex presentation, and the fetal heart must be observed frequently throughout labor. Meconium is often expelled during labor, due to downward pressure of the contracting uterus upon the fetus, but this does not have the same significance that it does in a head presentation. If the membranes are ruptured, meconium is seen draining from the vagina. If the presentation is a footling, one or both feet may prolapse through the vagina as labor progresses. This does not necessarily mean that the birth is imminent. The patient is often not ready for delivery when the feet appear, since they will prolapse whenever the cervix has dilated sufficiently to allow them to pass through, although it has not yet dilated enough to allow the largest part of the baby to be born. In vertex presentations the larger part of the baby, the head, is born first, and the rest of the body follows quickly, while in breech presentation labor is complicated by the larger part of the baby being born last. The head does not have time to mold, since it must pass through the birth canal quickly; it is often even slightly widened because it has been flattened somewhat in utero by pressure from the fundus. A deep episiotomy is often made to decrease the resistance from the pelvic soft parts as much as possible.

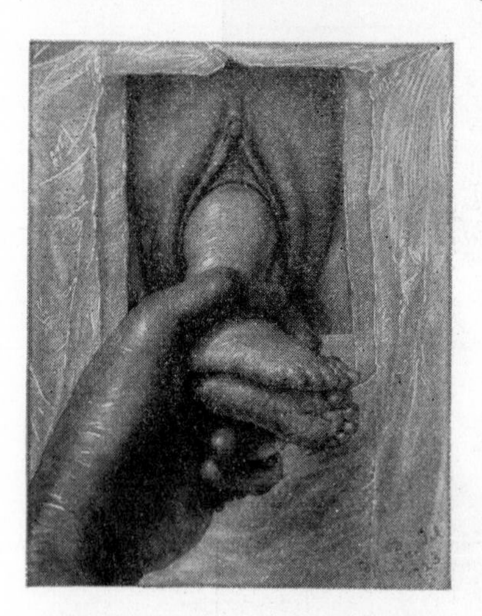

**Fig. 123.** Breech extraction; traction upon the feet. (From Eastman, N. J.: *Williams Obstetrics,* 11th ed. Courtesy of Appleton-Century-Crofts, Inc., New York.)

Breech extraction is not very dangerous for the mother, but the fetal mortality is slightly higher than with cephalic presentation.

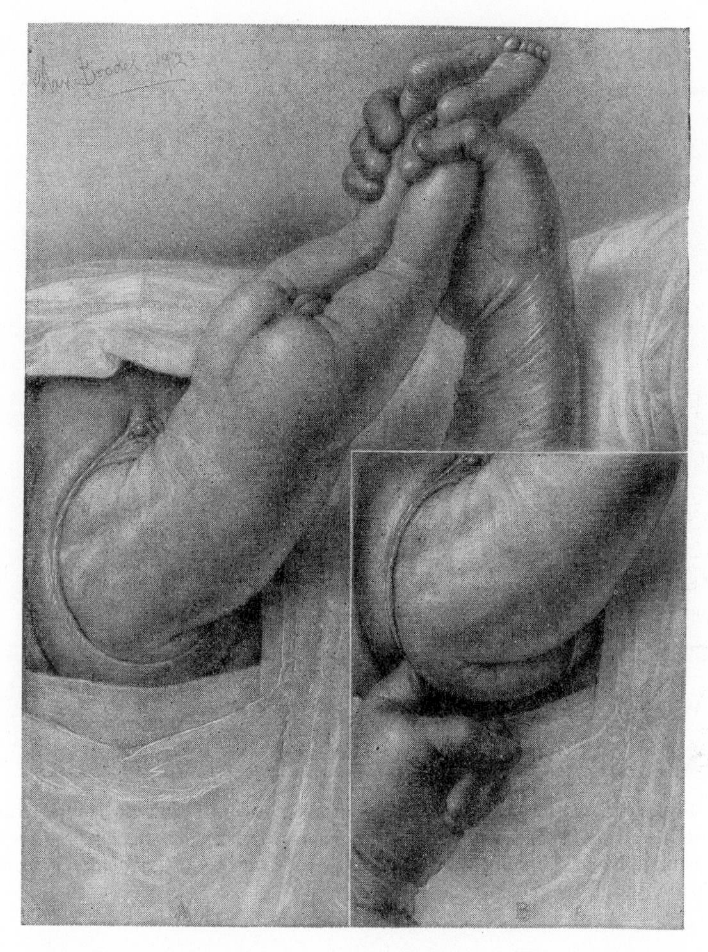

**Fig. 124.** Breech extraction; upward traction to effect delivery of posterior shoulder. (*Inset*) Freeing posterior arm. (From Eastman, N. J.: *Williams Obstetrics,* 11th ed. Courtesy of Appleton-Century-Crofts, Inc., New York.)

Part of this fetal mortality is due to the higher incidence of breech presentation in premature labors and in pregnancies where other complications, that may lead to fetal death, already exist. Babies which have been delivered by breech extraction have a larger incidence of intracranial hemorrhage or injury to the spinal cord, either of which may prove fatal. Fractures of the humerus and clavicle

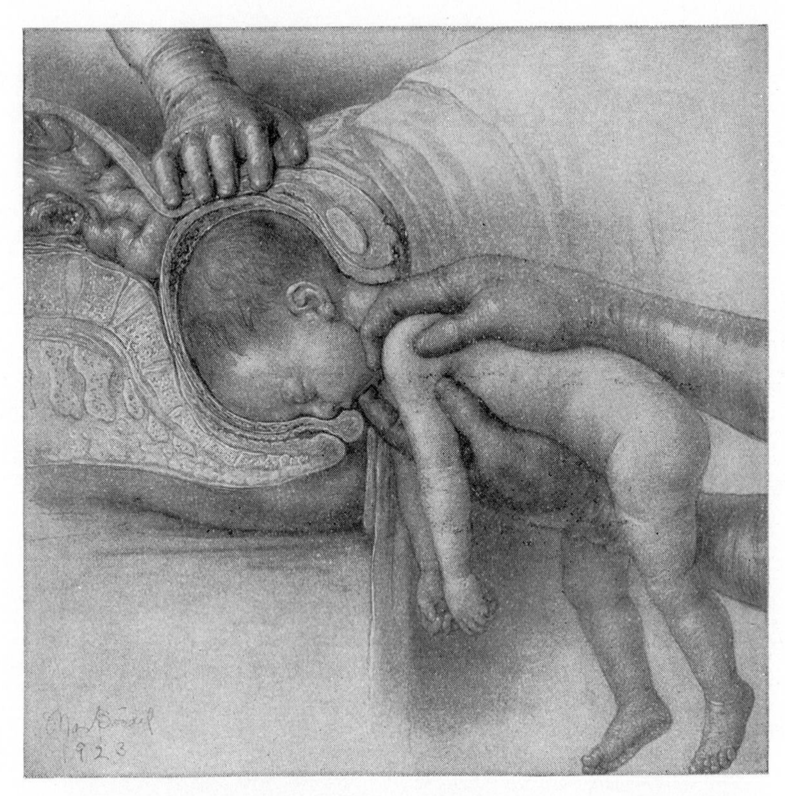

**Fig. 125A.** Breech extraction; suprapubic pressure and horizontal traction have caused the head to enter the pelvis. Mauriceau's maneuver. (From Eastman, N. J.: *Williams Obstetrics,* 11th ed. Courtesy of Appleton-Century-Crofts, Inc., New York.)

cannot always be avoided, but are not usually serious. Overstretching of the neck or too much pressure on the brachial plexus may be followed by paralysis of the arm, which must be carefully treated in the postnatal period. Hematomas of the sternocleidomastoid muscles may occur, but should disappear spontaneously and therefore are not serious.

**Version and Extraction.** By version is meant the turning of the child within the uterus so that the part which was presenting at the superior strait is replaced by another part in order to hasten or facilitate delivery. It is usually performed as the patient lies flat on

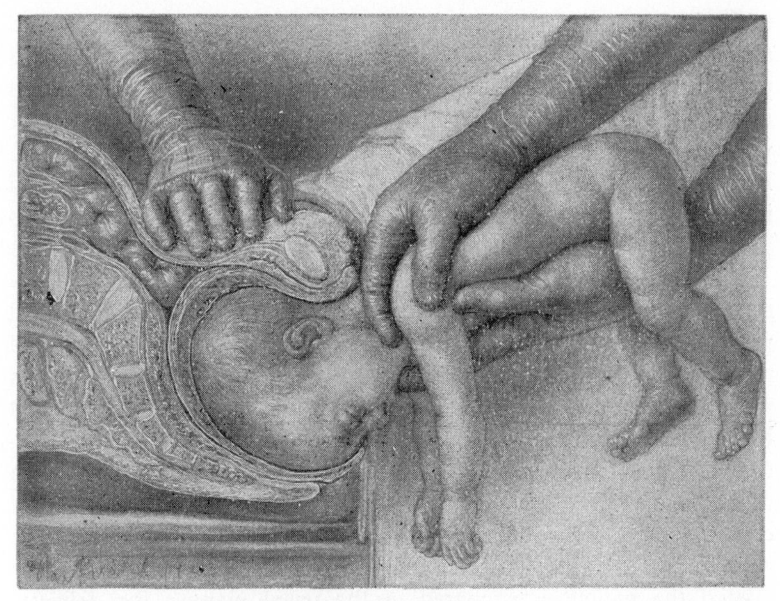

**Fig. 125B.** Breech extraction; Mauriceau's maneuver, upward traction. (From Eastman, N. J.: *Williams Obstetrics,* 11th ed. Courtesy of Appleton-Century-Crofts, Inc., New York.)

her back, and is done with great gentleness, for fear of rupturing the uterus. When the fetus is so turned that the head becomes the presenting part, the procedure is termed a *cephalic version;* if so turned that the breech presents, it is termed a *podalic version.* The methods of accomplishing these ends are described as *external version,* if the turning is done entirely with the hands working through the abdominal wall; *internal version,* if one entire hand is introduced into the uterine cavity; and *combined version,* when one hand is outside on the abdomen and two or more fingers are introduced through the cervix into the uterus.

External cephalic version is sometimes performed late in pregnancy, or early in labor, in transverse or in breech presentations to secure a vertex presentation. It cannot be done after the presenting part is engaged, when there is an insufficient amount of amniotic fluid to allow for easy movement of the child, or when the uterine muscle is very irritable. It is a procedure which should not produce pain and which may be performed with the patient on a bed or examining table. In external version the fetal poles are grasped with each hand and gently stroked toward their new position; the pole which should present is moved toward the pelvic inlet and the other pole is moved in the opposite direction. If the head does not engage soon after version is completed the fetus may turn back to its original position. If performed at the time of onset of labor the head may be pressed into the superior strait and held there until the uterine contractions push it down sufficiently to fix it.

Podalic version, or making the breech the presenting part, is sometimes performed in transverse presentations; in some abnormal head presentations when it is believed that delivery can be accomplished more easily by breech extraction; and on the second baby in twin pregnancy. Having converted the presentation into a breech the usual breech extraction follows. Internal podalic version is most easily performed when the membranes have not ruptured previously or when there is a sufficient amount of amniotic fluid left to make movements easy; it is very difficult or even impossible when the membranes have been ruptured for a long period of time. After the cervix is fully dilated the patient is prepared in the usual manner for delivery. Wearing a pair of long rubber gloves, known as gauntlet gloves, which reach to the elbow, the doctor introduces his hand and arm into the birth canal until the baby's feet are reached, and after grasping them and pulling them down delivery is completed by breech extraction. Deep anesthesia is necessary; there must be no disproportion between the baby and the pelvis as previously determined by pelvimetry.

If version is attempted when the uterus is tetanically contracted or when the lower segment is greatly stretched, there is danger of rupture of the uterus; otherwise the prognosis for the mother is good. The prognosis for the child is questionable; it is fairly good when the indications for performing the version are not serious and when no difficulty is encountered in the breech extraction. The commonest present-day indication for version and extraction is delivery of the second baby in a twin pregnancy.

**Cesarean Section.** This is an operation by means of which the child is delivered through an incision made in the abdominal and uterine walls. It is thought by some that the operation was named for Julius Caesar, who, it is believed, was delivered by this method, but this seems scarcely probable. The operation was almost always fatal in those days, and, moreover, as the uterine wall was not sutured after the child was extracted, a woman was not likely to have other children afterward even if she did live; Caesar's mother had several children after he was born. Another explanation for the name is that during the reign of Numa Pompillius a law, called Caesar's law, was passed, which required that the abdomen be opened and the child extracted in every case in which a woman died late in pregnancy, as one means of increasing the population. Thus it will be seen that a cesarean operation on a woman who has just died is a very ancient procedure. As performed today, such operations on the living woman are based on the most modern and scientific knowledge and methods. One common indication for the operation is contracted pelvis; other indications are a previous cesarean section scar, abnormal presentation of the fetus, tumors blocking the birth canal, some cases of toxemia, placenta previa, abruptio placentae, and certain medical complications, of which diabetes is one of the most common.

The pelvic indications for cesarean section are dependent upon the degree and character of the pelvic contraction and upon the size and moldability of the child's head in relation to the pelvis. This explains why in two women with pelves of the same size and shape one will have a spontaneous delivery and one will require a cesarean section. The former has a relatively small child which can pass through her pelvis; the second woman's baby is too large, or the head not sufficiently moldable, to pass through her pelvis. This illustrates the great importance of pelvimetry and of constant watching during pregnancy. In cases of borderline pelves, where the disproportion between the fetal head and the pelvis is not pronounced and where there is a question of whether or not the head will pass through the pelvis, a trial of labor is sometimes given. This means that the patient is allowed to start active labor; if after a few hours of fairly strong contractions the head does not progress through the pelvis, a cesarean section is done. When the pelvic inlet is abnormally small a trial labor would, of course, be of no value, and the cesarean section in such cases is planned in advance. X-ray pelvimetry is of great value in determining the type of pelvic contraction and also in estimating the relationship between the size of the fetal head and the space in the pelvis.

When delivery by cesarean section is definitely planned for a patient, the elected time is often about two weeks before the expected date of confinement. This allows the baby to have the longest possible intrauterine life, and yet makes it possible to perform the operation before the patient goes into labor. The wisdom of doing a cesarean section either before labor begins, or early in labor, has been explained by bacteriologic studies conducted by Drs. John W. Harris and J. Howard Brown.* They found that there were no bacteria in the uterus until after the patient had been in labor six hours. From this time on, the number of infected cases increased hourly. The danger of infection also increases with the length of time that the membranes have been ruptured. Although the use of antibiotics greatly reduces the hazards of infection in the present day, it is still best to plan for the elective cesarean section before the onset of labor.

A cesarean section is not performed when the child is dead, except in certain cases of antepartum bleeding, where it is necessary to do the operation to control hemorrhage.

There are several types of cesarean section; these are commonly known as the classical, the low cervical, which may be intra- or extraperitoneal, and the cesarean hysterectomy, which is also known as a Porro cesarean section. The *classical* operation consist of opening the abdomen in the midline between the umbilicus and the symphysis pubis, placing a packing around the uterus to keep amnotic fluid and blood out of the abdominal cavity, and making an incision through the anterior wall of the uterus. It may be necessary to cut through the placenta if it lies anteriorly. A hand is inserted into the uterine cavity and the baby is grasped by the feet and extracted. The cord is cut, and the baby is handed to an assistant for further attention. Ergonovine or oxytocin (Pitocin) is given just as the baby is delivered to aid in contracting the uterine muscle, and the placenta and membranes are immediately removed. The uterine and abdominal walls are then approximated with sutures. Some obstetricians prefer this method when there is a choice, but only if it can be performed before the onset of labor or in the early part of the first stage, because of the greater danger of infection after several hours; many are reluctant to undertake it even early in labor if the patient has been examined vaginally, particularly if the technic of the examination is open to question. In certain cases the classical cesarean section is easier to

* Harris, John W., and Brown, J. Howard: "The Bacterial Content of the Uterus at Cesarean Section," *Am. J. Obst. & Gynec.*, **13**:133–43, (Feb.) 1927.

perform than any other type and it is also much faster if haste is necessary in delivering the baby.

The *low cervical* cesarean section, also called a *laparotrachelotomy,* is regarded with increasing approval, especially if a section must be performed after six or more hours of labor. It consists of the same type of abdominal incision as in the classical section; after the abdomen is opened the bladder is dissected off the uterus, the lower uterine segment and upper part of the cervix are exposed, and the incision is made in the lower part of the uterus, behind the bladder, instead of through the fundus. An incision, sufficiently large to permit passage of the baby's head, is made in this area. The baby's head is delivered either by applying forceps to the head or by lifting it out of the incision with the hand while pressure is applied to the fundus. The uterine incision in this operation is, after closure, outside of the peritoneal cavity.

The low cervical cesarean section is easiest to perform after the patient has had contractions, which have stretched the lower uterine segment, but it may be done before labor begins and before a lower uterine segment is well formed. The operation may be longer and more difficult than the classical procedure, but there are certain important advantages. The outstanding of these being that the operation may be done quite safely on a patient who has been in labor for some time, even after the membranes have ruptured, since there is little exposure of the peritoneum during the operation. Another advantage is that rupture of the uterus may be less common in subsequent pregnancies if the patient has had a low cervical operation instead of a classical one.

If a cesarean section is contemplated for a patient who is already showing signs of infection, it may be best from the standpoint of the mother's condition to do an extraperitoneal cesarean section or possibly a hysterectomy following a cesarean section. The use of antibiotics in the patient who is potentially infected greatly reduces the danger of a cesarean section, but fever at the time of operation may still be a contraindication to any procedure other than the extraperitoneal or Porro cesarean section. In the *extraperitoneal cesarean section* the peritoneum is not opened; access is gained to the uterine wall by separating the bladder and the vesicouterine peritoneum until the lower uterine segment is exposed, into which an incision is then made. It is a difficult operation to perform. In the *Porro cesarean section,* or *ce-*

*sarean hysterectomy,* the abdomen and uterus are incised, the child and placenta are extracted, and a subtotal or total hysterectomy is performed.

Until recently, mortality in cesarean section was distressingly high. Today, however, it is a relatively safe procedure. This is due to increased knowledge about the times at which the operation may and may not be performed with safety, the type of operation to perform in each case, the improvement made in both operative and aseptic technic, and the use of blood transfusions and antibiotics. The mortality rate is low when the operation is performed for contracted pelvis, but rises when other obstetric complications or medical complications make the operation necessary. Conservative obstetricians feel that even with the improved technic it should be performed only when definitely indicated. The reasons in general are that mortality is still higher than in vaginal deliveries, except in seriously complicated cases, and also that the scar remaining in the uterus constitutes a weak point in the muscle wall which may rupture in subsequent pregnancies and labors. Danger of rupture is probably minimal if the incision has been well sutured and if it has healed without infection.

The fetal mortality following birth by cesarean section is higher than following vaginal delivery. Babies born by this route appear to need more stimulation to establish respirations and are subject to more respiratory complications than those born by the vaginal route. Aside from this danger the baby's life may have been threatened in utero by certain obstetric or medical complications which made the operation necessary.

Cesarean sections have been repeated 10, or possibly more, times in the same patient, but because of some danger of a weakened uterine wall the doctor may recommend that the patient not have more than three pregnancies when cesarean section is the only method by which she can safely be delivered. One delivery by cesarean section does not necessarily mean that all of the following deliveries must be by the same route. If the first operation was performed because of a contracted pelvis the subsequent pregnancies will necessarily have to be terminated in a similar manner, but if it was performed because of toxemia or antepartum bleeding and if the postoperative course was afebrile then a vaginal delivery may be considered for subsequent pregnancies, unless there is some possibility of dystocia or unless the uterus is greatly distended. However, the patient should be in a hospital and under close observation as soon as labor begins. Tenderness over the former operative site and any evidence of bulging of the area are danger signals. A number of physicians believe, however, that "once a cesarean, always a cesarean" is a good rule to follow to avoid the danger of uterine rupture.

When a patient dies undelivered during the latter months of pregnancy a cesarean section is often performed immediately after death with the hope of saving the child.

*Preoperative Preparation.* The nurse's duties in connection with a cesarean section are the same as those for any abdominal operation, plus making arrangements for receiving and caring for the baby. Should a patient go into labor before the scheduled day, haste in preparation is necessary so that labor does not progress too long. The nurses responsible for the preparation of the patient and the operating room must then work very quickly.

Ideally the patient is admitted to the hospital 24 hours before surgery so that she may rest and be properly prepared as for any other operation. This is possible when the cesarean section is planned in advance and a date set for the surgery, with the exception of those patients who go into labor long before the expected date of confinement. On admission, a complete physical examination and laboratory studies of the blood and urine may then be done. An x-ray of the abdomen is frequently taken, and the film examined for any fetal abnormalities which, if present, may alter the plans. Typing and crossmatching for blood transfusion should always be done before surgery. Blood should be on call or arrangements should be made for a donor to be immediately available during surgery in case a transfusion is necessary for excessive blood loss.

The patient is prepared by shaving the abdominal and pubic hair, withholding food and fluids the night before surgery, and evacuating the bowels. An enema given the morning of surgery cleans the bowel sufficiently. Any stimulation to the bowel earlier than this may stimulate contractions and thus make it necessary to perform the operation before the scheduled time. An indwelling catheter is inserted into the bladder before surgery and is left open and draining so that the bladder will be completely empty during the operation. The insertion of the catheter may be the responsibility of the nurse, and she should be sure that the bladder is empty just before the patient is taken to the operating room.

Preoperative medication ordinarily consists of scopolamine or atropine; any narcotic drug administered to the patient will narcotize the baby and make resuscitation difficult. Morphine, or one of the other opium derivatives, is usually given after the baby has been delivered.

*Preparations for operation* including the skin preparation and the sterile drapings are the same as for any abdominal operation. Equipment for resuscitation of the baby and a heated crib in which to transport it to the nursery must always be in readiness in the operating room. It is important to set up a separate sterile table with equipment for the infant and to have an experienced person available to resuscitate the baby, if necessary, and to tie and dress the cord so that the surgeon and his assistant may continue with the operation. As soon as the baby's breathing is well established he may be placed in the heated crib and taken to the nursery for further care and observation. (See pp. 334–41 and 771–72.)

Ergonovine and/or oxytocin (Pitocin) are administered just as the baby is born; it may be necessary to repeat these oxytocics later during the operation to control bleeding from the uterus. The nurse should have these medications ready to give immediately as ordered.

The anesthetic administered for the operation may be either inhalation or spinal anesthesia or local infiltration of the operative field. When inhalation anesthesia is used it is important that the baby is delivered as rapidly as possible to avoid depression of the baby's respirations. For this reason it is advisable to make all preparation, including skin cleaning and draping, before the anesthesia is begun and that no time is lost between its administration and the delivery of the baby.

*Postoperative Care.* The postoperative care of a patient who has had a cesarean section consists of both postoperative and postpartum care. Since the patient has had an anesthetic and an abdominal operation she must have the same care that any patient would receive following abdominal surgery. She must be closely watched until she has recovered from the anesthetic; the blood pressure, pulse, and respirations must be carefully checked at frequent intervals. Parenteral fluids will probably be administered on the day of operation, but may not be necessary the following day; the patient has had very little or no manipulation of the bowel during surgery and is ready to take food and fluids more quickly than the usual postoperative patient. Many doctors will allow the patient to drink water as soon as she recovers from nausea, to take solid food in 24 to 48 hours, and to resume a regular diet as soon as she can tolerate it. Many of these patients do not suffer much from gas pains and abdominal distention, but if they do have discomfort, a rectal tube and heat to the abdomen will usually give relief. Occasionally such serious complications as ileus and acute dilatation of the stomach occur, and these must be treated as quickly as possible. The nurse must always be alert to any signs of their development; vomiting and abdominal distention should always be reported to the doctor. The position of the patient may be any that is comfortable for her and should be changed frequently. Ordinarily she is up out of bed and walking a day or two after surgery. The indwelling catheter in the bladder is usually connected to a drainage bottle and left in place for one to two days. In most instances the patient has no difficulty in voiding after its removal. Antibiotics may be given for three to five days following surgery as a prophylactic measure against postpartum infection, this being particularly important if the patient were in labor or had ruptured membranes before surgery.

Postpartum hemorrhage must be guarded against, just as after vaginal delivery. Because of the abdominal dressing it may be difficult or impossible to palpate the fundus without disturbing the wound, but the blood pressure reading and pulse rate and the amount of vaginal bleeding that is present will help to determine whether or not there is excessive intrauterine bleeding. Ergonovine is administered every four hours for 24 hours to help keep the uterus contracted and control bleeding. The care of the perineum and the breasts is the same as for any postpartum patient and will be outlined in detail in Chapters 16 and 17.

**Fetal Destructive Operations.** Destructive operations have as their purpose the crushing or dismembering of the child in utero to decrease its size in order to effect delivery in cases of obstructed labor. In the early days such operations were resorted to fairly often in the presence of conditions that threatened the mother's life and which apparently could not be met in any other way. Today they are very rarely performed, although fetal destruction may be indicated in the delivery of a dead infant when termination of labor by other methods proves difficult or prolonged.

**Manual Removal of the Placenta.** Manual removal of the placenta becomes necessary when the placenta fails to separate from the uterine wall: either because of faulty uterine muscle action or adhesions between the placenta and the uterus; or when it is retained, after separation, by contraction of the uterus below the placenta. If the placenta is not expelled from the uterus in one-half hour after delivery of the baby, during which time several attempts at expression by downward pressure on the fundus are made, it is manually separated and/or removed. If, during an interval of waiting and attempts at expression, bleeding becomes profuse, due to partial separation, immediate removal is necessary.

When this operation is indicated, rigid aseptic technic must be used because there is great danger of infection following this procedure in which the blood loss may be great and in which the hand may be inserted between the placenta and the uterine wall, where it comes into direct contact with the blood sinuses. Before beginning the operation the external genitalia should again be cleaned with an antiseptic solution, fresh sterile draping sheets should be applied, and the operator should change into another pair of sterile rubber gloves, preferably gauntlet gloves. With one hand inserted into the uterus and the other hand grasping the fundus through the abdominal wall the placenta is peeled from its attachment to the uterus. It must be inspected carefully to make certain that fragments have not been left behind. Oxytocic drugs are given after removal, and a uterine packing may be inserted. Deep anesthesia may be necessary for this procedure. Whenever it becomes obvious that the placenta is not separating normally the patient should be typed and crossmatched for a blood transfusion, if this was not done earlier, in case the blood loss during or after the separation becomes profuse. Antibiotics are administered as a prophylactic measure against infection following this manipulative procedure.

**Artificial Termination of Pregnancy.** As was explained in Chapter 9, if it is sometimes deemed advisable to terminate pregnancy by artificial means, in the interests of the mother or child or both, the procedures are termed *therapeutic abortion* (see pp. 200–201) and *induction of labor.*

*Induction of Labor.* Various methods of induction of labor may be used in an attempt to terminate a pregnancy before, at, or after the expected time of delivery. Termination of pregnancy after the thirty-fifth week may be considered advisable to protect the mother and/or baby from a condition which might prove hazardous if it is allowed to persist. Several conditions may at one time or another be an indication for inducing labor, but the most frequent complication that indicates termination of pregnancy in the last weeks is pre-eclampsia. Some physicians elect to induce labor, at full term, on the patient without complications.

Induction of labor is usually attempted for conditions which would indicate that birth of the baby before long is desirable, but which are not severe enough to warrant a cesarean section. If delivery seems quite imperative and the condition of the cervix is such that induction of labor seems a likely possibility, it may be attempted; if conditions are not favorable for induction, a cesarean section may then be contemplated. Labor can usually be induced in patients near term, and sometimes even several weeks before term, if the cervix is soft and partially effaced and the canal is open sufficiently to admit one finger. When these conditions are not present labor ordinarily cannot be induced, or if contractions do begin with the induction the labor is slow and desultory. In any case it may be more prolonged and uncomfortable. Induction of labor is not always successful even when conditions for this procedure seem quite satisfactory. In general the farther away from term the more difficult it is to induce labor.

Induction of labor may be attempted either by the administration of medication or by artificial rupture of the membranes. Rupture of the membranes is a more certain method, but requires vaginal manipulation and makes it quite imperative that labor then proceed. One regimen for a medical induction is to give 30 ml (1 oz) of castor oil early in the morning and follow it by one or two soapsuds enemas in one to two hours. The enemas are most effective when given in large amounts and with the solution as warm as the patient can tolerate. (The castor oil is not difficult to take if it is given in 90 to 120 ml [3 to 4 oz] of orange juice with one-eighth to one-fourth teaspoonful of baking soda added and stirred well just prior to taking it.) Labor occasionally begins with only castor oil and enema stimulation, but ordinarily oxytocin (Pitocin) is administered by the hypodermic, intranasal, or intravenous route, beginning one to two hours after the enemas have been given. Oxytocin (Pitocin) may be given with only enemas preceding or without either of these preliminary procedures.

The initial dose of oxytocin (Pitocin) when administered hypodermically should not exceed 0.25 minim; this small dose is recommended in order to test the individual patient's reaction to the drug. This amount may be increased to 0.5 minim and then to 1.0 minim if a larger dose is necessary to stimulate contractions. It is not safe to increase the dosage over 1.0 minim, and the medication should not be repeated in less than 30 minutes. The drug may be injected every one-half to one hour for six doses or until labor is established, which may be after one or two doses.

When oxytocin (Pitocin) is to be administered intranasally a cotton pledget saturated with 10 units (15 minims) of solution is placed against the inferior turbinate bone. Nasal packs are changed every one-half to one hour until six to eight doses have been given, unless labor is well established earlier. Advantages of the nasal pack method are that the oxytocin (Pitocin) absorbs slowly through the mucous membrane of the nose, and the effect of the drug can be stopped quickly, by removing the nasal pack, if the uterine contractions become too hard and long. Once the drug has been injected hypodermically, oxytocic action continues until all of it has been absorbed.

Oxytocin (Pitocin) may be administered by a continuous intravenous drip method with good effect. It is believed that this route of administration produces more physiologic uterine contractions, because the patient is receiving a small dose continuously, whereas the hypodermic injection is intermittent and the intranasal method is unreliable as to rate of absorption. The intravenous route, in which the exact amount of oxytocin (Pitocin) that is administered can be measured, should thus eliminate some of the dangers and uncertainties of the other two routes. The intravenous solution to be administered is usually made by adding 10 units (15 minims) of oxytocin (Pitocin) to 1000 ml of a 5 per cent glucose solution. This is given by a continuous drip, and the rate of flow carefully regulated. The strength of the dilution must be known, and it must be dilute enough to be easily measurable. The drip is started with a rate of flow in which 0.25 to 0.5 minim of oxytocin (Pitocin) will be given in one-half hour; this is gradually increased to 0.5 to 1.0 minim per one-half hour. Contractions begin in 5 to 10 minutes after treatment is started and continue at a regular rate, although these may not be true labor contractions. If after several hours it becomes obvious that the induction is not successful, the treatment is discontinued. The patient must never be left alone during an intravenous injection of oxytocin (Pitocin), since there is danger that the speed of the drip may be increased if the clamp slips or as the patient moves her arm. As soon as contractions increase or become severe, the intravenous solution is slowed or discontinued.

Whenever oxytocin (Pitocin) is administered by any of these methods there is danger of tetanic uterine contractions, and it becomes necessary to observe and time the first few contractions after each dose is given to make certain that the uterus relaxes following a contraction. Severe and prolonged contractions may cause uterine rupture or produce hypoxia in the infant. If such contractions develop, the oxytocic drug must be discontinued immediately by stopping the intravenous injection or removing the nasal pack. It may be necessary to counteract violent prolonged contractions as a result of oxytocin (Pitocin) by the administration of ether anesthesia. The administration of medication for induction of labor is discontinued at any time that the patient develops regular uterine contractions and is apparently in active labor. If labor has not begun at the completion of the induction, there is still some possibility that it may begin at some time later in the day. When the induction has been unsuccessful and there is no urgency in delivery of the infant, it may be repeated after several days.

Artificial rupture of the membranes either before or after castor oil and/or enemas will almost always ensure good results and may be used whenever termination of pregnancy is somewhat urgent. This should be done only if the head is presenting and engaged. The membranes are loosened from their uterine attachment as far as it is possible to do so, with a finger inserted through the cervix, and they are then nicked with a membrane hook. Labor usually begins in a few hours; if it does not start, oxytocin (Pitocin) may be used. A medical induction may be used to induce labor in cases where the membranes have ruptured spontaneously and contractions have not begun in 12 to 24 hours.

## COMPLICATIONS OF LABOR

**Difficult labor,** also known as **dystocia,** may be due to poor uterine or abdominal muscle action, pelvic contraction, abnormalities of the pelvic organs, or abnormal fetal position or development; it may be caused by anything which interferes with the normal mechanical processes of labor. Whenever the contractions of the uterine or abdominal muscles are weak and infrequent, labor may be quite prolonged. A contracted pelvis causes dystocia whenever cephalopelvic disproportion exists. Pregnancy is usually terminated by cesarean section in cases of contracted pelves, but if labor does proceed in certain cases it may be prolonged in the first stage by slow cervical dilatation and in the second stage by the length of time required for molding of the head to fit the pelvic cavity. Abnormal presentation and position of the fetus may greatly interfere with labor. Excessive size of the fetus or fetal deformities increase the mechanical difficulties of birth. Dystocia due to fetal abnormalities and presentation will depend upon the size of the child, the type of malformation, and the kind of presentation. Sometimes labor, although prolonged, terminates spontaneously in these abnormal cases; at other times, operative interference is necessary.

Obstruction to the descent of the fetus may be caused by abnormalities of the reproductive tract or by uterine or ovarian tumors. Uterine fibroids may cause dystocia: either by obstructing the pelvic cavity if they are situated low or by causing an abnormal presentation of the fetus; or they may produce uterine inertia by interfering with muscle contractions. Spontaneous deliveries are frequently possible, but if the tumor obstructs the birth canal a cesarean section is necessary and may be followed by a hysterectomy. If the uterus is not removed it is important to watch the patient very closely for postpartum hemorrhage following delivery. Ovarian cysts may complicate labor by obstructing the pelvic canal or by rupture during labor. If a cyst is diagnosed early in pregnancy it may then be removed during the fourth month, but if it is not found until late nothing is done until labor begins, at which time treatment will depend upon whether or not the cyst is causing obstruction.

**Uterine Inertia.** Prolonged labor is frequently due to uterine inertia and is ordinarily not a serious complication. The uterine contractions in these cases are so weak and infrequent that cervical effacement and dilatation are very slow, and labor may last for days. Usually the contractions will become stronger and more frequent after a variable period of time has elapsed, and as soon as they do labor progresses normally and more rapidly. Except for increasing exhaustion, the patient may not be very uncomfortable with these weak infrequent contractions. In other cases of prolonged labor the patient may be quite uncomfortable due to frequent cramp-like pains which hurt, but are ineffective in producing cervical dilatation. This type of contraction also becomes more effective after some time elapses. In still other cases labor progresses normally for some time, and then the contractions become weak and ineffectual as the patient becomes tired. This is known as *secondary uterine inertia* as differentiated from *primary uterine inertia* in which the contractions are weak and infrequent at the beginning. There are also cases in which the cervical canal becomes completely obliterated quite readily, but the external os does not dilate easily. In these cases it is difficult to follow the progress of labor by rectal examination because the cervix becomes paper-thin and is difficult to palpate. If labor is very prolonged the cervix may finally become thick and edematous.

Poor uterine contractions may be due to a number of causes, one of which may be a loss of muscle tone when the uterus is distended an unusual amount as with a multiple pregnancy or with an excessive amount of amniotic fluid, or when several pregnancies have followed one another closely. In some instances it is believed that reflex nervous influences may be responsible for poor uterine contractions. Mechanical influences, such as uterine muscle tumors or a sagging forward of the uterus with a pendulous abdomen, may also be factors in producing poor uterine contractions.

A prolonged second stage is more frequently due to mechanical obstruction to the presenting part or due to weak contractions of the abdominal muscles than to weak uterine contractions. Ineffectual abdominal muscle contractions may be due to poor muscle tone, more common in multigravidous patients, or poor cooperation from the patient in contracting her abdominal muscles because of fear of pain or for other reasons. Patients who have attended prenatal classes are less fearful and thus better able to cooperate, and having practiced prenatal exercises they understand the directions for pushing and are able to use their muscles for bearing down to best advantage. Inhalation anesthesia, given for analgesic effect, may help the patient use her abdominal muscles more effectively by reducing the pain felt with the contractions and thereby increasing her ability to cooperate.

As long as the patient does not become exhausted and the fetal heart tones remain good, a prolonged labor is not dangerous. The contractions which are weak from the beginning will usually become effective with time, and the only treatment necessary is to reassure the patient and give her a hypnotic or an opiate for rest at night. If the contractions have been strong and effective at first and then decrease, the administration of a narcotic to allow the patient to get a few hours' rest will usually be sufficient to increase the effectiveness of the contractions later. Enemas, given after the rest period, and walking about the room may help to increase the intensity of the contractions. Since the food and fluid intake during labor is usually small, intravenous glucose solution is given to prevent dehydration and acidosis and to provide needed energy by supplying the carbohydrate that is used in the body with the muscular activity of labor. Sedatives or narcotics for rest and intravenous glucose for energy, at rather frequent intervals during a prolonged labor, will prevent maternal exhaustion and increase the effectiveness of the contractions until cervical dilatation is complete. The use of oxytocin (Pitocin) to stimulate contractions is often dangerous because it may produce useless tetanic contractions or produce contractions that are too forceful and prolonged, with rupture of the uterus or impairment of placental circulation the end result. In cases in which posterior pituitary extract seems indicated, it is necessary to make certain that there is no mechanical obstruction to delivery and that a faulty presentation is not present. The patient must be observed constantly during the administration of oxytocin (Pitocin); if the contractions become forceful at any time the drug must be discontinued immediately. On the other hand, if there is no improvement in the strength of the contractions after two to three hours of posterior pituitary extract stimulation it is useless to continue. Labor which is retarded in the second stage, unless it is due to disproportion between the child and the pelvis, can usually be safely terminated by forceps delivery.

Antibiotics, for the prevention of an intrapartum infection, may be administered during a prolonged labor, especially if the membranes rupture early. Bacteria from the vulva and vagina may multiply in the fluid which is in the vagina and gain access to the open amniotic sac.

One of the important functions of a nurse in caring for a patient with prolonged labor is to sooth and comfort the patient and make every provision possible for physical and mental rest. To eliminate worry and fear, insofar as possible, the nurse must give frequent reassurances and must help the patient to understand that although the labor is slow there is no need for concern for herself or her baby.

The patient will become anxious, discouraged, and irritable at intervals, especially when she becomes tired. There is less anxiety and less discouragement when the patient is not left alone, and continuous care by a calm, reassuring, and understanding person is of inestimable value.

The nurse can help the patient keep up her energy by urging the intake of food and fluid to the extent that the doctor wishes her to take them. Frequent baths, back rubs, changes of linen, and changes of position are refreshing and aid in improving the patient's general comfort. If the patient may be out of bed a shower bath and fresh bed linen often do much toward making her feel better and rest more comfortably for a few hours. Providing for proper ventilation and for quietness of the room, especially after sedation has been given, is important for maximum rest. In addition to providing the best of general nursing care it is, of course, necessary to give the special care the patient in labor requires, as discussed in Chapters 12 and 13, and to make observations on the progress of labor and for evidence of complications.

**Occiput Posterior Position.** When the vertex presents with the occiput in the posterior portion of the pelvis, a condition which is called an occiput posterior position, labor is usually prolonged. The mechanism of labor is the same as that previously described with the exception of the longer distance through which the occiput must rotate to reach the symphysis pubis. With the occiput in the anterior portion of the mother's pelvis it must rotate only 45 deg to reach the symphysis while the distance is 135 deg from the posterior position (Fig. 68). This internal rotation may take place as the head is descending during the first stage of labor, or it may not begin until the head has reached the perineum. In some cases rotation does not take place at all, or it takes place only partially, that is, to a transverse position, known as a *deep transverse arrest,* or to an obliquely anterior position. With enough time complete rotation of the head and spontaneous delivery will occur in many of these patients. When it becomes apparent that the head is arrested and little or no progress is made within an hour or two of second-stage labor, rotation may be completed manually or with the aid of forceps; forceps then is used to complete delivery of the head.

In some cases the occiput spontaneously rotates to a posterior position so that it lies directly over the sacrum instead of under the symphysis pubis. During delivery from this position, called a *direct occiput posterior position,* that part of the head near the large fontanel stems itself under the symphysis pubis, and the head becomes more and more flexed until the occiput slips over the perineum. Spontaneous delivery occurs in many of these cases, but the second stage is prolonged. Episiotomies must be deeper, and perineal lacerations occur more frequently than with the direct occiput anterior position since a larger diameter of the head distends the vulva during delivery. Many obstetricians prefer to rotate the head from a direct occiput posterior position to an anterior position for delivery, provided it can be accomplished quite readily.

**Face Presentation.** In face presentations the head is in extension as it descends into the pelvis instead of the usual position of flexion. In these cases the occiput points toward the back and the face enters the pelvis first (Fig. 69). On abdominal palpation the cephalic prominence is found on the same side as the back instead of on the side of the small parts, and on rectal or vaginal examination the features of the face may be differentiated. Diagnosis by palpation is sometimes difficult, and an x-ray may be necessary to establish it. X-ray pelvimetry is also important to rule out pelvic contraction, which, if present, would change the method of delivery. Face presentations are rare, but the fetal mortality rate is greatly increased in this abnormal presentation.

Spontaneous delivery cannot occur unless the chin rotates anteriorly so that it lies under the symphysis pubis, and this rotation may not occur until late in labor. When the chin lies anteriorly the neck can slip around the short symphysis pubis without difficulty, but if the chin lies posteriorly the neck is too short to allow the chin to travel the relatively long distance along the anterior surface of the sacrum, and delivery is impossible without a change in position, unless the child is small enough to allow the shoulders to enter the pelvis also. When the chin lies posteriorly, spontaneous rotation to the anterior position often takes place after the face reaches the pelvic floor. If this does not occur, serious difficulties are encountered, and it becomes necessary to change the presentation or perform a cesarean section, depending upon various circumstances.

During delivery of the head, after the chin has rotated anteriorly, the mouth appears at the vaginal opening, the chin stems against the symphysis pubis, and the head flexes so that the nose, eyes, brow, and finally the occiput slip over the perineum. The face usually becomes edematous due to effusion of serum under the skin during labor, and the skull becomes markedly molded.

**Transverse Presentation.** In a transverse presentation the longitudinal axis of the fetus lies at right angles to the longitudinal axis of the mother, and a shoulder is usually over the superior strait of the pelvis. This is called a shoulder, or acromion, presentation. Delivery is impossible in this position unless the child is very small. If labor progresses with the child presenting transversely, the shoulder usually becomes wedged in the pelvis and the arm frequently prolapses into the vagina. If the uterus continues to contract hard, a thinning and even rupture of the lower uterine segment may occur. Fortunately a transverse presentation occurs in only a small percentage of all cases.

Spontaneous version to a longitudinal presentation occasionally occurs after onset of labor, but if it does not take place, interference is always necessary for delivery. In the primigravidous patient a transverse presentation should lead to the suspicion that a pelvic contraction is present and x-ray pelvimetry is indicated. Even when the pelvis is normal a cesarean section is usually considered the method of delivery for the primigravida if the position is transverse at the onset of labor. In the multigravida, external cephalic version is usually attempted if this abnormal presentation is diagnosed before labor, or early in labor with the membranes still intact; if this is not successful, internal podalic version and breech extraction may be done at the end of the first stage, provided the membranes have not been ruptured so long that the uterus fits too tightly around the child. If the membranes rupture early a cesarean section is usually performed.

**Tetanic Contractions.** A patient has a tetanic contraction of the uterus when it does not relax at regular intervals, but instead stays contracted continuously. This condition usually occurs during the second stage of labor, but may be present in the first stage and is found mostly in prolonged labors that are due to a mechanical obstruction to the advancement of the child. These contractions are very painful; there is danger of rupture of the uterus, and danger of asphyxia of the child due to interference with the placental circulation. It may be possible to relax the uterus by administration of a sedative or an anesthetic, and then labor should be ended as soon as it can safely be accomplished.

**Pathologic Retraction Ring or Bandl's Ring.** Normally there is a retraction ring between the upper and lower uterine segments during labor. In obstructed labors this may become more pronounced and therefore pathologic. An excessive amount of thinning of the lower uterine segment and a thicker, more tightly contracted than normal, upper segment are found. The retraction ring rises to the umbilicus or above and can be seen as a depression across the abdomen. The patient may have intense pain above the symphysis pubis and may go into a state of shock. Due to the tetanic state of the uterus labor does not progress, and there is considerable danger of rupture of the uterus. Treatment will depend upon the condition of the mother and baby and the cause of the retraction ring. If delivery can be completed vaginally, careful manipulation and deep anesthesia are important; a cesarean section may be necessary.

**Ruptured Uterus.** A ruptured uterus results from a splitting of the uterine wall at some point that has become thinned or weakened and is unable to stand the strain of further stretching, or force of uterine contractions; it is accompanied by an extrusion of all or a part of the uterine contents into the abdominal cavity. There are two types of rupture of the uterus, the spontaneous and the traumatic. *Spontaneous rupture* of a normal uterus is a rare accident and usually occurs only in prolonged labors, obstructed labors, or certain faulty presentations. As has been stated, rupture of the uterus at the site of a scar from a previous cesarean section sometimes occurs because of the presence of a weakened wall. When *traumatic rupture* occurs, it is usually during an obstetric operation, although a blow or fall on the abdomen may cause rupture. The uterus may rupture at any time during pregnancy or labor. In cases of rupture before labor begins the tear is usually found in the upper part of the uterus, while rupture during labor occurs in the lower segment.

In obstructed labors the lower uterine segment becomes thinner and thinner as the contractions pull the retraction ring higher. Finally the lower segment becomes very sensitive, the contractions become harder and may become tetanic, the contraction ring becomes very prominent, and the pulse becomes rapid. These signs indicate that rupture of the uterus is imminent. The common symptoms when rupture occurs are sudden and acute abdominal pain during a contraction, which the patient describes as being unlike anything she has ever felt and as though "something had given way" inside of her.

There is immediate and complete cessation of labor pains because the torn uterus no longer contracts. Sooner or later the patient has signs of shock because of the hemorrhage, which is usually internal, although there may be vaginal bleeding as well. Her face becomes pale and drawn and covered with perspiration; her pulse is weak and rapid; she appears exhausted and may complain of chilly sensations and air hunger. Abdominal palpation shows that the uterus is more sensitive than formerly and that the presenting part has slipped away from the superior strait while at the side of the fetus the contracted uterus, partly or entirely empty, may be felt as a hard mass. In some cases there is an incomplete rupture, which may extend into the broad ligament; the blood loss is then slower than in a complete rupture. The signs of shock may be delayed for several hours, especially if the baby is not completely extruded from the uterus, or if the rupture is incomplete. Pain and abdominal tenderness are always present with rupture.

As a preventive measure, the patient in whom there is some possibility of obstructed labor must be carefully observed for ballooning out of the lower uterine segment or rising up of a retraction ring, since these are signs of impending rupture. Prompt termination of labor is necessary. Abdominal tenderness and pain should lead to the suspicion that rupture may have occurred; it may be possible to institute treatment before shock develops. First a laporotomy is done to remove the baby, and then a hysterectomy is usually performed. Occasionally the laceration in the uterus is sutured, but it may be subject to rupture in case of subsequent pregnancies. Blood transfusions are of inestimable value to overcome the effects of blood loss. Antibiotics are administered to prevent infection to which the traumatized tissues are very susceptible.

A ruptured uterus is a very grave accident; the baby nearly always dies, due to placental separation, and the maternal mortality rate has been high in the past. However, early diagnosis, immediate treatment, and the present easy availability of blood for transfusions and antibiotics for combating infection should improve maternal prognosis.

**Cervical Lacerations.** Small lacerations of the cervix always accompany delivery, but they heal rapidly and without complications. These lacerations change the shape of the cervix so that it is no longer round. Sometimes the tears of the cervix are deep; these deep lacerations may even extend into the vagina or into the lower uterine segment. Extensive tears are most apt to occur during operative deliveries, especially if delivery is attempted before the cervix is fully dilated. They may also occur during a violent labor and precipitous delivery. Profuse bleeding accompanies deep lacerations.

Whenever bleeding during or after the third stage is excessive and the fundus remains well contracted, lacerations of the cervix or vaginal wall must be suspected. The cervix and vagina are very flabby following delivery, and direct inspection around the entire circumference of the cervix is necessary to make a diagnosis and to repair lacerations. For an examination of the cervix the vaginal walls must be separated by retractors and the cervix brought into view; this is done by grasping the cervical lips with ovum or sponge forceps and applying traction while at the same time making downward pressure on the fundus of the uterus. Forceps with teeth should not be used to grasp the cervix because the tissues are very vascular and friable. As lacerations are discovered the bleeding can be brought under control quickly by approximating the lacerated edges of the cervix or vaginal wall with sutures. Although some doctors do not consider inspection of the cervix necessary in all cases, many doctors inspect it after all operative deliveries and some examine it following all deliveries; this is done to detect lacerations which may bleed later.

## BIBLIOGRAPHY AND STUDENT REFERENCES

Bill, Arthur H.: "Forceps Delivery," *Am. J. Obst. & Gynec.,* **68**:245–49, (July) 1954.

Bookmiller, Mae M., and Bowen, George L.: *Textbook of Obstetrics and Obstetric Nursing,* 2nd ed. W. B. Saunders Co., Philadelphia, 1954.

Davis, M. Edward: "The Modern Role of Cesarean Section," *S. Clin. North America,* **33**:101–23, (Feb.) 1953.

Davis, M. Edward, and Sheckler, Catherine E.: *DeLee's Obstetrics for Nurses,* 15th ed. W. B. Saunders Co., Philadelphia, 1951.

Dorr, Edward M.: "Breech Presentation in Pregnancy and Labor," *S. Clin. North America,* **33**:77–85, (Feb.) 1953.

Eastman, Nicholson J.: *Williams Obstetrics,* 11th ed. Appleton-Century-Crofts, Inc., New York, 1956.

Eller, William, and Mengert, William: "Recognition of Midpelvic Contraction," *Am. J. Obst. & Gynec.,* **53**:252–58, (Feb.) 1947.

Garnet, James D.: "Rupture of the Uterus in Pregnancy," *S. Clin. North America,* **34**:1513–22, (Dec.) 1954.

Greenhill, J. P.: "Prolonged Labor," *Obst. & Gynec.,* **1**:476–85, (Apr.) 1953.

——— (ed.): *Obstetrics,* 11th ed. W. B. Saunders Co., Philadelphia, 1955.

Gustafson, Gerald W.: "Management of Occiput Posterior Position," *J.A.M.A.*, **139**:280–85, (Jan. 29) 1949.

Harris, John W.: "The Use and Abuse of Forceps," *Postgrad. Med.*, **2**:81–84, (Aug.) 1947.

Hellman, Louis M.: "Uterine Inertia," *M. Clin. North America*, **35**:791–804, (May) 1951.

Hellman, L. M.; Harris, J. S.; and Reynolds, S. R. M.: "Intravenous Pituitary Extracts in Labor with Data on Patterns of Uterine Contractility," *Am. J. Obst. & Gynec.*, **59**:41–48, (Jan.) 1950.

Klingensmith, Paul O.: "The Clinical Management of Dystocia," *S. Clin. North America*, **34**:1579–89, (Dec.) 1954.

McCall, Milton L.: "Surgical Complications of Pregnancy," *S. Clin. North America*, **28**:1507–18, (Dec.) 1948.

McNally, Hugh B., and Fitzpatrick, Vincent de P.: "Patients with Four or More Cesarean Sections," *Obst. & Gynec. Survey*, **11**:516–21, (Aug.) 1956.

Maternity Center Association: "Test of Labor—Is It Passé?" *Briefs*, **15**:2–4, (Dec.) 1951.

———: "Social Causes of Difficult Labor," *Briefs*, **16**:12–13, (Autumn) 1952.

Pattison, D. Stanley: "Induction of Labor, Indications and Methods," *Am. J. Obst. & Gynec.*, **68**:233–39, (Feb.) 1955.

Paxson, Newlin F.: "Modern Indications for Cesarean Section," *S. Clin. North America*, **28**:1487–1506, (Dec.) 1948.

Stone, Melvin L.: "The Intravenous Use of Dilute Pituitrin for the Induction and Stimulation of Labor," *Am. J. Obst. & Gynec.*, **59**:49–57, (Jan.) 1950.

Thoms, Herbert: *Classical Contributions to Obstetrics and Gynecology*. Charles C Thomas, Publisher, Springfield, Ill., 1935.

Woodward, H. L.; Gardner, B.; Bryant, R. D.; and Overland, Anna E.: *Obstetric Management and Nursing*, 15th ed. F. A. Davis Co., Philadelphia, 1955.

Zabriskie, Louise, and Eastman, Nicholson J.: *Nurses Handbook of Obstetrics*, 9th ed. J. B. Lippincott Co., Philadelphia, 1952.

# PART V. THE CARE OF THE MOTHER

## *Chapter 15*

## Physiology of the Puerperium

The puerperium * is ordinarily regarded as comprising the five to six weeks immediately following delivery, although strictly speaking it extends from the onset of labor to the return of the reproductive tract to normal. During this period the mother's body undergoes various changes which restore it very nearly to its nonpregnant state, leaving the patient in a normal, healthy condition. The most important of these changes are involution of the uterus, loss of weight, and improvement in the tone of abdominal and perineal muscles. The alterations which produce this restoration are normal physiologic processes, but mismanagement or lack of care while they are taking place may result in serious complications; these may be immediate, for example, hemorrhage and infection, or remote, possibly even chronic complications. Recognition of these dangers, as well as the possibility of preventing them, is responsible for the present custom of obstetricians to observe their patients during the puerperium. This is in sharp contrast to the old practice of the doctor visiting the puerperal woman only when there was a complication so apparent that he was summoned.

The precautions and care which the doctor desires for his patient before and after delivery involve intelligent and watchful nursing. In order to give such care the nurse must understand something of the normal physiology of the puerperium, just as she did of pregnancy

* From *puer,* child, and *parere,* to bring forth.

and labor; otherwise she may not be able to distinguish evidences of normal change from the signs and symptoms of pathology.

## ANATOMIC CHANGES

**Involution of the Uterus.** Considerable attention is centered in the remarkable atrophic changes that take place in the uterus during the puerperium, since the patient's recovery and future well-being may depend upon their being normal. Immediately following delivery the uterus is a solid mass of tissue with a flattened cavity and presents a pale appearance due to the compression of the blood vessels by the contracted muscle fibers. The inner surface, where the placenta was attached, is raw and bleeding. After delivery the uterus weighs about 1000 gm (2.2 lb), is from 17.5 to 20 cm (7 to 8 in.) high, about 12.5 cm (5 in.) across, and 10 cm (4 in.) thick; the top of the fundus can be felt at or slightly below the level of the umbilicus. It remains about the same size for two days and then decreases so rapidly in size that by the tenth day it usually cannot be palpated above the symphysis pubis. Its weight is decreased to 454 gm (1 lb) at the end of one week, and at the end of six to eight weeks the uterus has descended into the pelvic cavity and resumed approximately its original position and size, as well as its former weight of 60 gm (2 oz).

This rapid diminution in the size of the uterus is termed *involution* and is accomplished by means of a process of self-digestion or *autolysis*. The protein material in the uterine walls is broken down into simpler components which are absorbed and eventually cast out, largely through the urine. This greatly increases the nitrogen content of the urine for several days. The change and absorption of uterine tissues are similar to the resolution that takes place in a consolidated lung in pneumonia.

There is evidently a close relation between the functioning of the breasts and of the uterus during the puerperium, and involution usually progresses more rapidly in women who nurse their babies than in those who do not.

The decidua which remains in the uterus after the placenta and membranes have been separated becomes differentiated into two layers within two or three days. The outer layer is cast off in the discharge from the uterus, and the inner layer which contains the fundi of the glands and a small amount of connective tissue remains to regenerate new endometrium. The entire endometrium is regenerated in three weeks with the exception of that over the placental area which is not completely restored for six to seven weeks. The blood vessels of the placental area become either compressed or thrombosed after delivery of the placenta. It is believed that the large vessels present in the uterus during pregnancy then become obliterated and that new smaller vessels develop.

**Changes in the Cervix and Vagina.** The cervix, vagina, and perineum, which have become stretched and swollen during labor, gradually regain their tone during the puerperium. The cervix and lower uterine segment form a flabby, collapsed, hollow tube immediately after delivery and contract slowly. The cervical canal will admit the hand immediately after delivery, two fingers for a few days thereafter, and only one finger at the end of a week. During pregnancy an increase in muscle cells in the uterus and a decrease in muscle fibers in the cervix took place; during the puerperium the exact opposite occurs in both of these organs—a decrease of muscle in the uterus and an increase in the cervix.

Small lacerations which occurred in the cervix during labor heal during this period, but it does not return to the exact size and shape it had before delivery. The external os instead of being a smooth round opening now becomes an irregular transverse slit.

Changes in the vagina occur slowly, and it never returns entirely to its original state. It gradually diminishes in size, and the rugae begin to reappear in three weeks. The hymenal ring is replaced by numerous ragged edges of tissue known as *carunculae myrtiformes*. The external genitalia which have been somewhat distended during pregnancy become smaller and more flabby. The stretched uterine ligaments become shorter as they recover their tone, finally regaining their former state. Until the ligaments, the pelvic floor, and the abdominal wall are restored to normal tonicity, the uterus is not adequately supported and therefore may be easily displaced.

**Abdominal Wall.** The abdominal wall is tightly stretched during pregnancy, and, therefore, when the tension is removed, immediately after labor the skin is very loose and the entire wall is soft and flabby. The normal and desirable course is for the muscles gradually to regain their tone and the wall to approach its original state in the course of two to three months. Exercise is usually necessary to improve the muscle tonus, but even with exercise these muscles sometimes fail to regain good tone. This is especially true when pregnancies follow each other in rapid succession, when there has been excessive distention, and in the asthenic type of individual who does not have good muscle tone at any time. In such cases there is likely to be the pendulous abdomen so often seen in multiparas, and a diastasis, or separation, of the recti muscles. The striae remain, but change to a silvery appearance.

**Urinary Tract.** The bladder becomes a pelvic organ again, and the dilatation of the kidney pelves and ureters, which is frequently present during pregnancy, disappears within four to six weeks. Some edema and hyperemia of the bladder are present for a short time following delivery, and there may be some submucosal extravasation of blood.

**Breasts.** In discussing puerperal changes of the breasts it is well to review breast anatomy and gestational development. It will be remembered that each breast contains 15 to 20 lobes; each lobe is made up of several lobules, which in turn consist of many acini. The lobular ducts unite to form one large duct for each lobe. These larger ducts then open to the outside through the nipple. The size and shape of the breast are largely due to the amount of fatty tissue it contains.

The acini, which are the functional units of the breasts, are composed of a single layer of epithelium from which the milk is formed. There are many small capillaries beneath this layer of epithelium.

It is believed that the ovarian and placental hormones and the pituitary gland hormones regulate the growth and development of the breast tissue during pregnancy and the initial secretion of milk during the puerperium. Most of the hyperplasia takes place during the first half of pregnancy with both the duct and the alveolar systems increasing in size and area. This development of breast tissue during pregnancy is necessary for lactation during the puerperium. At about the middle of pregnancy the alveolar cells show secretory activity, and there may be further breast hypertrophy due to the accumulation of these secretory products.

For the first two or three days after the birth of the baby the breasts remain much the same as during pregnancy. They secrete a small amount of yellowish fluid called *colostrum,* which differs from milk chiefly in that it contains less fat and sugar, but more salts and protein than milk and also in the fact that it coagulates upon boiling.

The lactogenic hormone of the pituitary gland, *prolactin,* released after parturition, then stimulates milk secretion, and the meager amount of colostrum is replaced by milk which rapidly increases in amount. The breasts enlarge considerably on the second, third, or sometimes as late as the fourth day and quite suddenly become firm, hard, and painful. This tenseness of the breasts is partly due to a fullness with milk and partly due to venous and lymphatic stasis. Sometimes this turgidity of the breasts is relieved by emptying, but many times the breasts will remain firm and tense even after nursing, during this period of engorgement. The engorgement will disappear in 24 to 48 hours, and although the milk supply is increasing, the breasts become softer and more comfortable.

It was formerly widely held that engorgement produces fever, but lactation is not an inflammatory process and if there is fever at this time some other cause (with rare exceptions) should be suspected.

The secretion of milk is definitely stimulated by regular emptying and will not continue for more than a few days without this stimulation. The amount of milk produced varies in different individuals. Some mothers will be slow to produce an adequate supply but may be able to nurse more satisfactorily after several weeks. The well-developed breast of moderate size usually produces an adequate supply while the pendulous breast which is made up of much fatty and less glandular tissue may not produce well. Ideally the breasts secrete a quantity and quality of milk which will adequately nourish the baby for six to eight months, the supply being automatically adjusted to the demand.

## CLINICAL ASPECTS

**Postpartum Chill.** The patient may have a severe shaking chill within a few minutes after delivery or soon after she awakens from the anesthesia; this may be a nervous reaction or may be due to vasomotor changes. It is not followed by an elevation in temperature and is not significant. A chill later during the puerperium and especially when followed by fever is a sign of infection somewhere in the body and must be considered serious.

**Temperature.** The temperature may rise to 38° C (100.4° F) immediately after a long labor, but it should drop to normal in 24 hours and remain practically so. For various causes, some of which are unexplained, the temperature will not infrequently be slightly above normal at times during the first few days of the puerperium, without the patient seeming to suffer any ill effects. A temperature of 38° C (100.4° F) is the upper limit of normality, and the patient is considered to have a morbid temperature if it reaches that point on any two days after the first 24 hours. It was formerly believed that a fever on the third or fourth day was due to the beginning of lactation but this is now known not to be true; its cause should be considered an infection somewhere in the body.

**Pulse.** The normal pulse rate is often slow during the puerperium, being about 60 to 70 beats a minute or even as low as 40 to 50 beats; this is referred to as puerperal bradycardia. It is thought that this is due to the decreased strain upon the heart after the birth of the baby and the reduction of the vascular bed with the contraction of the uterus. In 7 to 10 days the rate is usually back to normal. There may, in some cases, be an increase in the pulse rate, which usually follows a long hard labor or a large blood loss at the time of delivery.

**Blood.** The blood chemistry may be altered slightly late in pregnancy and in the early puerperium, but it soon returns to the nonpregnant level. Anemia may be present due to blood loss during delivery, but any anemia tends to be magnified by the hemodilution of pregnancy, and this must be taken into consideration in evaluating the blood picture. With the large quantity of fluid eliminated from the tissues during the early days of the puerperium the blood will soon return to its normal concentration. Much change is seen in one week, and the normal concentration is reached in two to six weeks. A leukocytosis is present during and just after labor and sometimes with the beginning of lactation, but the reading falls back to normal rapidly.

**Loss of Weight.** One of the striking changes during the puerperium is the loss of weight, due largely to the elimination of normally increased fluid in the tissues, the decrease in the size of the uterus, and the escape of vaginal and uterine secretions, termed *lochia*. There is, of course, the initial body weight loss of 5 to 6 kg (11 to 13.2 lb) with the expulsion of the uterine contents. Usually the patient will return to approximately her nonpregnant weight by the end of the sixth to eighth week.

**Skin.** There is frequently profuse perspiration, especially at night, during the first few days, while the elimination of fluid is most active, but this gradually subsides and becomes normal by the end of a week. The perspiration sometimes has a strong odor, and there is frequently an appreciable amount of desquamation.

**Urine.** Some patients find it difficult, even impossible, to void during the first several hours after delivery because of the removal of intra-abdominal pressure, the recumbent position, and the swelling and bruised state of the tissues about the urethra. The bladder is likely to be less sensitive than it ordinarily is, and the patient will be able to retain an abnormally large amount of urine for several hours without discomfort or desire to void.

The output of urine during the first few days is greater than normal, and there is also a considerable increase in the amount of nitrogen excreted, beginning two or three days after delivery. This is evidently derived from the broken-down proteins in the uterine wall; the excess gradually subsides as involution progresses, and disappears by the time the uterus descends into the pelvis, about the tenth postpartum day.

**Digestive Tract.** Some patients may be nauseated and may vomit immediately after delivery, but this discomfort, if present, disappears in a few hours and they are hungry and are able to eat a normal amount of food in 12 to 24 hours. Many patients are able to eat within a couple of hours. Most patients are very thirsty and will start to drink a large quantity of fluid very soon after delivery.

The bowels may be constipated, at least during the early puerperium, because of the loss of intra-abdominal pressure, the relaxation of the abdominal muscles which makes them less able to aid in evacuation of the bowel, the intestinal sluggishness acquired during pregnancy, and the lack of exercise.

**Afterpains.** These pains are caused by the alternate contraction and relaxation of the uterine muscle and are more common in multiparas than in primiparas, because the muscle fibers of the former have somewhat less tone than the latter and therefore tend to relax and then contract, whereas the better muscle tone of the primipara helps to maintain a firm uterus.

These afterpains usually subside after the first 24 to 48 hours, although they may persist for three or four days. They may amount to little more than vague discomfort, but not infrequently they are so severe as to require the administration of analgesics. Afterpains are affected by nursing, being more severe as a rule when the baby is at the breast than at other times. Persistent afterpains may be due to retained blood clots.

**Lochia.** The vaginal discharge, known as lochia, consists of the uterine and vaginal secretions, blood, and the uterine lining that is cast off during the puerperium. During the first three or four days this discharge is bright red, consisting to a large extent of blood, and is termed *lochia rubra*. As the color gradually fades and becomes pinker and more serous it is called *lochia serosa*. After about the tenth day, if involution is normal, the discharge is whitish or yellowish and is designated *lochia alba*. The total amount of the lochial discharge is from 150 to 400 ml (5 to 13.3 oz), being more profuse sometimes in women who nurse their babies. Under normal conditions the discharge is profuse at first, gradually diminishing until it entirely disappears by the end of the puerperium. There may be small amounts of blood retained during the first day or two and expelled later as clots, without any serious significance, and there may be a more bloody discharge after the patient becomes more active; however, if the lochia is persistently blood-tinged, it may be taken as an indication that the uterus is not involuting as it should or that a piece of placental tissue has been retained. The normal characteristic odor is fleshy and much the same as menstrual blood. A foul odor is suggestive of infection.

**Menstruation.** In women who do not nurse their babies, menstruation will probably return within eight weeks after delivery; in those who do nurse the newborn, return of menstruation is ordinarily postponed until the fifth to sixth month, although the time is variable, since the function may begin in two months or may be suspended as long as 18 months. Menstruation returns before lactation has ended in 70 to 80 per cent of the patients. If it has not already returned it will begin in two months after lactation has stopped. The cycle and amount may be irregular for the first few months.

Ovulation is usually suspended during lactation, but a nursing mother may become pregnant and sometimes does so within a few weeks after delivery even though she has not menstruated.

**General.** Most patients recover very quickly and except for perineal discomfort feel very well; most are able to move about easily and eat and drink normally within a few hours after delivery. Multiparas usually recover from the exertion of labor and delivery more quickly than primiparas. This is probably due to the fact that the labor is shorter in the former than in the latter and that their tissues are less likely to be bruised and lacerated. Primiparas may have more muscle soreness from the harder work of the second stage of labor. Considering the many physiologic changes which have occurred in the past months, return of the body to its nonpregnant state is surprisingly rapid, especially if good care is given.

## BIBLIOGRAPHY AND STUDENT REFERENCES

Bookmiller, Mae M., and Bowen, George L.: *Textbook of Obstetrics and Obstetric Nursing,* 2nd ed. W. B. Saunders Co., Philadelphia, 1954.

Davis, M. Edward, and Sheckler, Catherine E.: *DeLee's Obstetrics for Nurses,* 15th ed. W. B. Saunders Co., Philadelphia, 1951.

Eastman, Nicholson J.: *Williams Obstetrics,* 11th ed. Appleton-Century-Crofts, Inc., New York, 1956.

Greenhill, J. P. (ed.): *Obstetrics,* 11th ed. W. B. Saunders Co., Philadelphia, 1955.

Woodward, H. L.; Gardner, B.; Bryant, R. D.; and Overland, Anna E.: *Obstetric Management and Nursing,* 5th ed. F. A. Davis Co., Philadelphia, 1955.

Zabriskie, Louise, and Eastman, Nicholson J.: *Nurses Handbook of Obstetrics,* 9th ed. J. B. Lippincott Co., Philadelphia, 1952.

*Chapter 16*

# Nursing Care during the Normal Puerperium

Many changes have taken place in the nursing care of the postpartum patient in the past 10 to 15 years. Some of this change has been the result of early ambulation in the puerperium and early discharge from the hospital; some has been due to an increasing realization of the importance of sending mothers home with adequate preparation to care for themselves and their babies. Before early rising the mother remained in bed for 7 to 10 days and stayed in the hospital another 4 or 5 days. Today she usually gets out of bed on the first day and many times goes home before the end of a week following the birth of her baby. Early ambulation has made the puerperium seem a more normal physiologic process. During this period the mother assumes responsibility for much of her own care. Formerly the nurse devoted most of her time to giving the mother physical care, but the amount of this care is now reduced considerably and much of it can be given by auxiliary personnel. This change, however, does not reduce the need for the well-prepared professional nurse, since it is essential for her to apply her knowledge and skills in many other ways than the actual giving of bedside care. Although physical care has been simplified the general principles of clean technic, watchfulness for complications, adaptability to the patient, and sympathetic understanding are just as important as formerly. Vigilance against complications of the puerperium, principally hemorrhage and infection, must be just as great as it always has been. In addition to guarding against these definite complications, the nurse must help to protect the patient from the less tangible effects of fatigue on mind and body. As many young mothers are in a more or less excitable condition after the baby's birth, the beneficial effect of promoting a tranquil and contented state of mind cannot be overestimated. The nurse will find that her understanding of the patient's emotional needs and her role as a teacher of the mother and her family have become increasingly important.

## EMOTIONAL ASPECTS

One factor influencing the young mother's state of mind, which the nurse must take into account, is that the entire scheme and purpose of the patient's life have been changed. She has very suddenly been plunged into a wholly new situation, and her reaction to this change will depend upon her temperament, disposition, and habits of adjustment. Nursing care during the puerperium is not complete unless the nurse helps the patient to make this adjustment easily.

Some women are forced to face the reality of increased responsibility very quickly, because they had not begun to appreciate this during their pregnancy. New mothers are frequently worried that they are not capable of giving their babies good care, and the nurse can help to relieve these fears by reassurances in many ways. Some women do not have their maternal feelings well developed immediately after the birth of the baby; they need encouragement and time to establish a satisfactory relationship to their child. Since they need help in appreciating that this lag in a feeling of closeness to the baby is not abnormal, an understanding attitude from the nurse will help to avert a feeling of guilt. Fortunately the majority of mothers are happy and comfortable in their outlook and may be kept so by the exercise of tact on the part of the nurse.

Although from a physical standpoint early ambulation is desirable, the mothers should not be expected to care for themselves until they are ready. Most mothers wish to do this very early, but some, because of fatigue or because of a need for dependency for a certain period of time, should be given physical care until they are ready to assume responsibility for their own care. The nurse must be willing to give this care. A good relationship between the mother and the nurse usually makes it possible for the mother to express her needs;

however, an observing and understanding nurse will recognize and meet these needs before the patient mentions them.

Many mothers wish to talk over their pregnancy, their labor, their own physical care, their baby and the care he will require, and their husbands' feelings toward the baby. Some have feelings of inadequacy regarding the care of their baby; others feel they were unusually difficult and uncooperative during labor; still others wish to express their anxiety over their children at home. Talking over these problems relieves tension—the nurse must be a sympathetic listener. The nurse must assure the mother that she can understand her feelings and give the mother ample opportunity to discuss them. Many mothers have questions regarding perineal care and breast care; they must be given intelligent and understandable explanations of the physiologic changes they should expect and the care they must give themselves.

The mother must have help in learning to care for her baby from a nurse who can put her at ease and give her a feeling of self-assurance. The nurse must never be critical of an inexperienced mother, but rather must be all the more ready to help her learn how to satisfy her baby's needs. To gain skill and confidence the mother not only needs help with the baby's physical care, but she must also be given opportunities to make her own decisions regarding his needs and an assurance that she can do well. Because she has been helped to find her own answers to her questions and has been reassured that her judgment is good, she becomes able to meet problems at home more easily.

Giving supportive care to mothers is essential in postpartum care. Such supportive care consists of helping them to understand their feelings, to know their own physical needs, and to learn how to care for their babies. The nurse who enjoys teaching mothers and who appreciates the value of emotional support will find great satisfaction in the care she gives during the postpartum period.

## PHYSICAL ASPECTS

**The First Hour after Delivery.** The care of the patient during the first hour after delivery has already been discussed in detail in Chapter 12, "The Nurse's Duties during Labor," but the importance of watching the consistency of the uterus should be emphasized once again. The nurse must stay with the patient for one full hour after the delivery of the placenta to observe the patient for postpartum hemorrhage. During this hour she must keep her hand on the patient's abdomen continuously to palpate the uterus and thereby note immediately any relaxation of the muscle (Fig. 112). If the uterus remains firm and below the umbilicus there is no danger of uterine hemorrhage, either visible or concealed, but if the uterus becomes relaxed it should be massaged, and frequently another dose of oxytocin (Pitocin) or ergonovine must be administered. The uterus should not be massaged, however, if it remains firm since unnecessary manipulation is painful and produces muscle fatigue; this in turn may cause relaxation of the uterus later. During this hour the perineal pad, or the large absorbent pad which may be used under the hips in place of a perineal pad, should be inspected frequently to discover excessive bleeding which may originate from the cervix or vaginal wall. A perineal pad, held in place by a T binder is frequently put on the patient before she leaves the delivery room. Some doctors object to the use of a perineal pad immediately; instead they prefer to have a large sterile absorbent pad placed under the hips for the first 12 to 24 hours after delivery.

If the blood pressure was elevated during labor it should be checked during this period, and whenever any cardiac or respiratory disease is present the pulse and respiration must be watched carefully.

It is important for the patient to see her husband immediately after delivery and for both parents to see the baby as soon as possible. There is a mounting anxiety when the interval between the birth of the baby and seeing the baby is prolonged. If the mother is responsive before she leaves the delivery room she should see her baby at that time or he may be shown to her and her husband as he is taken to the nursery. Although the parents have seen the baby as he is taken to the nursery they will wish to see him again when he has been weighed, cleaned, and dressed. The nurse will find that taking the baby back to the parents at this time and allowing the mother to hold the baby for a few minutes is well worth the extra time it may take. Unless the baby is a premature or has some complication which requires immediate nursing care he will not suffer from being taken to the parents for a brief period before he is placed in his warmed crib.

Unless the patient is under the influence of drugs given during labor, she is usually nervous and exhausted and may complain of generalized discomfort, and perineal pain in particular. To ensure adequate rest and relaxation she is frequently given an analgesic drug when she returns to her room or as soon as she awakens from an anesthetic, if she has had one. Unless anesthesia has been deep the patient is awake almost immediately upon leaving the delivery room. Morphine up to 10 mg (1/6 gr) or meperidine (Demerol) up to 100 mg (1½ gr) is often used to relieve discomfort and promote rest. If the patient is then allowed to lie in a comfortable position, if the room is darkened and visitors are restricted, she will be able to get a few hours of rest. The patient will often expect to sleep immediately, but may find that sleep is not possible for several hours and sometimes not possible for 8 to 12 hours, because of the physical and nervous exhaustion and the excitement that follows the birth of the baby. The nurse should explain this and advise the patient that if sleep is not possible she should try to lie quietly and get some rest.

**Temperature, Pulse, and Respiration.** The temperature, pulse, and respiration should be checked every four hours during the day and also at night if indicated. A fever and a rising pulse rate are the first signs of an infection; the uterus, the breasts, the urinary tract, and the respiratory tract being most frequently affected. A fever of 38° C (100.4° F) and a pulse rate about 100 should always be reported to the doctor. Fever occurring on the same day that the breasts become engorged should not be passed off lightly as a "milk fever," or believed to be caused by the normal breast engorgement, because engorgement does not produce an elevation of temperature except in rare instances of extreme engorgement when the temperature may be elevated for a few hours. However, if the temperature has been normal for several days or a week and then very suddenly rises to 38.3° C (101° F) or even 39.4° C (103° F) it is frequently due to a breast infection.

**Involution.** The progress of involution of the uterus can be noted by observing its size and consistency and the character, amount, and odor of the lochia. In describing the consistency of the uterus the terms soft and boggy or firm and round are frequently used. Its size can be indicated by its height and is measured by the number of fingerbreadths the top of the fundus lies above or below the umbilicus. Immediately after delivery the top of the fundus is usually several fingerbreadths below the umbilicus, on the following day it is at the level of the umbilicus, and then the uterus slowly descends into the pelvis and decreases in size (Fig. 126). It is best to measure the height of the fundus when the bladder has recently been emptied because the uterus, due to its stretched ligaments, can easily be moved about and a distended bladder may push it up or to one side. It is difficult to be exact as to the rate at which the fundus descends because of the great variations, which are still within normal limits, in different individuals, but it is usually not palpable above the symphysis pubis after the tenth day.

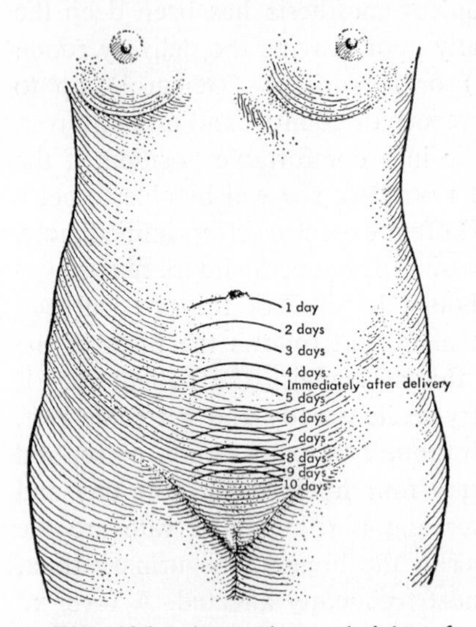


**Fig. 126.** Approximate height of the fundus on each of the first ten days after delivery.

If the uterus is involuting properly the lochia will gradually decrease in amount and change from rubra to serosa within a few days and on approximately the tenth day change to lochia alba.

Ergonovine in 0.2-mg ($\frac{1}{320}$-gr) doses is frequently given every 4 hours for the first 24 hours to keep the uterus well contracted or it may be given 3 or 4 times a day for several successive days to hasten involution. If the uterus remains soft and large and the patient continues to have a large amount of bright red lochia, both of which are signs of subinvolution, ergonovine may be repeated after several days for another 24-hour period. Bright red vaginal bleeding or the expulsion of blood clots may be due to retention of a small piece of placenta or some of the fetal membranes. Involution is usually more rapid when the baby nurses as nursing stimulates uterine contractions.

**Afterpains.** Afterpains, caused by alternate contraction and relaxation of the uterine muscle, occur in about 75 per cent of multiparas. They become particularly severe at nursing time due to stimulation of the uterus at this time, but usually do not last for more than 48 hours. Unless the primiparous patient has had her uterus distended more than the normal amount, she ordinarily has no afterpains. If these pains persist for much longer than 48 hours or if they are severe in the primipara, the possibility of retention of secundines or blood clots must be considered. Relief of the discomfort caused by these contractions can be given by administering drugs for pain relief; codeine 30 to 60 mg (½ to 1 gr) and aspirin 0.30 to 0.60 gm (5 to 10 gr) given together usually control this discomfort. An ice bag, placed over the lower abdomen, may help to keep the uterus contracted and promote comfort.

**Care of the Perineum.** Technics of perineal care vary greatly in different hospitals, but the purposes of perineal care and the general principles of care are always the same. Special attention to the perineal area of the postpartum patient is necessary because of the continual drainage of lochia during the first 7 to 10 days after delivery. The purpose of this care is to keep the area clean and dry, to eliminate odor, and to increase the comfort of the patient. Healing is promoted by keeping the episiotomy repair clean and dry.

The technic of the perineal care that is given in the hospital has been simplified, and the amount of nursing time spent on this aspect of puerperal care has been greatly reduced since early ambulation of the postpartum patient. This simplification has made it much easier for the patient also. She is now taught to give her own care almost as soon as she is ambulatory; this adds to her comfort and makes it possible for her to learn a procedure, early in her hospital stay, which she may use at home.

The frequency of perineal care varies in different hospitals. Some doctors recommend that the perineum is washed only once or twice a day while others prefer that some type of care be given approximately every four hours or at least after each voiding and defecation. Many times patients decide upon the frequency of care themselves after they begin their own care. At the present time nurses give perineal care to all patients who, for some reason, must stay in bed and to all patients for the first 12 to 24 hours after delivery, or longer if the patient does not feel able to care for herself. In some hospitals the patient may be instructed to wash her own perineum at bath time, but is given a perineal irrigation by the nurse in the afternoon. This is especially the case if the patient feels the need of having a nurse do the care from the standpoint of carefully cleaning the sutured area.

Regardless of the technic used it is important for the nurse to protect the patient against infection conveyed from her hands, or from equipment, or from another patient. The perineal area should be treated as a wound, and precautions must be just as rigid when there is no perineal repair as when sutures are present, because it is the uterine cavity itself that must be protected against infection. There is danger that pathogenic organisms brought to the perineum will ascend to the uterine cavity, which is an open wound. The minimum requirements are that each patient has her own bedpan to prevent contamination from another patient and that the nurse wash her hands carefully with soap and water before she gives perineal care or changes pads. All equipment and all pads should be sterilized before use.

In caring for the perineum the nurse must remember also the danger of the patient infecting herself with her own fingers and should caution her against this risk. The patient should be told that if she feels uncomfortable, or thinks she is bleeding, she must lie quietly and summon a nurse, but on no account to try to discover what is wrong. There is little doubt that cases of severe infection have been caused by the introduction of organisms into the vagina by means of the patient's own fingers, after the most scrupulous precautions had been taken by doctors and nurses.

There are many minor variations in procedure; in some instances the cotton balls used to wash the patients are handled with forceps and the nurses' hands never come in contact with the equipment or the vulva, while in others the nurse is directed to scrub carefully and then use her hands to handle the cotton pledgets. The nurse should, of course, wash her hands carefully even when she uses the forceps technic because her hands must be clean to apply the pad. To wash the patient, boiled water or tap water is adequate, although in most instances a diluted soap solution is used. Sometimes a saline solution or an antiseptic solution may be used. The solution that is used must always be mild and diluted enough to avoid irritation and burning of the skin and mucous membrane. In all cases it is well to remember that the care should be an external irrigation only and that it is best not to separate the labia or to pour the solution over the vulva if the introitus is very relaxed, in order to prevent any solution from running into the vagina. It is important to wash the perineum from front to back and never to bring the cotton balls up over the vulva once they have touched the anal region.

The care of the perineum is the same whether or not there are sutures, except that special attention must be given to removing all of the lochia from the sutures when they are present and this is sometimes a little difficult. It is important, however, that the nurse removes this lochia very gently in order not to pull on the sutures, since tension on them causes the patient distress. The nurse must also be careful not to pull apart the approximated skin edges of the episiotomy repair while she is washing the perineum. A suggested procedure for perineal care is as follows:

## POSTPARTUM PERINEAL IRRIGATION (Perineal Care)

Object:

1. To keep the vulva and perineum clean of lochia
2. To promote the comfort of the patient

Precautions:

1. Use strictly aseptic technic
2. Do not touch the vulva or perineum with the hands
3. Always discard the cotton ball after it has touched the anal region
4. Avoid unnecessary exposure of the patient

Equipment:

1. Bedpan
2. Newspaper for waste
3. Sterile cellucotton pad—12 in. square or larger
4. Tray with the following equipment:
    a. Small basin containing 8–10 cotton balls in a green soap solution (30 ml [1 oz] green soap to 500 ml [1 pt] water)
    b. 180–240-ml (6–8-oz) pitcher with warm sterile water
    c. 8–10 dry cotton balls
    d. One Pean forceps

Procedure:

1. Wash hands
2. Take equipment to the patient's room
3. Place the patient in the dorsal recumbent position
4. Spread the newspaper out at the foot of the bed
5. Remove the soiled cellucotton pad from beneath the patient and wrap it in newspaper
6. Place the patient on the bedpan
7. Drape
    a. Fan upper bedding down to the thighs, covering the part of the body thus exposed with a cotton blanket
    b. Bring the fanned bedding well in between the legs

8. Take cotton balls from the green soap solution with forceps and wash (Fig. 127A)
   a. Each thigh beginning in the groin and washing as far out as there is any lochial discharge

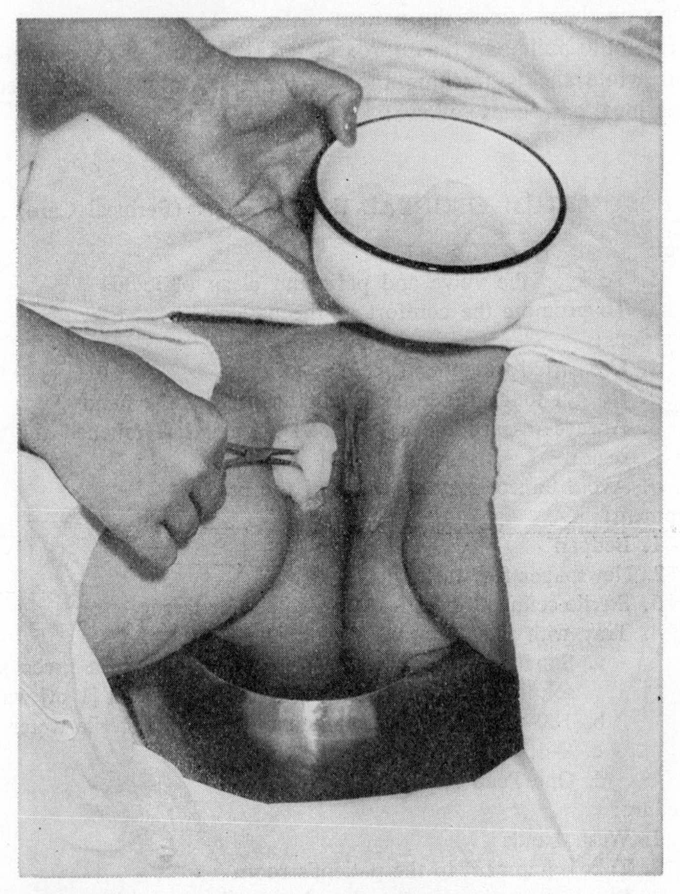

**Fig. 127A.** Washing of the vulva, perineum, and inner aspect of the thighs following delivery. This washing is done with sterile cotton balls which have been removed from a diluted green soap solution and which are held with sterile forceps. All washing is from above downward, and each cotton ball is discarded when the anal region is reached. With the patient on the bedpan, the soap solution can be removed by pouring sterile water over the vulva and inner aspect of the thighs. Cotton balls are used to dry the area.

b. Over the vulva and perineum, wiping from above downward

9. Discard the cotton balls on the newspaper
10. Pour most of the remaining soap solution over the vulva unless the introitus is gaping
11. Pour sterile water from the pitcher over the thighs and vulva to wash off the soap
12. Dry the thighs and vulva in the same manner in which they were cleaned, using the dry cotton balls held with the forceps
13. Remove the bedpan, having the patient turn on her side at the same time
14. From the remaining soap solution squeeze a cotton ball as dry as possible against the side of the basin and wash from the perineum back over the anus (Fig. 127B)
15. With another cotton ball squeezed as dry as possible wash the buttocks
16. Wash off the soap by repeating this same procedure with cotton balls squeezed as dry as possible from the sterile water
17. Dry this area with sterile dry cotton balls
18. Place a sterile cellucotton pad against the buttocks and have the patient turn on her back

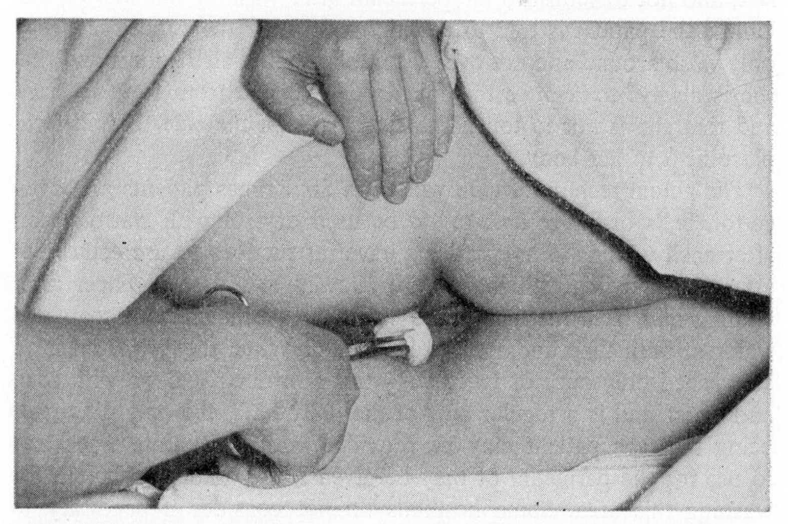

**Fig. 127B.** The patient lies on her side for completion of the perineal care; this makes it possible to clean the anal region and the buttocks. Sterile cotton balls held in sterile forceps are used as in Fig. 127A, and again each cotton ball is discarded after it has touched the anal region.

19. Adjust the covers
20. Remove the equipment to the service room, where it is washed, and resterilized by boiling or autoclaving; dispose of the waste

Charting:

1. The amount and kind of lochia
2. The healing of the perineum
3. Patient's discomfort, if any

Instructions for the patient's own care vary in different hospitals, but a few principles are always the same. The patient must be given detailed and clear instructions as to her care and she must be provided with sufficient equipment. She must be instructed to wash her hands before she begins her care and that she must always place all supplies—cotton balls, washcloth, towels, and pads—on a clean surface. Adequate provision must be made for disposal of soiled cotton balls and pads and washcloths and towels. She must be told exactly when and how she is to do this care—whether it is to be done only at bath time and after a defecation or after each voiding. The patient must always understand very clearly that she is to wash the vulva and perineum first (including the sutured area), the anal region last, and not to return to the perineum after washing the anal region. Unless the patient is told to actually wash over the sutures she may only wash around and not over them. She should also understand that she is always to remove the soiled perineal pad from front to back and that she is not to touch the clean pad on the side that she will place next to her body.

The actual technic of care will vary. Sometimes patients are given cotton balls or gauze sponges to be used dry, or with warm water, after each voiding. Some patients have instructions to use celluwipes after each voiding. Still others are allowed to use toilet paper after voiding and have instructions to wash the perineum with soap and water at bath time and after a defecation. When the perineum is to be washed only once or twice daily this is ordinarily done with soap and water and is a regular part of the daily bath, the only difference being that the patient may be provided with a separate washcloth to use for the perineum or may be given a disposable washcloth for washing this area. Some hospitals do not consider it necessary to provide the patient with a separate washcloth for perineal care, this care merely being a part of the daily bath. This method seems to be entirely satisfactory when the patient is provided with a clean washcloth and towel each day and is given proper instructions. Regardless of the method employed it is important for the patient to be given a procedure that she can carry out at home.

In regards to the use of pads some obstetricians believe that a perineal pad should not be used while the patient is in bed, since it slips and moves about, and thus may transfer infective material from the anus to the vagina. Accordingly, they advise that large, sterile, absorbent pads should be used under the patient's hips to receive the lochia, the pads being changed as often as necessary. In these cases the use of a perineal pad, held in place by a T binder or the patient's own belt, is begun when the patient gets out of bed. Whenever the patient gets into bed, and particularly when she plans to stay in bed for several hours, she may remove the perineal pad and again use the large cellucotton pad under her hips. Some patients find this method more comfortable than continuous use of the perineal pad, especially if the pad irritates the sutured area. Once the patient begins to get in and out of bed frequently she may find that it is too much trouble to change from one type of pad to another. When perineal pads are worn they should be applied so that they will be snug enough to prevent sliding back and forth over the perineum, but not so tight as to be uncomfortable.

Perineal sutures cause some patients considerable discomfort, sometimes for as long as seven or eight days; others do not complain of pain. Occasionally the entire vulva and perineum may be edematous for the first day or two due to excessive stretching of the tissues at the time of delivery. The edema of tissues is ordinarily not painful, but if it places tension on the sutured area there is pain. Dry heat, applied by the use of a heat lamp for 20 to 30 minutes two or three times a day, frequently gives some relief of perineal pain (Fig. 128). Analgesic ointments or sprays, applied to the sutured area, may give relief from perineal discomfort. If the patient experiences pain while sitting she may be somewhat relieved by sitting on a large rubber air ring, which is inflated with just enough air to relieve pressure on the perineal area. If the perineum causes the patient much discomfort it may be necessary to administer analgesic medication for pain relief for a few days after delivery. Perineal sutures are usually absorbable; if nonabsorbable ones are used they are removed in approximately one week. A patient who has experienced considerable perineal pain is usually more comfortable when the sutures begin to absorb or when they are removed.

The nurse should inspect the perineum daily for any redness or swelling and report it to the doctor. Daily charting should include the appearance of the perineal repair, the degree of pain the patient experiences, and the effects of treatment given.

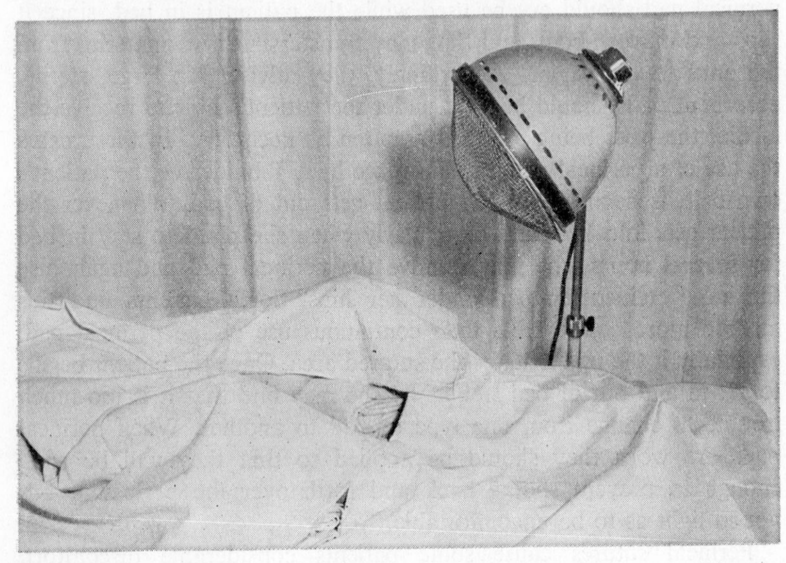

**Fig. 128.** Application of dry heat to the perineal sutured area. Adequate draping and a comfortable position are important.

**Douches.** In connection with perineal care, it is well to caution the nurse against giving douches without explicit orders. To prevent carrying infective material up into the uterus, douches are not given early in the puerperium. They may be started any time after the seventh day, but many doctors prefer to have them withheld until the twelfth or fourteenth day or even for the first six weeks. If begun early they are usually ordered to be taken once or twice daily until the patient returns for her six-weeks' postpartum examination. By cleaning the vagina of discharges, douches make the patient more comfortable and also aid in healing of the perineum and cervical lacerations. The patient may need instructions for taking douches.

**Hemorrhoids,** which may develop (or, if present, enlarge) during pregnancy because the pressure of the enlarged uterus interfered with circulation in the pelvic veins, may become more edematous with the straining of the second stage of labor. They are sometimes very painful for a few days post partum, but gradually decrease in size and cause less discomfort as the circulation improves. The nurse should do what she can to keep the patient comfortable by the application of either heat or cold, whichever gives most relief, in the form of a heat lamp or ice compresses, or by the application of an analgesic ointment or spray or rectal suppositories. If hemorrhoids were present before pregnancy they subside to their usual size during the puerperium; if they were not present before pregnancy they will probably disappear completely.

**The Bladder.** Some patients, particularly primiparas, have difficulty in voiding after delivery. This difficulty is due in part to impaired tone of the bladder wall and in part to decreased sensitiveness of the bladder following the pressure and trauma during labor. Retention may also be due to swelling of the tissues at the base of the bladder and around the urethra which is caused by the trauma of delivery, especially in long labors and instrumental deliveries. A weak abdominal wall may add to the difficulty the patient has in emptying her bladder. Because of the increased capacity and lessened sensitivity of the bladder following delivery, it may become greatly distended without discomfort and can fill with 1000 or even 1500 ml of urine without giving the patient a feeling of fullness. This overdistention may add to the loss of bladder tone and may make it even more difficult for the patient to empty her bladder later, and it may also cause abrasions in the bladder wall which increase the danger of cystitis. The nurse must bear in mind then that a distended bladder or residual urine may easily occur during the puerperium unless the patient is carefully watched; any evidences of either should be reported to the doctor promptly, and a record should be made on the patient's chart.

A distended bladder may be recognized by watching the abdominal contour. It can be seen as a mass distending the lower abdomen or it may be palpated above the symphysis pubis. As it fills, it pushes the uterus up higher into the abdomen or toward one side, and unless the nurse palpates the abdomen carefully she may mistake the distended bladder for the uterus. Some patients complain of discomfort and constant desire to void while others have neither discomfort nor desire to empty their bladder.

To prevent the bladder from becoming greatly distended the nurse should urge the patient to use the bedpan within a few hours after delivery even if she has no desire to void. She should not catheterize, however, until the full bladder can be palpated in the lower abdomen, which may not occur for 8 to 12 hours (or it may occur much earlier), and only after having resorted to various expedients in order to help the patient empty her bladder. Some doctors prefer that the patient sit straight up in bed or get out of bed and sit on a bedpan placed on a chair before resorting to catheterization. In some instances the patient may even be allowed to walk to the bathroom, with assistance, if the bathroom is nearby and if she feels able to walk.

The nurse should watch for residual urine by measuring the amount of each voiding for the first few times, remembering that because of increased urinary output and bladder capacity the new mother should void considerably more than the average amount. Small amounts voided at frequent intervals are an indication of the presence of residual urine. It is probably not necessary to catheterize after the first small voiding because the patient who has been able to empty her bladder partially the first time she voids may be able to do so more completely in another few hours. Catheterization for residual urine is indicated, however, after several small frequent voidings and especially when the bladder can be palpated above the symphysis pubis.

If the nurse is ordered to catheterize the patient, she must observe strict asepsis and extreme gentleness throughout the procedure. To prevent contamination of the vulva she should wear sterile gloves when possible and if they are not available, she must be very careful to wash her hands thoroughly just before beginning the procedure. The cotton balls which are used to wash the area around the meatus should always be squeezed dry enough to prevent the cleaning solution from running into the vaginal meatus because it may be a source of contamination to the birth canal. In catheterizing the postpartum patient the nurse must always be very careful to separate the labia gently to prevent pulling on the perineal sutures, which causes the patient considerable pain, but she must separate them far enough to be able to see the meatus which is frequently difficult to find due to small lacerations and edema of the tissues of this area. A good light must be directed on the area. With the postpartum patient there is always some danger of carrying lochia into the bladder unless the procedure is done quickly; the catheter must be inserted before the lochia, which usually flows freely, covers the urinary meatus. A cotton ball placed over the vaginal orifice immediately after cleaning the area between the labia minora will help to keep the vaginal secretions from spreading upward.

Some doctors prefer to insert an indwelling catheter for one to two days if the patient is unable to void. This allows the bladder to rest completely and also eliminates the necessity of frequent catheterization. Others believe that there is no more danger of cystitis from frequent catheterizations than there is with an indwelling catheter and that the muscle may regain its tone more quickly if the bladder fills and is emptied with some regularity.

An accurate record of the intake and output is ordinarily not kept on the normal postpartum patient, but when there have been complications during pregnancy or if they arise during the puerperium the nurse should keep an accurate record. Even when a complete record of the output is not necessary the amount of the first few voidings should be noted to help in determining the adequacy of the urinary output. The nurse should expect the postpartum patient to have a large output the first few days because she eliminates the fluid which has been stored in her tissues during pregnancy.

**The Bowels.** The puerperal patient is often constipated and needs assistance in regaining regularity in the movements of her bowels. The use of cathartics and enemas varies, but it is usual to give an enema on the second or third morning after delivery if the patient has not had a bowel movement at the end of this time. Thereafter mild cathartics or soapsuds, sodium bicarbonate, or saline enemas are given often enough to produce a bowel movement daily or at least every other day, if this is not accomplished by diet and activity. Mineral oil given daily, or milk of magnesia in some instances, often eliminates the necessity of enemas. If the mineral oil is given at bedtime it will not interfere as greatly with the absorption of vitamins in the diet taken during the day.

The abdomen may become very distended with gas on the first or second day post partum because of the increased space for the intestines. This distention will soon disappear, but if the patient becomes uncomfortable a rectal tube may give relief or an enema may be given unless contraindicated this early.

In cases of third-degree tears, catharsis is often delayed for four to five days in order that the torn edges of the rectal sphincter may become well united before being strained by a bowel movement. In these cases an enema of 120 to 180 ml (4 to 6 oz) of warm oil is often given as the first enema, and the patient encouraged to retain it overnight or for several hours, in order to soften the feces and lessen the strain and irritation of evacuation. In other cases, daily cathartics are given, and the bowel contents kept soft and moving freely.

**The Daily Bath.** During the first week or two following delivery the patient's skin must aid in excreting fluid from the tissues throughout the body and metabolic products from the involuting uterus. She should, therefore, have a soap and water bath every day to remove the material that will very readily accumulate on the surface of the skin. Daily baths are also an important measure in promoting the patient's comfort since the profuse perspiration may have a strong odor, and the breasts may feel uncomfortable due to leakage of milk. Showers are usually permitted on the second or third day following delivery, and tub bathing may be resumed during the third or fourth week post partum. Some doctors permit tub bathing after the second week post partum.

**Care of the Breasts.** The care of the breasts is designed to accomplish certain ends which may be summarized as follows: First is the promotion and maintenance of a milk supply that is adequate to nourish the baby; other important factors include promotion of the mother's comfort and prevention of breast infection, facilitating the baby's nursing by attempting to bring out flat nipples, and preventing cracked or fissured nipples. It may be stated in general that the promotion and maintenance of an adequate milk supply are accomplished by giving the mother encouragement and help in her efforts to nurse her baby, and by regular and complete emptying of the breasts (see Chap. 17).

As has been explained in Chapter 15 there is little change in the breasts for the first two or three days after the birth of the baby; colostrum is present, but the breasts do not secrete much milk and therefore do not become uncomfortable with fullness. Although there is little milk in these first days the baby should be started on breast feeding so that the breasts may be stimulated to produce and so that the baby may learn to suck well at the breast. All babies do not nurse well when first put to the breast and if time can be spent during these first days to teach them to take the mother's nipple they probably will be ready to nurse vigorously when the breasts do begin to secrete a large amount. Early breast feeding is important to the establishment of an adequate supply of milk, and the baby may be started nursing in four to six hours. In some hospitals the baby is not put to breast for 24 hours for the sake of giving the mother an opportunity to rest after delivery and giving the baby a chance to spit up excessive mucus before he starts feeding.

Ordinarily alternate breasts are nursed approximately every three to four hours during the first days; later both breasts may be nursed at each feeding if necessary for further stimulation to produce milk. In some hospitals the 2 A.M. feeding is omitted so that the mother will have several hours of undisturbed sleep each night; others believe that emptying the breasts frequently is important for adequate milk production, and the 2 A.M. feeding is omitted only the first night or two, before the breasts become very full.

If a baby sucks vigorously it is often considered unwise to leave him at the breast for more than 5 minutes the first few times that he nurses. This time is then gradually increased to 10, 15, and 20 minutes. Limitation is placed on the nursing time at first because the nipples are sensitive, especially in women with a delicate skin, and if the baby is allowed to nurse too long at the beginning, the nipples may become very irritated and cracked.

*Breast engorgement* usually develops sometime between the second and fourth day. The breasts become heavy, distended, and painful. Engorgement on the second day usually indicates that the mother will have a large amount of breast milk early, whereas engorgement as late as the fourth day is frequently followed by a slower increase in the amount. Occasionally the breasts will produce a large amount of milk without previous engorgement. It used to be customary to massage engorged breasts and apply pressure bandages and various kinds of lotions and ointments, but these measures are now considered unnecessary and dangerous. During this period of engorgement the patient should be kept as comfortable as possible by supporting the heavy breasts, by applying ice bags which relieve the pain, and by the use of analgesic drugs if necessary. Codeine and aspirin constitute the analgesic most frequently used. Since the breasts do not remain uncomfortable long, this medication need not be repeated more than once or twice and therefore will not be dangerous for the baby.

Engorgement of the breasts makes it difficult for the baby to nurse; sometimes the baby cannot grasp the nipple well because of the tenseness of the breasts, and the nipple may become sore quickly during the baby's attempts to nurse. If the baby cannot grasp the nipples it becomes necessary to empty the breasts by the use of a breast pump until the engorgement decreases. The breasts do not always become soft with nursing during this period of engorgement; this is true even when the baby is able to nurse well. If he has sucked vigorously, it is not necessary to use a breast pump to attempt to empty them further; this is a tedious and uncomfortable process and may injure the nipples.

Some doctors feel that engorgement of the breasts at the beginning is due to a filling of the breasts with blood; this may interfere with emptying of the breasts, and engorgement increases as they fill with milk. Engorgement with milk may lead to secondary lymphatic and venous stasis. Michael Newton and Niles Newton believe that engorgement "begins with retention of milk in the alveoli. The alveoli become distended and compress surrounding milk ducts. This leads to obstruction of the outflow of milk, further distention of the alveoli, and increased obstruction. If unrelieved this may lead to secondary vascular and venous stasis." *

Newton and Newton believe that milk may be retained in the alveoli when the mechanism by which the milk is discharged into the ducts is not functioning well and that insufficient sucking at the breast, either because the mother or the hospital restricts the time, may inhibit the mechanism. "The importance of suckling before 'the milk comes in' is minimized. All too often the coming of milk is equated with the beginning symptoms of engorgement, and thus thorough attempts to empty the breast begin only after the vicious cycle of engorgement has started." *

Sometimes during this interval of engorgement a hard tender mass is felt in one or both axillae. This mass is glandular breast tissue which also becomes engorged and filled with milk. The congestion decreases in one to two days, and the lump gradually disappears as the milk in it dries up. An ice bag applied to the axilla will help to relieve the discomfort.

The patient should be reassured that the discomfort of engorgement will subside in 24 to 48 hours because she may believe that the breasts will remain uncomfortable during the entire time that she nurses her baby and may become discouraged. When the breasts

* Newton, Michael, and Newton, Niles: "Postpartum Engorgement of the Breast," *Am. J. Obst. & Gynec.,* **61**:666, (Mar.) 1951.

do become soft and comfortable the mother may think that her milk supply has decreased unless she is again assured that the breasts are normally comfortable even when they are functioning adequately.

A breast support should be applied as soon as the breasts become engorged and heavy. There are several methods of supporting heavy breasts; any method is adequate providing it lifts the breasts, suspending their weight from the shoulders, and does not make pressure at any point. One widely used support is a muslin binder, with adjustable shoulder straps, that is fitted to the patient by the use of safety pins (Fig. 129). The breasts are pulled upward and inward as the binder is fitted in such a way that it does not make pressure anywhere. The shoulder straps should be adjusted so that the breasts are held up and that their weight is suspended from the shoulders. Another very satisfactory support is the breast sling (Fig. 130). These slings can be adjusted to all patients and will not put pressure on the nipples, but they are difficult to apply and are not comfortable unless adjusted with great care. The nurse must remember that the slings should fit similarly to a brassiere, give adequate support under the breasts, but not be so snug as to pull over the shoulders or around the neck.

After the engorgement subsides the breasts may be heavy because they are filled with milk, but they will not be uncomfortable if adequately supported. Very full breasts, especially when large, often give rise to discomfort and even pain, because of their weight. Therefore, unless the breasts are small or very soft, a breast support should be continued even after the engorgement has subsided. All patients should be urged to obtain well-fitting brassieres, preferably a nursing brassiere, to wear after they leave the hospital. A nursing brassiere is not absolutely essential if a well-fitted uplift brassiere is worn, but most patients prefer a nursing brassiere because it opens in the front, which makes it more convenient for nursing, and it is usually made with a piece of moistureproof material in front to prevent any milk which leaks out of the breasts from soiling the clothing (Fig. 131). Some patients prefer to wear a nursing brassiere in the hospital in place of the other types of breast support, and in most instances this is very satisfactory if the brassiere fits well. A brassiere is frequently not entirely comfortable during the period of engorgement because the breasts are a little larger at that time than they will be later and the brassiere may fit too snugly. Usually it is necessary to wear a clean cloth inside the breast binder or brassiere to absorb the milk that leaks out of the breasts between nursing periods. While in the hospital the patient may be given squares of sterilized gauze to use for this purpose.

After four or five days post partum, when the engorgement has

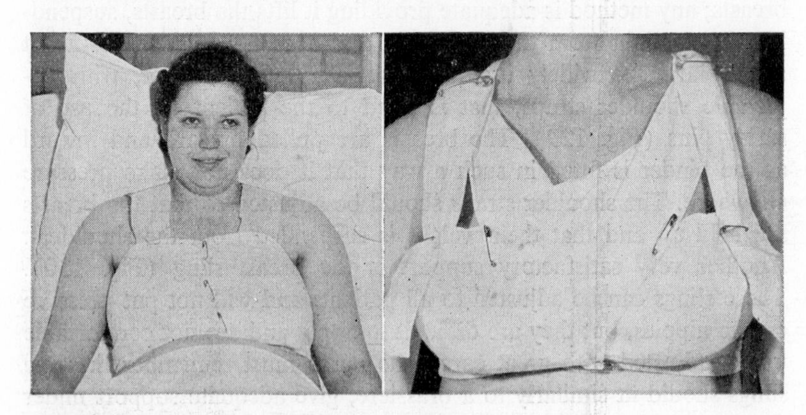

**Fig. 129 (left).** Supporting heavy breasts with a muslin binder. The breasts are pulled upward and inward and the binder fitted so as to avoid pressure at any point. The shoulder straps should be adjusted so that the breasts are lifted upward and their weight suspended from the shoulders.

**Fig. 130 (right).** Supporting breasts with breast slings. To make the breast slings, triangular pieces of heavy cheesecloth are folded twice so that they form a strip of material 6 in. wide and 5 ft long. Two of these strips may be placed into a pack and sterilized for future use. The steps in application of breast slings are as follows:

1. Standing on the right side of the patient, place one sling under the left breast and pin over the right shoulder.
2. Place the second sling under the right breast and pin over the left shoulder.
3. Do not pull these slings snugly since they become tighter with further pinning.
4. Pin the two slings together in the back in the same place that a brassiere is ordinarily hooked.
5. Pin the two strips together in the front by drawing them together snugly so that they make a straight line under the breasts—similar to the fit of a brassiere.
6. Pull up the front of the slings so that a cup is formed to give support to the breasts. The cupped part is pinned to the shoulder straps for added support. The slings should fit so that there is support to the breasts without pressure and they should not pull over the shoulders.

subsided and the baby is nursing well, the breasts should normally be comfortable except for some feeling of fullness just before nursing time. If at any time the patient complains of a *sensitive area* in the breast, there is a possibility that a section of the breast is not being emptied completely. Usually a hard lump or nodular area, known as a *caked breast,* can be palpated under the sensitive portion. As ab-

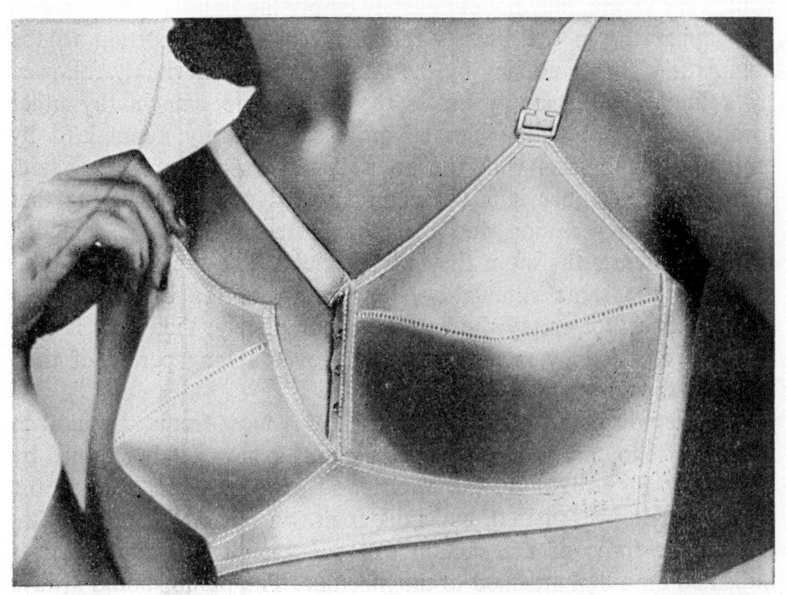

**Fig. 131.** Regular nursing brassiere #7035. The brassiere unhooks in the front for nursing, and each shoulder strap is detachable. Each cup has a moistureproof flannel-lined pad and holders for gauze. (Courtesy of Maiden Form Brassiere Co., Inc., 200 Madison Ave., New York, N. Y.)

scesses may result from caked breasts, particularly if the nipples are sore, it is of great importance that the nurse watch closely for the first evidence of painful lumps and notify the doctor immediately. The application of breast slings and an ice bag as soon as any discomfort appears is important. To attempt to empty the breast more completely the doctor will usually want the breast pump used after the baby nurses. It may take several days for this hard area to soften, but if the patient does not develop a fever it is ordinarily not serious. The nurse must on no account massage caked breasts on her own responsibility, and she instructs the patient not to do so, since massage may bruise the breast tissue and render it more susceptible to infection.

**Methods of Emptying the Breasts.** The natural method of emptying the breasts is by the baby's nursing, but sometimes a frail baby is unable to accomplish this without help, and even a robust baby, while very young, may not completely empty the breasts. As the secretory apparatus in the breasts functions only in proportion to the stimulation, feeble nursing by the baby is almost inevitably followed by a limited milk supply unless the breasts are emptied by other means. Milk production can be quite satisfactorily maintained by emptying the breasts with the breast pump or manual expression. One must remember it is the complete and regular emptying that stimulates the secretion and that the more milk that is removed from the breasts the more they will produce. The breast pump does not have the same stimulation, however, that the baby's sucking has and does not empty the breasts as completely; therefore, if they must be emptied by means of a pump over a long period of time the milk supply may decrease.

The electric breast pump is the apparatus most frequently used in the hospital to empty breasts which cannot be completely emptied by the baby (Fig. 132). By the application of intermittent suction the baby's nursing is imitated, and milk is drawn out of the breast. The amount or force of the suction can be carefully regulated and is indicated on a dial attached to the machine. The pump should always be started with low suction which is gradually increased until the milk flows freely; it is a shock to the patient and painful if the suction is strong at the beginning. The amount of suction can be regulated to suit each individual patient, but unless otherwise specified it is wise not to use more than 6 to 8 lb of pressure.

It usually takes from 10 to 15 minutes to empty the breast and it is not necessary to continue with the pumping much longer even if the breast does not become soft, because the pump is not as effective as the baby and in some instances the milk cannot be drawn out readily. Nothing more is accomplished in a longer period of time.

The water-suction breast pump (Fig. 133) is just as effective as the electric pump and has the added advantage of being cheaper. It is easy to use in the home; however, it is possible to rent an electric breast pump, and the patient may find this more convenient

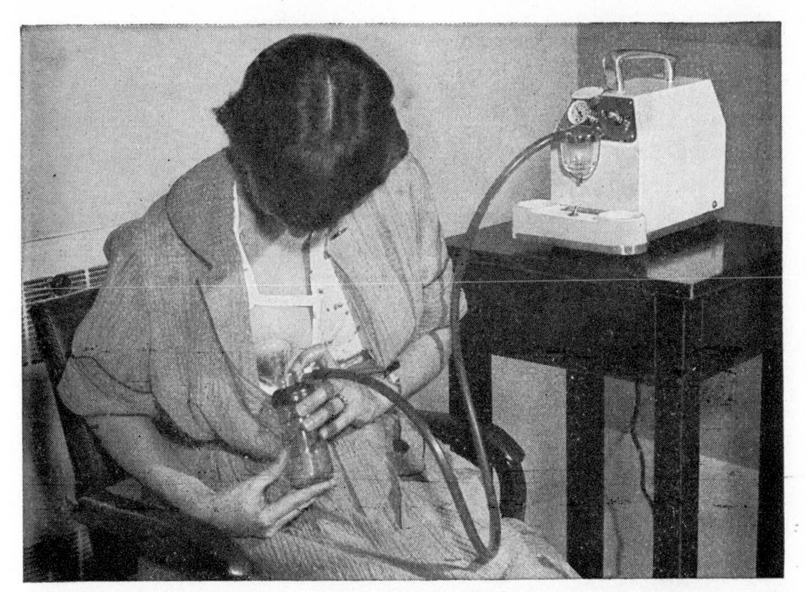

**Fig. 132.** Emptying the breasts by means of an electric breast pump. The patient may be taught how to adjust the amount of suction to her needs and tolerance, and to apply the intermittent suction that is necessary to draw milk out of the breasts.

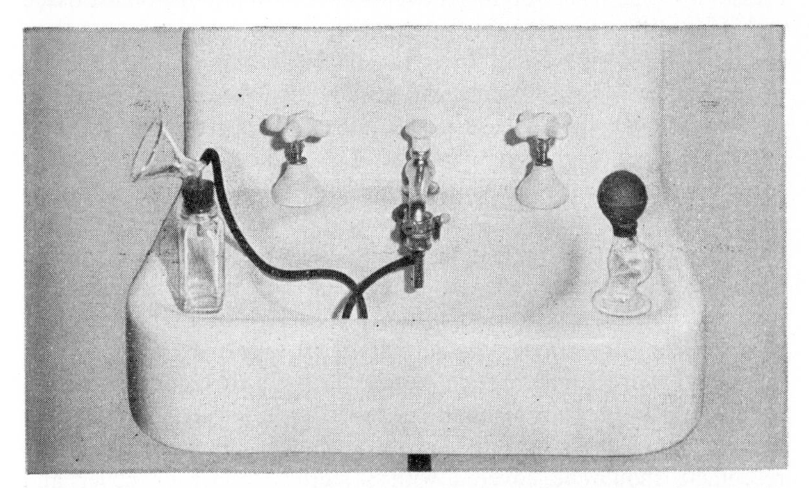

**Fig. 133.** (*Left*) The water-suction pump attached to the faucet. The pressure is obtained by running water. Suction is made and broken by closing and opening the valve on the breast shield. (*Right*) The hand breast pump with which suction is obtained by alternately collapsing and releasing the rubber bulb.

to use at home. The water pump can be attached to any faucet, the pressure being obtained by running water, and the suction can be made and broken by alternately closing and opening the valve on the breast shield with the thumb or finger.

It may be necessary for the mother to use one of the above kinds of breast pumps after her discharge from the hospital if she has to supply breast milk for a premature baby still too weak to nurse. A hand breast pump (Fig. 133) working on the same principle as an Asepto syringe has also been used at times, but its use is a slow process and it is not very satisfactory. The suction is obtained by collapsing the rubber bulb, placing the end of the syringe over the nipple and the areolar area, and then releasing the bulb. If it is impossible to use either the electric or water-suction pump, manual expression may be used.

In preparation for manual expression, the nurse should trim her nails, scrub her hands thoroughly with soap and warm water, and dry them on a sterile towel. The nurse places her hand on the breast with her fingers below as a support and the thumb above, directly opposite the first finger, both being about 1 to 1½ in. from the nipple; she presses the thumb and forefinger deeply backward into the breast tissue and then without moving them forward or in any way changing their position on the skin brings them together well behind the nipple. If properly done this movement will send the milk from the nipple in a stream, which should be directed into a sterile receptacle without coming in contact with anything else. This milking motion should be repeated rhythmically 30 or more times per minute and continued until the breast is empty. In endeavoring to increase or re-establish the milk supply the rhythmical back-and-together motion should be continued for some minutes after the milk has ceased to flow. The mother may be taught to empty her breasts in this way herself and thus stimulate them to increased activity or supply milk for a baby unable to nurse at the breast satisfactorily. Scrupulous cleanliness should be observed throughout any procedure used for emptying the breasts, and if the milk is not given to the baby at once the sterile receptacle should be covered with a sterile stopper or cover and placed in the refrigerator.

Although the normal and most satisfactory method of emptying the breasts is by a robust baby's nursing, there are many circumstances in which artificial emptying is of benefit to both mother and child.

Some babies have to learn to nurse and often do not suck vigorously enough during the first few days of life to stimulate the breasts to secrete an adequate amount of milk; or, after a feeble baby has extracted all the milk he can by nursing, the breasts may be completely emptied by expression and his feeding then complemented by the breast milk thus obtained. This complete emptying has the additional advantage of further stimulating the breast tissues to secrete. When a baby is feeble or immature, it may be given the advantage of breast feeding by having the milk expressed into the sterile receptacle and fed from a nursing bottle. Besides emptying the breasts if the baby does not nurse well, artificial means of emptying may be used to prevent and relieve caked breasts, and to allow fissured nipples to heal by emptying the breasts with less irritation to the nipples than they may receive by vigorous nursing.

**Care of the Nipples.** In the care of the nipples it is important for the nurse to always wash her hands well before handling anything that comes in contact with the breasts or nipples and especially before applying breast slings or dressings. The mother should also be instructed to wash her hands before each nursing time; they will then be clean not only for handling the baby, but also for the necessary handling of the breast slings or dressings. She should be requested not to touch her nipples with her fingers or anything unsterile, and certainly not to examine fissures.

If the nipples are given special care before and after each nursing, they are washed with sterile water using sterile cotton pledgets or applicators. Antiseptic solutions are not recommended, and boric acid is dangerous since the baby may receive a toxic dose. The trend at the present time is to wash the breasts and nipples only once daily, at bath time, using mild soap (sparingly) and water. The skin of the nipples may appear dark because it alters in appearance and it may become crusty; attempts should not be made to wash off these crusts. The breasts should be washed first when the bath is taken, and a clean washcloth and towel should be used each day. More frequent washing is not done; further care consists only of keeping the nipples covered with sterile gauze, breast support, or towel. Niles Newton in *Maternal Emotions* says that:

The standard advice to mothers is to keep their nipples clean. Nipples in our society are well protected by clothing from outside soil so that the "dirt" mothers wash off is mostly the natural accumulation of sweat, sebum, and milk.

These nipple secretions are probably very important to the health of the nipple skin by preparing it to withstand vigorous sucking.[24] Sweat with sebum has antibacterial properties. Sebum is an important contributor to the protective covering of the skin, and helps to keep the skin pliable. Sweat may also help to keep the skin pliable and normally acid. The breast milk itself may also contribute to the health of the nipple skin. Newly secreted human milk is very rich in lysozyme—an antibacterial substance.

The result of keeping the nipples "clean" is damaged nipples and excruciating pain in some instances. An experimental study [24] found that mothers washing their nipples with soap solution had more nipple pain on all five days of their hospital stay than the control group who used only water. The pain was both more frequent and more extreme. Nipple pain in turn caused a limitation of sucking and the failure of breast feeding.*

In the hospital, between nursing periods, the nipples are covered by some sort of protective dressing. Sterile gauze is probably the most common of all breast dressings and may be held in place by the breast binder, sling, or brassiere. If milk does not leak from the breasts the gauze is not necessary when sterile slings or binders are worn. Sterile towels pinned inside the nightgown may be used by the patients who do not wear a breast support. These precautions will protect the nipples from becoming contaminated from the patient's hands, clothing, or bedding.

After the mother leaves the hospital she will find it necessary to use breast pads to protect her clothing against the milk which often leaks out of the breasts. Disposable breast pads, which may be worn inside a brassiere, are available for this purpose and prove very satisfactory. If the mother feels that their cost is prohibitive she may use pieces of cloth from worn towels or other absorbent material; these are washed with care, and ironed if sterilization seems necessary, and used over and over. Squares of cellucotton may also be suggested.

Nipple pain and *cracked* or *fissured nipples* are common early in the lactation period, especially between the third and fifth day. Although adequate nursing is important to the stimulation of milk secretion, the nipples must be protected against prolonged use in the beginning of the lactation period to prevent irritation. Since the

* Newton, Niles: *Maternal Emotions.* Paul B. Hoeber, Inc., New York, 1955, p. 45.

nipples will at first naturally be somewhat sensitive to a baby's sucking, the baby is allowed to nurse for only 5 to 10 minutes during the first two days; this time may then be gradually increased as it becomes evident that the nipples can tolerate longer periods of sucking. Nipples are very apt to become sore when the baby cannot grasp them well; he may then chew at them in his efforts to suck. The nurse must try to help the mother get the entire nipple, and part of the areolar area, into the baby's mouth during the early days of sucking, when he may have difficulty in grasping the nipple. It is often very difficult for the baby to get the nipple into his mouth during the period of engorgement when the breasts are tense; flat nipples are likewise hard to grasp. If the nipples are flat or somewhat retracted, the mother may attempt to nurse her baby and to pump the breasts after nursing as necessary; some babies can suck from a flat nipple, but if, after several days' trial, it is found that the baby cannot grasp the nipple easily, it is usually advisable to discontinue the breast feeding. The nurse must watch the condition of the nipples very carefully, and if they begin to appear even slightly irritated or if the mother complains of pain while nursing, measures should be taken to prevent fissures. Small cracks or fissures cause much discomfort and provide an entrance for bacteria; sometimes these begin as small blisters. It is well to check again on the length of time the mother is nursing her baby because some, in spite of previous instruction, will nurse their babies for 25 to 30 minutes, since, if the baby is willing to nurse, they think he must surely be getting milk. It may even be necessary to decrease the time of nursing to five minutes when the nipples become sore. The mother can be told that she may lengthen the time and satisfy the baby's desire to suck after her nipples become toughened.

A widely employed method of treatment for sore nipples is to apply an ointment after each nursing and then squares of sterile wax paper to keep the ointment from being absorbed by the gauze or towel placed over the breasts (Fig. 134). These squares of wax paper are pressed into place and held for a moment by the hand, the warmth of which softens and molds them to the breast so that they remain in place. The ointments most frequently used are a vitamin A and D mixture, a lanolin ointment, or one of the preparations for treatment of sore nipples which is on the market, such as Massé nipple cream. The ointment can be removed from the nipple with a sterile gauze square before the baby is nursed. Sometimes the nipples are exposed to the air for short periods of time for purposes of drying them.

With the above treatment the nipples usually heal, become toughened, and cause no more trouble. They must be watched carefully,

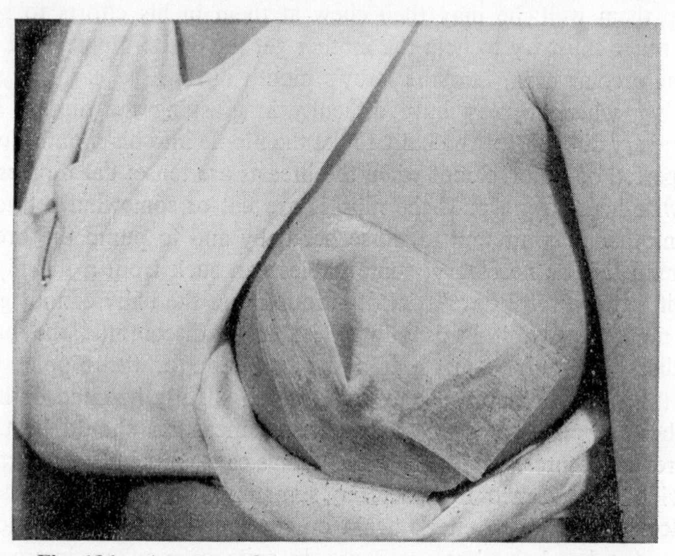

**Fig. 134.** A square of sterile wax paper placed over the nipple to which an ointment has been applied. The wax paper prevents absorption of the ointment onto the sling or brassiere. This picture also shows how the breast sling may be folded down for nursing the baby, thus making it unnecessary to remove the entire sling at that time.

however, because they may become cracked and the abrasion may become extensive enough to cause bleeding; even a fissure which is barely visible may be deep enough to bleed, and the baby may swallow blood while nursing. Severe fissures or abraded areas are sometimes painted with an astringent or antiseptic; compound tincture of benzoin, balsam of Peru, mild protein silver (Argyrol), or 2 to 5 per cent silver nitrate solution being most frequently used. The application of ointment is also continued, but the most important treatment is temporary discontinuance of nursing, which gives the nipples rest and allows them to heal. When they are cracked and bleeding, one can easily understand that continued suckling would only aggravate the condition and increase the danger of infection. A nipple shield is sometimes used as a protection during the nursing, but it is not very satisfactory because most babies cannot empty the breast through the shield; then the breasts will either never be completely emptied or the pump must be used afterward, and this only prolongs the irritation. When the nipples must be given a rest from the baby's sucking it is better to use the breast pump or manual expression than to use the nipple shield. Either of these will rest the nipples and give them an opportunity to heal, while at the same time the baby is supplied with breast milk and the breasts are stimulated to continue their secretion. With 24 to 48 hours of rest the nipples will heal sufficiently to allow the baby to nurse again. After they have healed they are usually quite tough and seldom become cracked a second time. In a few cases, however, the nipples do not heal or become very sore again when nursing is resumed, and it may be necessary to discontinue nursing entirely.

The nurse will appreciate the reason for all this painstaking care if she will call to mind the fact that the breast tissue is highly vascular and at this time very active metabolically and therefore particularly susceptible to infection. The baby's sucking may be very vigorous and is sometimes accompanied by a good deal of chewing and gnawing of the nipples. Since some patients have a particularly sensitive skin, the skin may become abraded or cracked as a result of the baby's sucking, and a portal of entry for pathogenic organisms is created in addition to that of the milk ducts which lead back into the breast tissue. Sound, uninjured nipples, then, are to be kept clean and protected from pathogenic organisms. Those that are abraded or cracked are to be handled as little as possible, kept clean, and when necessary protected against further injury by means of manual expression or the breast pump.

**Drying Up the Breasts.** This becomes necessary when the baby is stillborn or dies, or a mother does not wish or is unable to nurse her baby. Formerly lotions, ointments, and binders were employed and often a breast pump as well. Various drugs were given by mouth, and the patient was put on a rigid diet; cathartics were given and fluids were restricted. It is true that some of these measures are still employed and are followed by a disappearance of the milk, but at the same time the breasts dry up quite as satisfactorily when none of these things is done, provided the baby does not nurse. The breasts may be engorged and very uncomfortable for a day or two, but the secretion of milk will subside when activity of the breasts is not stimulated by the baby's sucking. For this same reason the breast pump should not be used because emptying the breasts merely stimulates them to secrete more milk. During the day or two that the patient is uncomfortable with engorgement, the discomfort should be relieved as much as possible. Some doctors want the patient to wear slings to support the heavy breasts, which gives relief from pain, while others prefer a tight binder. The application of ice bags and the administration of analgesic drugs will also help to relieve the discomfort. Naturally, the nurse will not press the patient to drink an extra amount of milk or other fluids if it is not desirable to promote the activity of the breasts, but, unless otherwise ordered, there is no necessity for placing restrictions upon the patient's fluid intake.

The breasts become soft and comfortable in 24 to 48 hours, and the secretion becomes less and almost disappears in one week; but a small amount of milk may be present in the breasts for several weeks, and a few drops will drain out occasionally.

Estrogens or androgens, or a combination of both, are used by many physicians to suppress lactation. It is believed either to inhibit the development of the lactogenic hormone or to prevent the hormone from stimulating the breasts to function. They must be started as soon as possible after delivery to be effective and are not used once the breasts have begun to lactate. Lactation is not always entirely suppressed, and the engorgement may appear on the tenth day or even later; but it is not as severe as it would have been without the use of these substances and it disappears more quickly. It is well to warn the patient that she may have some filling of the breasts after she leaves the hospital. These preparations are sometimes given in fairly large doses over a period of one week or in a lower dosage for 10 to 15 days. Diethylstilbestrol was one of the first estrogenic substances used for this purpose and it is still quite frequently used; others are now available. Some physicians do not use any of these substances to suppress lactation; some do not use diethylstilbestrol because it stimulates growth of the endometrium, and if this is excessive it may cause postpartum bleeding, which in some cases may be profuse.

**Diet.** Opinions as to diet vary slightly with different doctors and in different hospitals, but, in general, a patient in good condition may be given light food the first 12 to 24 hours followed by a general diet or she may be offered a general diet immediately after delivery. In planning the patient's diet the nurse must keep in mind that the function of her breasts must be promoted to produce milk of a quality and quantity adequate to nourish the baby.

The best producer of such milk is a diet which includes calories, proteins, minerals, and vitamins above the normal requirements for the patient. The nurse will do well to convince the patient of this, in addition to bearing it in mind herself, and to place little reliance on so-called milk-producing preparations. If the patient has had a toxemia of pregnancy, a high-protein, sodium-poor diet may need to be continued for at least a few days during the puerperium. In addition to her food the nursing mother should have an abundance of water to drink, and to facilitate this it is a good plan to keep a pitcher or Thermos bottle of water on the bedside table and replenish it every four hours.

The diet of the nursing mother is discussed in greater detail in Chapter 17, "The Nursing Mother."

**Drugs.** There is little need for the use of drugs in the care of the postpartum patient, and their use should be limited whenever possible. Many drugs are excreted through the milk and may affect the baby in the same way as though they were administered directly; for example, salicylic acid, potassium iodine, lead, mercury, iron, arsenic, atropine, chloral hydrate, alcohol, opium, and various cathartics. Opium derivatives are sometimes used for the control of pain the first day or two, but are usually not necessary after the baby begins to obtain milk, and cathartics can be avoided by proper diet, exercise, and the use of mineral oil at night. Various drugs, known as galactogogues, have been recommended from time to time as stimulants to milk production, but have not proved of value. Vitamins, either as multivitamins or as concentrates of A and D, are usually prescribed for the mother while she is nursing her baby. Iron may be ordered if she is anemic.

**Position in Bed.** After the first few hours following delivery, during which time the patient should lie quietly to rest, she should be allowed and urged to move about freely in bed and to sit up. Sometimes the patient is encouraged to lie first on one side and then on the other, and then face downward at intervals, in order to change the position of the uterus and thus tend to prevent backward displacement.

**Visitors.** Restriction of visitors, except for the immediate family, during the first few days of the puerperium is recommended, and some hospitals allow only members of the immediate family throughout the entire hospital stay. The limitation of visitors for the first four or five days gives the mother more opportunity to rest and prevents her from being disturbed during the time that she may be uncomfortable from either perineal pain or breast engorgement. Certainly no one with a cold or other infection should be allowed to visit in an obstetric nursing unit. Children are not permitted to visit in order to prevent an outbreak of contagious diseases.

**Abdominal Binders.** There is considerable difference of opinion about the advantage of using abdominal binders for the puerperal patient, and the nurse will accordingly care for the patients of some doctors who use them and for those of others who do not. The application of a moderately snug binder for the first day or two is a fairly common practice, since multiparas, particularly, may be made uncomfortable by the sudden release of tension on their flabby abdominal walls, a discomfort which a binder will relieve. During the first few days after the patient gets up and walks about, she is sometimes given great comfort by a binder that is put on as she lies on her back and is adjusted snugly about her hips and the lower part of her abdomen. The binder often relieves a feeling of emptiness in the abdomen.

The continued use of a binder after the first day or two is not as general as it formerly was. Some women ask for binders in the belief that they help to "get the figure back" to its original outline, and some doctors feel that the use of the binder is helpful in restoring tone to the abdominal muscles, which amounts to about the same thing. Both the straight swathe and the Scultetus binder are used for this purpose, and they are put on in the usual manner, snugly and with even pressure, but not uncomfortably tight.

Those doctors who disapprove of the binder believe that it interferes with involution and by making pressure tends to push the uterus back and cause a retroposition, in addition to retarding, instead of promoting, a return of normal tone to the abdominal muscles. Accordingly, these doctors instruct their patients that exercise, instead of binders, will restore muscle tone.

**Ambulation.** The time for getting the puerperal patient out of bed has changed considerably during the past 10 to 15 years. It had been customary before this time to keep all patients in bed for 7 to 10 days, get them up gradually, perhaps only an hour the first day, over a period of several days, and allow them to go home between the twelfth to fourteenth day. At the present time patients are allowed up within 24 hours. Getting up may be done gradually by sitting on the edge of the bed at first and on the same or following day sitting up in a chair or walking around the room, or it may be done more quickly by having the patient get up and walk as soon as she is allowed to be out of bed. Some doctors prefer that the patient walk rather than sit when she first gets up because walking has a favorable effect on circulation, whereas sitting may promote venous stasis in the legs. The patient should be assisted by a nurse the first time she gets out of bed.

Early rising dates back to ancient times and has varied widely in the customs of different people. Some writers even early in the nineteenth century said that the earlier a patient got out of bed the better and that an upright position helped to expel blood. Others believed that these patients should be kept in bed three weeks because of danger of prolapse of the uterus. There have been all variations between these two extremes. Difficulty encountered in keeping the patient delivered at home in bed first called attention to early rising, and a shortage of hospital beds stimulated an interest in attempting to get patients up early. The time that a patient remained in bed was gradually decreased until the present regimen of getting up on the first to second day post partum was determined.

Early rising means controlled ambulation. Activity is usually increased quite rapidly, but there should be frequent rest periods. Because this is best controlled in the hospital and because it is still considered necessary to give postpartum care to the breasts and perineum, the patient is usually not discharged from the hospital before the fifth to eighth day after delivery.

Many good effects have been noticed with early ambulation. Involution is hastened, lochia decreases rapidly, the episiotomy heals well, and it helps to prevent pulmonary complications and thrombophlebitis. The patient has a general feeling of well-being with less debility and less depression and in general has a more rapid and comfortable convalescence than she did when she stayed in bed a week or more. It is too soon to know the end results of early rising, especially in regard to prolapse and relaxation, complications which were most expected, but thus far no harmful effects have been noted. Cases of retroversion of the uterus have apparently not increased.

**Exercises.** The general purpose of exercise is to strengthen the abdominal muscles, thus helping to prevent a large pendulous abdomen; to strengthen the perineal muscles; to increase the patient's

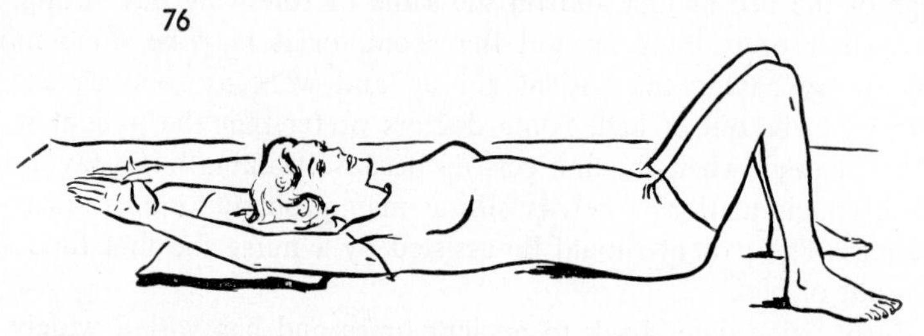


**Fig. 135.** Stretching main trunk muscles. (Reproduced from the *Reminder Sheets for Exercises, Rest Positions, Breathing and Relaxing Techniques,* published by Maternity Center Association, New York City, with their permission.)

general tone, just as exercise benefits the average person; to promote involution; to prevent retroversion; and to prevent thrombophlebitis. To accomplish these much-to-be-desired ends the exercise must be taken with moderation and judgment, started slowly, increased very gradually, and constantly adapted to the strength of the individual patient.

Some doctors do not recommend regular early exercises, but instead only encourage the patient to be as active as she feels able; others recommend that certain prescribed exercises be started on the second postpartum day. When exercises are prescribed to be started early they are usually light exercises which do not require much exertion; more strenuous exercises are begun later, approximately two to three weeks after the baby is born.

The main trunk muscles may be stretched by *extending the arms* well above the head while lying on a flat surface (Fig. 135). In the *knee-to-chest exercise* the back muscles from head to coccyx are stretched by touching the knees to the chin. This also aids in strengthening the abdominal muscles. In this exercise the patient lies on a flat surface, flexes her knees on the abdomen and the legs on the thighs, and then attempts to touch her knees and chin by bringing her knees up and her chin down (Fig. 136). A *leg-raising exercise* is frequently prescribed to strengthen the abdominal muscles. While lying on the back one leg is raised, without bending the knee, and let down slowly; then the other leg is raised and lowered slowly. Later both legs are raised at once, starting by lifting the heels off the floor, and increasing this distance until the legs are raised com-

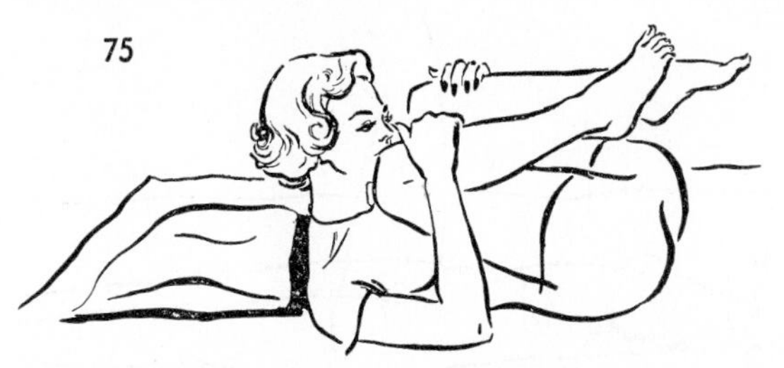


**Fig. 136.** Stretching back muscles from head to coccyx. (Reproduced from *Reminder Sheets for Exercises, Rest Positions, Breathing and Relaxing Techniques,* published by Maternity Center Association, New York City, with their permission.)

pletely (Fig. 137). The abdominal muscles may also be strengthened by *raising from a recumbent to a half-sitting position.* While lying on the back, without a pillow, the arms are crossed on the chest. In the beginning the head and shoulders are raised just enough to clear the floor; later this exercise is carried to a sitting position while the feet are crossed and the hands are clasped behind the head (Fig. 138). As these exercises require much effort they must be increased very gradually. They may be done only once or twice on the first day, two or three times on the second day, and so on, if the patient is not fatigued, until they are repeated up to 10 times each morning and evening. These exercises should be continued for several months; the results will depend upon the amount of stretching during pregnancy and the ability of the muscles to regain their tone, as well as how faithfully the patient carries out these exercises.

The pelvic floor muscles may be strengthened by alternately contracting and relaxing them slowly and smoothly. To carry out this exercise the patient usually lies on a flat surface, her breathing should be natural, and her abdominal muscles should be relaxed (Fig. 139).

To help the uterus return to a good position the woman may lie in a prone position, with her abdomen and her feet resting on pillows, while she is resting and relaxing (Fig. 140). The *knee-chest position*

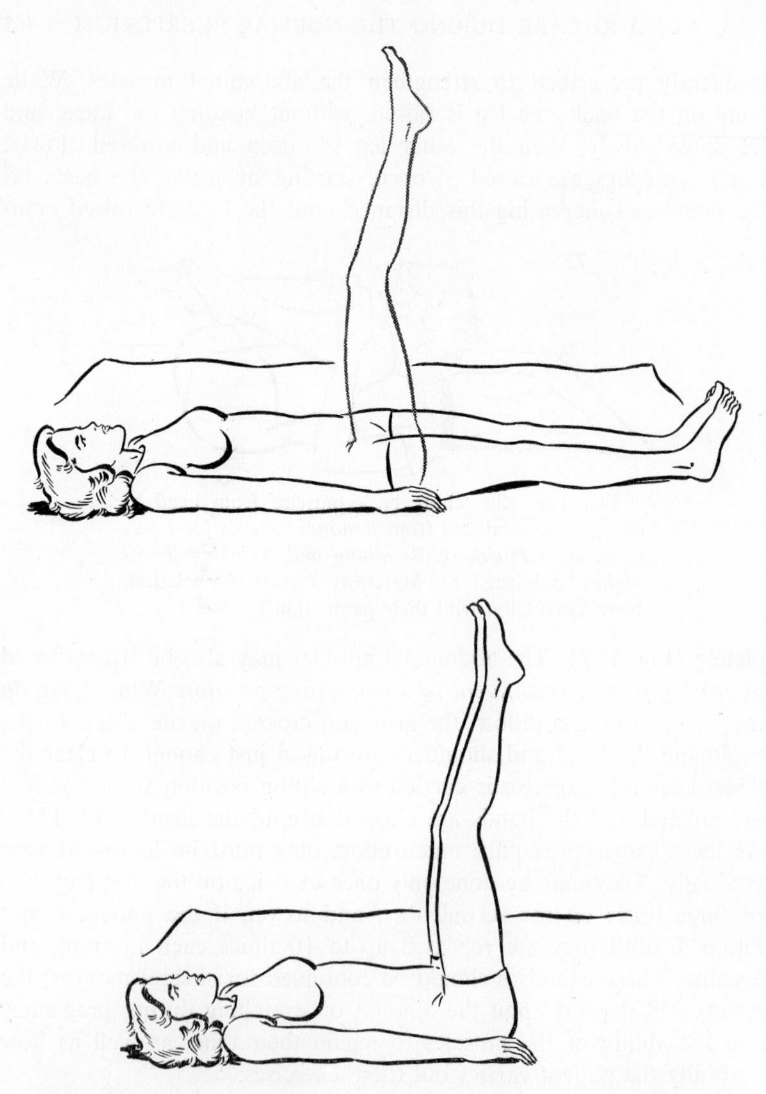

**Fig. 137.** Strengthening the abdominal muscles by raising and lowering the legs. While lying on the back the right leg is raised, without bending the knee, and let down slowly. Next the left leg is raised and lowered slowly. Later both legs are raised at once, beginning usually by merely lifting the heels off the floor and increasing this distance until the legs are raised completely.

is used in some cases for several months after delivery to correct a retroversion of the uterus (Fig. 141). The patient rests on her knees and chest for a few minutes, being particularly careful while assuming this position that the thighs are perpendicular to the floor and that

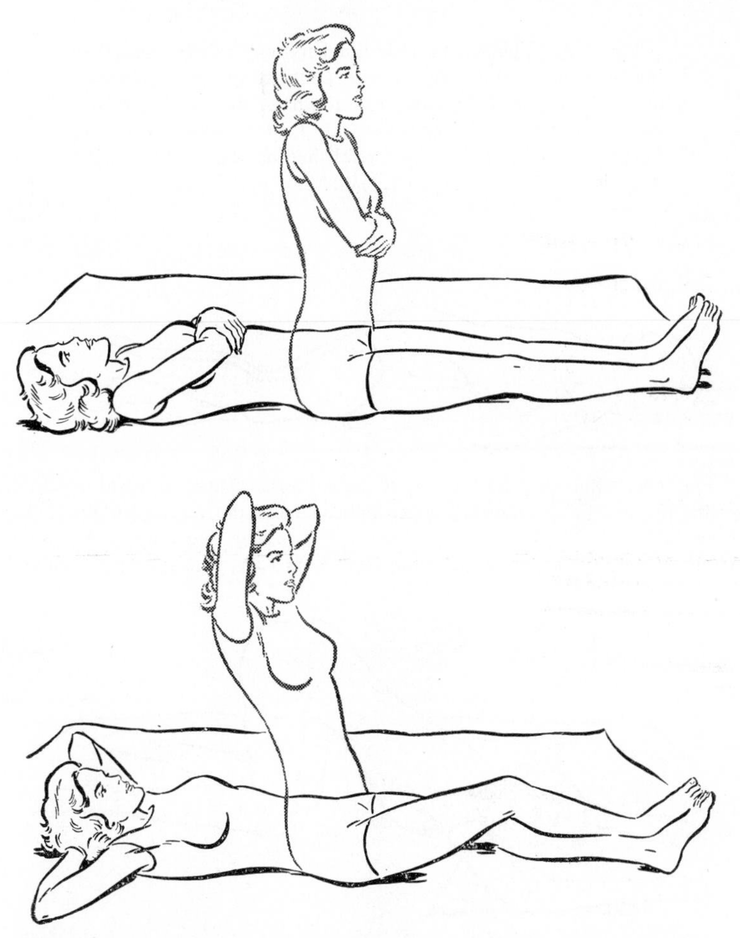

**Fig. 138.** Strengthening the abdominal muscles by raising from a recumbent to a half-sitting position. This exercise is started while lying on the back, without a pillow, and crossing the arms on the chest. At first the head and shoulders are raised just enough to clear the floor. Later this exercise is carried to the sitting posture while the feet are crossed and the hands are clasped behind the head.

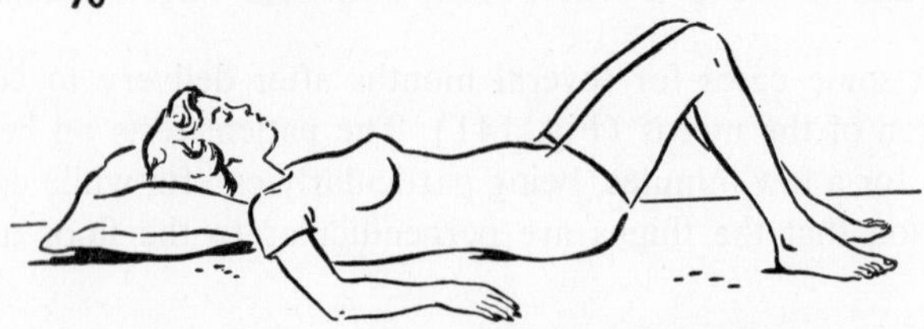

**Fig. 139.** Lying with abdominal muscles relaxed, breathing naturally while alternately contracting and relaxing pelvic floor muscles slowly and smoothly. (Reproduced from the *Reminder Sheets for Exercises, Rest Positions, Breathing and Relaxing Techniques,* published by Maternity Center Association, New York City, with their permission.)

**71**

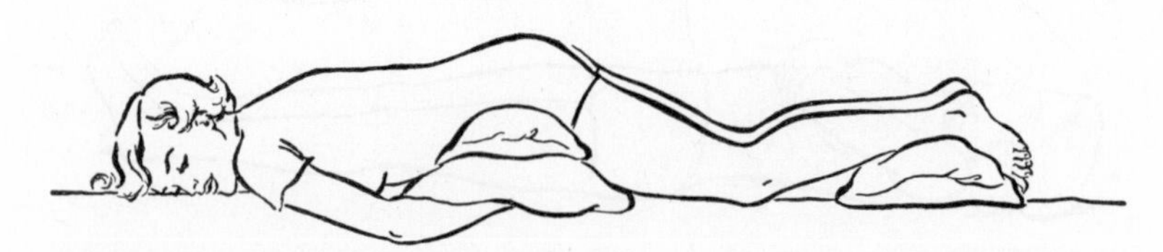

**Fig. 140.** Relaxing face down to help uterus return to good position, palms up, breathing naturally. (Reproduced from the *Reminder Sheets for Exercises, Rest Positions, Breathing and Relaxing Techniques,* published by the Maternity Center Association, New York City, with their permission.)

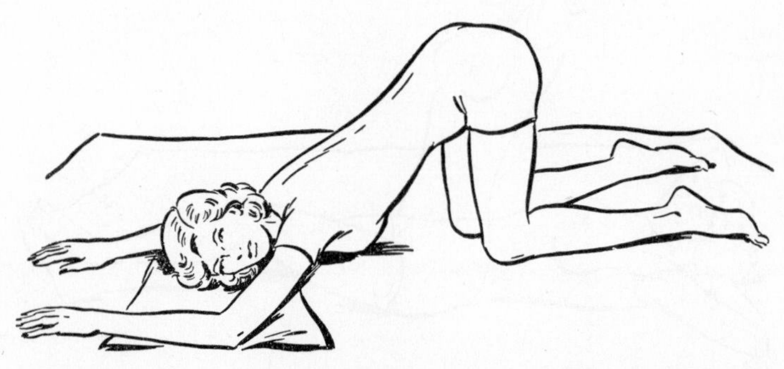

**Fig. 141.** The knee-chest position. The body rests on the knees and chest. The thighs must be kept perpendicular to the floor, the upper part of the body should rest on the chest, which must be brought down to the floor, instead of resting on the elbows, and the back must not be allowed to sag. With the body in this position the uterus gravitates forward.

the upper part of the body rests on the chest instead of the elbows. The back must not be allowed to sag. The position is most effective when there is no constriction around the waist from clothing and when the vagina is opened after the position is assumed to allow air to enter. This exercise is usually taken twice daily for one minute at first and gradually increased to as long as 10 minutes. While this position is maintained the pressure of the abdominal viscera on the pelvic organs is relieved, the uterus falls forward into its normal position, and the circulation to the pelvis is improved.

## DISCHARGE EXAMINATION AND INSTRUCTIONS

When the patient leaves the hospital she is given a thorough examination and instructions as to her care for the next few weeks. At this time the doctor inspects the breasts for areas of caking and the nipples for fissures; he examines the perineum to determine how well the repair has healed and the abdominal wall for relaxation. Also, the uterus is examined for position and amount of involution, the cervix for healing of lacerations, and the vaginal wall for degree of relaxation. If the patient leaves the hospital before the seventh to eighth day the pelvic checkup may be omitted, and she may be instructed to return in one to two weeks for the completion of the examination. Before she leaves she is given instructions as to her care for the next four to six weeks or until she sees the doctor again. If the uterus is not well involuted or is retroverted, she may be given an order to take more ergonovine and may be told how to carry out exercises to help the uterus return to a good position. She may be instructed in taking douches, is given exercises to strengthen the abdominal wall, and is instructed in the rate at which she may resume her normal activities. She is usually told not to go up and down stairs for the first week at home and to limit her work to feeding and bathing the baby during this time. After the first week she may gradually return to her usual work and may go outdoors for a longer period of time. It is best for her not to resume all normal activities before six weeks after delivery, but due to financial reasons some women do all their own work earlier. The time at which the doctor allows the patient to take tub baths varies from two to four weeks. All patients are instructed to have no sexual intercourse for six weeks. If the mother is nursing her baby, the care of her breasts and nipples and the diet and vitamins that she should take are discussed with her. It is important to relieve her of as much worry as possible over the care of her baby by making certain that she is well informed about his care. Referral to a visiting nurse agency is extremely important since the public health nurse can make a valuable contribution in helping the mother apply her knowledge of her own and her baby's care to the home situation and can give assistance with other problems that may arise.

Quite evidently, then, some ill health and certain gynecologic problems may be prevented by good care during the first few days and weeks after the baby's birth.

In addition to this sustained, general care, it is a customary preventive measure for the doctor to make a thorough pelvic examination from four to six weeks after delivery. By this time the reproductive organs have usually returned to their normal state. Again the condition of the breasts, nipples, perineum, uterus, cervix, abdominal wall, and support to the rectum and bladder are observed. A slight abnormality, if detected at this time, can usually be corrected with little difficulty, but if allowed to persist it may result in a more serious problem and prolonged treatment. If the uterus is not properly involuted, for example, or the perineum is not well healed, douches and sitz baths may be ordered; a uterine displacement, which seems to be present in about one-third of all cases, may be treated by postural exercises or a pessary. If the cervix is red and eroded and an irritating discharge is present, a cauterization of the involved areas may be necessary. All cervical lesions should receive careful treatment to prevent the possibility of these areas predisposing to gynecologic problems sometime later. At this six-weeks' examination the blood pressure and the weight are checked, a urinalysis is done, and a blood count may be taken (Fig. 142).

The pelvic examinations are usually repeated in six months and one year. This will sometimes reveal abnormalities which were not present at the six-weeks' examination; cervical erosion may need treatment at this time or follow-up examinations on complications of pregnancy, such as the toxemias, may be indicated. Adequate postpartum care over a period of a year may prevent or cure many conditions which would otherwise cause trouble in later years.

In summarizing the nursing care of the patient during the puerperium it is evident that this includes both physical and emotional care. Physical care includes meeting all of the mother's bodily needs, relieving physical discomforts, helping to prevent postpartum complications, and making observations of the patient's physical status. In order to inform the doctor promptly of any departure from the normal in the patient's condition, the nurse's watchfulness should embrace regular observations and recording upon the following:

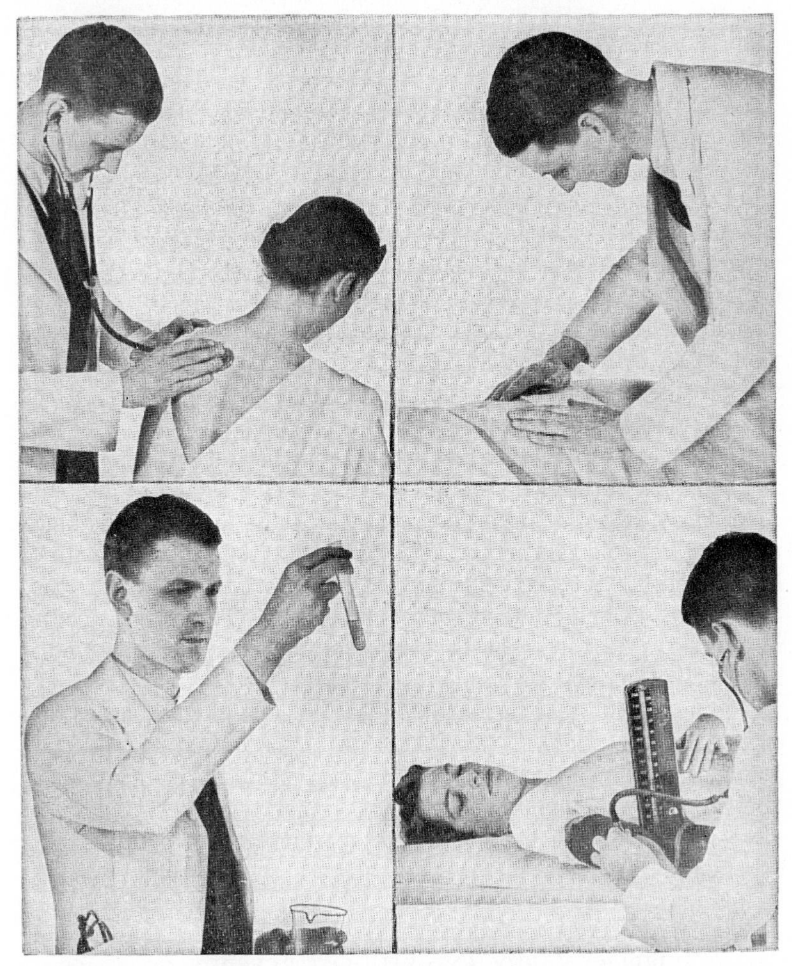

**Fig. 142.** A check-up six weeks and three months after the baby comes, for follow-up evaluation and instruction. (Reproduced with the permission of Maternity Center Association, New York City.)

1. The patient's general condition, the amount and character of her sleep and activity, her appetite, and her nervous and mental condition
2. The temperature, pulse, and respiration
3. The height and consistency of the fundus
4. The quantity, color, and odor of the lochia
5. The persistence and severity of afterpains
6. The condition of the perineum
7. The condition of the nipples and breasts
8. The functions of the bladder and bowels

As has been mentioned previously, postpartum nursing care consists not only of providing for the mother's physical care, but also includes meeting her emotional needs. Physical needs are usually quite obvious and easily met. The physical needs of many postpartum patients are minimal because the new mother is primarily a well person who is soon able to care for herself. Unless the nurse recognizes her role in giving emotional support to the mother, and in teaching the new mother, she may not find the care of postpartum patients an entirely satisfying experience. Giving emotional support will provide the nurse with satisfactions that she would miss if she saw the mother only as a person who needed physical care, and perhaps not much of that. The new mother may have dependency needs, and the nurse must recognize these needs and be willing to give care accordingly. She may need guidance in working through her adjustments to her role as a mother; she needs instructions in the care of herself and her baby; and she needs an understanding of the physiologic processes that are taking place in her body. The mother needs a nurse who is friendly, shows warmth and understanding, and who is interested in her and her family.

The nurse who sees the mother's less obvious physical needs and cares for them, and who has a concept of the postpartum patient's potential emotional needs, recognizes these needs when they appear (perhaps in an intangible way), and then makes every effort to meet these needs will find nursing the postpartum patient a challenging experience.

## BIBLIOGRAPHY AND STUDENT REFERENCES

Benedek, Therese: "The Psychosomatic Implications of the Primary Unit: Mother–Child," *Am. J. Orthopsychiat.*, **19**:642–54, (Oct.) 1949.

Bookmiller, Mae M., and Bowen, George L.: *Textbook of Obstetrics and Obstetric Nursing,* 2nd ed. W. B. Saunders Co., Philadelphia, 1954.

Casper, Thelma A., and Cawley, Marie: "Early Ambulation and Postpartum Care," *Am. J. Nursing,* **52**:1210–11, (Oct.) 1952.

Davies, Velma, and Pratt, J. P.: "The Stimulation and Maintenance of Lactation," *Am. J. Nursing,* **46**:242–44, (Apr.) 1946.

Davis, M. Edward, and Sheckler, Catherine E.: *DeLee's Obstetrics for Nurses,* 15th ed. W. B. Saunders Co., Philadelphia, 1951.

DeClue, Jayne F.: "Early Ambulation in a Postpartum Unit," *Am. J. Nursing,* **54**:295–96, (Mar.) 1954.

Eastman, Nicholson J.: *Williams Obstetrics,* 11th ed. Appleton-Century-Crofts, Inc., New York, 1956.

Greenhill, J. P. (ed): *Obstetrics,* 11th ed. W. B. Saunders Co., Philadelphia, 1955.

Haufrecht, Fred: "A Procedure to Reduce Perineal Discomfort in the Puerperium," *Am. J. Obst. & Gynec.,* **70**:205–7, (July) 1955.

Javert, Carl T.: "The Immediate Postpartum Period as a Fourth Stage of Labor," *Am. J. Obst. & Gynec.,* **54**:1028–32, (Dec.) 1947.

Kline, Carl L.: "Emotional Illness Associated with Childbirth," *Am. J. Obst. & Gynec.,* **69**:748–57, (Apr.) 1955.

Leithauser, Daniel: "Early Ambulation," *Am. J. Nursing,* **50**:203–6, (Apr.) 1950.

Lesser, Marion S., and Keane, Vera R.: *Nurse–Patient Relationships in a Hospital Maternity Service.* C. V. Mosby Co., St. Louis, 1956.

Mahoney, Viola: "Perineal Irrigation Simplified," *Am. J. Nursing,* **44**:145–46, (Feb.) 1944.

Maternity Center Association: "Long Range Effects of Early Ambulation," *Briefs,* **18**:10–11, (Nov.) 1954.

Miller, Norman F.: "Why Mothers Go Home," *Mod. Hosp.,* **79**:81–82, (Nov.) 1952.

Newton, Michael, and Newton, Niles: "Postpartum Engorgement of the Breast," *Am. J. Obst. & Gynec.,* **61**:664–67, (Mar.) 1951.

Newton, Niles: "Nipple Pain and Nipple Damage: Problems in the Management of Breast Feeding," *J. Pediat.,* **41**:411–23, (Oct.) 1952.

———: *Maternal Emotions.* Paul B. Hoeber, Inc., New York, 1955.

Peck, Elizabeth: "Perineal Care," *Am. J. Nursing,* **47**:170–71, (Mar.) 1947.

Rosenblum, Gordon; Melinkoff, Eugene; and Fist, Harry S.: "Early Rising in the Puerperium," *J.A.M.A.,* **129**:849–53, (Nov. 24) 1945.

Wiedenbach, Ernestine: "Safeguard the Mother's Breasts," *Am. J. Nursing,* **51**:544–48, (Sept.) 1951.

Woodward, H. L.; Gardner, B.; Bryant, R. D.; and Overland, Anna E.: *Obstetric Management and Nursing,* 5th ed. F. A. Davis Co., Philadelphia, 1955.

Zabriskie, Louise, and Eastman, Nicholson J.: *Nurses Handbook of Obstetrics,* 9th ed. J. B. Lippincott Co., Philadelphia, 1952.

*Chapter 17*

# The Nursing Mother

From the standpoint of survival of the newborn, breast feeding is no longer the necessity that it was before the development of satisfactory artificial feeding, but there are many other advantages to breast feeding which should be given careful consideration.

## FACTORS IMPORTANT TO SUCCESSFUL BREAST FEEDING

**Advantages of Breast Feeding.** Breast milk is still the best food for the normal newborn; it is more readily digested and assimilated than cow's milk. Breast-fed babies have fewer and less serious gastrointestinal disturbances and less respiratory infections than the artificially fed babies and also have a greater immunity to some of the childhood diseases. Breast-fed babies seem to show more general body activity. Some studies have shown that breast-fed babies have a lower morbidity and mortality rate than the artificially fed, although this depends upon the environment and culture in which artificial feedings are given. When a mother is breast feeding satisfactorily the milk is always clean, available, and of the proper temperature, and there is no need for sterilization and refrigeration of formula.

Breast feeding helps to meet the baby's emotional as well as his physical needs. It gives him a feeling of security, providing closeness to his mother. The milk flow is well regulated, and he can suck until he is satisfied and take the amount of food that he wishes without being regulated as to amount. Breast feeding is also satisfying to the mother who really wishes to breast-feed her baby; it meets the mother's need for a continued close relationship to her baby and thus helps to satisfy her maternal emotions.

**Factors Affecting Breast Feeding.** Psychologic, sociologic, and physical factors enter into whether a mother breast-feeds her baby successfully or unsuccessfully or makes no attempt to breast-feed. Some mothers honestly wish to breast-feed their babies; some nurse their babies, but do not feel that it makes much difference to the baby if they must change to artificial feeding; some try to breast-feed even when they prefer to give an artificial feeding; and some are definitely opposed to breast feeding. Some mothers do not seem to be emotionally ready to breast-feed their babies; to others the idea of breast feeding is distasteful. To some the idea of breast feeding seems rather primitive or they feel that it may be disfiguring or too tiring. Some mothers do not breast-feed because the custom in a community is to give bottle feedings, especially since artificial feedings have become safer and easier in recent years. We must admit that with the complexity of modern life and the general home and social circumstances, to which many women are accustomed before their babies are born, breast feeding may present a problem. Some of these mothers may wish to breast-feed, but believe they may be criticized by friends and relatives who do not particularly approve of this method of feeding. The husband's feelings regarding breast feeding also enter into a woman's decision. Some women feel that they can leave the care of the baby to others more easily when he is fed by bottle. Some express the belief that their milk may not be good for the baby or they think they will worry if they do not know just how much milk the baby is taking at each feeding.

If the idea of breast feeding is unpleasant to a woman, attempts to induce her to breast-feed often lead to unsuccessful nursing and mental conflict; feelings of guilt should not be injected or increased. These women should, therefore, not be urged to breast-feed their baby, but where minor objections are given it may be well to discuss them. The mother who eats adequately will usually not become exhausted by feeding her baby nor will she gain weight from the extra food she eats. If she does show signs of exhaustion later or loses weight the decision can then be made for her to stop nursing her infant. Breast feeding is not necessarily confining, since a bottle feeding can be given when the mother wishes to be away. To the woman who is planning to return to work it might be well to explain the advantages of nursing the baby for at least the first six weeks. Then if her hours of work are not too long or irregular she may be able to nurse her baby most of the time and have someone else offer him a bottle feeding when she is away.

Certain physical conditions of the mother or baby make breast feeding inadvisable or impossible. Tuberculosis and certain acute infectious diseases, especially those to which a baby is particularly susceptible, such as whooping cough or typhoid fever, are definite contraindications to breast feeding. Other complications in the mother, such as heart disease, kidney disease, or syphilis, may be contraindications, but are not absolute, as they will depend upon the mother's condition; epilepsy and mental illness may well be contraindications, but will depend entirely upon how well the mother can be watched. The return of menstruation is not an indication for weaning, but the baby may have some colic, vomit, or have loose stools on the first day of the period. Pregnancy in itself does not render the milk unwholesome, but it is not considered wise for the mother to continue nursing the baby during a subsequent pregnancy because of the strain it may place on her. Flat or inverted nipples may make it impossible for the baby to grasp the nipple well enough to nurse. An immature baby or one with an abnormality, such as cleft lip or palate, may be unable to nurse; in these cases the breasts can be emptied by artificial means if breast milk is desirable for the infant.

Successful breast feeding depends to a large extent upon the attitude of the mother; those who really wish to nurse their infant are generally more succesful in having an adequate supply than those who are indifferent or those with negative feelings. A mother must want to breast-feed her baby for it to be a satisfactory experience for both herself and her baby. The mother who breast-feeds her baby when she does not wish to, but because it is expected of her, may provide the baby with breast milk, but not necessarily with the comfort and security that should accompany breast feeding. Artificial feedings may then be much more satisfactory to both mother and baby; the mother must not be made to feel that bottle feeding her baby deprives him of essential emotional needs since a feeling of security and affection can be given to a bottle-fed baby.

When a mother is undecided about breast feeding her baby and does not express adverse feelings, she can often be encouraged to do so. Many mothers can nurse a baby successfully with help and encouragement; they often need the sanction of doctors and nurses to be motivated to do so and they need considerable support in their attempts. These mothers need information about breast feeding, but explanations concerning its value should be such that the mother still feels free to make her own decision.

In any discussion concerning breast feeding the advantages should not be stressed to the extent that the mother who does not want to breast-feed her baby, or cannot for some physical reason do so, will develop a feeling of inadequacy or guilt. These mothers must be helped to realize that they can satisfy their babies' and their own emotional needs in many other ways and that a good mother–child relationship can be established without breast feeding.

**Factors That Influence the Secretion of Breast Milk.** Since emotions may influence the secretion of milk in a number of ways, it seems that the first essential toward successful breast feeding is a mother's real desire to nurse her baby. Success depends to a very large extent upon this attitude. A desire to nurse, a state of good nutrition, adequate rest, and exercise are important factors in establishing breast feeding and in maintaining the secretion of an adequate supply. The psychic influence on the production of breast milk is so significant that contentment and freedom from worry are especially important. Women who wish to nurse and have happy cheerful dispositions usually nurse their babies satisfactorily, while those who do not have a great desire and who worry and fret are likely to have an insufficient supply of milk. In addition to this sustained influence, the temporary effect of fright, grief, anxiety, or any marked emotional disturbance may result in a decrease in a quantity of milk that previously has been satisfactory. A mother's lack of faith in her ability to nurse may be detrimental in its effect; therefore, a woman who is willing to nurse must be assured at frequent intervals that she can nurse her baby if she will persevere. If the nursing does not seem very satisfactory at first she must not give up, but continue to put the baby to the breasts regularly. The mother who is really anxious to breast-feed does not ordinarily worry whether or not her milk will be good for the baby nor does she worry about the amount he will get at each feeding. She usually assumes that the feedings will be successful. Niles Newton in *Maternal Emotions* explains that:

There are two major mechanisms involved in breast feeding. One is the secretion of milk; the other is the expulsion of milk. The breast can be distended with milk but if the expulsion mechanism fails, the baby fails to get enough milk.

Another name for the expulsion mechanism is the let-down reflex. A series of experiments by Petersen [9, 31, 32] in cows indicated that sucking stimulation causes the posterior pituitary to discharge oxytocic hormone which acts on the smooth muscle fibers near the alveoli. These contract and thus the milk is pushed out into the larger ducts where it is available to the milking machine. The experiments of Waller and of Newton and Newton [20, 27] have demonstrated that the let-down reflex also exists in human beings.

The importance of this let-down reflex lies in the fact that it is very sensitive to the emotions. . . . Newton and Newton found that the baby got significantly less milk when the mother was subjected to pain or emotional disturbance.

Breast feeding failure is related to let-down reflex inhibition. Newton and Newton [27] found that women who needed to give their babies supplemental formulas actually kept almost 50 per cent of their milk in their breast. Neither the sucking baby nor the breast pump could remove it. However, it could be removed by setting off the let-down reflex artificially with injections of oxytocic hormone. . . .*

The let-down reflex is stimulated by the baby's sucking and by other factors, such as the sight of the baby, the baby's cry, and the anticipation of a feeding time. Sometimes the mother will notice that milk begins to drip from her breasts at a time when she is anticipating giving a feeding or when she hears the baby cry; often she will notice milk dripping from the breast opposite to the one from which the baby is sucking. Pain, emotional conflicts, or other distractions interfere with the let-down reflex, and the baby gets less milk than he could if it were functioning well. Nipple pain and painful uterine contractions sometimes make nursing difficult. To help prevent inhibition of the let-down reflex the mother must be given adequate pain relief if she is uncomfortable, must be provided with a quiet and

* Newton, Niles: *Maternal Emotions*. Paul B. Hoeber, Inc., New York, 1955, pp. 45–46

undisturbed atmosphere while she is nursing her baby, and must be given encouragement that the breast feeding will be satisfactory.

The breasts must be stimulated in order to secrete. Sucking stimulation is very important in establishing and maintaining an adequate milk supply, and whenever possible the number of times that a baby nurses should not be limited by the use of regular feeding schedules nor should the duration of a feeding be so limited that the let-down reflex is not adequately stimulated.

It is fairly safe to say that if the mother and the doctor and the nurse all want the baby to nurse at the breast, and do everything they can to make this possible, the feeding will be successful except under quite unusual conditions. An important part of the nursing care of mother and baby is the help the nurse gives in making breast feeding successful.

## INSTRUCTION AND ASSISTANCE TO THE NEW MOTHER

**The Feeding Schedule.** The baby is put to breast for the first time anywhere between 4 and 24 hours after he is born. Some doctors believe that the breasts should be stimulated as soon as possible and recommend starting the baby on breast feeding as soon after birth as the mother's and baby's condition permits; others believe that a longer interval between birth and the first nursing is advisable. The doctors who recommend postponing nursing until the baby is approximately 24 hours old feel that this period gives him an opportunity to spit up mucus which may cause difficulty during the first day, particularly if feedings are offered. This interval also gives the mother an opportunity to rest and sleep, and the baby may be benefited by being kept warm and quiet. His need for food is not yet great, nor is there much nourishment available for him.

During the first two or three days the baby obtains mainly colostrum while nursing, but the regular sucking is extremely important, not alone for the sake of giving him this time to learn to nurse but for the sake of stimulating the breasts to secrete milk. Moreover, suction on the nipples definitely promotes involution of the uterus, and this change usually progresses faster in women who nurse their babies than in those who do not. For the first few times a baby nurses it may be wise to limit the nursing time to 5 to 10 minutes to allow the mother's nipples gradually to become accustomed to the irritation of sucking. This time is then gradually increased to 15 to 20 minutes as tolerated by the nipples.

Until the breasts produce an adequate supply of milk, which may take from four to seven days or even longer, it is usually necessary to offer the baby a bottle feeding immediately after the breast in order to give him an adequate fluid intake and to satisfy his hunger. This complemental feeding may be a full-strength formula, a dilute formula, a 5 per cent glucose solution, or boiled water. Some doctors prefer to give the low-caloric feeding or nothing but water for the complemental feeding because they believe the baby will nurse better if he is hungry. Others believe he will suck better when he is well satisfied between feedings than he will if he gets very restless due to hunger, and therefore order a full-strength formula. After the first day or two, or as soon as the baby takes the bottle feeding without accumulating mucus or without much regurgitation, it is wise to let the mother offer the baby his complemental feeding so that she may learn to feed him with the bottle also.

In most hospitals it is customary to weigh the baby before and after each nursing to determine how much milk the mother is producing. For accuracy the scales must be graduated in ¼ or at least ½ oz, or in grams, and the baby must be weighed in exactly the same clothes after nursing as before nursing. A wet diaper or dress must not be changed until after the weight has been taken. As soon as the mother is producing what seems to be an adequate amount of breast milk the bottle feeding may be omitted, although it is probably best to let the baby decide when he does not want it because he seems to be a good judge of his needs. Sometimes the mother or the nurse thinks he has not taken enough from the breast and offers him a bottle which he will refuse if he has had adequate breast milk, and no amount of urging will make him take more. At other times he has taken so much breast milk that it seems he should surely be satisfied, but if he fusses and cries after the feeding he is probably still hungry and needs to be offered the second breast or a bottle. He may need only 15 ml (½ oz) of formula to satisfy him, but if he wants several ounces they can be given, because there is little or no danger that he will overeat. Allowing the baby to nurse from the other breast at this time may give him the additional food he needs and help to stimulate milk secretion.

A four-hour schedule is often used for the average-sized baby, and a three-hour schedule for the smaller one. Some babies will conform to this plan, while others will eat well only when fed on a self-demand schedule, which means the interval between feedings may be from three to six hours in the very young baby and may even vary from every two hours to every eight hours. The individual baby will also vary his schedule from day to day, but ordinarily all babies will take from six to eight feedings in 24 hours. The best time to feed the baby is when he cries with hunger. The contractions of the empty stomach cause pain and make the baby cry. If he is allowed to eat when he has hunger pains he will soon learn that food in his stomach brings about relief of pain and that eating is a pleasant experience. When he is allowed to cry until a certain approved time he may not eat well because he has lost his feeling of hunger and has also become exhausted. If a sleeping baby is awakened to be fed he may not eat well because he is not hungry enough to eat, and the whole process is made unpleasant for him by spanking or snapping his feet in an effort to wake him. Some babies may be sleepy the first few days of life, possibly due to medication given the mother during labor or due to a long difficult delivery. When these babies are allowed to wake up completely before each attempt is made at nursing, the whole process is more pleasant for everyone concerned. At first they may want to eat only every six to eight hours, but within a few days they are ready for more frequent feedings and may soon go on approximately a four-hour schedule.

The baby's feedings should be carried out the same at night as in the daytime. Many people are anxious to omit the 2 A.M. feeding almost immediately, but this cannot be done without discomfort to the baby until he is ready for it. It is not a habit which must be changed; rather, it is his hunger that wakes him until he gets enough calories from the feedings taken during the day to satisfy him during the night. When this time comes he will omit the 2 A.M. feeding himself.

**Starting the Baby to Nurse.** An important skill that the nurse must develop is to help the mother to nurse her baby successfully. In preparing to nurse her baby the mother should be instructed to wash her hands and assume a comfortable position. At first it will probably be easier for her if she lies on her side with the bed flat. Later she may want to sit up and hold the baby in her arms. Some babies do not nurse well in the beginning, and it is easier for the nurse to assist the mother when she is flat in bed than when she is in an upright position (Fig. 143). When the nurse takes the baby to the mother it is important to make certain that she is well over on her side so that the baby does not have to reach up to grasp the nipple. The mother may

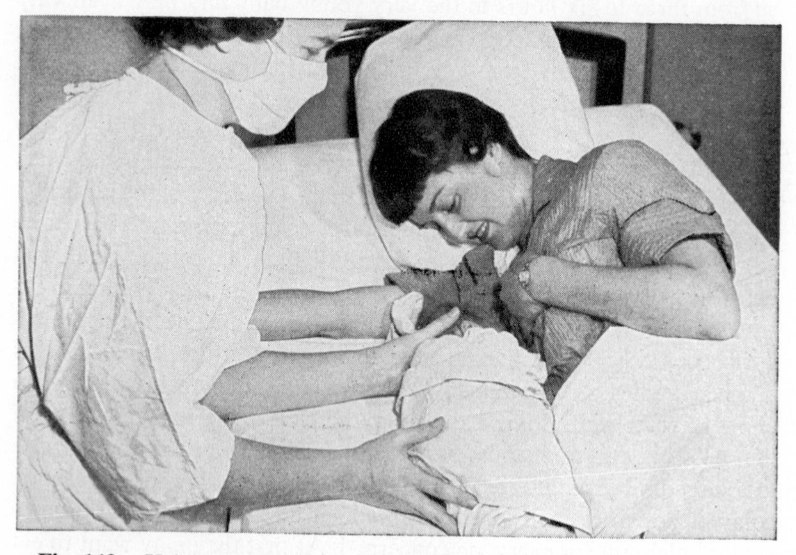

**Fig. 143.** Helping the mother nurse her baby. The nurse assists the mother and baby in assuming a comfortable position, helps the baby to grasp the nipple, and suggests to the mother other ways of making the feeding pleasant for both herself and her baby.

want to hold the baby in the curve of her arm but this usually places him in a cramped position and he is probably more comfortable if he lies flat on the bed. When both mother and baby lie in a comfortable and relaxed position the baby will be able to take into his mouth not only the nipple but the areola as well, so as to compress the base of the nipple with his jaws as he extracts the milk by suction (Fig. 144).

After the baby has been placed on the bed beside the mother no attempt should be made to force him into eating immediately. His rooting reflex is well developed, and he will hunt for the nipple himself if given a few minutes' time. He will either smell the milk and hunt for it or hunt for any object that touches his cheek; therefore, if the mother's nipple is touched to the baby's cheek he will instinctively turn his head, open his mouth, and grasp it. It may be necessary for the nurse to put her hand on the back of the baby's head to direct him to the nipple, but she should be very careful not to place her fingers on his cheeks because he will feel the pressure and turn his

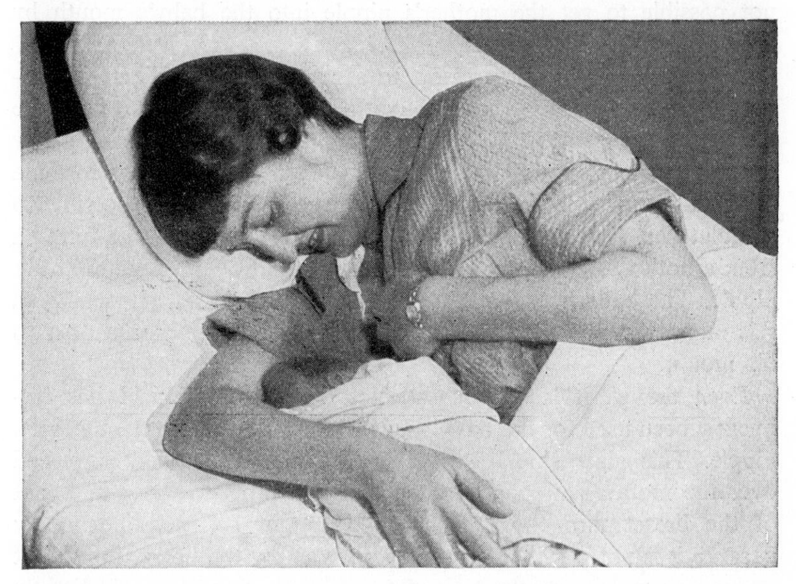

**Fig. 144.** Nursing the baby while lying in bed. Mother and baby are in a comfortable position. A pillow is propped under the mother's head so that she can observe the baby without strain. The mother places her arm around the baby to hold him securely. The baby's head is in a comfortable position, and the mother is turned toward him sufficiently so that he does not have to reach for the nipple. Note that the mother is holding the breast away from the baby's nose with her finger to permit him to breathe without losing a grasp on the nipple.

head toward them. She should not try to force his head in the proper direction because he may fight against it and begin to cry hard. The baby may put his hands to his mouth while he is attempting to grasp the nipple; they may be moved away gently, but he does not like to have them held down to his sides. It may be necessary for the nurse to put her other hand on the mother's breast and compress the areolar area between her thumb and forefinger to make the nipple more prominent or light massage of the nipple may make it stand out better. Therefore, if she has one hand on the mother's breast bringing out the nipple and the other hand on the back of the baby's head, she can bring his mouth up to the nipple quickly when he opens it and is ready to grasp, or she can touch the nipple to the baby's cheek and when his head turns toward it be ready to put it in his mouth. It is not possible to get the mother's nipple into the baby's mouth by trying to gently pry it open.

The nurse may have to resort to a number of expedients in persuading the baby to begin to nurse, since he does not always take the breast eagerly at first. Moistening the nipple by expressing a few drops of colostrum or milk or by placing a few drops of formula on it may prompt him to take it more eagerly. It may be possible to stimulate his sucking by letting him take a few swallows of formula from a bottle and then removing the bottle and offering the mother's nipple. The baby gets the taste of food and the idea of sucking in this manner and is more willing to suck at anything placed next to his mouth.

Even though it is very unsatisfactory, a nipple shield has frequently been used for the baby who refuses to suck from the mother's nipple. This glass shield with a rubber nipple attached is placed over the mother's nipple, and the baby attempts to draw milk out of the breast through it. The shield cannot be used indefinitely because it is not possible for the baby to empty the breast through it and it only postpones the task of teaching the baby to suck directly from the mother's nipple.

If the baby gets angry and begins to cry hard while efforts are made to get him to nurse it is best to pick him up and comfort and quiet him and then start again. He will not take the mother's nipple while he is crying even though his mouth is wide open and the nipple can easily be placed into it.

If the baby does not nurse after approximately 10 minutes of effort it is best to stop and try again at the next feeding or at any time that the baby seems hungry. It may be necessary to offer a bottle in place of the breast feeding he is refusing, but if he does not seem hungry he can be put back in his crib without a feeding. It is permissible to omit one or even more feedings to allow the baby to get hungry, but if he is particularly resistant to breast feeding, starving him will not help solve the problem. He will simply have to be offered a bottle when he does not nurse and tried at the breast each feeding time until he does suck. A baby that is difficult to start on breast feedings should not be taken out to nurse until he is hungry and fully awake; the self-demand feeding schedule is found particularly valuable with these infants. Some will refuse to nurse at the breast for several days or even a week; during this time the mother's breasts must be emptied with a breast pump.

The mother must be prepared for meager results from the early attempts to induce the baby to nurse, but perseverance will usually meet with success. When the baby once begins sucking and especially if he gets the nipple well back into his mouth, he will continue without any more difficulty because as soon as he has the nipple in his mouth his sucking reflex functions, he draws milk from the breast, and is anxious to continue. If he takes only one or two sucks and stops again he undoubtedly is trying to nurse but is not getting the nipple back into his mouth far enough. The nurse must then try to get more of the areolar area into his mouth as he opens it to grasp the nipple again. The infant's first grasps on the nipple are uncomfortable to the mother; she will have less discomfort if he gets the nipple well back into his mouth early so that he does not have to make many attempts to obtain a good grasp.

After the baby has sucked well for a minute or two and is quite obviously swallowing milk it is safe to assume that he will continue without assistance. He should be supported close to the breast so that he will not have to work hard to hold onto the nipple, but the nurse must instruct the mother to hold her breast away from the baby's nose by pushing her forefinger into the breast tissue closest to his nostril; this permits him to breathe freely, otherwise he must let go to take a breath. She must also be told to expect the baby to stop nursing and take a rest every few minutes and that when he rests he stops sucking and appears to fall asleep, but keeps the nipple in his mouth. Usually after a moment he will start sucking again, but if it seems that he is resting for too long a period it is well for her to gently wake him by patting him on the back. She should be instructed not to stroke his cheek to restart sucking because he may release the nipple to hunt for the object that is touching his cheek. If the baby does let go of the nipple while he rests he may grasp it again without any difficulty unless he has finished nursing. When he has sucked for 5 to 10 minutes and appears to be satisfied, no attempt should be made to force him to eat more. He has probably emptied the breast during this time or satisfied his hunger and his desire to suck.

The mother should be instructed to hold the baby up after his feeding and pat him on the back gently to get up the air bubble he has in his stomach (Fig. 145). It may be difficult for her to do

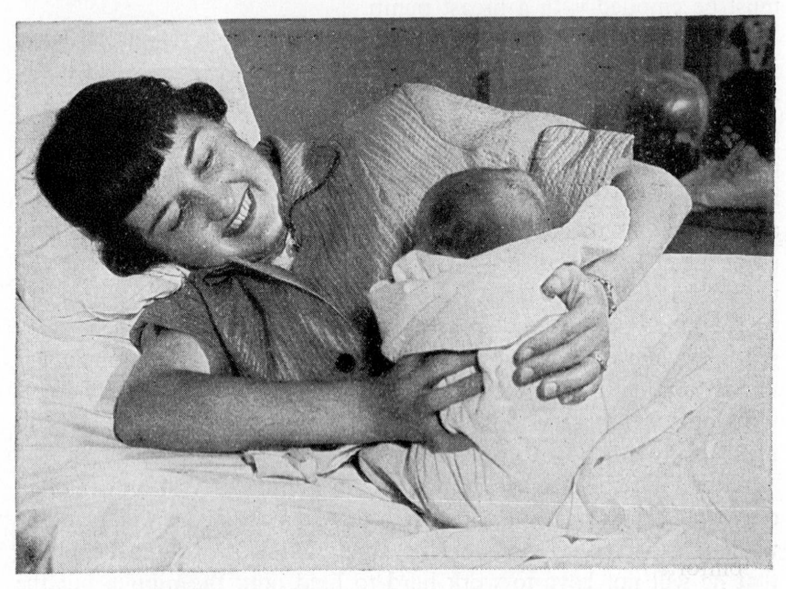

**Fig. 145.** Bubbling the baby during a breast feeding in bed. The mother is holding the baby upright after his feeding and patting him gently on the back to raise the air bubble in his stomach.

this the first few days if she does not move around easily and she may need assistance from the nurse. Some mothers like to stop the baby's nursing for an air bubble halfway through a feeding, but this is not necessary with all babies, and if a baby has been difficult to start at the breast it is wise to wait until the end of the feeding.

The nurse must realize that many babies do not nurse well the first week of life and that if nursing is to be made a pleasant experience the baby must not be forced to take the nipple or urged to nurse longer than he wishes. The baby that takes the breast feeding reluctantly may be a problem for several days, but he usually improves with each feeding and in many cases offers no resistance after the first time he sucks well. Even the baby who sucks eagerly may have trouble grasping the nipple during the period of engorgement and may need some assistance from the nurse who compresses the breast so that he can grasp the nipple.

**Length of Nursing Time.** Most of the milk is emptied from the breast in the first five to six minutes of sucking, and the baby may stop nursing and fall asleep after this time, but he may want to continue much longer. Many people are under the impression that a baby must nurse 20 minutes and if he falls asleep in less time they try to wake him to make him continue. The mother should be taught that the baby who falls asleep after five minutes of vigorous sucking is satisfied and need not be urged to continue nursing. If he continues for 20 minutes or more he does so because the breasts are not secreting adequately and he is hungry, or because he nurses slowly and intermittently and thus takes a longer time to obtain the milk, or because he enjoys sucking. If the mother's nipples are sore, as they may be during the first four to five days, she may have to take the baby off the breast at the end of 5 to 10 minutes to avoid irritation; this may, however, interfere with complete emptying of the breasts. After the nipples have become toughened she may let the baby nurse as long as he wishes to satisfy his desire to suck.

**Increasing the Supply of Breast Milk.** The mother should not become discouraged too easily if her milk supply does not increase rapidly because it may take from two to three weeks, or even longer, to develop an adequate supply. Certainly nursing must be continued for more than six or seven days to determine how much the breasts will produce. The amount may increase after the mother leaves the hospital because she is in more natural surroundings at home, provided, of course, that she rests sufficiently, eats adequately, drinks plenty of fluid, and does not have too many social obligations or household worries.

As a rule, the baby nurses from only one side at each feeding in the beginning, emptying the breasts alternately, but if there is not enough milk in one breast for a complete nursing both sides may be used later. If after five to six days, therefore, one breast is not supplying an adequate amount and if the nipples are not sore the mother may try nursing both breasts at each feeding, or the baby may be satisfied on a three-hour schedule on either one or both breasts. This frequent emptying may stimulate them to produce more milk. When the baby is nursed from both breasts the first one should be nursed approximately 10 to 15 minutes and the second one for 5 to 10 minutes, depending upon when the baby is satisfied. It is important to alternate the side from which the baby starts each time.

Nursing the baby from both breasts every time may stimulate them so much that it becomes necessary to change back to one side, and the full breasts may cause discomfort until the supply of milk again becomes adjusted to the baby's need. A problem that may present itself is irritation of the nipples from frequent use. Efforts to stimulate milk production should not be carried to the point where the nipples become cracked or the mother becomes too tired. If the baby does not receive an adequate amount after several days' trial of nursing on both sides he may be nursed for 5 to 10 minutes on each side and offered as much formula as he wishes immediately afterward. Nursing from both breasts should not be started if the milk decreases after four or five months, as it is then better to wean the baby.

**Fluid and Calorie Requirements.** A baby needs about 2½ oz of fluid per pound of body weight and 50 calories per pound. Therefore, a 10-lb baby will need 2½ oz times 10 or 25 oz of fluid, and 50 calories times 10 or 500 calories in 24 hours. When calculating the fluid and caloric requirements it is always necessary to do so over a 24-hour period. Since there are 20 calories in 1 oz of breast milk, a 10-lb baby taking 25 oz of breast milk in 24 hours will receive the 500 calories which are his approximate needs. A breast-fed baby will therefore have both his fluid and caloric requirements fulfilled if he takes 2½ oz of breast milk per pound of body weight in a 24-hour period. This is only a method of determining if the baby is getting his approximate requirements when there is some doubt and need not be strictly followed. It is not necessary to figure the baby's food intake unless there is some question about his feedings. The normal healthy baby will know the amount of milk he wants to take at each feeding and he should be allowed to eat as much as he needs to be satisfied and not forced to take more than he wants.

**Breast Feeding at Home.** Many mothers find it easier to let the baby nurse when he wishes during his first few weeks at home than to insist on a regular feeding schedule. The entire family is less disturbed and the home more peaceful if the baby is fed when he cries. When kept on a strict schedule he may wake up and cry hard before his next feeding; this causes much unnecessary worry. The baby may only be hungry, but the mother may think he has colic or is ill. Along with the worry her breast milk supply is likely to decrease.

It might appear that an irregular feeding schedule would make it difficult to plan either a hospital or home "routine," but some babies cannot conform to a regular schedule with comfort. Often a baby will develop a schedule of his own after the first few days, and the mother can usually depend upon him to eat at approximately the same time each day. If she is too much disturbed by a self-demand feeding schedule she can be assured that her baby will conform to a more regular schedule within a few weeks.

It is well to plan on giving the baby his 2 A.M. feeding until he is ready to discontinue it. He will not do this suddenly, but will gradually sleep for longer periods of time during the night and be ready to sleep through entirely when he weighs between 10 and 11 lb or by the age of six to eight weeks.

The amount of breast milk may decrease temporarily the first day or two at home, particularly if the mother gets too tired and worried. During these few days the baby may be satisfied with the breast feeding alone if he is nursed frequently or nursed from both breasts each time. If he is not satisfied or if the breasts do not produce an adequate supply very soon, he will need complemental feedings.

When the mother is tense at nursing time the baby may not get an adequate amount of milk at an individual feeding. She may find it easier to relax and feel more restful if she lies down while she nurses her baby; but if she has a tendency to fall asleep, there is some danger of injuring him and it is better for her to sit in a chair. This is especially true during the night feedings (Figs. 146 and 147).

If the amount of breast milk is insufficient when the mother leaves the hospital she should plan on partially feeding the baby at the breast for at least a few weeks because the amount of milk will probably increase at home. It may take from two to three weeks for the breasts to secrete an adequate amount, and if the milk does not increase the baby can be weaned as easily at home as in the hospital. Some doctors consider breast feeding worth while as long as the mother secretes at least 10 oz a day.

When the baby does not get enough breast milk a complemental feeding must be offered, and many mothers are quite reluctant to give both breast and bottle because they feel it makes too much work and that it prolongs the feeding. This method will not be too difficult if it is planned carefully and if she has the bottle of formula warming during the time that she is nursing so that it is ready to offer to the baby as soon as he has emptied the breast.

Normally it is not necessary for the mother to weigh the baby before and after each breast feeding to determine how much milk he is

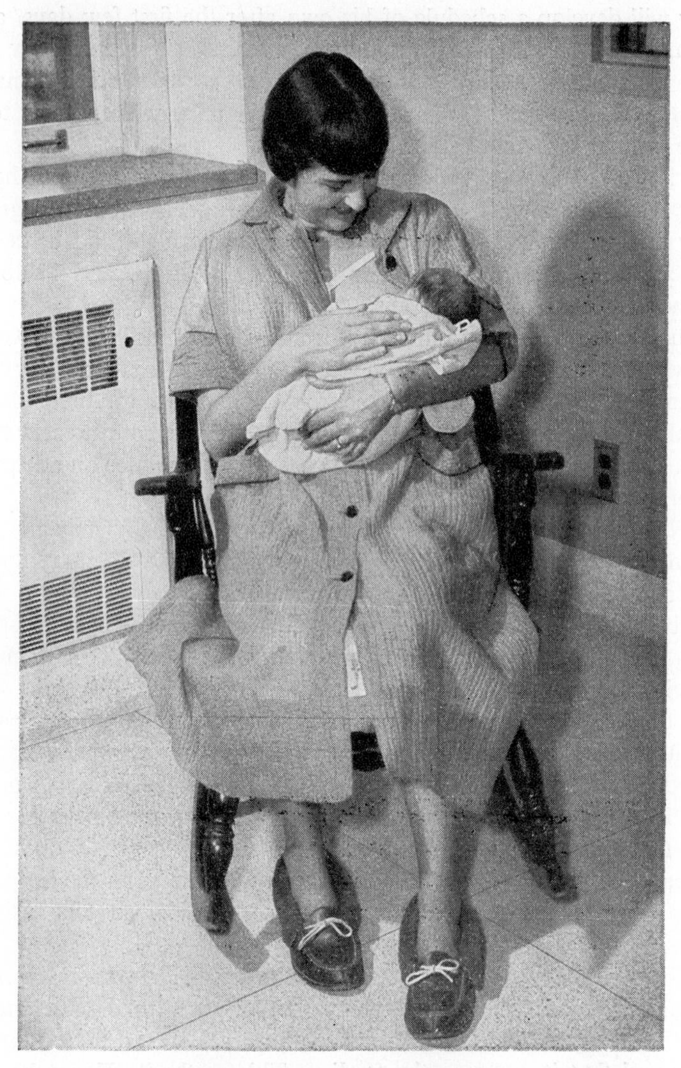

**Fig. 146.** Nursing the baby while sitting in a chair. The mother should be in a comfortable chair (preferably a rocking chair) and with her feet touching the floor easily or placed on a stool. The baby is held in her arm in such a position that the upper part of his body is higher than the lower part.

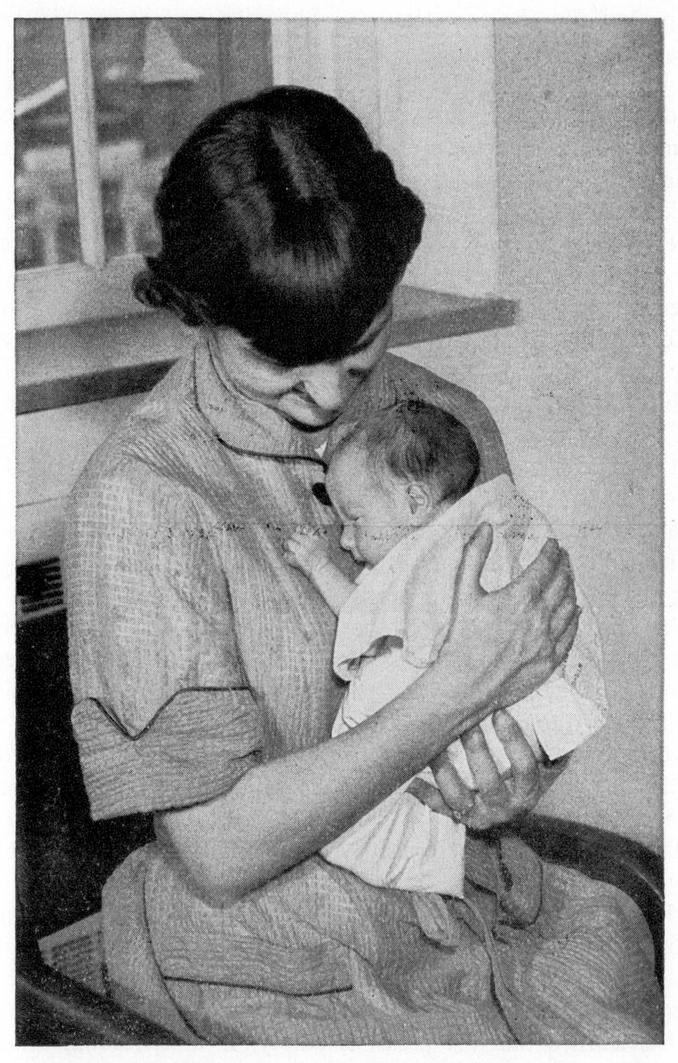

**Fig. 147.** Bubbling the baby while sitting in a chair. The mother's body is helping to support her infant in this upright position for bubbling.

taking because she can determine his satisfaction from his general behavior. If he is getting enough to eat he will be contented after nursing and will sleep for two to four hours; he will seem generally good-natured and comfortable while awake; he will have good color, normal stools, and gain weight steadily. If he is being inadequately nourished he will usually be unwilling to stop nursing and will give evidence of being dissatisfied when taken from the breast. He may be listless or fretful and will not gain weight as expected. When the baby seems to be insufficiently nourished the mother should find out how much milk he is getting in a 24-hour period. As each fluid ounce of food will increase his weight 1 oz, the amount of each feeding may be ascertained by weighing him, in his clothes, before and after each feeding. The doctor must then be consulted to decide the kind and amount of artificial feeding that the baby needs.

It is permissible for the mother to omit a breast feeding and give a bottle of formula in its place if she plans on being away from home for more than four hours. In fact, many doctors believe it is advisable to give the baby a bottle in place of a breast feeding two to three times a week to keep him accustomed to formula and a rubber nipple. Some babies become so accustomed to breast feeding that they refuse a bottle when offered one and present a serious problem if they must be weaned because of a decreasing milk supply or illness of the mother. Instead of an artificial feeding several times a week some doctors recommend offering the baby water from a bottle once or twice a day to keep him used to sucking from a rubber nipple.

There are no idiosyncrasies to mother's milk, but breast-fed babies may have disturbances from underfeeding, overfeeding, or colic. Underfeeding in early infancy is usually due to an insufficient quantity of breast milk. The baby does not gain weight, wakes up hungry in two hours, cries, sucks on his hands, and wants to stay at the breast a long time. Finally he gives up early or does not nurse at all because he has learned that the breast is empty. If underfeeding continues the stools and urine decrease in amount, and the baby may become very quiet instead of being fretful. As a means of self-protection he sleeps for long intervals.

A baby with colic may behave much the same as a hungry baby, but colic usually occurs at the same time each day while the hungry baby will fuss at any time of day. The baby with colic continues to gain weight, whereas a hungry baby does not.

Overfeeding is not common in the breast-fed baby because he is not likely to get too much food on a four-hour schedule, or he will vomit the excess, or will not eat often. This may happen, however, when the baby is nursed from both breasts or more frequently than at four-hour intervals. He becomes fussy due to indigestion, and the mother may mistake the fussiness to be hunger and feed him frequently. With overfeeding the baby usually gains weight very rapidly, he may regurgitate some of his food, and he will usually have many loose acid stools which irritate the buttocks. Some babies have a tendency to be fussy without the presence of any of these disturbances.

**Weaning.** One advantage in giving the baby a supplementary bottle once a day is that it paves the way for weaning when the time comes to make this change. Under ordinary conditions, the mother begins to wean her baby any time from the second to the twelfth month, depending upon her ability or desire to nurse her baby. The end of lactation is usually forecast by a decrease in the quantity, and sometimes by a decrease in the quality of the breast milk. Having started by replacing one breast feeding daily with a bottle feeding, she should gradually increase the number of daily artificial feedings until all of the breast feedings are discontinued. There are exceptions to this general rule, of course, and under any conditions the weaning should be directed by a doctor. The middle feeding is usually dropped first; that is, the 6 P.M. feeding if the baby is still being fed at 10 P.M. or the 2 P.M. feeding if his last meal is at 6 P.M. Finally the baby is given only a 6 A.M. and 10 P.M. or a 6 A.M. and 6 P.M. feeding from the breast, depending upon whether he is on four or five meals a day. The 6 A.M. breast feeding should be the last one omitted because there is more milk in the early morning than later in the day.

The rapidity of the weaning usually depends upon the amount of breast milk being secreted. It may be done over a period of four to five days or four to five weeks. The mother is ordinarily not uncomfortable if she weans the baby slowly enough to give the breasts a chance to adjust to the decreased demand and to stop their function.

If the mother's milk is satisfactory and the baby is doing well, it is considered wiser not to discontinue the breast feeding during the hot summer months.

An erroneous belief, widely current, is that the return of menstruation is an indication for prompt weaning because of the milk being made unfit or unwholesome. Although this is not true, the baby may have some colic, vomiting, or loose stools and may be slightly upset the first day or two of the menstrual period.

Ovulation is usually suspended during lactation, but a mother may become pregnant while nursing a baby and this sometimes occurs within a few weeks after delivery. Contrary to the prevailing idea, pregnancy does not render the mother's milk unwholesome and is not, therefore, an indication for immediate weaning of the nursing baby. It is, however, a great strain upon the average woman to attempt to supply nourishment to a baby in utero and one at the breast. All three may suffer as a result of such an effort, but if the mother and nursing baby do well the weaning may be accomplished gradually.

If it should become necessary to wean the baby suddenly, the breasts may become very full and painful. In this case the use of a brassiere to give support, the application of ice to the breasts, and the use of drugs for pain relief will promote the mother's comfort. The secretion of milk stops when the breasts are not stimulated, and the discomfort disappears in one to several days.

## PERSONAL HYGIENE OF THE NURSING MOTHER

**Diet.** The diet demands special consideration during the lactation period, just as it did during pregnancy, since the normal physiologic processes are now also altered and additional demands are placed upon the body. Nutritional requirements are considerably elevated above the normal needs. Throughout the entire nursing period the mother's diet must be such that it will nourish her adequately and also aid in producing milk. The mother should be advised early in the postpartum period in regard to the foods that she must include in her daily intake for an optimum diet. If she has been on a restricted caloric intake during pregnancy it is difficult for her to realize that it now becomes necessary to increase the calories in her diet as well as other food essentials, and she needs a careful explanation.

The diet during lactation must include calories, protein, minerals, and vitamins above normal requirements (Chart II, p. 128). Energy requirements of the mother during the period of lactation may be increased to as much as 50 per cent above her normal requirements.

Her diet must be sufficiently high in calories to meet the needs of her own body, to meet the caloric value of the milk secreted, which is 20 calories per ounce, and to furnish the energy that is used in the actual production of milk. Thus a mother who is secreting 30 oz of breast milk per day would need 600 calories above her own needs to meet the caloric value of the milk secreted plus the calories needed to produce this milk, which is about 10 per cent of the caloric value of the milk produced. Some authorities place the caloric needs for milk production higher. Fairfax T. Proudfit and Corinne H. Robinson in *Nutrition and Diet Therapy* state that: "Approximately 130 calories are required for each 100 ml of milk, and thus the daily production of 800 ml of milk would necessitate an additional 1000 calories in the diet." *

The value of a high-protein diet during pregnancy as an important factor in preparation for successful lactation has been discussed in Chapter 6. During the lactation period itself it is necessary to increase the protein intake even more than it was increased during pregnancy since the protein in the food must both cover the mother's needs and be converted to milk protein. "The mechanics of converting protein of food into milk protein is only about 50 per cent efficient, and thus about 2 gm of food protein is required to produce 1 gm of milk protein." *

The recommended daily protein requirement is 100 gm, or approximately 2 gm per kilogram of body weight. Much of this should be in the form of animal protein since a suitable intake of all of the essential amino acids is important.

The mother's mineral and vitamin intake should also be high because it is through her food that the breast-fed baby gets some of the materials that are necessary for the growth which takes place during the first few months of life. The calcium and phosphorus requirements are increased during lactation; the calcium requirement is approximately 2 gm daily, and the phosphorus requirement is correspondingly high. Since breast milk is low in iron, the iron requirement is apparently not increased, but the mother should have a sufficient intake for her own needs.

The vitamin requirements during lactation are not definitely known, but certain recommendations are made. Because the vitamin

* Proudfit, Fairfax T., and Robinson, Corinne H.: *Nutrition and Diet Therapy,* 11th ed. The Macmillan Company, New York, 1955, pp. 236 and 237.

A content of breast milk is high, it is recommended that the mother increase her vitamin A intake to 8000 international units daily. The recommended thiamine intake is 2 mg daily, an intake which is only slightly higher than that recommended during pregnancy. Thiamine is apparently poorly transferred from the mother's body to the breast milk, but an adequate diet is important to assure this transfer. Although the amount of riboflavin and nicotinic acid that is necessary during lactation is not definitely established, it is known that women who have a high intake of these vitamins produce breast milk with a higher concentration than the women who take a lesser amount. Since breast milk has a high vitamin C content the ascorbic acid recommendation during lactation is as high as 150 mg daily. Vitamin D is recommended in amounts of 400 to 800 international units each day.

If the diet that the mother had during pregnancy was adequate and well planned the only change that is now necessary is a few additions. If the milk intake is increased to 1½ qt daily the additional protein, calcium, phosphorus, riboflavin, and thiamine requirements are quite well fulfilled and some of the additional vitamin A and caloric intake is furnished. The ascorbic acid requirement will be fulfilled if the amount of citrus fruit recommended during pregnancy is continued and liberal amounts of other fruits and vegetables are used. Even when the vitamin content of the food ingested is high, it is always well to supplement it with vitamin D in a concentrated form to make absolutely certain that all of the calcium in the food is well utilized. Bread, cereal, potatoes, and desserts will increase the caloric intake, but this intake must be adjusted to each individual mother's needs and is regulated according to her weight. If her weight remains stationary, her caloric intake is considered adequate; but if she loses or gains weight, the amount of carbohydrate and fat in her diet should be increased or decreased accordingly. It is often advisable to augment the food provided by her three regular meals by taking a glass of milk, cocoa, or some beverage made of milk, during the morning, afternoon, and evening. A fluid intake up to 2500 or 3000 ml is important for adequate milk production.

Milk production will not be good if there is any marked deficiency of protein or caloric intake.

The mother may eat any food that agrees with her. The old and widespread belief that certain substances from highly flavored vegetables such as onions, cabbage, turnips, and garlic are excreted through the milk to upset the baby's digestion is not given general credence today. Some doctors believe that cabbage and members of the cabbage family have a tendency to give the baby colic; others think that chocolate or certain berries may produce signs of allergy, such as rashes. Ordinarily the mother may eat any kind of food she wishes unless she finds that her baby is disturbed by any particular one. Any food, of course, which causes her to have indigestion should be avoided.

Many drugs are excreted in the milk, but mineral oil, milk of magnesia, and aspirin can safely be taken by the nursing mother. Smoking and alcoholic beverages in moderation are not considered harmful.

**Bowels.** The nursing mother's bowels should move freely and regularly every day. She will usually be able to establish the habit of a daily movement by taking exercise, eating bulky fruit and vegetables, drinking an abundance of water, and regularly attempting to empty her bowels every day, preferably immediately after breakfast. Mineral oil or milk of magnesia may occasionally be necessary, but strong cathartics should be avoided.

**Rest and Exercise.** The nursing mother will not produce a good supply of breast milk without adequate rest and sleep, and a moderate amount of daily exercise in the open air is beneficial. Because fatigue has such an injurious effect on the amount of milk secreted, the average mother should have eight hours of sleep at night and an afternoon nap.

Her exercise will have to be adjusted to her tastes, customary habits, circumstances, and physical endurance, and it must always be stopped before she is tired. Walking is often the best form of exercise that the nursing mother can take, although she may engage in any mild sports that she enjoys. Violent exercise is inadvisable because of the exhaustion that may follow.

**Recreation.** Part of the value of exercise lies in the pleasure and diversion which it gives, since a happy, contented frame of mind is practically indispensable to the production of milk. In addition to some regular and enjoyable exercise, therefore, the mother needs a certain amount of recreation and change of thought and environment. If her life is monotonous and dull, the average woman is likely to become irritable and depressed, to lose her poise and perspective, to worry and fret, and, then, no matter what she eats or how much she sleeps, her breast milk will decrease. This, of course, reminds us that her emotional stability is a determining factor in the mother's ability to nurse her baby successfully.

For the sake of giving the mother an opportunity for recreation as she desires, it is a good plan to suggest that she replace one breast feeding with a bottle feeding sometime in the course of any day that she wishes to do so. The freedom which this long interval between two nursings gives the mother for recreation will usually have a very favorable influence upon breast feeding.

## BIBLIOGRAPHY AND STUDENT REFERENCES

Aldrich, C. Anderson: "Ancient Processes in a Scientific Age," *Am. J. Dis. Child.,* **64**:714–22, (Oct.) 1942.

———: "The Advisability of Breast Feeding," *J.A.M.A.,* **135**:915–16, (Dec. 6) 1947.

Barnes, George R., Jr.; Lethin, Anton N., Jr.; Jackson, Edith B.; and Shea, Nilda: "Management of Breast Feeding," *J.A.M.A.,* **151**:192–99, (Jan. 17) 1953.

Blake, Florence G.: *The Child, His Parents and the Nurse.* J. B. Lippincott Co., Philadelphia, 1954.

Bookmiller, Mae M., and Bowen, George L.: *Textbook of Obstetrics and Obstetric Nursing,* 2nd ed. W. B. Saunders Co., Philadelphia, 1954.

Burke, Bertha S., and Stuart, Harold C.: "Nutritional Requirements during Pregnancy and Lactation," *J.A.M.A.,* **137**:119–28, (May 8) 1948.

Davis, M. Edward, and Sheckler, Catherine E.: *DeLee's Obstetrics for Nurses,* 15th ed. W. B. Saunders Co., Philadelphia, 1951.

Eastman, Nicholson J.: *Williams Obstetrics,* 11th ed. Appleton-Century-Crofts, Inc., New York, 1956.

Greenhill, J. P. (ed.): *Obstetrics,* 11th ed. W. B. Saunders Co., Philadelphia, 1955.

Hill, Lee F.: "Breast Feeding and Mixed Feeding," in McQuarrie, Irvine (ed.): *Brennemann's Practice of Pediatrics,* Vol. I. W. F. Prior Co., Inc., Hagerstown, Md., 1948, Chap. 25.

———: "Is Breast Feeding Worth Salvaging?" *J. Pediat.,* **45**:502–4, (Oct.) 1954.

Holt, L. Emmett, Jr., and McIntosh, Rustin: *Holt Pediatrics,* 12th ed. Appleton-Century-Crofts, Inc., New York, 1953.

Lyon, Robert A., and Wallinger, Elgie M.: *Mitchell's Pediatrics and Pediatric Nursing,* 4th ed. W. B. Saunders Co., Philadelphia, 1954.

Nelson, Waldo E. (ed.): *Textbook of Pediatrics,* 6th ed. W. B. Saunders Co., Philadelphia, 1955.

Newton, Niles: *Maternal Emotions.* Paul B. Hoeber, Inc., New York, 1955.

Newton, Niles, and Newton, Michael: "Recent Trends in Breast Feeding: A Review," *Am. J. M. Sc.,* **221**:691–97, (June) 1951.

———, and ———: "Relation of the Let-Down Reflex to the Ability to Breast Feed," *Pediatrics,* **5**:726–32, (Apr.) 1950.

———, and ———: "Relationship of Ability to Breast Feed and Maternal Attitudes toward Breast Feeding," *Pediatrics,* **5**:869–75, (May) 1950.

Ogden, Kathleen, and MacKeith, Ronald: "Good Nipples Promote Successful Breast Feeding," *J. Pediat.,* **46**:210–14, (Feb.) 1955.

Proudfit, Fairfax T., and Robinson, Corrine H.: *Nutrition and Diet Therapy,* 11th ed. The Macmillan Company, New York, 1955.

Sage, Letitia L.: "The Battle of the Bottle," *Am. J. Nursing,* **47**:395, (June) 1947.

Spock, Benjamin: *The Common Sense Book of Baby and Child Care.* Duell, Sloan, and Pearce, New York, 1946.

Trainham, Genevieve, and Montgomery, John C.: "Self-demand Feeding for Babies," *Am. J. Nursing,* **46**:767–70, (Nov.) 1946.

U.S. Department of Health, Education, and Welfare: *Infant Care,* Publication No. 8. U.S. Government Printing Office, Washington, D.C., 1955.

Wolff, Ilse S.: "Mothers' Views on Breast Feeding," *Nursing Outlook,* **1**:145–48, (Mar.) 1953.

Woodward, H. L.; Gardner, B.; Bryant, R. D.; and Overland, Anna E.: *Obstetric Management and Nursing,* 5th ed. F. A. Davis Co., Philadelphia, 1955.

Zabriskie, Louise, and Eastman, Nicholson J.: *Nurses Handbook of Obstetrics,* 9th ed. J. B. Lippincott Co., Philadelphia, 1952.

*Chapter 18*

# Complications of the Puerperium and Nursing Care

The most important of the complications of the puerperium are hemorrhage, puerperal infection, thrombophlebitis, mastitis, and cystitis and pyelitis. The importance of these to the nurse lies in the possibility of their prevention by means of the careful and intelligent care which she helps to give during pregnancy, labor, and the early weeks after the baby is born.

## POSTPARTUM HEMORRHAGE

Maternal deaths due to hemorrhage, trauma, and shock have decreased considerably during the last two decades, but these factors are still major causes of maternal mortality, comprising close to one-third of the total deaths (Fig. 148). Although many deaths due to these causes occur in the prenatal period following abortion, tubal pregnancy, and antepartum bleeding, a considerable number are due to hemorrhage during or after delivery. Blood transfusion is as valuable in the treatment of hemorrhage as antibiotics are in the treatment of infection; a major factor in the decrease of maternal deaths due to hemorrhage is the easier availability and greater use of blood for transfusion in the present day than in former years.

Postpartum hemorrhage is a blood loss, from the birth canal, of 500 ml or more following delivery of the baby; this loss has at times even been as high as 2000 to 2500 ml. Although the postpartum period does not begin until labor is completed, excessive blood loss during the third stage is also ordinarily considered when postpartum hemorrhage is discussed. Normally the patient should bleed very little either before or after the placenta is expressed, slight blood loss coming with its expulsion, but at times the bleeding is profuse throughout the

| | 1935 | | 1952 | |
|---|---|---|---|---|
| Cause | Per cent of total deaths | Rate per 10,000 live births | Per cent of total deaths | Rate per 10,000 live births |
| Sepsis | 41 | 24.0 | 19 | 1.3 |
| Toxemia | 22 | 12.7 | 35 | 2.3 |
| Hemorrhage, Trauma, Shock | 31 | 18.2 | 30 | 2.0 |
| Others | 6 | 3.3 | 16 | 1.1 |
| TOTAL | 100 | 58.2 | 100 | 6.8 |

**Fig. 148.** Maternal mortality by causes, United States, 1935 and 1952. (Kirkwood, Samuel B.: "Twenty Years of Maternal Care," *Children,* **2**:134, 1955.)

third stage. The blood loss at the time of delivery should normally be less than 200 ml, but the average patient, if in good health, can lose considerably more than this amount without suffering marked ill effects. The amount of bleeding should, however, always be kept at a minimum, because blood is the first line of defense. When bleeding occurs later than 24 hours after delivery it is termed a *late postpartum hemorrhage*.

**Causes.** The most frequent cause of postpartum hemorrhage is *uterine atony,* or impaired tone of the uterine muscle. There are many sinuses or blood spaces between the muscle fibers directly underneath the placenta; as separation takes place the uterine muscle normally contracts, and the sinuses are closed off with eventual thrombus formation. When the muscle fibers fail to contract and the vessels are not constricted, hemorrhage takes place.

*Uterine atony* is frequently due to exhaustion of the muscle. This exhaustion may follow a prolonged labor; overdistention of the uterus with a multiple pregnancy, a large baby, or hydramnios; or it may be caused by too much massage of the fundus in the third stage of labor. Sluggish muscle, as evidenced by poor contractions during the first stage of labor, can also be expected to contract poorly after the third stage. Whenever any of these conditions have been present during labor the nurse must be particularly careful to check the state of contraction of the uterus during the first few hours after delivery. The uterine muscle may also fail to contract well when there has been premature separation of the placenta, which allowed bleeding into the muscle, or when fibroid tumors are present.

Pieces of *retained placental tissue* or blood clots, or incomplete separation of the placenta during the third stage, comprise a second important cause of blood loss by keeping the muscle from constricting the blood vessels adequately. As long as the entire placenta is attached there is no danger of hemorrhage, but if partial separation occurs or if even a small piece of the placenta remains adherent the torn vessels at the point of separation may bleed, because the part that is still attached interferes with complete constriction of the sinuses. Incomplete separation may be due to poor uterine muscle contractions or defective decidua or early manipulation of the uterus during the third stage of labor.

*Tears in the reproductive tract* constitute the third major cause of bleeding. Perineal and low vaginal wall tears usually do not bleed profusely, but those which occur in the cervix or high in the vaginal vault may be so deep and extensive that they open large blood vessels. Cervical or high vaginal wall tears are most likely to follow operative deliveries, especially if the cervix is not completely dilated, but they occur occasionally even with spontaneous births. In some cases the labia become torn, and if these lacerations extend into the clitoris they may also cause profuse bleeding.

When bleeding occurs during the third stage it is more likely due to partial separation of the placenta or to deep tears in the birth canal than uterine atony. Late hemorrhage, more than 24 hours post partum, is probably due to the retention of a small piece of placental tissue which has not interfered with contraction of the uterus and has therefore not caused bleeding early but which later undergoes necrosis, is cast off, and is followed by bleeding from the area of separation. The blood vessels are usually thrombosed by this time, and bleeding is not common, but if it does occur it may be severe.

**Symptoms.** The bleeding in postpartum hemorrhage may be visible externally immediately, may be entirely internal, or may be present both externally and internally. Ordinarily there is a steady flow of blood from the vagina (it is important to recognize that this slow loss may be adding up to an excessive amount), but if the cervix is closed with a clot a large amount of blood may be collected in the uterus with only a serous discharge draining from the vagina. When the uterus is palpated through the abdominal wall it is found to be large and boggy, and if pressure is applied large amounts of blood clots and of fresh blood can often be expressed through the vagina. For this reason it is particularly important to palpate the fundus continuously for the first hour after delivery. Other symptoms are those associated with hemorrhage; however, the pulse and blood pressure may not vary much from normal until a large amount of blood has been lost, and then change quite suddenly. Then when signs of the effect of blood loss appear the patient will have: a weak rapid pulse, low blood pressure, rapid shallow respirations, a pale color, cold perspiration, dizziness, faintness, air hunger, restlessness, and anxiety, and progress to a state of profound shock.

**Prevention.** To make certain that the patient is in good condition for labor, the blood cell count and hemoglobin level should be checked during pregnancy and anemia corrected if present. Bleeding should be anticipated when the uterus is sluggish or overdistended; thus it is wise to type and crossmatch the patient for blood transfusion on the slightest indication. Avoiding early operative interference whenever possible is a good preventive measure. No effort should be made to express the placenta until the uterus changes from a flattened to a globular shape, but when the placenta does show signs of separation it should be expelled immediately and inspected carefully to ensure its being intact. Since anesthesia sometimes has a relaxing effect on the uterus, speed in completing any operative procedure and repair of lacerations, thus allowing the patient to awaken as soon as possible, may prevent blood loss. The loss of blood from an episiotomy should be kept at a minimum since this loss added to that lost from the uterus may bring the total amount close to 500 ml.

After labor is completed the danger of hemorrhage is greatest during that critical hour immediately following; it is practically routine the country over to watch the patient closely during this period, both for the sake of preventing bleeding and for the early detection of hemorrhage, making prompt treatment possible.

**Treatment.** If bleeding occurs during the third stage and is thought to be coming from the uterine cavity, efforts should be made to expel the placenta as soon as possible; it may become necessary to remove it manually. The hemorrhage may, of course, be due to deep lacerations which must be sutured as quickly as possible.

When bleeding occurs after the placenta is delivered, uterine atony, which is the most common cause, must be considered first. The fundus can very readily be palpated; if it is found to be relaxed the bleeding most likely is due to failure of the muscle fibers to constrict the blood vessels. If the fundus is firm, the bleeding is probably not from an intrauterine source, and it becomes necessary to look for and repair lacerations. When the cervix is to be inspected it is necessary to draw it down and into view because the entire birth canal is so relaxed that either a speculum or digital examination is unsatisfactory. Retractors are necessary to hold the vaginal walls apart, and a sponge or ovum forceps is used to grasp and expose the cervix; any sharp instrument will tear the soft cervical tissues. A good light must be provided for this procedure. Some doctors routinely inspect the cervix following operative deliveries; others believe that small lacerations will heal spontaneously and that the added manipulation is unnecessary, and they inspect the cervix only when there is excessive bleeding. Suturing the bleeding edges controls hemorrhage due to tears of the reproductive tract.

Obviously, when atony of the uterine muscle is present, the first step in controlling hemorrhage from this cause is stimulating the muscle to contract; this is done by means of massage and the administration of oxytocic drugs. The fundus should be compressed against the symphysis pubis or between the hands, and vigorously massaged (Fig. 111). Oxytocin (Pitocin), 10 oxytocic units (international standard), is used intramuscularly, and ergonovine 0.2 mg ($\frac{1}{320}$ gr) intravenously. If abdominal massage and oxytocics are not effective in controlling bleeding, bimanual compression of the uterus may be employed. In performing this procedure the doctor pushes one hand quite deeply into the abdomen and massages the posterior aspect of the uterus while at the same time he inserts the other hand (gloved) into the vagina and massages the anterior aspect of the uterus by rubbing his fist against the uterine wall. This procedure provides considerably more stimulation to the uterine muscle than can be given with abdominal massage alone, and it also compresses the venous sinuses of the uterus. The uterine muscle may soon contract sufficiently to control bleeding, but if it does not quickly do so bimanual compression may need to be continued for an indefinite period of time.

Since the retention of even a small piece of placental tissue will prevent the uterus from contracting firmly, the treatment of hemorrhage from this cause is immediate removal of the retained fragment. It is to avert this occurrence that the placenta is carefully inspected after its expulsion. If the placenta is not intact, the obstetrician may introduce his gloved hand into the uterus and remove the retained portion, making it possible for the muscle to contract properly to close the open blood vessels. If gauntlet gloves are available, they are worn for this procedure.

If bleeding is not controlled after the above treatment, preparation may be made to pack the uterus and must be made to give supportive therapy for the accompanying shock. While blood is being obtained for transfusion, intravenous fluids of an isotonic glucose solution, plasma, or plasma expander are given to maintain an adequate blood volume; plasma is preferred when available, as it maintains the blood volume more effectively. Elevation of the foot of the bed will also help to prevent shock. If time permits, the vulva should be reprepared before a packing is inserted, and the gloves should always be changed.

A uterine packing applies pressure to the open blood vessels and mechanically stimulates the muscle to contract. Plain gauze, 2 in. wide and 5 to 8 yd long, is used. (All the raw edges must be folded in before the pack is prepared for sterilization.) The doctor inserts the packing either by placing his hand into the uterine cavity and feeding the packing in along his hand, or by means of an instrument known as a packer. In 1902, Holmes devised a packer, which is a tubular instrument with an obturator (Fig. 149). This packer can be introduced through the vagina and cervix and up to the top of the uterus. When the obturator is removed the packing can be inserted through the metal cylinder by means of a metal plunger. Regardless of the method used it is very important to carry the packing to the top of the uterus, but great care must be taken not to go through the uterine muscle which is soft and can be easily punctured. As the packing fills the uterus, the packer or the hand is gradually pulled out until the vagina is also packed with the gauze.

While the packing is in place the nurse must watch the patient closely for bleeding through the pack and check the pulse rate and blood pressure frequently. The patient is given ergonovine orally or intramuscularly every 4 hours for the next 24 hours, and an ice bag is applied to the lower abdomen. This will help to keep the muscle contracted. An indwelling catheter is frequently inserted into the bladder because the pressure of the packing against the urethra may make it impossible for the patient to void. In carrying out perineal

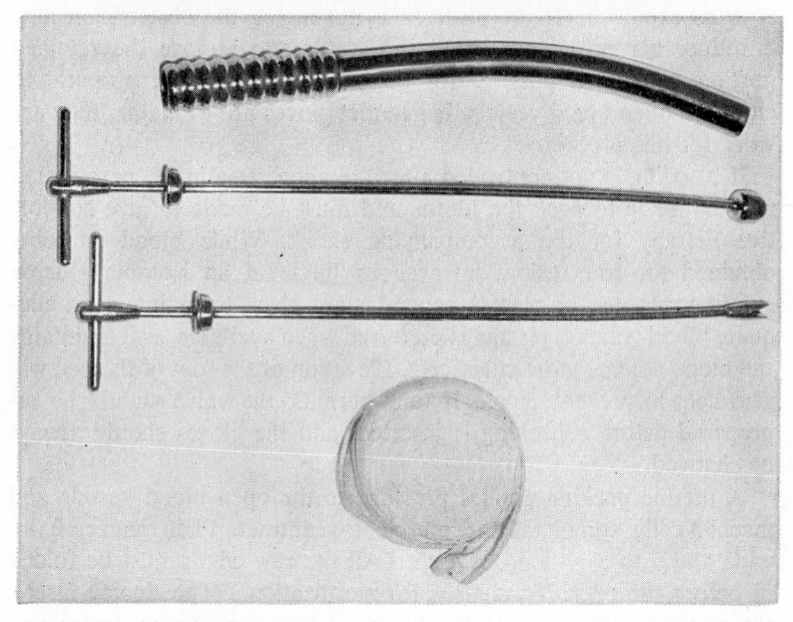

**Fig. 149.** Holmes uterine packer and gauze packing for use in the control of postpartum hemorrhage. *From top to bottom:* tubular packer, which may be obtained in several sizes; obturator, which is used while the packer is inserted; fork, which is used to insert the gauze through the packer; roll of four-ply folded gauze packing, 2 in. wide and 5 yd long.

care the nurse must be careful to keep the gauze, which may protrude from the vagina, from becoming saturated with the irrigating solution and thus add to the possibility of infection of the uterus.

The packing is seldom left in place for more than 24 hours because of the danger of infection. Immediately after its removal ergonovine is given intramuscularly or intravenously, and the nurse must watch the fundus carefully for a few hours for any evidence of relaxation. Some doctors believe that packing of the uterus is unphysiologic and prefer to use bimanual compression of the uterus instead of a uterine packing. They believe that the packing may not permit the uterine muscle to contract sufficiently to constrict the blood sinuses and may even distend these sinuses. They also believe that in some cases blood may accumulate above the packing and that further bleeding may then not be recognized early.

Sometimes a dilute solution of oxytocin (Pitocin) (1 ml which equals 10 oxytocic units [international standard] in 1000 ml of a 5 per cent glucose solution) is administered for several hours after delivery if the uterine muscle has a tendency to relax. Its oxytocic stimulation should help to maintain the muscle in a state of contraction. This solution is given slowly (20 to 30 gtt per minute) over a period of one to several hours; it is continued until the uterus remains well contracted without massage.

If all measures fail to stop the bleeding it may become necessary to remove the uterus. When much blood has been lost, transfusions are given for several days in succession. Although the blood loss is restored, a patient who has had a postpartum hemorrhage may not recover as quickly as one who has had no complications. Since a patient who has had considerable blood loss is very susceptible to infection and since there is increased danger of infection following the manipulation necessary for a cervical repair or other procedures, antibiotics are administered for several days post partum whenever there has been excessive bleeding.

The patient is more or less in shock by the time the bleeding has been controlled and needs the rest, quiet, and supportive therapy that is ordinarily employed in such cases. She should be well covered with blankets, surrounded with hot-water bottles, and urged to drink large amounts of fluid.

Should bleeding become profuse during the doctor's absence, after the termination of the third stage, *the nurse must stay with the patient and massage the fundus; some one else must elevate the foot of the bed* (on the seat of a straight chair or upon firm blocks) *and summon the doctor.* In anticipation of such an emergency the nurse should always have an understanding with the doctor regarding the administration of oxytocin (Pitocin) and ergonovine since a single dose of one of these drugs upon the occurrence of a profuse hemorrhage due to uterine muscle relaxation may be very effective in controlling the bleeding. Postpartum hemorrhage is an emergency, fortunately a rare one, and the nurse who is confronted with this serious situation will have to be quick-witted and use her best judgment in caring for the patient until the doctor arrives.

Above all, the nurse must remember that severe hemorrhage from a relaxed uterus can almost always be prevented if the fundus is kept hard, by massage when necessary, during the first hour or so after delivery.

### DELAYED POSTPARTUM HEMORRHAGE

This ordinarily occurs a week or more after delivery and is due to retention of a piece of placental tissue or failure of some of the decidua to go through regressive changes; thus proper uterine involution is hindered. Sometimes the administration of an oxytocic drug is adequate treatment, but it may also be necessary to remove instrumentally the piece of placental tissue and to give a blood transfusion, if warranted by the amount of blood loss.

### BLOOD CLOTTING ABNORMALITIES

In some pregnancies, especially those complicated by a premature separation of the placenta to a severe degree, there may be a great reduction in the fibrinogen level of the blood. When this occurs the blood clotting mechanism fails, and bleeding may be uncontrollable by the usual means. Transfusions of plasma or whole blood replace fibrinogen, but it may take a very large amount of these substances to restore the blood clotting mechanism. In cases of bleeding due to a low serum fibrinogen level the administration of fibrinogen (fractionated from human plasma) is very valuable in raising the level sufficiently to restore the clotting mechanism; it should thereafter be possible to control hemorrhage by arresting the bleeding at its source.

### HEMATOMAS

A hematoma may develop in the connective tissue of the vulva or under the vaginal mucosa as the result of injury to a blood vessel in these tissues. Injury to a blood vessel may occur during delivery (without laceration of the superficial tissues of the vagina or vulva) or the injury may be due to puncture of a vessel during repair of an episiotomy. Bleeding into the tissues may be slow, but continuous. These tissues become very distended, and the patient experiences a great deal of pain. The hematoma may not be visible, especially if the bleeding is under the vaginal mucosa. Intense pain in the perineal region, due to stretching of tissue, may be the only evidence of a hematoma for some hours, and the nurse must always notify the doctor of such pain. A vulvar hematoma becomes visible as a swelling develops on one side of the vulva; later a purplish discoloration of the skin over the swollen area appears. A vaginal hematoma may not be detected until pressure symptoms lead to an examination; a soft mass is then found to protrude into the vagina or the rectum. Even with an examination the amount of blood lost is hard to determine since the hematoma may extend upward into the broad ligament; blood loss into such a hematoma may be excessive.

Treatment consists of incision of the hematoma, removal of blood clots, ligation of the bleeding vessel, blood transfusion to combat the effects of blood loss, and antibiotics for prophylaxis against infection. If the hematoma is small it can usually be left untreated, slow resorption taking place.

## PUERPERAL INFECTION

Puerperal infection results from the entrance of pathogenic bacteria into the female reproductive tract before or during labor or in the puerperium. It is one of the most destructive and most dreaded of the complications which may develop in the puerperal patient, and has evidently been so considered since the days of Hippocrates. Until the last century this veritable scourge was so utterly baffling that it was regarded as a dispensation of Divine Providence and was therefore accepted with the same philosophic resignation as earthquakes and cyclones.

In dramatic contrast to this unresisting attitude is the present knowledge concerning the cause and prevention of this disease: it is now known to be a wound infection and therefore practically preventable; it is to be ascribed to the carelessness of mankind rather than to the indifference of Providence. This change in attitude was due very largely to the devoted work of three men who were deeply stirred by the tragic frequency with which young women laid down their lives in so-called "childbed fever." These men were Ignaz Semmelweis, Oliver Wendell Holmes, better known to Americans as poet and humorist, and Louis Pasteur, each contributing his own special observations to the sum total of knowledge which was to mean so much to mothers of today. Also the teachings of Lister concerning antisepsis and the introduction of sterile rubber gloves by Dr. Halsted, of Johns Hopkins Hospital, have had the same lifesaving effect upon obstetric patients as upon all surgical patients.

Within the last few years the treatment of puerperal fever has become more satisfactory. Chemotherapeutic agents have appeared in rapid succession. Sulfanilamide was developed in Germany in 1935. Since that time other sulfonamides have come into use. Penicillin, which was developed by British scientists, has been followed by a host of antibiotics making therapy ever more specific. While formerly treatment of puerperal infection could be directed merely toward helping the patient build up general resistance to the disease, these medications now aid in preventing or overcoming infection by their bacteriostatic power over many types of bacteria.

In 1843, Oliver Wendell Holmes read a paper before the Boston Society for Medical Improvement, entitled "The Contagiousness of Puerperal Fever." In this paper he presented striking evidence that in many instances something was conveyed by doctor or nurse from an ill person to a maternity patient, with puerperal fever as a result. He was attacked and ridiculed for his theories, and some of the leading obstetricians declared that it was an insult to their intelligence to expect them to believe that an agent invisible to the naked eye could work such havoc.

In 1847, Ignaz Semmelweis, of the Vienna Lying-In Hospital, decided as a result of some of his investigations that puerperal fever was a wound infection, and that septic material was introduced into the birth canal on the examining finger of the doctor or nurse, after contact with an infected patient or cadaver. Accordingly, he required that all vaginal examinations be preceded by washing the hands in chloride of lime, after which precaution the mortality from infection dropped from 10 per cent to less than 1 per cent. In 1861, Semmelweis offered his theories and conclusions in a masterly work on this subject, the title of which may be translated as "The Etiology, Conception, and Prophylaxis of Child-Bed Fever," but the actual cause of the disease was still unknown.

About 1879 Pasteur demonstrated what is now known as the streptococcus, in certain patients suffering from puerperal fever. Pasteur Vallery-Radot wrote:

Pasteur does not hesitate to declare that that microscopic organism (a microbe in the shape of a chain or chaplet) is the most frequent cause of infection in recently delivered women. One day, in a discussion on puerperal fever at the Academy, one of his most weighty colleagues was eloquently enlarging upon the causes of epidemics in lying-in hospitals; Pasteur interrupted him from his place. "None of those things cause the epidemic; it is the nursing and medical staff who carry the microbe from an infected woman to a healthy one." And as the orator replied that he feared that microbe would never be found, Pasteur went to the blackboard and drew a diagram of the chain-like organism, saying: "There, that is what it is like!" His conviction was so deep that he could not help expressing it forcibly. It would be impossible now to picture the state of surprise and stupefaction into which he would send the students and doctors in hospitals, when, with an assurance and simplicity almost disconcerting in a man who was entering a lying-in ward for the first time, he criticised the appliances, and declared that the linen should be put into a sterilizing stove.*

Slowly, but very slowly, the teachings of these earnest men were adopted by the medical profession, with the result that in well-conducted hospitals the precautions which have been described in preceding chapters are rigidly observed.

Adding the use of antibiotics, either prophylactically or as treatment, to these precautions has dramatically reduced the death rate, and today one woman in about 10,000 births dies of puerperal infection, instead of 1 in 10, as in much earlier days. In the year 1864, 23 per cent of the patients at the Maternité, in Paris, died of puerperal infection. Among the deaths associated with childbirth less than one-fifth are now due to sepsis as compared with over one-third as late as 1935 (Fig. 148).

To the nurse there is considerable significance in Pasteur's characterization of the infected young mother as an "invaded patient," since the nurse's preparation for the patient's labor and her care of the patient during the puerperium should be enormously influential in preventing this "invasion." In this connection she may well ponder Florence Nightingale's assertion that: "The fear of dirt is the begin-

* Vallery-Radot, Pasteur: *The Life of Pasteur*. New York, 1923, p. 291. (Quoted in *Classical Contributions to Obstetrics and Gynecology* by Herbert Thoms, p. 191.)

ning of good nursing." Certainly the obstetric patient cannot be well cared for unless the nurse has this "fear" in her heart.

Puerperal infection, then, in the light of present information, is regarded as a wound infection, the placental area being invaded by pyogenic bacteria which are introduced into the reproductive tract before, during, or after labor. This is true in cases of abortion as well as in term deliveries. The warm, dark, moist uterine cavity with its rich supply of blood and serum and a reduced amount of oxygen offers the optimum growth conditions required by most bacteria.

Infection of the raw and bleeding placental site may occur at any time during labor or the 10 days following, although the danger of infection decreases steadily after the first day post partum.

Puerperal infection may be due to many kinds of bacteria, either singly or in various combinations; the streptococci, staphylococci, colon bacilli, gonococci, and gas bacilli being some of the causative agents. Of these, the streptococcal infections, either aerobic or anaerobic, are most frequently seen and are also the most serious. Infection may sometimes develop even though bacteria are not brought in from outside sources. It is then produced by organisms already present in the reproductive tract and is known as *autogenous infection*. Many bacteria are normally harbored in the vagina, living there as saprophytes and ordinarily doing no harm, but with vaginal examinations or operative deliveries or in instances where the membranes have been ruptured for a long period of time before delivery these organisms may ascend or be carried to the uterine cavity and an infectious process may thus originate. This autogenous infection is more likely to occur when the tissues are bruised by prolonged labor or operative delivery than when birth has been spontaneous. It is rarely as serious as an infection due to an outside source.

**Diagnosis.** A diagnosis of puerperal infection is made when the patient's temperature rises to above 38° C (100.4° F) on the third or fourth postpartum day and remains elevated for over 24 hours if no other explanation can be given for the fever. Morbidity has been defined by the Joint Committee on Maternal Welfare as a temperature of 38° C (100.4° F)—if taken at least four times daily—on any two of the first 10 postpartum days, with the exception of the first 24 hours.

**Symptoms.** The symptoms vary greatly according to the infecting organism and according to the site and extent of the inflammation.

The area of involvement may vary from a small lesion, or simply an infection of the perineal incision, to a generalized infection. If the streptococcus is the causative organism the local reaction may be slight, but these bacteria sometimes pass into the lymphatic system and blood stream, causing a septicemia.

In mild types of infection, the patient's course may be entirely normal for the first three or four days, after which she may complain of chilliness or even have a chill; her temperature will be elevated, ranging between 38° C (100.4° F) and 38.3° C (101° F), and it may remain elevated for a few days, after which it will drop again to normal as the patient recovers.

The severe type of puerperal infection, formerly so dreaded, is characterized by an abrupt rise of temperature, sometimes as early as the second or third postpartum day, reaching 39.4° C (103° F) or 40° C (104° F) or even a higher level. The pulse is usually rapid and weak, and chills are not uncommon. There is likely to be abdominal tenderness and even distention with nausea and vomiting, since the severe form of puerperal infection frequently involves the peritoneum as well as the uterus. Headache, malaise, deep pelvic pain, and weakness are frequent. The condition of the lochia depends upon the infecting organism. In infection by some organisms the lochia may be greatly decreased in amount and almost odorless, while with others it may be profuse and have a foul odor. The attack may be very acute and result fatally in a few days, or it may gradually subside and the patient recovers.

**Areas of Involvement.** Infection during the puerperium occurs most often in the uterus, and, if mild, may amount to nothing more than an *endometritis,* or inflammation of the uterine lining. It causes slight chills followed by fever and a rapid pulse; the uterus will be found to be somewhat relaxed and tender. The infection may remain limited to the uterus because there is apparently an increased defense built up by the body during pregnancy and labor to hinder its spread. More severe infections, however, leave the uterus by way of the lymphatics or veins to involve progressively the parametrial tissues, the peritoneal cavity, and the entire body with the production of a generalized systemic infection. If the uterine musculature is involved, the infection is known as a *metritis;* when it spreads through the lymphatics or blood stream to the connective tissues around the uterus, it is termed a *parametritis,* or a *pelvic cellulitis.* Involvement of these tissues may also occur following infected cervical tears. The symptoms vary from only mild chills and fever to severe chills, high temperature, rapid pulse, and general malaise. Sometimes abscesses develop in the involved tissues. In some cases the infection manifests itself as a *salpingitis,* but this is common only when the gonococcus is the causative organism. Another manifestation is a *peritonitis;* the infection spreads from the endometrium to the peritoneum, usually by way of the lymphatics, but sometimes by the blood stream or by surface extension through the fallopian tubes. Included among the symptoms are pain and abdominal distention, vomiting, chills, fever, rapid pulse, and restlessness and anxiety. This infection may remain localized in the pelvic peritoneum or may spread to the entire peritoneal cavity where the rapid absorption of toxins into the blood may have serious effects. Bacteria may gain entrance into the blood stream through the lymphatics or veins and thus cause a *septicemia.* A *thrombophlebitis,* which will be discussed later, is another form in which the infection manifests itself.

**Treatment and Nursing Care;** *Preventive.* Puerperal infection is such a serious complication that the greatest effort should be made to prevent it. The nurse's part in preventing this complication is an important one and consists of so preparing for labor that it may be conducted with asepsis; she must maintain the same sterile procedure during delivery as she would throughout a major surgical operation and protect the perineal region from infection after delivery. This means that all linen, dressings, instruments, and gloves—anything coming in contact with the patient—must be sterilized by steam under pressure. The hands should be properly prepared by careful scrubbing, and sterile gloves must always be worn. Since the upper respiratory tract is a reservoir for streptococci, it is absolutely essential that a mask be worn at all times during the delivery to prevent droplet infection. Some hospitals insist on the use of masks in the labor room as well as in the delivery room. Routine periodic throat cultures of all persons employed in the obstetric unit are important to eliminate streptococci carriers. Anyone who has an upper respiratory infection or a skin lesion should not be allowed to care for obstetric patients; this also holds true for any person having recently cared for an infectious patient, especially one having a streptococcal infection.

Precautions in the delivery room alone are not adequate, however, because infection can be carried to the patient during labor or the early puerperium. Individual bedpans should be provided to prevent organisms which are nonvirulent for one patient from being carried to another in whom they might cause an infection. While shaving the patient the nurse must be careful to prevent hair and soapsuds from entering a gaping introitus; during the postpartum care the solution used for washing the perineum should not be allowed to flow into the vagina. It is important for the nurse to instruct the patient not to touch or examine her perineum. Infection with organisms from the intestinal tract can be prevented by taking special precautions during perineal care not to wipe from the anal region toward the vagina.

Treatment of a vulvitis, vaginitis, or other local infection during pregnancy is another factor in the prevention of puerperal infection. The patient should also be instructed in proper hygienic care of herself and in the importance of avoiding contact with persons who have a contagious disease. She is also instructed not to have intercourse during the last four to six weeks of pregnancy since this may become a source of infection should she go into labor soon thereafter.

It can be seen then that good aseptic technic during labor and delivery is absolutely essential for prevention of infection, but there are also other factors predisposing to puerperal infection which should, insofar as possible, be prevented or treated. Early rupture of the membranes (which ordinarily act as a barrier to the entrance of bacteria into the uterus) and vaginal examination during labor (which may carry organisms already present in the vagina into the uterine cavity) may increase the possibility of infection. When these procedures are indicated great care must be taken to perform them with aseptic technic, and antibiotics are frequently administered during and following labor for prophylactic reasons.

A patient who has had a long, hard labor, who has injury to the birth canal, or who has anemia due to blood loss is less able to resist infection than one who has had an easy, normal delivery. It is therefore important to keep up the patient's resistance during a long labor with adequate rest and fluids, and to prevent blood loss or to replace it when necessary. Tears of the reproductive tract and entrance into the birth canal during the third stage of labor add to the dangers of infection. The placenta must be carefully inspected to discover if fragments are missing; retention of pieces of placental tissue or membranes predisposes to infection and should be avoided if possible. The uterus must not be bruised by too vigorous massage. Profuse bleeding, toxemias of pregnancy, acute or chronic systemic diseases, prolonged labor, difficult operative deliveries, manual manipulation in the third stage of labor, and precipitous deliveries for which preparation has been inadequate always predispose to infection. Antibiotics are usually administered prophylactically during labor and/or the first two to four days post partum when any of these complications develop.

Although puerperal infection is easier to treat at the present time than it was in former years, prevention remains a very important factor. The ready availability of antibiotics for prophylaxis is not enough; it is still important to conscientiously employ aseptic technic in every instance. A few patients continue to die of infection in spite of much more effective treatment than formerly was available.

*Curative.* The treatment of puerperal infection has been revolutionized since the discovery of the antibiotics. Penicillin is the antibiotic that is commonly used because it is effective against many types of organisms. Other antibiotics are frequently used, however, and in most instances a combination of antibiotic drugs is administered since the use of more than one agent may be more effective than any single one alone.

The curative treatment is also directed toward increasing the patient's resistance to infection. Increased fluid intake is of great importance, some doctors ordering from 3000 to 4000 ml or more in 24 hours. If the patient cannot obtain the necessary amount by mouth, the fluid intake is maintained by parenteral administration of glucose solution and physiologic saline solution. Easily assimilable food with high-caloric and high-vitamin content is given at frequent intervals. The patient should be kept warm and quiet in a light airy room and have adequate rest and sleep. She must not be allowed to exert herself any more than is necessary, and if she has pain adequate analgesic medication should be given.

If abdominal distention or vomiting occur, the use of nasal catheter suction-siphonage may give relief. The bowels should move freely, but the nurse must be careful not to give an enema without an order from the doctor. As in all wound infection, drainage is important. Accordingly the patient is usually placed in a semisitting position or the head of the bed is elevated to promote free drainage of the lochia; Fowler's position also impedes upward extension of the infection.

In an effort to limit the infection to the uterus, measures are usually employed that tend to maintain the uterine muscle in a state of contraction, such contraction tending to prevent extension of bacteria through the uterine walls and also the absorption of toxins. Probably the commonest treatment to this end is the administration of ergonovine over a period of 24 to 48 hours; this also aids in the expulsion of blood clots and/or pieces of membrane from the uterine cavity. If abscesses form as a result of the infection it may be necessary to drain them when they become localized.

Blood transfusions are widely employed to aid in increasing the patient's resistance. They help overcome the toxic effects of the disease and the anemia which develops. Many doctors place such high value upon blood transfusions in puerperal infection that they give this treatment very early in the disease, somewhat in the nature of a preventive measure.

A patient with a puerperal infection should be promptly and completely isolated, preferably in a room off the obstetric unit. If the nurse who cares for her must come in contact with other patients, she should wear gloves and a gown while attending the infected woman and thoroughly scrub her hands after each attention. She must not care for a patient in labor or for one in the early postpartum period.

### GONORRHEAL INFECTION

In a postpartum infection due to the gonococcus, some patients have a moderately elevated temperature, usually not over 38.9° C (102° F) and may develop abdominal tenderness; others remain afebrile and asymptomatic. The infection usually spreads by surface extension from an endometritis to a salpingitis, oöphoritis, and/or pelvic peritonitis. The gonococcus has a special affinity for the fallopian tubes and is very likely to produce an inflammation of the tubes which may result in closure of the fimbriated openings. Accordingly, it may be impossible thereafter for ova to enter the tubes and gain access to the uterus; hence the patient may not again become pregnant. Unlike other infections, gonorrhea is not conveyed to the patient during or soon after labor on instruments or examining fingers, but is previously present in the vulvovaginal glands and from them may



cautioned against this for fear of
and causing an embolism elsew
same reason, the patient must
violent movements for some tin
about, but to walk and move r

Since thrombophlebitis is a
administered until the tempera
such as heparin and bishydrox
the formation of further thromb
because they may increase the
from the uterus may result. Bl
one of the spinal anesthetic ag
spasm and improve circulation
hasten resolution of the inflam

The patient is usually kept
perature has returned to norn
wear an elastic bandage, som
of the leg. The chances of a
pregnancy or following pelvi
plication has once occurred.
the circulation and may be
formation.

MASTITIS (INFLA

Mastitis is always due to
organisms. These may be b
patient or her attendants or
which are ordinarily presen
the tissue until it is injured
by way of the subcutane
by massage or other manip
those bacteria already pres
tissues. Stasis of milk in a
does not in itself cause inf
bacteria to enter more rea

Various kinds of orga
tions, but the causative a
The infection may develo

most frequently seen between the first and fourth weeks post partum. The patient who has been feeling well suddenly develops chills and fever; the temperature rises to 39.4° C (103° F) or 40° C (104° F) very quickly, and the pulse rate increases. On inspection of the breast one of the lobes is found to be red and painful and feels hard to palpation. Formerly this infectious process progressed until the patient became chronically ill and progressively weaker and frequently developed abscesses which in some instances had to be incised and drained. Healing was often slow and painful, and destruction of breast tissue sometimes extensive. With present-day treatment the patient almost always recovers quickly.

**Treatment and Nursing Care;** *Preventive.* Breast infections can largely be prevented by caring for the nipples during the latter months of pregnancy as described in Chapter 6 and by the use of an appropriate technic in the care of the breasts and nipples during the puerperium (pp. 444–57). Frequent occurrences of infection may mean neglect on the part of those caring for the patient. The nurse's part in preventing this complication has been outlined in the care of the breasts and consists of cleanliness and gentleness, unremitting watchfulness, prevention of fissured nipples, treatment of fissures if they do occur, proper care of engorged breasts, and prompt reporting to the doctor if any signs of infection develop. She must never massage the engorged breast.

*Curative.* Treatment generally consists of breast support, application of ice bags while the breast is indurated and painful, and the administration of penicillin, or occasionally a combination of antibiotics. (An essential part of the nursing care is early and proper application of an adequate support to the heavy painful breasts as described in Chap. 16.) If treatment is instituted early the infection usually subsides in a day or two. With the present-day use of antibiotics the inflammation almost always resolves without abscess formation, and if incision is necessary it is only to drain out a small amount of pus.

Some doctors discontinue breast feeding immediately and dry up the breasts when a patient develops a mastitis, because they believe that the less stimulation there is to the breast the more quickly the infection will disappear; they also believe that the patient may have trouble with mastitis again, later on, if she continues to nurse. Others are not in favor of stopping lactation because they wish to avoid the distention of breast tissue that occurs when emptying of the breast is suddenly discontinued. In addition the baby has the benefit of continued breast feeding. When lactation is to be continued the nursing is temporarily stopped and the breast is emptied by means of a breast pump, and the milk is discarded during the time the patient has a fever. Breast feeding is again resumed in one to three days unless recovery is slow.

## CYSTITIS AND PYELITIS

The slight lesions which are generally present in the bladder mucosa following delivery favor the development of cystitis, especially when catheterization is necessary or when residual urine, which becomes infected easily, is present. There is always stretching and trauma of the base of the bladder during labor and delivery; this causes mucosal edema and hyperemia. There is also a temporary loss of bladder tone, due to pressure and minor injury, that makes the patient less sensitive to bladder fullness and gives her an increased capacity, which may result in overdistention of the bladder, in complete inability to void, or in residual urine, thus predisposing to cystitis. The urethra is also subject to trauma during delivery with the result that voiding may be difficult or impossible. Primiparas and women who have had operative deliveries usually have more difficulty in completely emptying their bladder than women who previously have borne children, or whose labor has terminated spontaneously.

As a preventive measure against cystitis it is important to observe the patient closely for evidences of a full bladder or residual urine. The distended bladder may sometimes be palpated above the symphysis pubis or the uterine fundus may be felt laterally, having been pushed aside by the full bladder. Some patients complain of discomfort and constant desire to void, some void small amounts frequently, and others have neither discomfort nor desire to void. With residual urine the patient frequently voids in small amounts, and, in a number of cases, the residual urine may be of sufficient quantity to make the bladder palpable. It may happen, however, that since the bladder is less sensitive after delivery than under normal conditions the patient will retain an undue amount of urine and suffer no discomfort.

Catheterization should be deferred until the patient has been given adequate time to void spontaneously; if it does become necessary the procedure must be done very carefully since the chances of introducing bacteria from the vulva are great. When a patient is unable to void some doctors recommend that an indwelling catheter be left in the bladder to avoid catheterization every few hours, while others feel that the indwelling catheter is as irritating as the frequent catheterizations and that the patient will regain tone more quickly if the bladder is allowed to fill.

Cystitis, then, is due to bladder trauma, stagnant residual urine, and bacteria which have gained entrance into the bladder. Symptoms usually begin several days post partum. These patients often have suprapubic or perineal discomfort, frequent and painful urination, or a feeling of not having emptied the bladder completely. The temperature may rise to 37.8° C (100° F) or even to 38.3° C (101° F). Microscopic examination of a catheterized specimen will show pus cells, bacteria, and even red blood cells.

Treatment consists of making certain that the bladder is emptied completely, of bladder irrigations if an indwelling catheter is present, of forcing fluids, and of the administration of drugs to cure the bacteriuria. A culture of the urine is taken to determine the causative organisms, and one of the sulfonamide derivatives or an antibiotic is administered for a few days with excellent results.

*Postpartum pyelitis* is neither as frequent nor as serious as pyelitis of pregnancy. The onset of symptoms is usually about the third day post partum, but may occur as late as the twenty-first day. The most frequent complaints are pain in the flank, frequency of urination, dysuria, chills, and fever. Microscopic examination of the urine shows pus cells and bacteria, most commonly the colon bacilli. The symptoms are similar to those occurring in antepartum pyelitis but are not as severe.

Treatment consists of increased fluid intake, bland diet, rest in bed, and the administration of one of the sulfonamide derivatives or an antibiotic. Cultures of the urine are taken every two to three days to determine when it becomes free of bacteria.

## SUBINVOLUTION

When the uterus does not return to its usual size and consistency as rapidly as is normal the condition is known as subinvolution. The uterus is larger and softer than it should be for the particular postpartum period, and the lochia is more profuse and brighter red in color. This condition may be due to retention of placental fragments or a part of the fetal membranes, or it may be caused by an endometritis. Treatment consists of the administration of ergonovine and of giving warm vaginal douches daily after the first to second week post partum.

## RETROVERSION OF THE UTERUS

Retroversion, or a tipping backward of the uterus, may be due to excessive relaxation of some pelvic structures, or simply a recurrence of a uterine position which was present before pregnancy. It may produce no symptoms, but in some cases it causes backache and an increased and persistent lochia. Treatment consists of instructing the patient to carry out knee-chest exercise (Fig. 141) and insertion of a pessary. The pessary is inserted some time between the third and sixth week post partum and is left in place for several months, being changed at approximately four-week intervals.

## MENTAL DISTURBANCE

A word about extreme mental disturbance during the puerperium is worth while at this point because the nurse will hear of this condition, and will almost inevitably come in contact with it at some time. It was formerly believed that there were certain mental disorders which were peculiar to pregnancy and the puerperium, but this belief has been dispelled by the present-day knowledge of psychiatry. The puerperal patient is sometimes delirious and violent for longer or shorter periods of time; these conditions are sometimes due to toxemia or fever. If the excitement or delirium are of toxic origin, they are relieved by treating the cause; from the nurse's standpoint the care would be the same as for any delirious patient. The patient should not be left alone and should be protected against harming herself.

In other cases mental unbalance, ranging from neurosis through psychosis, results from the patient's reaction to the idea of motherhood, just as it might have resulted from an equal strain of some other character. A mental disturbance which is due to the patient's inability to adjust herself to the state of motherhood, and all that that implies to her, is discussed in Chapter 7, "Mental Hygiene of the Expectant Mother." Acute schizophrenia is occasionally observed during the puerperium; it requires the customary therapy and does not differ essentially from schizophrenia developing at any other time.

## BIBLIOGRAPHY AND STUDENT REFERENCES

Ball, Otho F.: "Ignaz Philipp Semmelweis," *Mod. Hosp.*, **75**:73–74, (Sept.) 1950.

———: "Oliver Wendell Holmes," *Mod. Hosp.*, **80**:87–89, (Jan.) 1953.

———: "Oliver Wendell Holmes," *Mod. Hosp.*, **80**:81–82, (Feb.) 1953.

Bauer, Gunnar: "Combating Thrombosis and Pulmonary Embolism," *Am. J. Nursing,* **47**:589–91, (Sept.) 1947.

Bookmiller, Mae M., and Bowen, George L.; *Textbook of Obstetrics and Obstetric Nursing,* 2nd ed. W. B. Saunders Co., Philadelphia, 1954.

Burdon, Kenneth L.: *Textbook of Microbiology,* 3rd ed. The Macmillan Company, New York, 1947.

Davis, M. Edward, and Sheckler, Catherine E.: *DeLee's Obstetrics for Nurses,* 15th ed. W. B. Saunders Co., Philadelphia, 1951.

Eastman, Nicholson J.: *Williams Obstetrics,* 11th ed. Appleton-Century-Crofts, Inc., New York, 1956.

Findley, Palmer: "Ignaz Philipp Semmelweis," *Am. J. Obst. & Gynec.*, **55**:700–710, (Apr.) 1948.

Greenhill, J. P. (ed.): *Obstetrics,* 11th ed. W. B. Saunders Co., Philadelphia, 1955.

Jensen, Julius, and Jensen, Deborah MacLurg: *Nursing in Clinical Medicine,* 4th ed. The Macmillan Company, New York, 1954.

Kennan, Alfred L.: "Coagulation Defects in Obstetric Accidents and Disorders," *Am. J. M. Sc.,* **229**:695–703, (June) 1955.

Kohl, Richard N.: "The Psychiatric Aspects of Obstetric Nursing," *Am. J. Nursing,* **48**:422–25, (July) 1948.

Lynch, J. Edward: "Venous Thrombosis in Obstetrics and Gynecology," *S. Clin. North America,* **28**:1469–76, (Dec.) 1948.

Stanton, Joseph R.: "Venous Thrombosis and Pulmonary Embolism," *Am. J. Nursing,* **55**:709–11, (June) 1955.

Thoms, Herbert: *Classical Contributions to Obstetrics and Gynecology*. Charles C Thomas, Publisher, Springfield, Ill., 1935.

Weber, Lennard L., and Paxson, Newlin F.: "The Management of Afibrinogenemia," *S. Clin. North America,* **34**:1601–13, (Dec.) 1954.

Willson, J. Robert: "Prevention and Treatment of Postpartum Hemorrhage," *S. Clin. North America,* **34**:1591–99, (Dec.) 1954.

Woltz, John H. E.: "Puerperal Infection," *Am. J. M. Sc.,* **211**:743–51, (June) 1946.

Woodward, H. L.; Gardner, B.; Bryant, R. D.; and Overland, Anna E.: *Obstetric Management and Nursing,* 5th ed. F. A. Davis Co., Philadelphia, 1955.

Zabriskie, Louise, and Eastman, Nicholson J.: *Nurses Handbook of Obstetrics,* 9th ed. J. B. Lippincott Co., Philadelphia, 1952.

# PART VI. THE MATERNITY PATIENT IN THE COMMUNITY

*Chapter 19*

## Beginnings of Prenatal Care*

To make adequate maternity care available for all who need it at a cost which they can afford and to teach them the urgency of seeking it early is one of the important social and health problems of a community. Many agencies and individuals are engaged in the task. The student nurse herself is one of the individuals and she is already familiar with one of the agencies—the hospital, as well as with antepartum and postpartum clinics and mothers' classes. It is important for her to know about community facilities at the same time that she is learning the fundamentals of obstetric nursing and participating in the care of the patient in the hospital, lest that portion of the care that is given by the hospital may be exaggerated in her mind and her picture of the whole remain incomplete or distorted. She will see her work with each individual patient as part of a great nationwide effort to improve maternity care and will have some conception of the difficulties to be overcome in securing adequate care for every maternity patient when she understands how the community facilities for that care came to be what they are today.

* Historical data in this chapter originally prepared by Anne A. Stevens, R.N.

## THE MATERNITY PATIENT IN EARLY TIMES

From the earliest times the birth of a baby has been followed by some form of tribal, racial, or familial ceremony. Among primitive peoples birth, like other mysteries, became the subject of many superstitions. Some of them persist to this day, and others have become the basis of customs which are still followed. These early ceremonies for the most part included no real care of the mother but were feasts or festivals of thanksgiving, sacrifice, or dedication to propitiate the gods or to ward off evil spirits.

In primitive society many women undoubtedly delivered themselves, but women have helped each other since the beginning of society and the skillful, or perhaps the more willing ones, became set apart as midwives—women who habitually and for gain assist women in childbirth. Experience and exchange of experiences constituted the only training of these early midwives. When delivery was difficult, priests and medicine men were sometimes called on to help with prayers and incantations.

In early civilizations physicians controlled the practice of the midwives and helped with difficult deliveries, although the physician who undertook midwifery was generally looked down upon. Hippocrates and Soranus did much to improve medicine and midwifery in Greece and Rome. During the Dark Ages in Europe much of this advance was lost. Midwives were of a low type, and executioners and barbers were called in to help with difficult deliveries.

About 1500 the first lying-in wards were opened where midwives delivered the poor and outcast. Then in the sixteenth and early seventeenth centuries Ambroise Paré of Paris and the Chamberlens, who migrated from France to England, stimulated medical men again to take an interest in obstetrics. The first school for midwives was established at Paré's instigation at the Hôtel Dieu in Paris. In the eighteenth century state and national regulation of the education and practice of midwifery was begun, and the whole maternity situation in Europe was greatly improved. Puerperal fever, however, was a veritable pestilence during the seventeenth, eighteenth, and nineteenth centuries. It was so great in the hospitals that the public attempted to abolish them. There was no place but hospitals in which poor women could be delivered, and so puerperal fever raged until after 1847 when Semmelweis, in Vienna, demonstrated that the washing of hands in chloride of lime solution before examining women in labor would reduce its incidence. This plague had interfered greatly with the advance of obstetrics. A few years later (1853), after much opposition from clergy and doctors and the general public over a period of time, Dr. James Y. Simpson of Glasgow succeeded in introducing the use of chloroform anesthesia as an aid in obstetrics. Thus the period of modern obstetrics may be said to have begun.

## MATERNITY CARE ABOUT 1900

In this country at the beginning of this century the teaching of obstetrics was based on a thorough understanding of the mechanics of labor and on the acceptance of the teachings of Semmelweis, Holmes, Pasteur, Lister, and Simpson. It included the aseptic technic of normal delivery as well as the technic for various operative procedures and the details in the care of certain abnormalities. As in other fields of human activity the teaching of the leaders was far in advance of the average practice.

Supervision during pregnancy was hardly begun. Except in the practice of the best obstetricians, of the most advanced general practitioners, and in a few hospitals, maternity care began when labor began and ended a few days later, seldom more than 14 days.

The institution of modern nursing had improved the general care and comfort of patients in hospitals and in their own homes when they were nursed by privately employed or visiting nurses, although there were still many of the untrained kind. Some of the latter gave excellent care, but many knew little of real nursing and less of asepsis; and their work was in no way standardized.

An unknown number of midwives, mostly untrained and unsupervised, were caring for an unknown number of patients. There are no records to tell how many, and estimates varied tremendously because of the great differences in different localities.

In those sections of the country where houses were far apart, population sparse, and doctors scarce, neighbors did what they could to help each other, but many women delivered themselves.

Poor mothers used the lying-in wards and hospitals in the cities. The semiprivate and private maternity services were not yet available. Private maternity patients used hospitals only for operative deliveries or in dire emergencies.

In connection with some maternity hospitals, outpatient services had already been organized whereby doctors and medical students from the hospitals delivered patients in their own homes. The patients were previously examined at the hospital and registered for home care. These services were popular among mothers who could not go into the hospitals because they would have to leave their homes and children with no supervision.

Although there are no records on which to base an exact statement for the whole country, it is undoubtedly true that, except among the foreign-born mothers, the family doctor was the preferred attendant at delivery.

The attitude of the general public about maternity was the result of false modesty and ignorance. The need for a doctor and perhaps a nurse when the baby came was understood, but the less said about it the better. Pregnancy was mentioned only in whispers, baby clothes were made in seclusion, maternity patients were desirous of concealing their condition as long as possible, and any suggestion of care during pregnancy was frowned upon as an unnecessary and unwarranted interference with nature. Prolonging the care or any special consideration for the mother after the baby came was regarded as pure pampering and was seldom indulged.

Obstetricians knew, because it became apparent when large numbers of patients were cared for, that the deaths incident to maternity were tragically many and often preventable, but maternal mortality rates for any considerable part of the country were not known until after 1915.

## THE BEGINNING OF PRENATAL CARE

About the beginning of this century a new light began to shine upon the problems of the maternity patient and little by little the light grew brighter, and gradually more and more doctors and patients participated in the new program of care.

A new idea often comes to several of those working on the same problem at about the same time, and it is not always possible to know who first promoted it. We do usually know who were the early leaders. One of these, in this case, was Dr. John William Ballantyne, of the Royal Maternity Hospital in Edinburgh, who cared for and studied a great many abnormalities of pregnancy and labor. He emphasized in the early years of this century the importance of supervising all maternity patients throughout pregnancy instead of giving them no attention before labor unless they became ill. He insisted that much that had been accepted by the maternity patient as sent by God, to be endured with no thought of cure, was preventable by intelligent care. Dr. Pierre Budin was another one of the leaders. He had initiated, in 1892, in Paris, consultations for nursing mothers, and later consultations were open for pregnant women too.

Outstanding obstetricians, here and there in this country, learned to prevent among their private patients several of the complications, abnormalities, and untoward results of pregnancy that so often occurred. Then these doctors began to urge the patients who registered at their hospital clinics, as well as their private patients, to come earlier in pregnancy and to return for periodic examinations. Their initial examinations included more and more attention to the history of previous illnesses. More consideration was given to the general physical condition. The importance of exact pelvic measurements was emphasized. Frequent urinalyses were made. The importance of changes in blood pressure was recognized, and many studies of the symptoms of beginning complications and the results of treatments were conducted.

Finally antepartum clinics that were more than mere registrations for care at delivery became an integral part of the maternity services directed by these obstetricians. Later, antepartum clinics became a part of all hospital maternity services, but even in 1918 many hospitals were unwilling to assume responsibility for patients before the seventh month of pregnancy.

Some time before this it had been learned that the deaths of babies less than one month old were caused in large measure by the condition of the mothers before the infants were born. After this relation between maternity care and neonatal mortality was recognized, the same kind of work which had been begun by a few obstetricians because it could help to save *mothers'* lives was undertaken in connection with baby hygiene work because it was thought it might save *babies'* lives too. This difference in emphasis was the beginning of a great increase in the attention given to the needs of the pregnant mother for her baby's sake. Unfortunately it was not apparent to any but obstetricians for several years that the real need for the sake of mother and baby was better maternity care during the whole child-bearing process, not prenatal care alone.

Prenatal clinics or prenatal nurses were added to the baby health station work of the Bureaus of Child Hygiene, Settlement Houses, Church Houses, etc. Many nonofficial health agencies privately financed, whether organized for family work, for baby work, or for special maternity work, participated in the early development of prenatal care.

The detail of the work in the new clinics was much the same as that being developed by the outstanding obstetricians in the ante-partum clinics of their hospitals and included a health history, an initial complete physical examination with pelvic measurements, weight, urinalysis, a blood pressure reading, and frequently a Wassermann test; return visits at varying intervals for observation and search for signs and symptoms of beginning abnormality, with special care for the patient who suffered these signs or symptoms or any other discomforts. Often there was some sort of home visiting by a nurse or hospital social worker, at least to the patients with apparent social problems. Sometimes the home visiting was done through co-operation between hospitals and visiting nurse societies. Where there was no provision for regular home visiting it was not unusual for an interested and enterprising young intern to go himself to the home of a patient to persuade her to come to the hospital when her symptoms were ominous and she had failed to return to the clinic as advised. All the hospital facilities for consultation and treatment were open to these clinics, and the care of the patients had the continuity that is possible when the complete service of clinics, delivery rooms, nursing units, outpatient service, and nurseries is given. These clinics were closed to all patients except those who were to be delivered in the inpatient or outpatient service of the respective hospitals.

In some instances obstetricians examined the patients in the un-attached clinics. More often young doctors interested in maternity or public health work made the clinic examinations with little or no supervision from an obstetrician. The health station nurses, visiting nurses, or special prenatal nurses did the home visiting. When these patients were ready for delivery or needed hospital care it was necessary to refer them to another doctor entirely unfamiliar with their problems during pregnancy. The unattached clinics gave supervision to a wide variety of patients—those who could not or did not decide until the last minute where they would be delivered, those who were to be delivered by midwives, and those by hospitals or private doctors not offering supervision early in pregnancy.

The development of the unattached prenatal clinics not connected with hospitals or staffed by the doctors and nurses doing the other maternity work in the community divided the responsibility for the medical, and often for the nursing, supervision of the patient. This was a disadvantage, since childbearing is a single process from the beginning of pregnancy to the cessation of lactation, and any break in the direction of the mother's care is a distinct loss. However, it was not then a question of continuous or broken care, but a question of separate prenatal care or no prenatal care for all but a few hospitals' and doctors' patients.

The different ways in which prenatal work was begun are illustrated by the following instances. As early as January, 1901, the Instructive District Nursing Association of Boston began an affiliation with the South End Branch of the Boston Lying-In Hospital. In early reports it is recorded that the obstetric nurse received from the hospital the "list of the cases to be visited, of those who have already been confined and of those *who are going to be.*" The nurse visited 174 prenatal patients in 1901 and taught them to get ready for delivery, to make their layettes, and to prepare other necessary articles. "In abnormal or threatening acute cases the nurse takes the temperature and reports all symptoms to the doctor in charge." In 1902 with a second obstetric nurse added to the staff the first maternity work was done for private doctors and included one prenatal patient and 37 postpartum patients. From then on this work increased.

Visiting nurses going about the districts caring for sick and postpartum patients in several cities and towns had probably always given more or less advice to the pregnant women they met, but had not heretofore (so far as records obtainable today show) taken them under their care as registered patients and attempted to visit them with regularity.

The insistence of the demands for actual physical care of the sick was frequently so urgent as to interfere with the development of this new prenatal nursing service. It was natural to defer visits which seemed to have no urgency when compared with the care of those who were in bed and really ill. Prevention was a new gospel in those days. Besides each nurse was more or less feeling her way in learning how to do the most for these patients. They were not sick and did not know they needed care. They were interested in clothes for the baby, in planning for care at delivery, and in talking over their fears and questions with someone who would listen with sympathetic understanding, but not in the least interested in the nurse's suggestions about taking better care of themselves. This was especially true of those who felt well or were convinced that their discomforts were the lot of all pregnant women and if left alone would take care of themselves.

Although that first prenatal nursing was a minimum of what is now known to be effective, the nurses undoubtedly discovered abnormalities and were able to secure treatment for patients who otherwise would have had none; probably an equally important contribution to the patients was the sympathetic understanding and all it did to allay fear and promote a wholesome mental attitude.

In July, 1907, The Association for Improving the Condition of the Poor in New York City—a social work agency that became interested in health work because of the relation between poverty and illness—employed two "teacher-nurses" to visit the pregnant women in the families under its care. This work was undertaken in connection with a rest house for mothers which was opened in March, 1907. A report the next year contains this statement: "Teaching mothers before confinement reduces the infant death rate. In 202 cases visited *before* and *after* confinement, there were 9 infant deaths —4.9 per cent. In 135 cases visited *after* confinement only, there were 22 infant deaths—17 per cent. What would happen to the Infant Death Rate if all mothers were taught and cared for *before* confinement as well as *after*." The Association for Improving the Condition of the Poor also assured extra rest for those pregnant women in its care who needed it by supplying cleaning women, or working housekeepers, regularly for help with the housework. This agency continued and increased its health services for expectant mothers.

In 1909 the Women's Municipal League of Boston, under the guidance of Mrs. William Lowell Putnam, supplied to the Boston Lying-In Hospital "a trained-nurse for social service among the hospital's patients. Cases referred to this nurse have been visited during pregnancy, and instructed in the lessons of personal cleanliness and hygiene. Cases requiring medical advice have been referred to the hospital, and some of these cases have been admitted for observation and treatment. Serious complications of labor have thus been prevented." (From the Annual Report of the Boston Lying-In Hospital for 1909.)

Beginning in January, 1917, The Metropolitan Life Insurance Company—which offered visiting nurse service to holders of industrial policies—contracted to pay visiting nurse associations for two prenatal visits to maternity patients having these policies. This was a real stimulus to the spread of prenatal nursing. The number of visits increased and came to include postpartum visits also. The example of this insurance company was followed by others. Dr. Louis I. Dublin, of the Metropolitan Life Insurance Company, has made many studies of maternity records and is therefore one authority quoted in support of the lifesaving value of prenatal and other maternity care.

In 1917, stimulated by the late Dr. Ralph W. Lobenstine, the Women's City Club of New York, under the guidance of Mrs. Irene Osgood Andrews and Miss Annie W. Goodrich, established the first maternity center in this country. Through the center it was planned to secure medical supervision and nursing care for every woman in the district served from the beginning of pregnancy until her baby was one month old by coordinating the maternity work of every hospital, private physician, midwife, and nursing agency in the community and by stimulating the development of additional facilities as a need was indicated. A register was kept of the patients being cared for and of those in need of care. A nurse employed by the center did the home visiting and teaching for these latter patients. Every effort was made to help them arrange for immediate care. A clinic was opened at the center where patients under no other medical care might be examined by an obstetrician and supervised until they could register with a doctor or hospital for care at delivery. Patients to be delivered by midwives were also given medical supervision here.

Classes were developed for the mothers, and a teaching exhibit of baby clothes and mother's supplies was displayed at the center. One of the nurses had office hours every afternoon, and the patients learned to visit the center freely. To give mothers needed rest a working-housekeeper service was established with a special fund and used with the greatest satisfaction. A list of women known to be good housekeepers and willing to do several hours' work a day was kept at the center. When the need arose one of the women was sent to the patient's home, paid for out of the fund, and the patient paid the center such proportion of the cost as she could.

"Every woman in the district" was never reached, but the work of the various agencies was coordinated and the amount of service thereby increased. Each nurse learned all that any of the other nurses knew as the records, routines, and printed "Advice for Mothers" were developed in the nursing conferences. Excellent working relations were established with the hospitals, the doctors, and the midwives in the district.

In connection with the opening of the center, the Visiting Nurse Service of Henry Street Settlement established a 24-hour delivery nursing service and gave a month's supervised experience to the students at the Manhattan Maternity Hospital. This was the first complete maternity nursing service in the city, including prenatal, delivery, and postpartum nursing that served private physicians as well as the outpatient service of the hospital.

Finally the Maternity Center of the Women's City Club became a part of the Maternity Center Association—a voluntary organization formed to establish centers throughout Manhattan.

These different ways of beginning this work encourage one to believe that a need, once it is recognized, *can* be met—if not in one way, then in another.

There was little uniformity in the home visiting connected with prenatal work in the early days. It ranged from the doorstep visit to urge the patient to return to clinic—to the friendly visit to allay fears and answer questions—to a visit for medical social work—to a real prenatal nursing visit. The latter included the friendly chat and help with everything that disturbed the mother's peace of mind or otherwise interfered with her care. It also included noting her temperature, pulse, respiration, blood pressure, and fetal heart rate; making a urinalysis; care of the breasts; advice about or care for discomforts as prescribed by the patient's doctor or by standing orders from the clinic doctor or medical board. Help was given in arranging for delivery and postpartum care with consideration for the economic situation, housing conditions, and family relationships. Instruction was given in personal and home hygiene, including nutrition, and in the preparations for the baby. Plans were made for fitting the baby's care into the home life, so as to give him what he needed without upsetting everyone else and taxing his mother to the point of overfatigue. Interpretation of the mother's condition and her needs was made to the family, and attention was given to the health needs of the other members of the family.

By degrees the nursing and clinic procedures became somewhat standardized. Record forms were improved. Routine technics were printed and distributed. Details, as well as principles, policies, and problems, were discussed at nursing conventions. In time the doorstep or purely advisory visit gave place in all good prenatal work to the more or less complete nursing and teaching visit. The content of the visit was adapted to the prevailing medical opinion or modified to suit individual doctors when caring for their patients.

Patients were encouraged by nurses to visit them in their offices when possible for a part of the nursing supervision. These visits did not supplant all home visits, but decreased the number necessary and were an economy in time and money. They were frequently combined with the visit to the doctor in the clinic or with attendance at mothers' classes.

In some instances prenatal nurses assumed the responsibility for reaching every expectant mother in the neighborhood, by a door-to-door canvass, because the mother who did not know enough about her need for care to seek it was no less the nurse's responsibility than the one who did. In fact, in the earliest days of prenatal work, the real task was to find the women who did not know that they needed care and to convince them that they did.

Organized prenatal work began in cities and was reasonably well developed there before much was done about it in rural districts, and yet this country had many maternity patients living in its vast rural areas. After World War I there was a great stimulation to all public health work. The American Red Cross Public Health Nursing Service, other voluntary agencies interested in health, and state departments of health and education encouraged the development of nursing services in counties and small towns throughout the country. Many of the nurses included some maternity work in their programs.

## BIBLIOGRAPHY AND STUDENT REFERENCES

See "Bibliography and Student References" for Chapter 20, pp. 574–77.

## *Chapter 20*

# Recent Trends in Maternity Care

### COMMUNITY HEALTH SERVICES FOR MOTHERS AND CHILDREN

The public health movement has from the very beginning stressed maternal and child health. The first *White House Conference on Children* was called in 1909 by President Theodore Roosevelt. The purpose of this meeting was primarily to discuss the needs of the dependent child, but out of this conference came many recommendations for meeting the problems of mothers and children. One of the most important of these recommendations was for the creation in the federal government of a special bureau for children. As a result the *United States Children's Bureau* was created by Congress in 1912 under the Department of Labor; since this time the federal government has undertaken to protect the welfare of children. Creation of bureaus of maternal and child health in various state and city health departments quickly followed the establishment of the federal Children's Bureau. In 1946 this federal bureau was transferred from the Department of Labor to the Federal Security Agency, and in 1953, when the former agency became the Department of Health, Education, and Welfare, was transferred to that department.

As a result of recommendations from other White House Conferences, which have followed the first at 10-year intervals, there has been much federal and state legislation to promote maternal and child health. Among other standards formulated at the second conference were those for the protection of the maternity patient as listed on page 544. The Children's Charter with 19 provisions was formulated by the third conference (Fig. 150). The fourth conference recommended that the local community should provide care for mothers and children as needed; that the states should set standards of care, give leadership, financial assistance, specialized service, and supervision to the local services; and that the federal government should help the states by giving financial support, research and consultation service, and set up standards of care on a national basis. It also recommended better training of doctors and nurses and more appropriations for research. The fifth or Mid-Century White House Conference, held in 1950, was called to obtain more facts about the emotional and social development of children and to consider what must be done to give every child an opportunity to develop the mental, emotional, and spiritual qualities necessary for individual happiness. This was the first time that the future parents of this country had an opportunity for active participation; youth was represented by delegates from its own group at this Mid-Century Conference.

A real impetus came to rural maternity work in 1921 with the passage by Congress of the Maternity and Infancy Act. This act, administered by the federal Children's Bureau, stimulated the formation of bureaus of child hygiene in state departments of health and made funds available for maternity and infant hygiene work, the plans for which were approved by the federal board created in the act.

The work that developed as a result of the passage of the act has included studies of causes of maternal mortality, neonatal mortality, stillbirths, analyses of mortality rates, and studies of conditions in maternity homes. It provided institutes and practice in well-established clinics so that nurses and doctors might learn the new methods, demonstration prenatal clinics, and classes and nursing services to convince localities of their value and inspire their permanent continuance. Included also were instruction and supervision of midwives, campaigns to improve birth registration, traveling child health and prenatal clinics, parental education by group instruction and by the distribution of letters and pamphlets, classes in infant care for girls, and many other related activities.

Federal appropriations ceased in 1929, but the states continued

[*Text continued on p. 538.*]

## THE CHILDREN'S CHARTER

1. For every child spiritual and moral training to help him to stand firm under the pressure of life.

2. For every child understanding and the guarding of his personality as his most precious right.

3. For every child a home and that love and security which a home provides; and for that child who must receive foster care, the nearest substitute for his own home.

4. For every child full preparation for his birth, his mother receiving prenatal, natal, and postnatal care; and the establishment of such protective measures as will make childbearing safer.

5. For every child health protection from birth through adolescence, including: periodical health examinations and, where needed, care of specialists and hospital treatment; regular dental examinations and care of the teeth; protective and preventive measures against communicable diseases; the insuring of pure food, pure milk, and pure water.

6. For every child from birth through adolescence, promotion of health, including health instruction and a health program, wholesome physical and mental recreation, with teachers and leaders adequately trained.

7. For every child a dwelling-place safe, sanitary, and wholesome, with reasonable provisions for privacy, free from conditions which tend to thwart his development; and a home environment harmonious and enriching.

8. For every child a school which is safe from hazards, sanitary, properly equipped, lighted, and ventilated. For younger children nursery schools and kindergartens to supplement home care.

9. For every child a community which recognizes and plans for his needs, protects him against physical dangers, moral hazards, and disease; provides him with safe and wholesome places for play and recreation; and makes provision for his cultural and social needs.

10. For every child an education which, through the discovery and development of his individual abilities, prepares him for life; and through training and vocational guidance prepares him for a living which will yield him the maximum of satisfaction.

11. For every child such teaching and training as will prepare him for successful parenthood, homemaking, and the rights of citizenship; and, for parents, supplementary training to fit them to deal wisely with the problems of parenthood.

12. For every child education for safety and protection against accidents to which modern conditions subject him—those to which he is directly exposed and those which, through loss or maiming of his par-

ents, affect him indirectly.

13. For every child who is blind, deaf, crippled, or otherwise physically handicapped, and for the child who is mentally handicapped, such measures as will early discover and diagnose his handicap, provide care and treatment, and so train him that he may become an asset to society rather than a liability. Expenses of these services should be borne publicly where they cannot be privately met.

14. For every child who is in conflict with society the right to be dealt with intelligently as society's charge, not society's outcast; with the home, the school, the church, the court, and the institution when needed, shaped to return him whenever possible to the normal stream of life.

15. For every child the right to grow up in a family with an adequate standard of living and the security of a stable income as the surest safeguard against social handicaps.

16. For every child protection against labor that stunts growth, either physical or mental, that limits education, that deprives children of the right of comradeship, of play, and of joy.

17. For every rural child as satisfactory schooling and health services as for the city child, and an extension to rural families of social, recreational, and cultural facilities.

18. To supplement the home and the school in the training of youth, and to return to them those interests of which modern life tends to cheat children, every stimulation and encouragement should be given to the extension and development of the voluntary youth organizations.

19. To make everywhere available these minimum protections of the health and welfare of children, there should be a district, county, or community organization for health, education, and welfare, with full-time officials, coordinating with a state-wide program which will be responsive to a nation-wide service of general information, statistics, and scientific research. This should include:

(a) Trained, full-time public health officials, with public health nurses, sanitary inspection, and laboratory workers.

(b) Available hospital beds.

(c) Full-time public welfare service for the relief, aid, and guidance of children in special need due to poverty, misfortune, or behavior difficulties, and for the protection of children from abuse, neglect, exploitation, or moral hazard.

For every child these rights, regardless of race, or color, or situation, wherever he may live under the protection of the American flag.

**Fig. 150.** This charter includes the principles that were formulated during President Hoover's White House Conference, 1930, on Child Health and Protection; the conference recognized the rights of the child as the first rights of citizenship and pledged itself to the above aims for the children of America.

with a program for maternal and child health and a good cooperative relationship existed between the states and the federal Children's Bureau.

In 1935 the *Social Security Act* was passed. This included, among other programs, annual appropriations for grants to the states to improve their health and welfare service to mothers and babies. These grants have been increased several times. The sum of $22,-000,000 was originally appropriated. Of this amount $11,000,000 were set aside for maternal and child health services, and the rest was to be used for crippled children and child welfare services. All 48 states, the District of Columbia, Alaska, Hawaii, Puerto Rico, and the Virgin Islands received grants; they had to, however, give some financial aid. The federal Children's Bureau has the responsibility for the administration of such grants. This money is sent to the state agencies to improve the work of their public health and welfare departments. In recent years an increasing amount of the maternal and child health fund has been spent on professional training. Institutes for nurses have been held, grants have been made to universities for courses in obstetrics and pediatrics, and inservice training programs have been developed. A shortage of trained personnel has to some extent hampered the maternal and child health program.

A special White House Conference on "Better Care for Mothers and Babies" was called in 1938 by the Children's Bureau to consider the particular problems of maternal and infant care. Suggestions made at this conference included the appropriation of more money for maternal and child health service and the correction of weaknesses in the program. It was recommended that mothers have adequate supervision throughout pregnancy; that delivery care be given by a qualified physician in an approved hospital with facilities for handling complications, or in the home assisted by a specially trained nurse; that postpartum and postnatal medical and nursing supervision be given; and that consultation service be given by obstetricians and pediatricians to the general practitioner.

At the present time a wide range of professional people—doctors, nurses, social workers, nutritionists, trained in special branches of their profession—make up the staff of the Children's Bureau. This makes it possible to give expert advice to the state departments and to develop standards of good service. Among its many other responsibilities the bureau gives advice on adoption policies; there is now greater interest in improving the care of unmarried mothers and their children. A professional journal, *Children* (formerly *The Child*), is published by the bureau to report on all aspects of its work and all phases of child care. Besides functioning in an advisory capacity for all of the states the Children's Bureau cooperates in an international program for maternal and child care.

All states have a bureau or division of maternal and child health in their state health departments. With the help of the local health departments they provide health services for children through school age and for mothers during and after pregnancy. A limited amount of medical, nursing, and hospital care is given; services are directed primarily toward a preventive program by promoting health through increasing prenatal clinics, well-child conferences, projects for the care of premature infants, and public health nursing services.

The largest maternity care program ever undertaken in this country was a special wartime project known as the *Emergency Maternity and Infant Care Program* (E.M.I.C.) which was established by an act of Congress in 1943. Under this program the federal government, without state aid and without cost to the family, provided for maternity care for wives of enlisted men in the lower pay groups and for care of their children during the first year of life. The Children's Bureau was responsible for federal operation of the E.M.I.C. program, and the state health departments administered it. Private physicians and the hospitals throughout the country provided for this care. When Selective Service ended in 1947, the need for this program decreased, and liquidation began July 1, 1947.

The *World Health Organization* is also undertaking a program to improve maternity care. A Maternal and Child Health Section was established in 1948, and the first World Health Organization Expert Committee on Maternal and Child Health met in Geneva in 1949. A review of child health problems and general surveys of the basic requirements of various countries have been made by maternal and child health advisers. This is to make it possible to give advice on how the needs in these different countries can be met best.

## MIDWIFERY

Nurse midwifery has been practiced for a long time and is well established in Europe. It is a well-protected and carefully regulated profession in Great Britain where, in 1950, the midwives delivered 65 per cent of the maternity patients in or out of hospitals and attended at many others. In England and Wales 45 per cent of the women were delivered at home in 1950. The patient consults a doctor at the beginning of pregnancy, and if he advises that it is safe for her to have a home delivery she chooses a midwife unless her doctor plans to give her complete care. The doctor and the midwife examine the patient at regular intervals during her pregnancy. The midwife attends the patient at delivery and during the postnatal period, but she asks for medical assistance at any time that it is indicated, and there is a medical postpartum checkup.

From the earliest days there have been midwives in this country giving some part of the maternity care in many communities. Their work has been curiously limited by custom but more recently controlled and regulated by state laws. They practice in isolated regions and among the Negroes and the foreign-born. Some of the midwives are well trained; others are ignorant and untrained and have created an unenviable reputation for the whole group which is undeserved by the conscientious well-trained ones. Even the untrained ones who provide the only care available as they have seen it given by their predecessors are hardly to be censured since they have attempted to fill a need.

State, county, and city departments of health have been making increased efforts to control and regulate the work of midwives by registration and licensure; by limiting their practice to normal deliveries; by forbidding the use of instruments or drugs to produce abortion; by requiring the reporting of births, the use of prophylactic medication in babies' eyes, the summoning of a doctor if an abnormality develops; and by providing classes and supervision to help them improve their work. Supervision has been difficult to provide because it has not always been possible to assign to this work either midwives with ability to supervise or qualified nurses with midwifery training.

Where the results of the work of a group of trained and supervised midwives doing normal deliveries have been studied, the maternal mortality rate among their patients has been below that for the community as a whole. This would suggest that the midwife is not a liability in the maternity situation, but that properly trained, restricted, and supervised she is an asset to the team, this being particularly true in communities where provision for other care is lacking.

Individual nurses have done heroic work in maternity nursing and in unavoidable midwifery in isolated regions. An impressive example of what one nurse alone could do is found in the work of Lydia Holman, for whom the Holman Association was named. Miss Holman worked for more than a third of a century in the mountains of North Carolina among the most isolated and often the most primitive conditions. She began by living alone in a tiny cabin and caring, herself, for the horse that provided her only means of travel, riding 25 to 30 miles over mountain trails, up the beds of streams, and fording rivers as she went from one patient to another. Later a hospital, with doctors and nurses caring for patients both within and without its walls, and teaching health and hygiene, was built. One of the babies she delivered became a doctor to work among his own people.

There was no school for midwives in this country until 1911 when the Bellevue School for Midwives was established in New York City through the combined efforts of the board of trustees of the hospital and a subcommittee of the New York Committee for the Prevention of Blindness, consisting of Miss Lillian D. Wald, Miss Carolyn C. Van Blarcom, and Dr. J. Clifton Edgar.

In 1925 a new type of midwife—nurses who had studied midwifery in England—was introduced into this country by Mrs. Mary Breckinridge as one practicable way to provide more adequate care for mothers in isolated regions. She established, in consultation with the State Department of Health of Kentucky, the Frontier Nursing Service in the mountain region of that state. The only attendants the mothers of that region had had up to this time were the "granny-women" whose only qualification for midwifery seemed to be that they were "too old to work but could still 'cotch' babies."

The nurse-midwives combine general public health nursing with midwifery and add to maternity care the nursing of the sick and injured, the prevention of communicable disease by immunization, and the promotion of the health of the family by teaching personal and home hygiene, nutrition, sanitation, and the like. The work, supported by voluntary contributions, has grown to include a hospital with a resident physician, several centers where the nurse-midwives live and hold clinics and classes, periodic clinics by visiting doctors and dentists; in reality it is a community health service of no small proportions.

One of the many obstacles to be overcome was the costly necessity of sending the nurses to England for the training in midwifery. Another was the poverty and inaccessibility of the patients. The long rides on horseback over steep mountain trails and through rocky creek beds sometimes flooded with "tides" to reach the isolated cabins where they live made it all but impossible to get doctors when abnormalities developed. In the face of these difficulties the first 1000 patients were delivered with no deaths from puerperal causes, and there was a reduction of one-third in the usual stillbirth and neonatal mortality rates.

In 1932, in New York City, the Association for the Promotion and Standardization of Midwifery, fostered by the late Dr. Ralph Waldo Lobenstine, opened at the Lobenstine Midwifery Clinic—a memorial to him—the first school in this country to train public health nurses in midwifery. The graduates are available as nurse-midwives to supervise and teach midwives under the direction of departments of health, to practice midwifery under medical supervision in out-of-the-way localities such as those served by the Holman Association or the Frontier Nursing Service, and to act as assistants to physicians practicing obstetrics.

Three years after its opening the Lobenstine Midwifery School was taken over by the Maternity Center Association. In 1942 the association increased its capacity for training nurses in midwifery by acquisition of the Berwind Free Maternity Clinic. Graduates receive a certified nurse-midwife diploma. The Frontier Nursing Service opened a school in 1939, and the Catholic Maternity Institute founded a school in Santa Fe, New Mexico, in 1945. Several others opened and closed in the interim.

The nurse-midwife must be a mature, resourceful person with an adequate educational background, a good knowledge of obstetrics, an appreciation of the psychologic factors involved in pregnancy, and an understanding of the people with whom she works. She may need to live in an area with few resources and may have to meet many obstacles that could interfere with good maternity care. In areas where doctors are few in number and hospital facilities are lacking, the nurse-midwife is indispensable and, therefore, she should be adequately trained and supervised; she should always have easy access to medical supervision. For a midwifery service to be successful, close cooperation must exist between the doctor and the nurse. The normal patient only should come under her care; any abnormality suspected or developing later requires the doctor's attention.

The number of deliveries by midwives in the United States has steadily decreased. It is estimated that before World War I approximately 40 per cent of the births were attended by midwives. Statistics show that in 1935 the number of deliveries by midwives was reduced to 10.7 per cent and by 1947 to 4.8 per cent. Most of the work of the midwives is concentrated in the rural areas of the South and particularly among the nonwhite population. In 1947 approximately 20,200 midwives, which is 93 per cent of the country's total number, were concentrated in 18 states of the South and Southwest where they performed 13.8 per cent of the total deliveries in these states, varying from 2 per cent in one state to 35.9 per cent in another. In the Northern and Western areas they attended only 1 per cent of the deliveries in 15 states and were not practicing or attended less than 0.05 per cent of the liveborn deliveries in another 15 states.

Although the number of deliveries by nurse-midwives is decreasing, they serve in many other areas of work. They act as consultants in federal, state, and local health departments, in the administration of maternal health programs, in conducting parents' classes, in arranging for and assisting with prenatal clinics, and in making prenatal and postpartum home visits. Some find that their duties consist mainly of the training and supervision of the untrained midwives, a program sponsored by state health departments to improve care; the planning of programs in the public health field; and the education of the community to the value of good obstetric care. The educational status of the plantation midwife is poor, and she may have been practicing for many years influenced by many superstitions. The trained nurse-midwife teaching the untrained may hold frequent meetings for demonstration purposes, and return demonstrations of technics. These meetings also include reviews of the danger signs during pregnancy, the essentials of prenatal care, nutrition, preparation for delivery, the contents of the midwives' bag, care during labor, care of the newborn, care of the premature, and postpartum care. Education of the people in the community to the value of good obstetric care, what they should expect of the midwives, and the way in which they can help the health departments to improve care is a part of this program.

## DEVELOPMENT OF COMPLETE MATERNITY CARE

Just about the time prenatal work was becoming standardized the emphasis began to shift from it to "complete maternity care." It was clear that the good accomplished by supervision and intelligent care during pregnancy could be entirely destroyed by poor care at delivery and greatly lessened by insufficient postpartum care. Medical and nursing care, no matter how good, are not enough without sufficient food of the right kind, adequate rest and recreation, attention to social and economic problems—family maladjustments, distorted mental attitudes, habitual emotional disturbances, inadequate income, and anything else which interferes with the normal progress of pregnancy, labor, and the puerperium.

As early as 1919 this idea of complete maternity care was formulated in the "Minimum Standards for Public Protection of the Health of Mothers," adopted at the Child Welfare Conferences of national and international authorities called by the federal Children's Bureau:

1. Maternity or prenatal centers sufficient to provide for all cases not receiving prenatal supervision from private physicians. The work of such a center should include:
   a. Complete examination by a physician as early in pregnancy as possible, including pelvic measurements, examination of heart, lungs, abdomen, and urine and the taking of blood pressure; internal examination before seventh month in primiparae; examination of urine every four weeks during early months, at least every two weeks after sixth month, and more frequently if indicated; Wassermann test whenever possible, especially when indicated by symptoms.
   b. Instructions in hygiene of maternity and supervision throughout pregnancy, through at least monthly visits to a maternity center until the end of the sixth month, and every two weeks thereafter. Literature to be given to mother to acquaint her with the principles of infant hygiene.
   c. Employment of sufficient number of public health nurses to do home visiting and to give instructions to expectant mothers in hygiene of pregnancy and early infancy; to make visits and to

care for patient in puerperium; and to see that every infant is referred to a children's health center.

d. Confinement at home by a physician or a properly trained and qualified attendant, or in a hospital.
e. Nursing service at home at the time of confinement and during the lying-in period, or hospital care.
f. Daily visits for five days, and at least two other visits during second week by physician or nurse from maternity center.
g. At least ten days in bed after normal delivery, with sufficient household service for four to six weeks to allow mother to recuperate.
h. Examination by physician six weeks after delivery before discharging patient.

Where these centers have not yet been established or where their immediate establishment is impracticable, as many as possible of these provisions here enumerated should be carried out by the community nurse, under the direction of the health officer or local physician.

2. Clinics, such as dental clinics and venereal-disease clinics for needed treatment during pregnancy.
3. Maternity hospitals, or maternity wards in general hospitals, sufficient to provide care in all complicated cases and for all women wishing hospital care; free or part-payment obstetrical care to be provided in every necessitous case at home or in a hospital.
4. All midwives to be required by law to show adequate training, and to be licensed and supervised.
5. Adequate income to allow the mother to remain in the home through the nursing period.
6. Education of general public as to problems presented by maternal and infant mortality and their solution.

Standards such as these express "what those who were devoting their lives to the study of maternity" considered to be the *minimum* requirements. Since these standards were formulated, the length of time after delivery at which it is safe to dismiss a maternity patient has been prolonged from six weeks to six months to a year. A gradual return to the usual activities and responsibilities, determined in each case by the patient's condition as a whole, is acknowledged as an essential element in good postpartum care. Much closer supervision is advocated for all patients who have or have had syphilis, tuberculosis, heart disease, chronic hypertension, diabetes, toxemia, infection, hemorrhage, or any postpartum complication. At one time it was enough to know that mother and baby were alive shortly after delivery, but now it is recognized that the effects of childbearing are sometimes not apparent until months later. Maternity care is not now considered complete until all subsequent care needed by mother and baby has been arranged.

In less than 50 years the concept of maternity care has grown from attendance at delivery and a few days' rest afterward to supervision, care, and help from the moment the patient thinks she may be pregnant until a year after the baby is born. The early care was given by a midwife or doctor and untrained assistant. Now a whole group of trained and supervised workers is needed—doctors, dentists, nurses, midwives, attendants, social workers, mental hygienists, occupational therapists, nutritionists, and household helpers —not all actually caring for patients but necessary as supervisors, advisers, or helpers to assure adequate care of all maternity patients in a community.

The emphasis today is on better teaching and practice in schools of medicine, midwifery, and nursing; increased supervision in hospitals; investigations of the circumstances of maternal deaths, and more recently fetal and neonatal deaths; refresher courses to increase information of changes and developments; regulation and control, by licensure and supervision, of doctors, nurses, midwives, and trained practical nurses. The need is stressed for supervised household workers to provide relief from housekeeping responsibilities during pregnancy when necessary and during the postpartum period, and for adequate hospital, laboratory, medical, dental, nursing, and social case work services. The coordination of all the work is urged so that each patient may have what she needs regardless of her economic status. The teaching of every man and woman why women need maternity care and what constitutes good care is included so that "women will seek it when they need it and citizens be willing to pay for it, both as individuals for personal service and as taxpayers for community services."

At the present time such complete care as outlined is not yet available for *all* mothers, but more and more are receiving excellent care, and there has been a very great improvement in maternity care during the last two decades. This is indicated by the great reduction in the maternal and infant mortality rate over the past 20 years. The maternal mortality rate which was as high as 6 to 7 deaths per 1000 live births in 1930 was reduced to 5.82 per 1000 live births in

1935, to 2.07 in 1945, and at the present is down to 0.53 deaths per 1000 live births (Fig. 151). This is a reduction of 90 per cent over the past 20 years. The three major causes of maternal deaths are still present, but a reduction in deaths due to these causes has played a large part in the lowering of the mortality rate. Improved prenatal care has reduced the deaths due to the toxemias of pregnancy, development of antibacterial drugs has greatly reduced deaths due to infection, and the increased use and availability of blood for transfusion has played a large part in reducing deaths due to hemorrhage and shock. In addition to the great decrease in the maternal death rate the morbidity rate has also fallen, and there has been a great improvement in the condition in which the mother returns to her nonpregnant state.

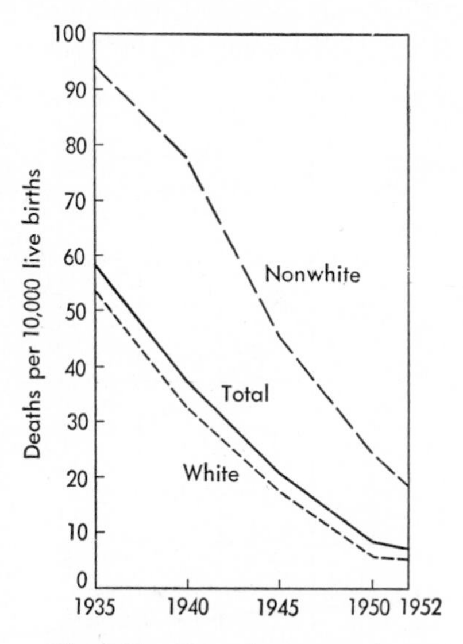


**Fig. 151.** Drop in maternal mortality 1935–52. Deaths of mothers in childbearing have dropped rapidly since 1935, but the death rate among nonwhite mothers is still more than twice as high as among white mothers. (Kirkwood, Samuel B.: "Twenty Years of Maternal Care," *Children,* **2**:135, 1955.)

This steady and rapid decline in maternal deaths is encouraging, but more can be done. That there is still much left to be done is indicated by the fact that the maternal deaths which occur among nonwhite mothers are still more than twice as high as among white mothers (Fig. 151). To further improve conditions, services must be spread to the people that do not yet have excellent care, and the depth of the service must be increased for those that are receiving good care. Every effort must also be made to further reduce morbidity and to reduce any adverse influences that certain social, economic, and psychologic conditions have upon the welfare of mothers and babies.

The infant mortality rate has also decreased considerably in the last two decades. In 1935 the death rate for infants under one year was 55.7 deaths per 1000 live births; in 1945 it was reduced to 38.3, and in 1952 the rate was 28.5 deaths per 1000 live births (Fig. 152). In spite of this reduction in the infant death rate it was estimated that in 1951 some 162,000 babies in the United States died before,

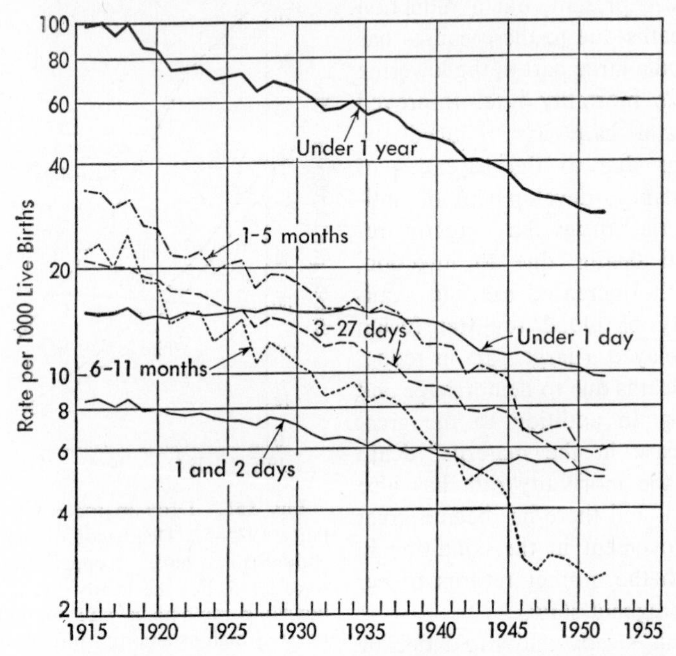


**Fig. 152.** Infant mortality rates by age: Birth-Registration States, 1915–52. (U.S. Department of Health, Education, and Welfare. National Office of Vital Statistics, Washington, D. C.)

during, or soon after birth. It is known that 75,192 of this number were neonatal deaths (under 28 days of life), and it is estimated that approximately 87,000 of this number occurred prior to, or during, birth in pregnancies which had reached 20-weeks' gestation.

Although the fetal death rate and the neonatal death rate have declined in the past two decades they have not decreased as rapidly as the death rate in infants between the first and twelfth month of life. Between the years 1945 and 1951 the post-neonatal death rate in the United States dropped 41 per cent, but neonatal deaths dropped only 18 per cent and fetal deaths per 1000 total births decreased only 21 per cent during this period. The smallest decrease has been during the first week of life (Fig. 190) and particularly in infants during the first hour of life. Between 1945 and 1951 the mortality rate for the first week of life declined only 11 per cent. More than two-thirds of the deaths in infants under one year of age occur in the neonatal period, that is, under 28 days of life, and more than one-third of the deaths under one year are in the first day of life. Approximately 10 per cent of all neonatal deaths occur during the first hour of life, these being largely due to immaturity, congenital malformations, birth injuries, and asphyxia and atelectasis.

The mortality among nonwhite infants is much greater than among white infants, with the relative difference being greater after the first few days of life than immediately after birth (Figs. 153 and 154). Some regions of the United States have a much higher fetal and neonatal mortality rate than others (Fig. 154).

[*Text continued on p. 552.*]

INFANT AND MATERNAL MORTALITY RATES:
BIRTH-REGISTRATION STATES, 1915–52

(Infant mortality rates are deaths under 1 year per 1,000 live births in each specified group. Maternal mortality rates are deaths from deliveries and complications of pregnancy, childbirth, and the puerperium per 10,000 live births in each specified group)

| | INFANT MORTALITY RATE (EXCLUSIVE OF FETAL DEATHS) | | | MATERNAL MORTALITY RATE [1] | | |
|---|---|---|---|---|---|---|
| YEAR | Total | White [2] | Non-white [2] | Total | White [2] | Non-white [2] |
| 1952 | 28.4 | 25.5 | 47.0 | 6.8 | 4.9 | 18.8 |
| 1951 | 28.4 | 25.8 | 44.8 | 7.5 | 5.5 | 20.1 |
| 1950 | 29.2 | 26.8 | 44.5 | 8.3 | 6.1 | 22.2 |
| 1949 | 31.3 | 28.9 | 47.3 | 9.0 | 6.8 | 23.5 |
| 1948 | 32.0 | 29.9 | 46.5 | 11.7 | 8.9 | 30.1 |
| 1947 | 32.2 | 30.1 | 48.5 | 13.5 | 10.9 | 33.5 |
| 1946 | 33.8 | 31.8 | 49.5 | 15.7 | 13.1 | 35.9 |
| 1945 | 38.3 | 35.6 | 57.0 | 20.7 | 17.2 | 45.5 |
| 1944 | 39.8 | 36.9 | 60.3 | 22.8 | 18.9 | 50.6 |
| 1943 | 40.4 | 37.5 | 62.5 | 24.5 | 21.1 | 51.0 |
| 1942 | 40.4 | 37.3 | 64.6 | 25.9 | 22.2 | 54.4 |
| 1941 | 45.3 | 41.2 | 74.8 | 31.7 | 26.6 | 67.8 |
| 1940 | 47.0 | 43.2 | 73.8 | 37.6 | 32.0 | 77.3 |

| YEAR | INFANT MORTALITY RATE (EXCLUSIVE OF FETAL DEATHS) | | | MATERNAL MORTALITY RATE [1] | | |
|---|---|---|---|---|---|---|
| | Total | White [2] | Non-white [2] | Total | White [2] | Non-white [2] |
| 1939 | 48.0 | 44.3 | 74.2 | 40.4 | 35.3 | 76.2 |
| 1938 | 51.0 | 47.1 | 79.1 | 43.5 | 37.7 | 84.9 |
| 1937 | 54.4 | 50.3 | 83.2 | 48.9 | 43.6 | 85.8 |
| 1936 | 57.1 | 52.9 | 87.6 | 56.8 | 51.2 | 97.2 |
| 1935 | 55.7 | 51.9 | 83.2 | 58.2 | 53.1 | 94.6 |
| 1934 | 60.1 | 54.5 | 94.4 | 59.3 | 54.4 | 89.7 |
| 1933 | 58.1 | 52.8 | 91.3 | 61.9 | 56.4 | 96.7 |
| 1932 | 57.6 | 53.3 | 86.2 | 63.3 | 58.1 | 97.6 |
| 1931 | 61.6 | 57.4 | 93.1 | 66.1 | 60.1 | 111.4 |
| 1930 | 64.6 | 60.1 | 99.9 | 67.3 | 60.9 | 117.4 |
| 1929 | 67.6 | 63.2 | 102.2 | 69.5 | 63.1 | 119.9 |
| 1928 | 68.7 | 64.0 | 106.2 | 69.2 | 62.7 | 121.0 |
| 1927 | 64.6 | 60.6 | 100.1 | 64.7 | 59.4 | 113.3 |
| 1926 | 73.3 | 70.0 | 111.8 | 65.6 | 61.9 | 107.1 |
| 1925 | 71.7 | 68.3 | 110.8 | 64.7 | 60.3 | 116.2 |
| 1924 | 70.8 | 66.8 | 112.9 | 65.6 | 60.7 | 117.9 |
| 1923 | 77.1 | 73.5 | 117.4 | 66.5 | 62.6 | 109.5 |
| 1922 | 76.2 | 73.2 | 110.0 | 66.4 | 62.8 | 106.8 |
| 1921 | 75.6 | 72.5 | 108.5 | 68.2 | 64.4 | 107.7 |
| 1920 | 85.8 | 82.1 | 131.7 | 79.9 | 76.0 | 128.1 |
| 1919 | 86.6 | 83.0 | 130.5 | 73.7 | 69.6 | 124.4 |
| 1918 | 100.9 | 97.4 | 161.2 | 91.6 | 88.9 | 139.3 |
| 1917 | 93.8 | 90.5 | 150.7 | 66.2 | 63.2 | 117.7 |
| 1916 | 101.0 | 99.0 | 184.9 | 62.2 | 60.8 | 117.9 |
| 1915 | 99.9 | 98.6 | 181.2 | 60.8 | 60.1 | 105.6 |

[1] For 1949–52, deaths are classified according to the Sixth Revision of the International Lists, 1948. For discussion of comparability between revisions, see text.

[2] Mexicans included with white each year except 1932, 1933, and 1934.

NOTE.—The birth-registration States increased in number from 10 States and the District of Columbia in 1915 to the entire continental United States in 1933.

**Fig. 153.** Infant and maternal mortality rates: Birth-Registration States, 1915–52. (U.S. Department of Health, Education, and Welfare. National Office of Vital Statistics, Washington, D.C.)

DEATHS UNDER 1 YEAR AND INFANT MORTALITY RATES, BY AGE AND RACE, FOR METROPOLITAN AND NONMETROPOLITAN COUNTIES: UNITED STATES, 1952

(By place of residence. Exclusive of fetal deaths. Rates per 1,000 live births in each specified group)

| ITEM | NUMBER | | | RATE | | |
|---|---|---|---|---|---|---|
| | All counties | Metropolitan counties | Nonmetropolitan counties | All counties | Metropolitan counties | Nonmetropolitan counties |
| ALL RACES | | | | | | |
| Under 1 year | 109,413 | 57,154 | 52,259 | 28.4 | 26.1 | 31.6 |
| Under 28 days | 76,252 | 42,165 | 34,087 | 19.8 | 19.2 | 20.6 |
| 28 days–11 months | 33,161 | 14,989 | 18,172 | 8.6 | 6.8 | 11.0 |
| Under 1 hour | 7,607 | 4,322 | 3,285 | 2.0 | 2.0 | 2.0 |
| Under 1 day | 37,412 | 21,415 | 15,997 | 9.7 | 9.8 | 9.7 |
| WHITE | | | | | | |
| Under 1 year | 84,752 | 45,679 | 39,073 | 25.5 | 23.9 | 27.7 |
| Under 28 days | 61,564 | 34,464 | 27,100 | 18.5 | 18.0 | 19.2 |
| 28 days–11 months | 23,188 | 11,215 | 11,973 | 7.0 | 5.9 | 8.5 |
| Under 1 hour | 6,289 | 3,616 | 2,673 | 1.9 | 1.9 | 1.9 |
| Under 1 day | 30,721 | 17,591 | 13,130 | 9.2 | 9.2 | 9.3 |
| NONWHITE | | | | | | |
| Under 1 year | 24,661 | 11,475 | 13,186 | 47.0 | 41.2 | 53.6 |
| Under 28 days | 14,688 | 7,701 | 6,987 | 28.0 | 27.7 | 28.4 |
| 28 days–11 months | 9,973 | 3,774 | 6,199 | 19.0 | 13.6 | 25.2 |
| Under 1 hour | 1,318 | 706 | 612 | 2.5 | 2.5 | 2.5 |
| Under 1 day | 6,691 | 3,824 | 2,867 | 12.8 | 13.7 | 11.7 |

NOTE.—For definitions of "Metropolitan counties" and "Nonmetropolitan counties," see Explanatory Notes.

**Fig. 154.** Deaths under 1 year and infant mortality rates, by age and race, for metropolitan and nonmetropolitan counties: United States, 1952. (U.S. Department of Health, Education, and Welfare, National Office of Vital Statistics, Washington, D.C.)

To help locate particular problems, work is underway, but much more is necessary, to discover the causes of and the means of prevention of fetal and neonatal deaths, of premature births, and of handicapping conditions which are associated with disturbances in fetal development and delivery. The prevention of premature births, which is the greatest cause of infant deaths, would reduce by one-half the neonatal mortality rate.

Results of poor maternity care which it is impossible to estimate are the periods of impairment which may follow complications or the mental trauma which sometimes accompanies a poorly supervised pregnancy. There are also the effects of the death of a mother which breaks up a home and leaves motherless children that cannot be estimated, but these effects are known to be great. Improvements, therefore, which cannot be measured but which, nevertheless, are very important are the decrease in the number of complications and periods of hospitalization with improved maternity care and, quite obviously, a decrease in the maternal mortality rate that leaves fewer broken homes and lessens the problems that follow this tragedy.

The improvement in maternity care over the past two decades can be attributed to several factors. The Children's Bureau, by emphasizing the high maternal and infant mortality rate and the preventability of many of these deaths, has laid the foundation for better care. Health agencies have made great effort to improve conditions. The public has shown more interest, and today the death of a mother is the concern of the community. Increased emphasis on obstetrics in medical schools and in postgraduate courses has raised standards of care by better preparation of the general practitioner and an increased number of specialists. Hospitals have increased their facilities for obstetric patients and have improved their care by segregation of the maternity patient from all other patients.

Good medical care (including the necessary consultations and laboratory tests)—continuous throughout pregnancy, labor, delivery, and the puerperium—is now available at hospital inpatient and outpatient maternity services.

Hospital insurance and an appreciation of the advantages of hospital care have induced more mothers to seek this care which makes available to them trained personnel and facilities for emergency treatment. Hospital deliveries in the United States have continued to increase in number over the past 20 years, rising from 37 per cent in 1935 to 79 per cent in 1945 and to 90 per cent at the present time. Over 99 per cent of the deliveries in highly urban areas now take place in a hospital.

The work of midwives is being supervised, and their patients are being examined by doctors in many cities and states. Nurse-midwives, supervised by a medical board and with medical consultation for abnormalities, are rendering a continuous service in some areas.

Nursing care and instruction, similarly continuous, are provided by visiting nurse services and other community nursing agencies for patients under medical care. Separate nursing services for the different periods of the maternity cycle are provided by many different agencies. Patients who do not know enough about their need for maternity care to seek it themselves are being sought and found.

Instruction in nutrition and help in planning meals and budgets are provided by social and by nursing agencies. A greater emphasis on nutrition has improved the general condition of the mother and the baby.

Advances in anesthesia and in the use of pain-relieving drugs have increased the chances of survival of the newborn. The use of antibiotics has greatly reduced the death rate due to infection, and the increased use and availability of blood and plasma have improved the treatment of excessive blood loss.

Dental care by individual dentists and by dental clinics is provided by health and social agencies.

Social case work service is provided by social agencies, by hospital social workers, by special case workers, and by mental hygiene supervisors in nursing agencies.

Occupational therapy, helpful in the treatment of maternity patients with chronic conditions that require long periods of rest and inactivity, is provided by hospitals, special agencies, and by nursing organizations.

Supervised household assistance by women who know how to give nursing care to a patient in bed, how to plan and dispatch housework properly, how to prepare and serve inexpensive balanced meals, and by neighbors who have had instruction in home nursing has been provided here and there in city and country.

Considerable teaching of the general public about maternity care is being done by official and voluntary agencies.

Services which support the social, emotional, and psychologic needs of the family are being added to maternal and infant care programs. As a part of complete care, responsibility is now being accepted for the recognition of the results of the stress and strain of a complex environment, and efforts are made to help reduce the effects of these pressures as much as possible.

In spite of these advances in the care of many obstetric patients, much remains to be done for others. There are some regions where care of the maternity patient is far from adequate. The mortality rate among nonwhite mothers is still more than twice as high as among white mothers (Fig. 153), and fetal and neonatal deaths among nonwhite infants are notably higher than among white infants (Fig. 153). Statistics also show that the risks in childbearing are considerably higher in nonmetropolitan than in metropolitan areas.

Providing the facilities to make complete maternity care available to every woman is a stupendous task. Believing that it is a possible achievement comes with the knowledge that each essential part of the care now known to be necessary has been provided somewhere, at some time, and is even now available to a large number.

The major obstacles to be overcome in making available to all mothers the facilities that are now enjoyed by many are (1) the individual ignorance of the need, (2) the inaccessibility of some mothers, (3) the difficulty in teaching others so as to influence their day-to-day living, and (4) the cost. These are sociologic as well as medical and nursing problems. The first obstacle is being overcome by every instance of good care as well as by the present efforts to teach the public why maternity care is necessary and what constitutes good care. Success is only a question of time.

Reaching mothers in their remote homes is a real problem. How to bring them the important supervision, teaching, and help month after month during the process of childbearing, as well as proper care at delivery, is the difficulty. The Frontier Nursing Service has shown one way to overcome some obstacles, even though there are others still to be solved.

To further improve the maternity situation and bring complete care to all it is necessary to provide good obstetric care to those living in the lower economic groups and in geographic areas that are not easily accessible. How to develop better maternal and child health facilities, more hospitals, or prenatal and home delivery service under the supervision of a physician, in some of the very remote areas, appears to be a problem which remains to be solved. An ideal program for all has not yet been found, but good ones have been developed by many communities and are being worked out by others. Some of the rural health programs which have been developed enlist the interest of all the physicians in the area, hold clinics and demonstrations for patients, make use of all of the public health facilities available, supervise the work of midwives in the area, and have a medical center and hospital to enable referral of patients with complications to the hospital and the specialist.

Today we must admit that there is a certain proportion of people that is poverty-stricken; these cannot afford adequate food, shelter, and clothing to keep them in optimum health. Many of these people delay adequate medical care because of the expense that it involves.

It does not seem an idle hope that in time the gaps between the areas of work now being done may be filled so that adequate care will be within the reach of all mothers.

To improve obstetric and pediatric care the American Committee on Maternal Welfare, the American Academy of Pediatrics, and the American Academy of Obstetrics and Gynecology have developed programs to serve all those concerned with the care of mothers and babies. The American Committee on Maternal Welfare held its first congress in 1939. Its meetings are designed to benefit both the general practitioner and the specialist. Meetings of special interest to the doctor, the nurse, the hospital administrator, the educator, and the public health worker have been scheduled. All aspects of obstetrics, practical and scientific, are considered. A mother's charter (Fig. 155), equivalent to the children's charter (Fig. 150), was adopted by this committee in 1941.

The American Academy of Pediatrics has a program for developing and improving facilities for the care of the newborn infant. It has published a manual of *Standards and Recommendations for Hospital Care of Newborn Infants—Full-term and Premature.* Its plans include the creation of state committees to sponsor this program of improving care and to serve as consultants to hospitals and health departments in solving problems concerning the newborn.

## TEACHING THE COMMUNITY ABOUT MATERNITY CARE

Teaching the community about maternity care is an important part of improving the maternity situation. No less an authority than the late Dr. J. Whitridge Williams is quoted as frequently having said:

"When the women of America recognize the value of and need for maternity care they will demand it, and then, and then only, will they get it."

This teaching began when individual doctors taught their individual patients about the hygiene of pregnancy. A few doctors used printed

## THE MOTHER'S CHARTER

THE DEFENSE OF MOTHERS IS THE DEFENSE OF NATIONS

*Every potential mother envisions the pleasures and obligations of creating and sustaining new life and is entitled to health and protection for the benefit of herself and humanity and should have:*

The inherent right to be well born without inherited or transmitted defect or disease.

The inalienable right to protection from disease and harmful influences during early infancy, infancy, and childhood, and to full development.

The opportunity to learn and know herself during adolescence and maturity and to acquire a knowledge of the origin and significance of human life.

The right to protection from pitfalls of married life and to a knowledge of its significance to herself and her potential family.

The privilege of proper premarital and preconceptional medical examination and advice and care for herself and her mate.

The right of proper and adequate care during pregnancy.

The right to receive adequate and necessary care during labor in her home or hospital.

The right to have appropriate care following labor in her home or hospital.

The right to secure proper and continuing subsequent care for herself and baby.

The right of preservation of health and life and happiness for herself and family.

(Courtesy of The American Committee on Maternal Welfare, Inc., Chicago, Illinois.)

**Fig. 155**

lists of supplies necessary for mother and baby and later expanded these to include some instructions about the hygiene of pregnancy and the symptoms to be immediately reported to the doctor. This individual teaching of the patient by her doctor is still being carried out by many and should be continued whenever possible. Classes and pamphlets can serve as supplements, but individual teaching is important in obtaining a good understanding of the patient and her problems, allaying her fears, and in establishing a good patient-doctor relationship. Its value cannot be overestimated. However, since the early beginning of prenatal teaching by the doctor, much literature has been printed and many classes for mothers and parents have been conducted which the doctor can use to supplement his instructions.

In 1912 *The Prospective Mother,** by Dr. Josiah Morris Slemons, was published, being one of the earliest books addressed to expectant mothers and emphasizing the hygiene of pregnancy. Many have been written since then, and in more recent years books directed toward the expectant father have also been published. Insurance companies added to the prenatal literature by printing instruction sheets for expectant mothers.

In 1913 the federal Children's Bureau published "Prenatal Care," the first of a series of pamphlets for parents. It is significant that the Children's Bureau, created in 1912 and charged with the responsibility for all matters pertaining to the welfare of children, should have begun its series of pamphlets with "Prenatal Care," thus endorsing the idea that the life of the child begins at conception, not at birth, and that welfare work for children begins with maternity care. This pamphlet has been revised at intervals since it was first published and was completely rewritten in 1949.

The first edition of "Infant Care," another Children's Bureau publication, was published in 1914. From the time that the first edition came out until 1952 more than 28,000,000 copies had been distributed. This publication has been revised, wholly or in part, many times and has been translated into eight languages. The tenth edition was published in 1955. Many other pamphlets and folders—among them "So You're Expecting a Baby," "Breast Feeding," "Diet and Development Wall Cards," "Your Premature Baby," "Your Child

* A fourth edition of this book was published in 1942 by Appleton-Century-Crofts, Inc., New York.

from One to Six," and "Your Child from Six to Twelve"—are distributed each year.

These bulletins are distributed largely on individual requests from parents, often at the suggestion of the doctor or the nurse. They are obtained through most state health departments or the representative of the Children's Bureau in the state, or they may be requested from the U.S. Government Printing Office.

Not only the patient but the family and the whole community need teaching if the public attitude toward maternity care is to be promoted. From the beginning prenatal nurses have taught patients and their families why women need supervision during pregnancy, and care afterward, and the reasons for each and every detail of their care.

Mothers' classes and mother-craft clubs were organized by the nurses so that prospective mothers might have the benefit of group teaching about their own and their babies' needs. Sometimes expectant fathers were included also. The outlines and briefs for these classes were printed by private agencies and by some departments of health and were used by nurses all over the country.

About 1916 some of the women's magazines that had long published articles on infant care began to concern themselves with maternity care in its individual and national aspects. They offered, gratuitously or for a small fee, letters and pamphlets of advice on the care of mothers and babies which were prepared by recognized authorities. State and city departments of health and various nursing and health organizations later prepared similar material for free distribution.

In 1930 the Maternity Center Association of New York City began a campaign to teach every man and woman in the country why maternity care is necessary and what constitutes adequate care. The campaign, culminating with an appeal to make Mother's Day, 1931, the beginning of better care for all mothers, was carried on through the newspapers, magazines, professional and trade journals, club-study programs, health-department bulletins, mayors', governors', and health officers' proclamations, sermons, radio broadcasts, and special local meetings to direct the attention of everyone to a consideration of the needs of his own community for increased or improved facilities for maternity care. The next year the campaign was repeated in conjunction with the state medical society and with special emphasis on what constitutes good care.

The general public was slow to learn the value of maternity care; however, a decided change in attitude gradually became evident. Pregnancy can be mentioned now, without apologies. The need for maternity care is discussed in the public press and the pulpit as well as in health journals and at medical meetings. People are learning that although childbearing is a natural process nature alone and unaided by medical science cannot be relied upon to keep the mother's body functioning normally under the stresses of certain situations. Many more patients are seeking care and seeking it earlier, but there still are others to be taught.

Mothers' classes increased from 1920 to 1930 and then interest fell off rapidly. Lack of enthusiasm in classes may have been due to a shortage of adequately prepared teachers and a decreasing interest in the material presented. These early mothers' classes placed much emphasis on preparation for home delivery and on the early diagnosis and care of the complications of pregnancy. Since World War II, however, the number of parents' classes has again increased. Classes now aim to give the parents an intelligent understanding of pregnancy and childbearing and they provide them with an opportunity to express their feelings and fears. In individual and group discussions many worries over the childbearing process are allayed; this should help to establish good family relations and provide a sound basis for child care. Unless these classes are conducted by a well-trained and enthusiastic instructor they may not be as beneficial as expected.

The teacher for parents' classes must have a good knowledge of obstetrics, be anxious to teach health, be emotionally stable, and have enthusiasm for the subject. The material presented should include more than a set of rules of prenatal hygiene and infant care. Scientific facts must be presented in a manner that will motivate the parents to follow the teaching through an understanding of changes that occur during pregnancy, a knowledge of the development of the baby, and an appreciation of how both mother and baby are benefited by continuous good care. Normal conditions should be stressed, and a sense of security developed. An important part of the subject matter is a development of attitudes which will help the parents to relate this pregnancy and the birth of the baby to the rest of their lives. The emotional needs must be given as much consideration as the physical care.

A well-qualified nurse and a doctor usually constitute the teaching staff for parents' classes. Assistance may be requested as desired and needed from a pediatrician, psychiatrist, social worker, and the parents themselves.

Classes for mothers and fathers alone, and combined, are being taught in some communities in connection with training for childbirth programs. These classes (Fig. 156) consist of lectures on the anatomy,

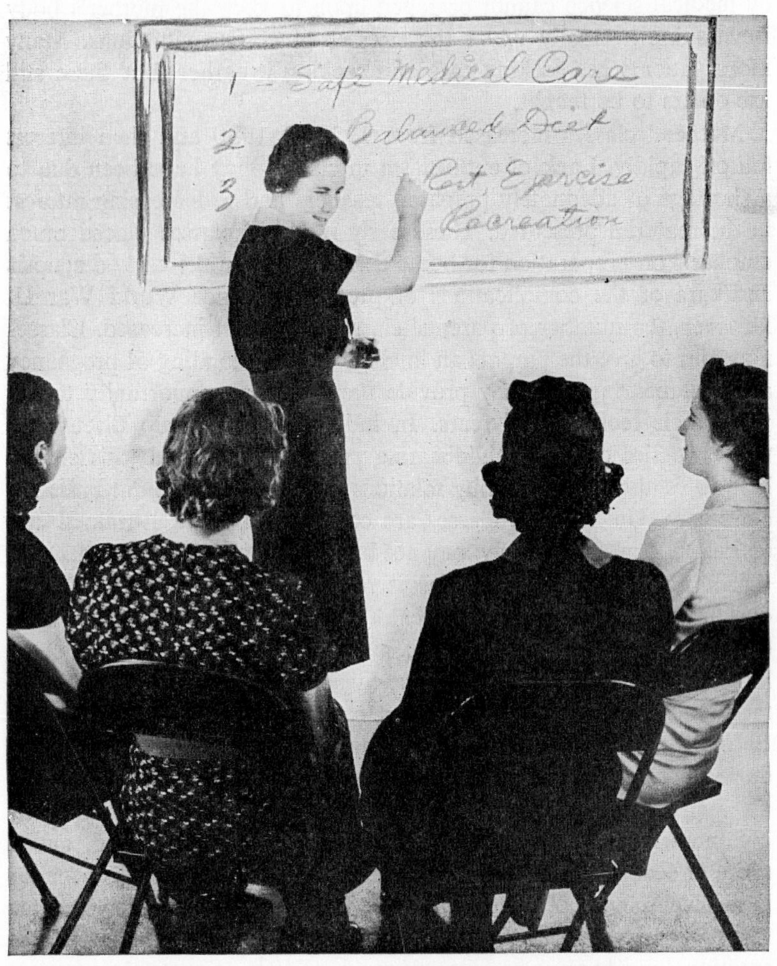


**Fig. 156.** Mother learns how to care for herself and baby at mothers' classes. (Reproduced with the permission of Maternity Center Association, New York City.)

physiology, and hygiene of pregnancy and labor with particular emphasis on the normalcy of pregnancy. Both the physical and the psychologic aspects are presented. Exercise classes which teach relaxation technics and aid in strengthening the muscles used during labor are conducted (Fig. 157). These classes may include a tour of the maternity unit and also the labor unit of the hospital in which the

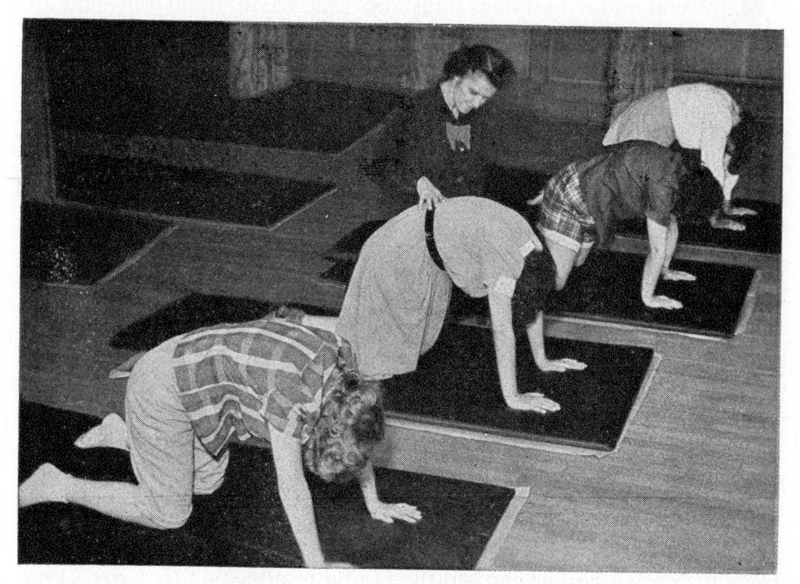

**Fig. 157.** Nurse teaching principles of posture to the prenatal patient; pelvic rocking exercise, quadruped position, and humped back exaggerated. (Courtesty of Visiting Nurse Association of Brooklyn, Brooklyn, N. Y. Medichrome, courtesy of Clay-Adams, Inc., New York, N. Y.)

patient will be delivered and an explanation of some of the procedures used during delivery. These programs, aside from having great educational value, help to strengthen the relationship and understanding between the prospective parents and the medical staff.

Education for raising a family should begin in the schools, where good attitudes and philosophies toward the responsibilities of parenthood can be taught. An important step in education has been the inclusion of the father in the teaching of maternity care. This stresses the importance of the entire period of pregnancy and childbirth as a family affair. This teaching helps both parents to understand the normal physical and emotional changes that occur, gives them more confidence, and helps them in making necessary adjustments in their lives.

## MEDICAL SOCIAL WORKER

Many community services must be utilized to fulfill our aim of complete maternity care. A medical social worker assigned to a prenatal clinic and/or hospital can be of great value to the mothers who need help with a variety of problems. A medical social service in a prenatal clinic allows for frequent interviews when an acute problem exists. The mother may need further help to obtain adequate care, need financial assistance, help in planning for care of the family while she is in the hospital, in planning for the baby's care if she must earn a living after he is born, in adjusting other members of the family to the new baby, or with innumerable emotional problems. The unmarried mother needs a great deal of assistance in making plans for herself and her baby and will surely need the guidance that the social worker can give in helping her to solve her problems. Another situation in which the social worker's help and guidance are of great value is that which arises with the birth of a premature baby; this brings with it additional expense and emotional stress.

By learning of the family's financial and physical setup and by an understanding of an emotional or psychologic problem that may arise, the social worker can aid the family in adjusting to a particular problem and give guidance in making the best use of available community resources. Community agencies, in turn, can learn from the medical social worker how they can be of most help to the family. By a recognition of the social, economic, or emotional needs of the mother and assistance in meeting these needs not only is her well-being greatly improved, but the child is born into a more secure situation which will contribute to his development as a well-adjusted individual.

## HOMEMAKER SERVICE

To give complete maternity care the homemaker service, which is still limited and mostly confined to cities, must be further developed. There are only a few such services in rural areas, but more interest is being shown. The homemaker is on the staff of a social service agency, is carefully selected and trained, and is supervised by a case worker. Essential qualifications are an ability to move from one family to another with ease and to adjust into any family situation.

The benefits from a homemaker are many. The family can be kept intact while the mother is in the hospital. It relieves her of the worry of the care of her family and of the dread of work she will have immediately upon returning home. The father does not have the worry of the care of his family while he is at work or the problem of finding competent help while his wife is away. The children have the security of remaining in their home environment. It is important for the homemaker to become acquainted with the mother and her family before the mother goes to the hospital; it is also important for the homemaker to remain in the home until the mother can resume her work (Fig. 158). She should be available to all families, but the lower income group usually need her services most.

## MATERNITY NURSING CONSULTANT

Many states now employ a maternity nursing consultant as a means of improving total maternal and child care. The consultant acts as a coordinator between public health agencies and hospitals and makes joint planning for patient care easier.

The maternal and child health consultant must be well prepared in the knowledge of basic nursing, have had obstetric and pediatric nursing experience as well as community nursing preparation and experience. She acts in the capacity of a hospital consultant by making studies and recommendations when problems arise in a hospital, such as problems regarding the care of premature infants or the control of epidemic outbreaks. She also makes studies to forestall difficulties in the nursing care of mothers and babies and to evaluate the good features of the nursing care. She makes an evaluation of the physical setup, the nursing procedures, the staff and student education program, the general nursing care, and concerns herself with anything else that contributes to the welfare of the mothers and babies. The consultant works with the public health agencies and assists with planning of staff education and health conferences. She may assist in a program of referral and follow-up care of mothers and infants and be particularly concerned with adequate teaching of the mothers and with good follow-up care in the home. She is in a position to correlate hospital with home care and with services offered by community public health nursing agencies.

This program probably had its beginning with inspection of hospitals under the Emergency Maternity and Infant Care Program. Im-

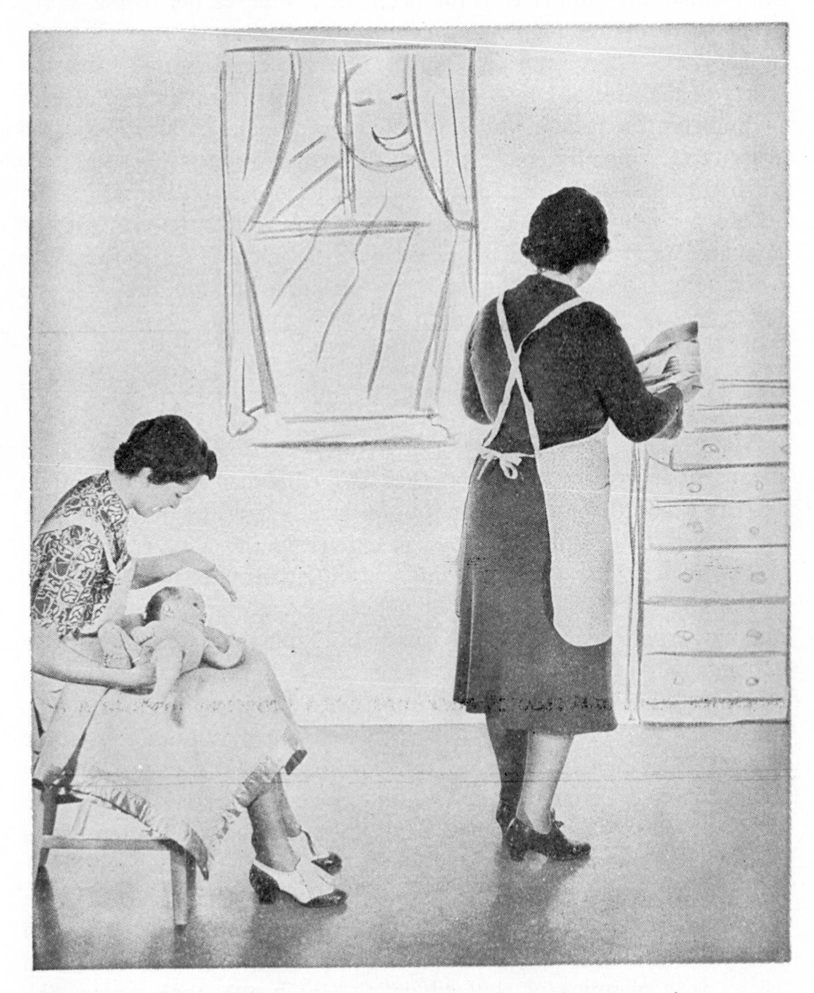

**Fig. 158.** Help with the housework gives the mother more time to care for her baby in a relaxed and carefree manner. (Reproduced with the permission of the Maternity Center Association, New York City.)

provements made under it created a desire for progress, and the value of the maternity nursing consultant was realized. Consultation in medical aspects is necessary at times, and as a result the team approach—doctors and nurses—has developed in the hospital consultation program.

## NATURAL CHILDBIRTH

A discussion of maternity care would not be complete without mention of natural childbirth and rooming-in, both of which have been instituted in hospitals in recent years. Dr. Grantly Dick Read, an English obstetrician, was first to use the term natural childbirth, and in 1933 published a book by that title in which he described the emotional aspects of pregnancy and delivery. In 1944, a book written largely for the lay public, was published in the United States under the title *Childbirth without Fear* and in England under the title of *Revelation of Childbirth.* Dr. Read came to this country in 1947 under the auspices of the Maternity Center Association to address audiences—professional and general public—on his interpretation of natural childbirth, a method based on the premise that childbirth is a normal physiologic process, but that misunderstanding and fear produce tension and pain. In the practice of natural childbirth fear must be overcome by education of the mother in the physiology of pregnancy and labor, by teaching the father to give emotional support, and by developing a change of attitude in patients and in the medical and nursing staff. It is essential for the medical staff to develop in the parents a feeling that everyone is really interested in them and to give reassurance to the patient in her ability to achieve a natural childbirth. The doctor, the nurse, and the parents must all work together.

Following Dr. Read's visit the late Helen Heardman, an English physiotherapist, who worked with patients being cared for by Dr. Read and other obstetricians, spent several weeks in the United States demonstrating to doctors, nurses, nurse-midwives, physiotherapists, and patients of the Maternity Center Association and the Grace–New Haven Community Hospital the controlled breathing, exercises, and relaxation technics used to prepare women for natural childbirth. She published a book under the title *A Way to Natural Childbirth,* in which she described exercises to be used during pregnancy, the controlled breathing and relaxation necessary during labor, and postpartum exercises for restoration of relaxed muscles.

The application of the principles of natural childbirth was instituted at the Grace–New Haven Community Hospital in 1948, under the auspices of the Yale University Schools of Medicine and Nursing and the Maternity Center Association, under the direction of Dr. Herbert Thoms. This program has worked out very satisfactorily and is being used in part or completely with patients in other hospitals and in home delivery services.

## ROOMING-IN

Trends in infant care have gone through complete changes over the past 50 years. At the beginning of this century babies were born in the home, mother and baby roomed together, and the mother cared for him instinctively; the baby was breast-fed and allowed to eat when he wished and he was held, rocked, and loved. The father had an important part in the care of mother and baby. Then early in the twentieth century infant care became increasingly strict, "especially in the scientific 1920's," when everything was done according to schedule. Babies were fed on an inflexible schedule, given artificial feedings according to the latest nutritional knowledge, and allowed to cry for long periods of time because picking them up would spoil them. All earlier methods of infant care were considered old-fashioned, and mothers were anxious to follow the latest scientific teachings. An era devoted to ultrascientific care had arrived. More and more babies were being born in hospitals. The busy hospital made schedules seem even more important. There was little time to teach the mother about the care of her baby; she went home inexperienced, but with a set of rules to follow. The father became unimportant, especially in the hospital situation.

Again a change has come about; a return to much of the earlier practice. This is a movement to "ancient processes in a scientific age." Schedules and routines are forgotten. The baby can receive loving when he desires it. His needs are recognized, and his rights as an individual are granted. Mother and baby rooming together is considered important for emotional security. Breast feeding becomes desirable; self-demand feeding schedule and picking the baby up when he cries, loving him and rocking him, are now considered important for the development of a well-balanced personality.

Thinking along these lines of less rigidity in the care of the baby began in the late 1930's. The first organized effort to improve infant care began in 1942 when the Cornelian Corner was organized in Detroit, Michigan. This group was composed of a psychiatrist, a pediatrician, an obstetrician, a nurse, and fellow workers in allied fields who planned to do research work and education in child development and family life. They emphasized the importance of allowing each baby to follow his own individual schedule since it is difficult for him to fit into a conventional one easily, and they stressed the value of early love to the development of a wholesome personality. Rooming-in, breast feeding, and self-demand feeding schedules were therefore given special emphasis by the Cornelians. They believed that the first step to the development of a well-balanced healthy adult was indulgent care as a baby.

Mothers began to request rooming-in, and professional support of this program increased. With growing concern over improving the care of the newborn infant, an attitude developed that at least the mothers who wanted their babies with them should have their requests granted. Separation of mother and baby and strict hospital nursery regulations had been instituted, at least in part, to improve infant health and reduce infant mortality. However, with overcrowding of nurseries and shortage of personnel danger of cross-infection became a threat. A return to rooming-in, with proper precautions, should restore the psychologic satisfaction of mother and baby and also give adequate protection against infection.

Rooming-in is a hospital arrangement by which the mother and baby room together, and the father has the privilege of caring for the baby as much as he wishes and thus becomes closely acquainted with him (Fig. 159). It provides the mother with all of the advantages of a hospital delivery and hospital care in as home-like an atmosphere as it is possible to provide. It is a program which focuses upon the family, providing a peace of mind which comes from close association of mother, father, and baby. The mother has the psychologic benefits derived from being allowed to handle, hold, or rock her baby any time he needs attention, from feeding him whenever he wishes to eat, and becoming well acquainted with his reactions. It also gives her the opportunity to learn how to care for her baby expertly with the nurses' help and guidance. The baby is much happier and has a greater sense of security than he has under a more strict nursery regime. Modern psychology teaches that this satisfaction—a sense of security, a feeling of being understood in infancy and throughout

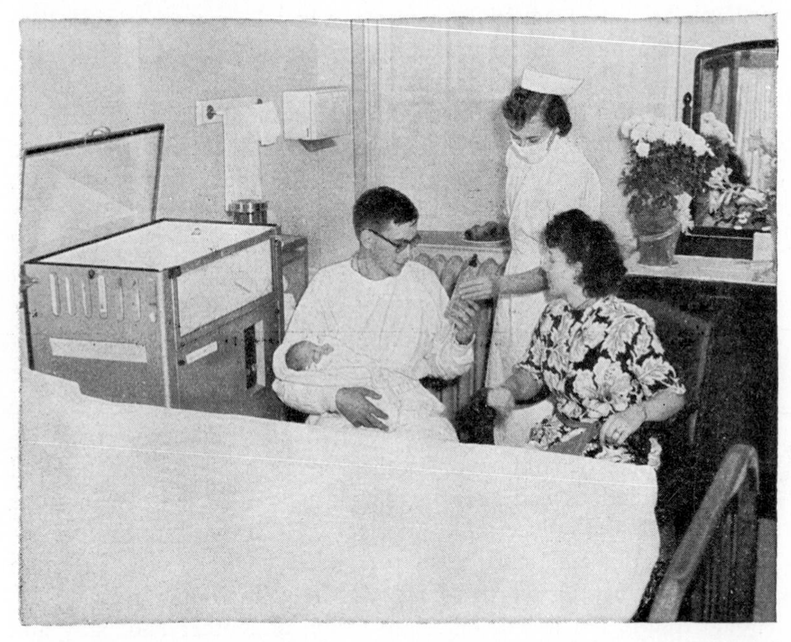

**Fig. 159.** Rooming-in. Mother and baby rooming together in the hospital allows for close association of mother, father, and baby. The parents learn to care for their baby with the nurse's help and guidance.

childhood—is important for the development of a well-balanced individual. This arrangement gives the father the privilege of becoming acquainted with his baby and participating in his care before he arrives home (Fig. 160). There is an atmosphere of democracy with no set rules and regulations which must be obeyed; mother, father, and baby can freely express their feelings. All this makes the adjustment in the home much easier by dispelling much of the lack of self-confidence and fear the parents would ordinarily have when they take a new baby home. They become well acquainted with him before he becomes their entire responsibility.

Rooming-in began with having the baby in the mother's room a part of each day. The George Washington University Hospital obstetric unit was designed to foster closer relationship between mother and baby. The mothers' rooms were planned around small nursery units. With the use of mobile bassinets which could be taken to the mother's bedside for certain periods of time and with the nursery

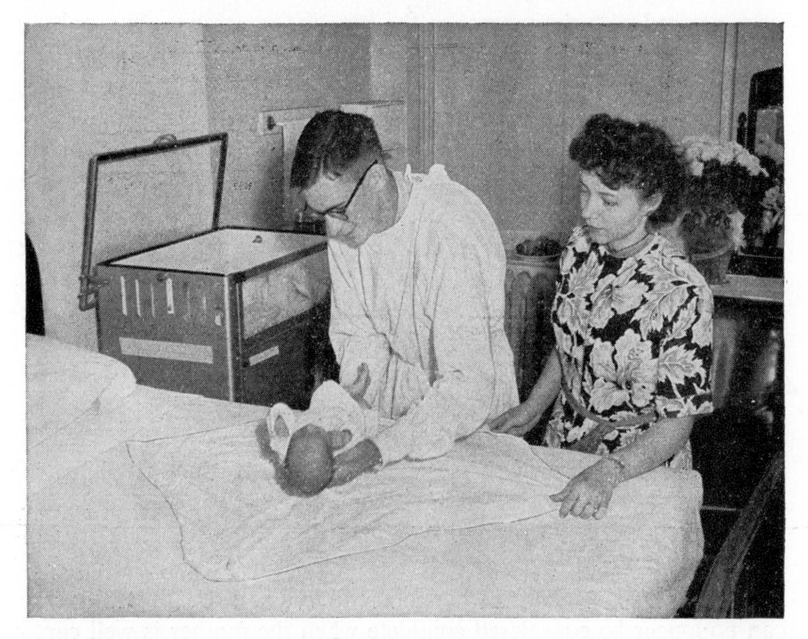

**Fig. 160.** When the baby is in the room with his mother, the father has the privilege of caring for his baby as much as he wishes and thus becomes closely acquainted with him.

close enough for the mother to observe her baby through the glass window, the teaching of mothers was greatly improved. Four hospitals in Detroit, Michigan, cooperated with the Cornelian Corner by having babies rooming-in in single-room arrangements for at least a part of each day and in some instances for the entire 24-hour period. In 1946 a four-bed rooming-in unit was established on the University Service of the Grace–New Haven Community Hospital for study purposes.

Since its early trial other hospitals have provided rooming-in; at least on a limited basis. Special room and equipment, when not available, are not too essential. A portable crib moved into the mother's room with a drawer space either below the crib or in the mother's dresser for baby clothes and a few of the essentials for his care are all that are needed for the physical setup. To be successful, interest and cooperation of the parents and hospital personnel are essential, and an adequate staff for nursing care is necessary.

Wherever it has been used, parents and hospital staff alike have been pleased with the success of the rooming-in arrangement and are fully satisfied that it serves its purpose well. It is not at all possible to arrange rooming-in for all mothers with the facilities available at the present time and all mothers do not wish to have this arrangement, but it is possible, in many instances, to provide it when requested. Since rooming-in must be limited it is, of course, of greatest value to provide it for the mother having her first baby who has the most to learn about infant care, but many times women with other children are eager to have rooming-in, and should have it, if possible, for the psychologic satisfaction derived from it and for the purpose of making breast feeding on a self-demand schedule easier.

Maternity care should be as all-inclusive as a good physical and mental health program; it should aim not only toward making maternity care safe, but also toward building a happy family life. At the National Health Assembly Meeting in 1948, at which all phases of public health were considered, a subcommittee on maternal and child health included in its recommendations for improving standards of maternal and child care not only the physical needs but the psychologic and social needs of mothers and children as well. Maternity care can no longer be considered complete when the mother is well cared for physically; it must now be considered in terms of the entire family. Parents' classes, better knowledge of the processes of childbirth, with less fear and tension, and more natural childbirth, and rooming-in of babies with their mothers are all directed toward this end. These services are limited to a relatively few number of families; the aim must be to make them available to many more.

## THE ROLE OF THE NURSE

Wherever maternity work is well done, there will be found the nurse responsible for some part of the care of each patient. The fundamental principles of obstetric nursing and the details of the care the nurse can give, as well as the privileges and responsibilities of the nurse, are presented in the other chapters of this book. A few of the important points in giving total patient care will be reviewed here.

The details of the work in the prenatal clinic may vary but should always include everything that will contribute to the comfort of the patient. Whatever else the nurse may do she will help the new patients most by putting them entirely at their ease. The young woman who goes to the doctor because she thinks she may be pregnant is often full of apprehension and vague fears as to what her examination will involve. If the nurse who greets her is glad to see her, interested in when her baby will come, and casually tells her what the doctor will do, she will have made a good beginning toward obtaining the patient's confidence and being able to help her in many ways as she returns during the following months.

Usually the patient will respond to a friendly approach by the nurse and be most grateful for her understanding. She may tell the nurse about symptoms or discomforts she would think too trivial to mention to the doctor, and so give the nurse an opportunity to interpret to the doctor the patient's needs and to the patient the doctor's instructions or preferences for her care. Much social work may be done if the nurse is prepared to help the patient solve any problems that interfere with her health and happiness, and to direct her to a social worker whenever this is possible.

The nurse conducting parents' classes must have a good knowledge of obstetrics and have enthusiasm for her subject. She must have the ability to present her material in an understandable language and in a manner that will make the subject matter become the personal concern of all of the parents. The emotional needs should be given full consideration, and a sense of security must be developed.

The nurse caring for the patient in labor finds that one of her important duties is a sympathetic understanding of the needs of the individual patient. With a good knowledge of the processes of labor and its emotional aspects she can be of great assistance to the doctor when she is with the patient during labor. She can help the patient apply the principles of relaxation and give invaluable emotional support by a sympathetic and confident approach. The care of the patient in labor provides the nurse with an excellent opportunity to give total patient care.

The nurse working in the rooming-in unit must be an excellent teacher, who has had experience in obstetric, pediatric, and psychiatric nursing and one who has the ability to do "the usual routine jobs in a non-routine manner." She must be adaptable enough to meet with ease any situation which may arise. She must be able to teach the parents the flexible schedule and the daily infant care with a technic which does not involve using the rigid "aseptic" nursery procedure that cannot be applied at home. A congenial and democratic atmosphere must exist in which everyone has an opportunity to express his feelings. The nurse must establish a good relationship with the family and realize that the success of the program depends upon her ability to teach the parents, to answer their questions, and dispel their fears and uncertainties. Success depends upon the help that she can give in applying that which they learn to their home environment. As in the care of the patient in labor the nurse is given an opportunity to do nursing of the highest caliber—she gives not only total patient care, but good family care.

The duties of the nurse in public health are many and varied. The associations' work is a "family health service." Whatever the reason for the initial visit to any home the plan is to give attention to every health and social need that is discovered, to teach personal and home hygiene, and not to dismiss the family until their needs have been met or are being cared for by another agency. Maternity nursing is a part of this family health service and is given to the pregnant and postpartum patients that apply or are referred for care and to those the nurses meet in their daily work.

In working with any one of these community agencies the nurse may be called upon to search for the patients who do not know enough about their needs for care to seek it themselves. It takes much more than instructions and a list of directions to inspire the nurse with a zeal to overcome the difficulties of finding and teaching patients and keeping them under care. That zeal will come from an overwhelming conviction in the nurse's own mind of the importance of adequate maternity care for every mother and of her responsibility as the nurse who knows the value of good care for finding and teaching the patient who has not yet learned its value. She frequently meets patients who have not consulted a doctor and to whom she can give information regarding maternity care and community services. Once the patient is receiving prenatal care the nurse can help the parents to carry out the medical advice they have received and she can explain and supplement the instructions given by the doctor. She has an excellent opportunity to discuss with them the many details of physical and mental preparation and help to dispel worry and fear. Very effective teaching can also be done in the field of nutrition. In her home visits and by group teaching she can re-emphasize the importance of regular visits to the doctor.

The patient with a problem is sure to be met often. Family relationships, the anguish of the unmarried mother, the distress of the deserted mother, the bitter resentment against the world and life because of an unwelcome pregnancy, troublesome in-laws, inadequate income, overcrowded apartments, the overwhelming difficulty of unaccustomed housework—all present problems. The nurse needs a knowledge of every community resource for social and recreational work and she needs wisdom and understanding; if she is to help these patients she must strike the right chord at the first meeting—otherwise there may not be a second one.

Good working relations must be established with all the social and welfare agencies in the community, such as family welfare departments, city and county welfare and relief agencies, and children's service societies. In this way the nurses can bring to their patients, by consultation or reference, every facility there is for overcoming the social conditions that interfere with health and happiness.

The nurse must learn something of the characteristics of the community, the nationalities of the residents and their traditions, the general economic status of the families, the common social and health problems, and the social and health agencies offering help regardless of whether she is employed in the hospital or by a community agency. With this knowledge the hospital nurse can give more effective care and bridge the gap between hospital and home care more completely. She will be in a position to help advise on referral to other agencies, making follow-up care of the mother and baby easier.

The public health nurse finds many opportunities to interpret hospital experience and learnings to the parents. Through her visits to the parents in their own home she is able to consult with them about the care of the mother, baby, and family living in general. Even the mother who has had the rooming-in arrangement in the hospital may need help in applying what she has learned and in making adjustments at home. With these mothers, the nurse has more time for the care she wishes to give beyond physical needs; instead of teaching the mother the fundamentals of infant care she can help her to apply her newly acquired knowledge to the home situation and give assistance with other problems that may have arisen.

The public health nurse may find that occasionally her various duties include the care of patients in labor, preparing for and assisting with home deliveries, and giving the mother and the baby nursing care in the postpartum period.

In any day's work the nurse who does obstetric nursing may find it among her duties to give to each patient health teaching, practical assistance, support for her fears and anxieties, aseptic care, skilled treatments, and help with other problems. To the doctor she gives dependable assistance, an assurance that his patients will be carefully watched, and discriminating reports. These reports are made in writing unless immediate communication is necessary in which case they may be made orally and the written report may follow. To the family she brings an understanding of the mother's needs, both physical and emotional, and offers help which will make the necessary adjustments easier. In all this she will find immense satisfaction.

Medical and nursing care, although very important, are not enough. All physical and emotional needs must be met, attention must be directed to solving social and economic problems, and care must be given to anything that may interfere with the mother's health and happiness and with the birth of a well baby into a happy and well-adjusted home.

## BIBLIOGRAPHY AND STUDENT REFERENCES

Adair, Fred L.: "The American Committee on Maternal Welfare, Inc.," *The Mother* (Quarterly Bulletin of The American Committee on Maternal Welfare), **1**:5–7, (Apr.) 1940.

American Committee of Pediatrics: *Standards and Recommendations for Hospital Care of Newborn Infants—Full-term and Premature.* American Academy of Pediatrics, Evanston, Ill., 1954.

Bauman, Elaine: "The Visiting Nurse Views Rooming-in," *Pub. Health Nursing,* **42**:263–66, (May) 1950.

Baumgartner, Leona: "The American Pattern for Child Health," *Briefs,* **14**:2–7, (Feb.) 1950.

Baumgartner, Leona, and Gold, Edwin: "Safer and Happier Motherhood," *The Mother* (Journal of the American Committee on Maternal Welfare, Inc.), **14**:7–11, (Autumn Quarter) 1953.

Blake, Florence G.: *The Child, His Parents and the Nurse.* J. B. Lippincott Co., Philadelphia, 1954, pp. 68–87.

Brackett, Alice F., and Price, Bronson: "Main Causes of Infant Mortality," *Nursing Outlook,* **1**:355–57, (June) 1953.

Brooksbank, Margaret: "Maternity Care in Great Britain," *Pub. Health Nursing,* **42**:650–51, (Dec.) 1950.

Caplan, Gerald: "Preparation for Healthy Parenthood," *Children,* **1**:171–75, (Sept.–Oct.) 1954.

Children's Bureau: "Parents Welcome New Edition of Infant Care," *The Child,* **16**:66–67 and 76, (Jan.) 1952.

"Children's Bureau Reviews a Year's Work," *The Child,* **12**:100–108, (Jan.) 1948.

Clifford, Stewart H., and Davison, Wilburt C.: "The Origin of Obstetric Nurseries," *J. Pediat.,* **44**:205–12, (Feb.) 1954.

Corbin, Hazel: "Maternity Care Today and Tomorrow," *Am. J. Nursing,* **53**:201–4, (Feb.) 1953.

Davis, M. Edward: "Trends in Maternal Health," *Pub. Health Nursing,* **40**:450–54, (Sept.) 1948.

DeLee, Sol T., and Duncan, Iva J.: "Training for Natural Childbirth," *Am. J. Nursing,* **56**:48–50, (Jan.) 1956.

Eastman, Nicholson J.: "Maternity Care Looks to the Future," *Children,* **1**:5–9, (Jan.–Feb.) 1954.

Eliot, Martha: "For the Health of the World's Children," *The Child,* **15**:44 and 53, (Oct.) 1950.

———: "New Horizons for Child Health," *Pub. Health Rep.,* **67**:169–71, (Feb.) 1952.

———: "A Twenty-Year Perspective on Services to Children," *Children,* **2**:123–26, (July–Aug.) 1955.

Faison, Jere: "Natural Childbirth," *Pub. Health Nursing,* **43**:120–25, (Mar.) 1951.

Galt, Edith: "Midwifery in China Today," *Briefs,* **16**:12–16, (Apr.) 1952.

Gibson, Mrs. George W.: "A Mother Speaks," *The Child,* **18**:19–21, (Oct.) 1953.

Goodman, Leonard: "Obstetrics in a Primitive African Community," *Am. J. Pub. Health,* **41** (Part II):56–64, (Nov.) 1951.

Gould, Lawrence: "How to Give Your Baby the Best Start in Life," *Child—Family Digest,* **1**:37–43, (June) 1949. (Reprinted from *Family Circle,* Jan., 1949.)

Gruener, Jeanette R., and Jensen, Deborah MacLurg: *Community Problems.* C. V. Mosby Co., St. Louis, 1954.

Hale, Minnie O.: "Arkansas Teaches Her Midwives," *The Child,* **11**:66–69, (Oct.) 1946.

———: "Arkansas Midwives Have All-day Graduation Exercises," *The Child,* **13**:53–54, (Oct.) 1948.

Harris, Antoinette: "A Public Health Nurse in Rooming-in," *Pub. Health Nursing,* **44**:580–84, (Oct.) 1952.

Heardman, Helen: *Relaxation and Exercise for Natural Childbirth.* Williams & Wilkins Co., Baltimore, 1950.

Heardman, Helen: *A Way to Natural Childbirth,* E. & S. Livingstone, Ltd., Edinburgh, 1950.

Hickcox, Verda: "Changing Maternity and Newborn Care in the Hospital," *Pub. Health Nursing,* **42**:435–39, (Aug.) 1950.

Hillard, Beatrice R.: "Teaching Patients in a Maternity Pavilion," *Am. J. Nursing,* **56**:324–26, (Mar.) 1956.

Hunt, Eleanor P.: "Getting at the Facts of Infant Losses," *Children,* **2**:15–21, (Jan.–Feb.) 1955.

Jackson, Edith: "New Trends in Maternity Care," *Am. J. Nursing,* **55**:584–87, (May) 1955.

Jackson, Edith, and others: "A Hospital Rooming-in Unit for Four Newborn Infants and Their Mothers," *Pediatrics,* **1**:28–43, (Jan.) 1948.

Jump, Dorothy: "Mothers' Classes for Preparation for Labor," *Pub. Health Nursing,* **43**:153–54, (Mar.) 1951.

Kirkwood, Samuel B.: "Twenty Years of Maternal Care," *Children,* **2**:133–38, (July–Aug.) 1955.

Losty, Margaret A.; Wallace, Helen M.; and Abramson, Harold: "What the Hospital Nursing Consultant Does," *Am. J. Nursing,* **48**:158–60, (Mar.) 1948.

McIntosh, Millicent C.: "Education for Maternity," *Briefs,* **14**:14–16, (June) 1950.

McLendon, Preston A., and Parks, John: "Nurseries Designed for Modern Maternity," *Mod. Hosp.,* **65**:46–49, (July) 1945.

Maternity Center Association: "A Review of the National Health Assembly," *Briefs,* **12**:8–11, (July) 1948.

———: "Special Parents' Class Number," *Briefs,* **12**:2–15, (Nov.) 1948.

———: "Yale Experiments with Natural Childbirth," *Briefs,* **13**:6–7 and 13–15, (Dec.) 1948.

———: "Motivation the Key to Health Education," *Briefs,* **13**:13–16, (Feb.) 1949.

———: "Rooming-in, Family Centered or Hospital Centered," *Briefs,* **13**:8–11, (May) 1949.

———: "Helen Heardman," *Briefs,* **14**:16, (Feb.) 1950.

———: "Pity the Poor Parent," *Briefs,* **14**:2–6, (Apr.) 1950.

———: "Rules That Didn't Work," *Briefs,* **14**:7, (Apr.) 1950.

———: "Maternity Care for the Community," *Briefs,* **19**:3–6, (Feb.) 1955.

———: "Twenty Years of Nurse Midwifery," *Briefs,* **19**:8–13, (Mar.) 1955.

Metropolitan Life Insurance Company: "Perinatal Mortality," *Statist. Bull. Metrop. Life Insur. Co.,* **37**:1–4, (Apr.) 1956.

Moloney, James C.; Montgomery, John C.; and Trainham, Genevieve: "The Newborn, His Family, and the Modern Hospital," *Mod. Hosp.,* **67**:43–46, (Dec.) 1946.

Morlock, Maud: "Homemaker Service to Mothers at the Time of Confinement," *Pub. Health Nursing,* **42**:282–86, (May) 1950.

Mustard, Harry S.: *An Introduction to Public Health,* 3rd ed. The Macmillan Company, New York, 1953.

Peck, Elizabeth: "Mothers' Classes Answer a Community Need," *Pub. Health Nursing,* **43**:616–19, (Nov.) 1951.

Read, Grantly D.: *The Birth of a Child.* William Heinemann, Medical Books, Ltd., London, 1947.

———: *Childbirth without Fear,* 2nd ed. Harper & Brothers, New York, 1953.

Rice, Elizabeth P.: "Prenatal Clinics Should Offer Medical Social Services," *The Child,* **14**:34–35 and 46–47, (Sept.) 1949.

Schlesinger, Edward R.: "Child-Health Services since 1935," *Children,* **2**:127–32, (July–Aug.) 1955.

Shepard, William P.; Smith, Charles E.; Beard, Rodney R.; and Reynolds, Leon W.: *Essentials of Public Health,* 2nd ed. J. B. Lippincott Co., Philadelphia, 1952.

Shoemaker, Sister M. Theophane: "Is Nurse-Midwifery the Solution?" *Pub. Health Nursing,* **38**:644–48, (Dec.) 1946.

Simmons, Leo W.: "Cultural Patterns in Childbirth," *Am. J. Nursing,* **52**:989–91, (Aug.) 1952.

Sinsarian, Frances P., and Taylor, Roberta W.: "Two Mothers Revolt," *Child Study,* **22**:45–52, (Winter) 1944–45.

Snoke, Albert W.: "Rooming-in and Natural Childbirth," *Mod. Hosp.,* **77**:98–110, (Sept.) 1951.

Taylor, Dorothy W.: "Evolution of British Maternity Services," *Am. J. Pub. Health,* **41** (Part II):35–41, (Nov.) 1951.

Thomas, Margaret W.: "Maternity Care—2000 A.D.," *Pub. Health Nursing,* **42**:259–62, (May) 1950.

Thoms, Herbert: "The Preparation for Childbirth Program," *Obst. & Gynec. Surv.,* **10**:1–6, (Feb.) 1955.

Thoms, Herbert, and Wyatt, Robert: "A Natural Childbirth Program," *Am. J. Pub. Health,* **40**:787–91, (July) 1950.

Wallace, Helen M.: "Current Trends in Health Services for Mothers and Children," *Pub. Health Nursing,* **44**:690–93, (Dec.) 1952.

Whitridge, John, Jr.: "Toward Better Care for Rural Mothers," *The Child,* **12**:98–99 and 109, (Jan.) 1948.

Wiedenbach, Ernestine: "Childbirth As Mothers Say They Like It," *Pub. Health Nursing,* **41**:417–21, (Aug.) 1949.

Worrell, Kathryn: "The Maternal and Child Health Consultant in the Hospital Program," *Pub. Health Nursing,* **42**:329–32, (June) 1950.

# PART VII. THE CARE OF THE BABY

## Chapter 21

# Characteristics and Development of the Normal Newborn Baby

Before beginning a discussion of the care of the newborn baby, the nurse will want to pause to consider this representative of the future. His importance to humanity defies estimation; his readiness for living can, however, be evaluated with considerable accuracy.

During the months immediately preceding birth, all physical structures necessary for independent life have functioned to a limited degree in utero. The incident of birth requires immediate adjustment to a vastly different environment and presents the newborn with hazards that can be anticipated—*must* be anticipated for each newborn if his optimum possibilities are to be realized.

In recognition of the unique dangers inherent in the first four weeks of life, students of obstetrics and pediatrics, of growth and development, and of biostatistics give them separate and important consideration. These four weeks are spoken of as the *neonatal period* and are characterized by the highest mortality rate of any period in infancy and childhood. The rapidity with which adjustments must be made decreases from day to day. The most drastic changes occur at the moment of birth; many important ones occur during the first day of life; and still many other adjustments are made, but continue at a somewhat slower rate during the next four weeks.

At the time of birth, the baby makes the most complete and abrupt change in his surroundings and condition that he will make during his entire lifetime. He has existed and evolved as a parasite for nine months, during which time he has been protected from injury, kept at the temperature which was best for him, and above all has been furnished with exactly the proper amount and character of nourishment necessary for his growth and development. Suddenly he emerges from this completely protective environment into a more or less hostile world, where he must begin life as a separate entity. The baby must not only continue the bodily functions and activities that were begun during his uterine life, but must also elaborate and establish others which were imperfect or were performed for him.

The nurse will recall that the fetus received its nourishment and oxygen, and gave up waste material, through the placental circulation; that the lungs were not inflated and that most of the blood flowed through the foramen ovale instead of through the pulmonary vessels, as it does after birth. The digestive tract, excretory organs, and nervous system were not needed during fetal life and therefore are imperfectly developed at birth. The respiratory system must function immediately after birth, and sudden changes in the circulatory system become necessary when oxygen must be obtained through the lungs. (See Figs. 36 and 37.)

The other functions are established more slowly, and the care of the baby must be such that the immature organs will not be overtaxed.

## WEIGHT

The average male infant weighs between 3300 gm (7¼ lb) and 3600 gm (8 lb) at birth. Female infants are usually somewhat smaller with an average between 3200 gm (7.1 lb) and 3330 gm (7⅓ lb). Negro babies tend to be lighter in weight than those of the white race. Approximately two-thirds of all full-term infants weigh between 2700 gm (6 lb) and 3850 gm (8½ lb), the other one-third being either above or below these figures. A baby weighing above 4500 gm (10 lb) is considered to be of an excessive size; this may cause dystocia and increases the risk of injury during labor and delivery. There is an unexplained tendency for all babies of some parents to be large; parents who were themselves large at birth tend to have large babies, and persons of large stature may be expected to have large infants. The first-born baby tends to be smaller than subsequent siblings.

All infants lose weight during the first few days of life. This decrease in weight, which ranges between 5 per cent and 10 per cent of the birth weight, is due to a loss of excess fluid from the body tissues and a relatively low food and fluid intake during this period. Forcing fluids may diminish, but will not prevent, this *physiologic weight loss.*

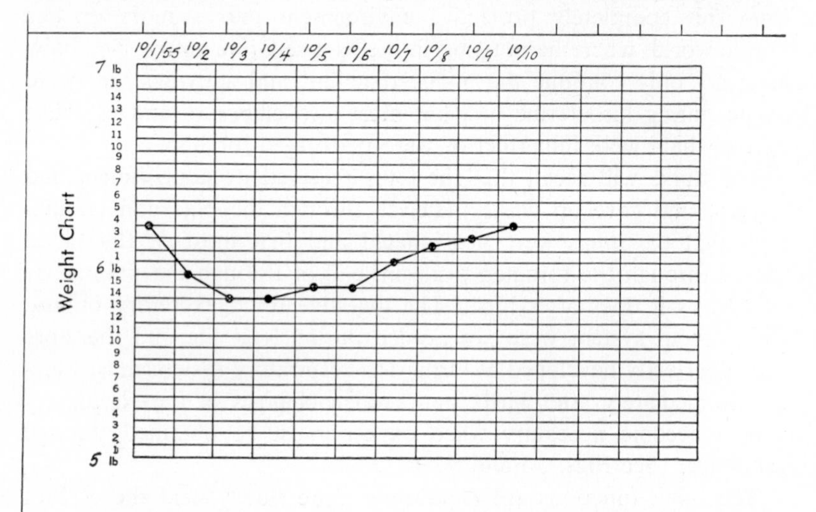


Chart VII. Weight chart of an infant weighing 6 lb, 3 oz, at birth, showing the physiologic weight loss on the first three days, a stationary weight on the fourth day, and a steady gain back to birth weight by the tenth day.

There is ordinarily no advantage in attempting to prevent it, and difficulties may be encountered when efforts are made to force food and fluids. The weight becomes stationary on the third or fourth day of life and then begins to increase. On some days it may remain stationary or even show a slight loss, but the general trend will be upward. Birth weight is usually regained in 10 to 14 days with approximately 25 per cent of the babies back to the original weight at the end of one week and 50 per cent by the tenth day of life (Chart VII). The birth weight is usually doubled by the age of five months which means that there will be a gain of 120 to 240 gm (4 to 8 oz) per week during this time.

## LENGTH

The average length of the newborn infant is 50 cm (20 in.) for boys and 49 cm (19.6 in.) for girls. The normal range is between

47.5 cm (19 in.) and 53.75 cm (21½ in.). Length is difficult to obtain because the baby normally lies tensely and with his legs flexed; to be measured accurately he must be placed flat on his back and extended as much as possible. The greatest increase in length occurs during the first three months of the baby's life.

## SKELETON

The young infant's body has a large amount of cartilage, the bones are soft because of the small amount of mineral deposit, and the joints are very elastic, especially during the first week of life. The great mobility of the joints which makes the body quite pliable offers mechanical advantages during delivery, and the flexibility of the skeleton allows the bones to bend rather than break if pressure is applied.

The head of the infant is much larger than an adult's in comparison to the rest of the body size, accounting for one-fourth of the body length in the infant as compared to one-eighth of the adult's body length. The cranium is large and the face relatively small compared to the adult head; the ratio of face to cranium being 1:8 in the infant and only 1:2 or 1:2.5 in the adult. The jaws are small, and the mandible, because of poor development, appears to recede; these bones develop further under the influence of mastication. The lower jaw grows more rapidly than the rest of the face. Asymmetry of the face, caused by intrauterine pressure, may be present at birth, but diminishes quite rapidly. The mandible may not be in the midline if it has been held against the shoulder in utero.

The bones of the cranium are loosely held together by membranes at the suture lines which allow for considerable molding of the head during labor and delivery, especially in the prolonged, difficult labor. This molding may make the head appear very elongated immediately after birth, but the distortion recedes rapidly, is much improved in 24 to 48 hours, and the head assumes its normal shape in about one week (Figs. 161 A and B).

A diffuse swelling, known as a *caput succedaneum,* may be present, at birth, in the soft tissues of the scalp which lie over the presenting part of the head. This swelling is due to edema produced by a difference in pressure on the tissues which are pressed directly against the cervix and those which lie over the dilated canal. Circulation is arrested in that part of the scalp which presents over the dilated cervical os. This edema is completely absorbed in one to two days, and the caput rapidly diminishes in size.

Sometimes a swelling, known as a *cephalhematoma,* appears on

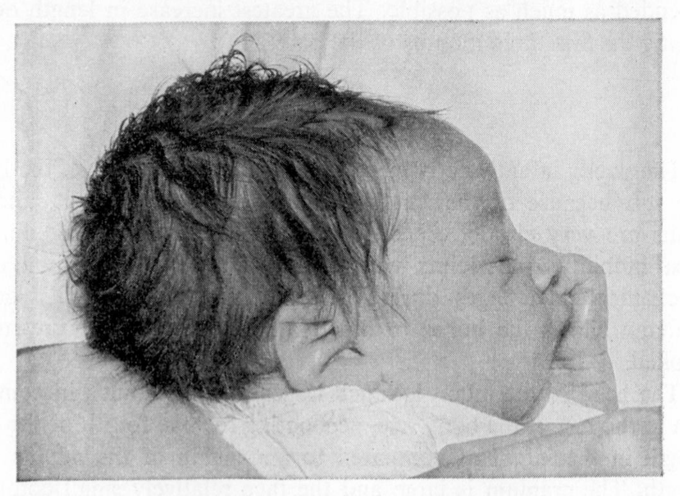

**Fig. 161A.** Elongation of the head immediately after birth due to molding during labor and delivery.

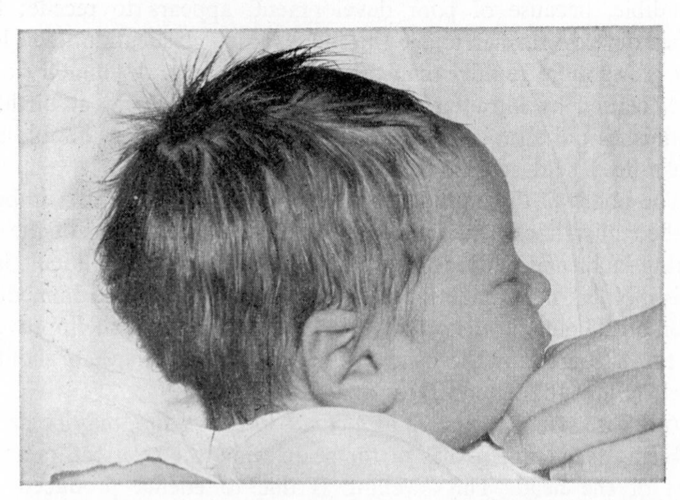

**Fig. 161B.** The same baby 24 hours later when the elongation has receded considerably and the head has assumed a more rounded shape.

the head soon after birth (Fig. 162). This swelling is a subperiosteal extravasation of blood due to rupture of a blood vessel and subsequent bleeding beneath the periosteum of one of the cranial bones.

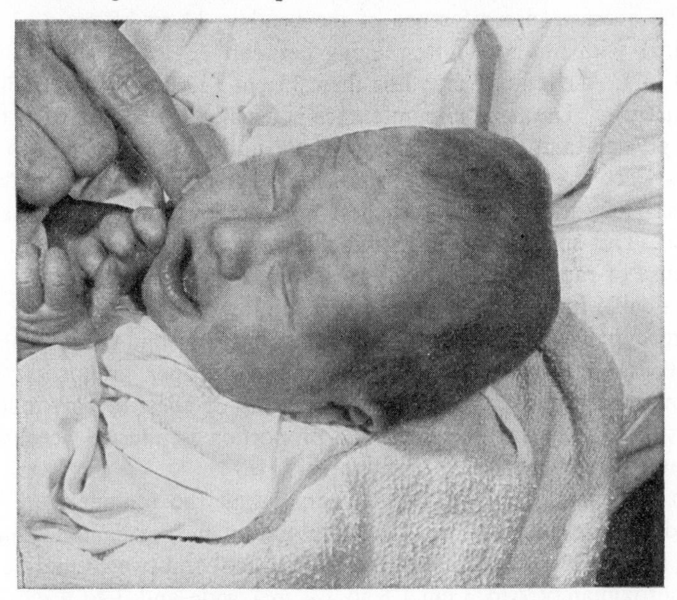

**Fig. 162.** A cephalhematoma over the right parietal bone.

It is most likely due to trauma of labor and delivery, this trauma probably caused either by friction of the skull against the mother's pelvic bones or by obstetric forceps. A cephalhematoma may occur following either spontaneous or instrumental delivery. The hematoma does not cross the suture line and is therefore limited to the surface of one cranial bone, but a hematoma may develop over more than one bone. The swelling varies in size depending upon the amount of bleeding; there may be an increase in size during the first few days of life. A superimposed caput succedaneum may obscure the swelling until the former has receded. Unlike the caput a cephalhematoma does not recede quickly and may require weeks for complete absorption. As the hematoma organizes, a hard border may be felt around a soft central area. Treatment is not necessary, since the hematoma will disappear spontaneously, but the area should be protected from further trauma.

The head of the infant born by cesarean section or by a breech extraction does not become molded during birth and is characterized by its roundness as compared to the usual elongated head of the vertex presentation with delivery through the birth canal.

The average circumference of the head is 34 to 35 cm (13.6 to 14 in.) with normal limits ranging between 33 to 37 cm (13.2 to 14.8 in.). A circumference less than 33 cm (13.2 in.) may indicate prematurity. The head circumference is usually 1.5 to 2 cm (.6 to .8 in.) greater than the chest measurement until the age of one to two years when they become the same size. A greater difference between the size of the head and the chest may be found in the premature infant. The size of the head increases considerably during infancy because of rapid brain growth; measurements taken at intervals may be valuable in making a diagnosis of failure of brain growth or of a hydrocephalus. The relationship between the head and chest measurements is important, since a disturbance in proper proportion may mean an abnormal development of the head or chest or may indicate chest or cardiac disease, unless the proportion is unusual because of malnutrition or a familial characteristic.

In the examination of the newborn infant the fontanels are palpated for size and tension. The anterior fontanel, a diamond-shaped area located at the juncture of the two parietal and two frontal bones, is approximately 2 to 3 cm (.8 to 1.2 in.) wide and 3 to 4 cm (1.2 to 1.6 in.) long. The posterior fontanel, which is triangular in shape and located between the occipital and parietal bones, is much smaller, and on palpation may be found closed, nearly closed, or wide open. The saggital suture, located between the parietal bones, can easily be palpated; it may vary in size from being wide open to being almost closed (Fig. 38). Much variation will be found in the size of the fontanels. Due to an overlapping of skull bones during birth, the size of the fontanels and also the circumference of the head will be smaller shortly after birth than a few days later. When the fontanels are palpated for size, their tension should also be noted. An increase in tension may indicate increased intracranial pressure or a hydrocephalus, while a decrease in tension may be found in the presence of dehydration or shock.

As compared to the head, the thorax and pelvis of the newborn infant are small. The abdomen is prominent due to weak muscles and rather large abdominal organs. The neck, arms, and legs are relatively short. The legs are abducted and flexed, and so markedly bowed that the soles of the feet may nearly face each other (Fig. 176.). The midpoint of the infant is at the umbilicus compared to the symphysis pubis in the adult, and the sitting height of the infant is almost 70 per cent of his total body length.

## THE RESPIRATORY SYSTEM

Some of the most profound physiologic changes which take place at birth occur in the respiratory system. Although the mechanism of respiration is established before birth, it is still necessary for radical changes to take place immediately after the baby is born. During fetal life pre-respiratory movements, which apparently begin during the fourth month of pregnancy and become more frequent as the fetus grows older, may move amniotic fluid in and out of the lungs, but oxygen is not obtained through the lungs until after birth. It is not until oxygenation through the placental circulation is lost that the respiratory system must function to maintain life. The hypoxia which follows the removal of placental circulation is an important factor in initiating breathing by carbon dioxide stimulation of the respiratory center. The physical stimulation produced by the birth process and the change of environment also act to stimulate active respiratory movements unless the hypoxia is severe enough to change the mechanism in such a manner that it does not function at all. The first breath, which should be taken within 30 seconds after birth, requires considerable exertion to expand the collapsed lungs and overcome the cohesive state of the alveoli. A spontaneous lusty cry is a good indication that this has occurred. Expansion is not complete for several days, however; time and effort are necessary to overcome the factors which prevent expansion of the alveoli. Included in these factors are a surface tension, which resists aeration, and also the incompletely developed elastic lung tissue and respiratory muscles. Patchy areas of atelectasis alternate with well-aerated areas; in most instances, however, there is an adequate gaseous exchange. Investigations have shown that arterial blood only 50 per cent saturated with oxygen at birth will become saturated up to 90 per cent or more of its capacity to carry oxygen in about three hours after birth.

An anatomic examination of the upper respiratory tract shows the nose to be small, shallow, and narrow; the openings into the nasal cavity are small. A delicate nasal mucous membrane causes the baby to sneeze vigorously and frequently which helps to clear the tiny passages.

The thorax is almost cylindrical in shape with the anteroposterior and lateral diameters the same size. This is due to pressure of the arms against it in utero. The xiphoid process is often prominent. The average circumference of the chest is 32 to 33 cm (12.8 to 13.2 in.), approximately 2 cm (.8 in.) less than the circumference of the head. If the chest circumference is less than 30 cm (12 in.) the baby is probably prematurely born. In the infant the ribs are placed horizontally, at right angles to the vertebral column, and almost at right angles at the sternum. They are soft, the attached muscles are weak, and little respiratory movement is carried out by the thoracic cage. Most of the respiratory movements are, therefore, accomplished by the diaphragm and the abdominal muscles. Pressure against the diaphragm from abdominal organs, especially in the horizontal position, may limit excursion and make the respirations shallow and rapid. When the baby sits up the ribs begin to slope, they become harder, the muscles become stronger, and breathing finally becomes thoracic.

Breathing in the newborn is characterized by an irregularity in depth, rate, and rhythm, which is easily altered by stimuli, and may also be irregular in sleep. Irregularity may be caused by a marginal state of hypoxia. Respiration should be quiet, accompanied by neither dyspnea nor cyanosis, although these conditions may be transitory during the first day or two of life. The average respiratory rate is from 35 to 50 times per minute, although it may vary considerably in the first few days of life without significance.

Breath sounds may be quite loud and harsh, especially at the lung bases, due to the patchy areas of atelectasis present during the early days of life. They usually cause little or no concern in the first few postnatal days. As the physiologic atelectasis decreases, the breathing becomes deeper and the rate slower. Because of a poor supply of elastic tissue the infant coughs feebly and is not able to expel secretions well.

## THYMUS

The thymus is normally large in the newborn and it continues to grow so rapidly that it triples its birth weight by five years of age. Thereafter little change in size takes place for about 10 years, when it finally decreases in weight. The thymus has frequently been considered a cause of difficulty in breathing or sudden death, but whether or not it is responsible for either respiratory obstruction or death is questionable. Another cause can usually be found for attacks of cyanosis or apnea.

## THE CIRCULATORY SYSTEM

Complicated and rather sudden changes in the circulatory system become necessary at the time of birth. The readjustments that take place when the circulation changes from a fetal to an independent one, with obliteration of the temporary structures used during fetal life, have been described in Chapter 4. Immediately after birth when oxygen must be obtained through the lungs, the pulmonary circulation becomes important and increases in volume. A rapid shift in circulation takes place; oxygenated blood is distributed similarly to that of an adult's circulation within a period of three hours or less after birth. Closure of the fetal openings, however, is a more gradual process, both functionally and organically. The foramen ovale will usually be closed by the third month of life, and the ductus arteriosus is occluded within a few weeks or at least by the fourth month. Transitory heart murmurs which disappear in a few days and have no pathologic significance are heard in some newborn infants. They are evidence of delayed closure of the fetal openings which ceased functioning at birth, the murmur being caused by leakage of blood through channels which have not yet been completely obliterated.

The heart and the blood vascular system are relatively large at birth. The heart is high in the chest and in a more horizontal position than it is later in life. Its rate of growth is slowed after birth. Although about 100 cm (40 in.) of vascular channels are removed at birth, with separation from the umbilical cord and the placenta, the cardiac output of an infant as compared to an adult is still large.

Comparatively, the *blood volume* at birth is approximately the same as the adult volume, about 10 per cent of the body weight. The volume is immediately affected by the amount of time which is allowed to elapse between birth and the clamping of the umbilical cord. Delay in severing the cord until pulsation has ceased will give the baby an additional 100 ml of blood because the contracting uterus can squeeze the blood out of the placenta and into the baby's circulatory system. Recovery of blood from the placental and umbilical vessels raises the volume to 11 or 12 per cent.

The *irregularity* of the *pulse rate,* varying between a marked bradycardia and tachycardia, is a manifestation of the immaturity of the cardiac regulatory center in the medulla and does not have the significance that it has in the older child. The pulse is labile, responding to all kinds of stimuli, physical and emotional, and is therefore under less environmental influence when counted during sleep. It is usually rapid with an average of 120 beats per minute. It may increase to 170 beats per minute with crying or other activity and may drop as low as 70 during sleep. The irregularity of rhythm may follow the same pattern as that of the respiratory system—when the respirations are slow the pulse is slow, and when the respirations become rapid the pulse becomes rapid also.

The *blood pressure* reading may vary with the size of the cuff that is used. With a cuff of 1-in. width, which is considered a proper size, the average systolic and diastolic readings are 80/46 at birth, 85/40 at one day of age, and 100/50 when the baby is 10 days old.

## THE BLOOD

The infant is born with a large number of *red blood cells,* 5,000,000 to 8,000,000 per microliter, and also a high *hemoglobin level,* 15 to 20 gm per 100 ml of blood. This extra number of red blood cells and high hemoglobin level, which are carry-overs of fetal life, were necessary to provide an adequate amount of oxygen in utero.

With improved oxygenation after birth they are not necessary, hemolysis takes place, and a rapid decrease in the number of erythrocytes and the amount of hemoglobin occurs during the first two weeks of life. However, before the decrease begins there may be a further slight increase in the red blood cells and hemoglobin in the first two postnatal days. Since the patchy areas of atelectasis which are present the first few postnatal days do not give the blood its full area for oxygenation, the increased number of erythrocytes and amount of hemoglobin during these early days aid in supplying an adequate amount of oxygen to the tissues.

**Physiologic Jaundice.** All infants have an excessive amount of blood bilirubin at birth; the breakdown of hemoglobin during the first two weeks of life increases this bilirubin level of the blood, and the immature liver which may not be excreting bile pigments well may also be unable to excrete bilirubin easily. As a result of these conditions jaundice manifests itself in the skin and sometimes in the sclera of newborn infants. This early jaundice, also known as *icterus neonatorum,* is considered physiologic jaundice because 50 to 75 per cent of all infants manifest it to some extent. It becomes visible in varying degrees on the second or third day of life, sometimes as early as 36 hours, increases for a few days, begins to decrease by the sixth or seventh day, and has usually disappeared by the fourteenth day without sequalae. The liver and spleen do not enlarge, anemia does not develop, and the stools remain normal. The urine may be darker than usual in color. If jaundice is marked, the baby may be a little sluggish and eat poorly. If jaundice appears to be pronounced or prolonged, it may become necessary to search for another cause. Some of the iron released by red cell destruction stays in the body and is very valuable as a source of iron during the early months when the baby does not receive iron in his diet.

**Immature Cells.** From 1 to 5 per cent of the *red blood cells* present at birth are *nucleated;* a number over 10 per cent is considered abnormal. These immature cells are due to the extramedullary blood-forming centers—the liver, spleen, and lymph nodes—which function in the fetus. Shortly after birth the bone marrow takes over the function of hematopoiesis entirely. These nucleated red blood cells decrease rapidly during extrauterine life and disappear within a few days.

The infant has only a small reserve of blood-forming tissue because all of the bone marrow in the baby is hematopoietic in contrast to only the ends of the long bones and certain flat bones in the adult. This means that in time of emergency the extramedullary blood-building sites must function, and the liver, the spleen, and the lymph nodes may become enlarged.

**Physiologic Anemia.** All newborn infants develop a neonatal physiologic anemia from which they recover spontaneously. During the first two weeks of life there is the rapid decrease in the hemoglobin concentration and the erythrocyte count, which brings about a drop to the normal adult level by the end of the two-week period. A slower decrease in red cells and hemoglobin then continues until a low point is reached at the age of three months with the red blood cells reduced to between 4,000,000 to 4,300,000 per microliter and the hemoglobin level between 11 and 12 gm per 100 ml of blood at this time. This drop in the hemoglobin and erythrocytes is termed physiologic anemia in the newborn; it does not produce symptoms and it does not need treatment, except in cases of infection or nutritional disturbances. After the third month a slow gradual rise takes place, more slowly in the amount of hemoglobin than in the number of red blood cells, until normal levels are reached by the seventh to ninth month of life.

**White Blood Cells.** A leukocytosis, with a count varying from 15,000 to 45,000 cells per microliter, is present at birth. This then decreases to between 10,000 to 16,000 in one week, but tends to remain somewhat elevated throughout infancy. As with the red blood cells, immature white cells are present at birth, but they rapidly decrease during the first few weeks of life. The polymorphonuclear neutrophils make up 45 to 55 per cent of the white blood cells at birth while there are only 20 to 30 per cent lymphocytes. This ratio is quite rapidly reversed, and between the first and eighteenth month of life the neutrophils constitute only 30 to 40 per cent of the total number of cells and the lymphocytes make up 50 to 60 per cent of the count. At the age of two years each of these types of cells constitute about 45 per cent of the leukocytes; a gradual increase in the ratio of neutrophils to lymphocytes continues until the adult level is reached at the age of six years.

**Physiologic Hypoprothrombinemia.** The prothrombin level decreases in all infants during the first few days of life, and blood clotting time is prolonged. Hypoprothrombinemia is most marked between the second and fifth postnatal day. This has been attributed to an insufficiency in the amount of vitamin K received in utero to maintain the prothrombin level during those first few days of life in which the bacterial flora in the intestinal tract, which are necessary to synthesize vitamin K, are not yet present. A low prothrombin level is largely prevented by administration of vitamin K to the mother during labor or to the baby soon after birth. Spontaneous recovery usually occurs in 7 to 10 days.

The **blood platelet count** and the **blood chemistry** of the infant are approximately that of adult levels. The nonprotein nitrogen is elevated up to 50 to 60 mg per 100 ml during the first 5 to 10 days of life. Blood sugar levels show a wide range; following an immediate drop after birth, the amount varies from 40 to 100 mg per 100 ml during the next few days. Symptoms of hypoglycemia do not develop, and it appears that a low blood sugar during this time is a physiologic condition.

## HEAT REGULATION AND BODY METABOLISM

The body temperature of the infant at birth is slightly higher than the mother's, but it drops from 1.1° to 2.8° C (2° to 5° F) almost immediately after birth, even when the baby is well protected with blankets and external heat. With chilling or insufficient covering, it may drop considerably and show a reading as low as 33.3° to 33.9° C (92° to 93° F). It begins to rise spontaneously soon after birth and returns to normal in approximately eight hours. The newborn infant's heat-regulating mechanism is imperfectly developed, and heat production is rather low; the application of external heat or adequate covering will, therefore, help to bring the temperature back to normal more quickly and easily. Great variations in external heat should be avoided, because the baby's temperature is relatively labile and responds quite readily to the environment. Due to an inadequate peripheral circulation the extremities are usually colder than the rest of the body.

A *dehydration fever,* also known as inanition fever or transitory fever, may manifest itself in some infants between the second and fourth day of life as a result of fluid loss from the body and a relatively low fluid intake. The temperature may rise to between 38.9° C (102° F) and 40° C (104° F); the skin feels quite dry, there may be a sudden weight loss, and a decrease in urinary output. It is most frequently observed in the babies that are satisfied with very small or infrequent feedings or in the ones that do not suck well during the first few postnatal days and as a result have a low fluid intake. The fever is easily reduced by increasing the amount of fluid taken. This can be accomplished by giving the baby water to drink in the intervals between his milk feedings or, if he does not take enough fluid in this manner, by the administration of parenteral fluids.

Although *basal heat production* rises rapidly during the baby's first year and the caloric requirements for basal metabolic needs are higher in infancy than at any other time during life, the basal metabolism remains quite low during the neonatal period. Approximately 80 calories per kilogram of body weight per day will fulfill the requirements during the early newborn period, but this amount will not suffice for more than several days. Although the basal metabolic needs do not change rapidly the caloric requirements do, because of the increased energy needed for growth and because activity increases daily during the neonatal period. To supply enough fuel for maintenance and for the rapid growth and the increased activity, a caloric intake of 110 to 120 calories per kilogram per day is soon required. This increased need is demonstrated by the daily increase in the amount of food necessary to satisfy the baby during his first few days of life. Caloric needs vary greatly for different babies of the same age and size. The active baby, because of his increased muscular activity, and the one who cries considerably use much more energy than the quiet infant, and thus have a much higher caloric requirement. Needs must be based upon weight gain, satiety, and general well-being.

The fluid requirement per kilogram of body weight is also greater in the infant than in the adult. His increased muscular activity, his greater caloric intake, and soon his increased basal metabolism—all place the demands for water above the needs later in life.

## THE GASTROINTESTINAL TRACT

Inspection of the mouth of the newborn infant reveals it to be shallow with a flat hard palate due to the absence of alveolar ridges. Glistening white raised areas, caused by an accumulation of epithelial cells, may be seen on the surface of the hard palate, and sometimes cysts are present on the gums. Neither of these are of any significance. The tongue is quite large. The frenum of the tongue is rather short and tight, a condition which does not affect nursing ability because it does not interfere with the use of the tongue in sucking. The newborn infant does not have the ability to move food from his lips to his pharynx, and must therefore receive his food on the back of his tongue to be able to swallow it. The salivary glands are immature, and the flow of saliva is minimal until the age of three months, at which time these glands become mature and the amount of saliva increases. The upper lip may be swollen for a short time after nursing, and sometimes a blister, known as the labial tubercle, appears in its center immediately following nursing.

Sucking, the only means by which the infant gets his food, is assisted by the presence of a series of corrugations in the anterior aspect of the mouth which aid in grasping the nipple and by strong sucking muscles. Deposits of fatty tissue called "sucking pads" are present in each cheek to prevent indrawing of the cheeks during nursing and to make the sucking effective. This mass of fatty tissue, so important to the method of obtaining food, remains even in cases of malnutrition when fat is lost from all other parts of the body; it disappears only when sucking is no more an essential means of obtaining food.

The capacity of the infant's stomach is quite difficult to measure; it has the ability to stretch very easily and it can readily empty its contents into the duodenum. With its physiologic capacity greater than its anatomic capacity, it is possible for the newborn infant to take more fluid at a feeding time than the normal capacity of the stomach would indicate that it could hold.

The intestinal tract is longer proportionately than in the adult. It has a large number of secretory glands and a large surface for absorption of food, but is poorly equipped with elastic tissue; the development of musculature is not complete, and nervous control is inadequate. Although the intestinal tract does not function in utero in the capacity of digesting and absorbing food, it has some opportunity to use its rather weak muscles. The fetus apparently swallows amniotic fluid as early as the fifth month of intrauterine life, and a fecal material known as meconium is formed quite early. This may be expelled in utero under hypoxic conditions. This gastrointestinal tract, which functions in a much more limited capacity in the fetus than either the circulatory or urinary system and has been active up to the time of birth only to the limited extent that swallowing and intestinal movements have taken place, is able, nevertheless, to assume its functions quite easily. It can digest and absorb a tremendous amount of food in proportion to body weight as compared to that of an adult, and apparently is quite capable of doing so even before full-term gestation, as is evident in the premature infant. Except for pancreatic amylase, which is deficient for several months, and lipase, which is deficient to a lesser degree, the digestive enzymes seem to be present fairly early in fetal life in an adequate amount to digest all of the simple foods very well with the exception of complex starches. Absorption of proteins and carbohydrates is very good; the ability to absorb fat is rather poor.

The character of the **stools** of the newborn infant changes each day during the first week of life. The stool passed during the first days consists of meconium, the fecal material which begins to appear in the intestine by the end of the fourth month of fetal life. *Meconium* is a sticky, black, odorless material made up of lanugo and vernix caseosa swallowed in the amniotic fluid, desquamated cells, digestive secretions, mucus, and bile pigments. Meconium may be excreted in utero under abnormal conditions; during the birth process, this being true especially in breech delivery in which case it is the mechanical result of pressure; or any time within the first 24 hours after birth. Some meconium is usually passed during the first 8 to 24 hours of life. The gastrointestinal tract, and therefore the meconium, is sterile at birth, but soon thereafter contains ingested bacteria.

The intestinal content changes from meconium to transitional stools and then to milk stools. During the first two to six days the color of the stool changes from black to greenish black, to greenish brown, brownish yellow, greenish yellow, and finally to the yellow color of milk stools. The transitional stools which appear sometime between the third and fifth day are rather loose, contain some mucus, and are greenish yellow in color. They consist partly of meconium and partly of milk stools. After the first four to five days the character of the stools depends upon the type of feeding. The breast-fed infant usually has yellow, semiformed, curdy stools which later change to a golden yellow with a pasty consistency and a characteristically sour odor. Formula feedings cause the stools to be drier, more formed, of a paler yellow or brownish-yellow color, and of a rather foul odor. The normal healthy infant may have greenish-yellow stools, and curds may be present in those of either the breast-fed or the artificially fed baby. Mucus, in small amounts, is not significant, especially in the breast-fed infant. A minute amount of blood, which follows bowel irritation caused by ingested food or bacteria, may be present in the stools during the first few days and is not significant if the baby does not show any other signs of hemorrhage. Frank blood, either fresh or old, is, of course, abnormal and requires investigation. Blood may be found in the stools if the baby has nursed from a bleeding nipple.

The number of stools per day varies a great deal, tending to be more frequent in the breast-fed than in the artificially fed baby. There may be only one stool daily, but more frequently they are passed from four to eight times a day. Constipation does not occur in the breast-fed infant and very rarely with artificial feedings. The ingestion of large amounts of milk during the first week or two of life may produce loose stools, but diarrhea of an infectious nature must always be considered a possibility.

Considerable **vomiting,** sometimes due to the swallowing of maternal discharges during passage through the birth canal, may occur during the first two to three days of life. The frequency of the vomiting should, however, decrease daily. A baby may vomit a feeding if the air he has swallowed during the feeding is not eructated. When the air leaves the stomach after he is placed in his crib, some of the formula may be expelled with the air. Air and food vomited at the same time make the volume appear to be many times the actual amount.

**Regurgitation,** or spitting-up, during or soon after a feeding is quite common in the newborn infant, because he has neither the valvular arrangement at the lower end of his esophagus that the adult has, nor the nervous control that develops later. Some of the feeding may, therefore, escape from the stomach during the first 20 to 30 minutes after a feeding; with the very active baby this may even continue at intervals for a period of 30 to 60 minutes.

**Colic,** or paroxysms of abdominal pain which last for several hours at a time, may start at the age of two weeks. The baby has cramps in his abdomen which produce pain, causing him to draw up his arms and his legs, clench his fists, and do considerable crying. These episodes of pain usually come at the same time each day and are most apt to appear between 6 P.M. and 10 P.M. The pain is due to distention of the intestines with gas and the ineffectual attempts which are made at its expulsion. The intestinal contents are not moved along well for several reasons: the musculature is inadequately developed, the amount of elastic tissue is deficient, and nervous control is rather poor. With the long periods of crying during these attacks of colic, the baby swallows air which may pass into the intestinal tract and exaggerate the condition by producing even more pain and more crying. The colic disappears at the age of three months, by which time the stomach and intestines have developed an adequate amount of elastic tissue and gained good nervous control.

## LIVER

The liver is relatively large, it occupies about two-fifths of the abdominal cavity, and its lower edge can be palpated somewhere between 2 to 5 cm (.8 to 2 in.) below the right costal margin. The liver has served as an important organ in blood formation in fetal life and it retains this function to some extent for a few months after birth. Along with its many other functions it is, therefore, one of the extramedullary centers of hematopoiesis, at least to a slight degree, in the newborn infant. Enough iron is stored in the liver, unless the mother's diet has been deficient, to carry the baby over the period in which his food, mainly milk, is iron deficient. This store of iron in the liver is used for hemoglobin formation during the first five months of life; after this period it is depleted, and foods furnishing iron must be added to the diet to prevent anemia.

## SPLEEN

The spleen is also relatively large. Ordinarily it is not palpable through the abdominal wall, but occasionally the tip can be felt at the costal margin.

## THE GENITOURINARY SYSTEM

The genitourinary system begins to develop early in fetal life and is ready to function quite adequately at birth. The kidneys are relatively large; they extend below the crest of the ilium and can be palpated through the abdominal wall. After several years they assume the adult position. The bladder is an abdominal organ, because the pelvic cavity in the newborn infant is too small to contain it. The external genitalia definitely show sex characteristics by the time the fetus is 16 weeks old and they are quite well developed at birth. The size of the scrotum and penis varies considerably. The scrotum may be edematous and contain some fluid at birth, but this condition is usually not a true hydrocele and disappears in a few days. The testes have, in most instances, descended into the scrotum by the eighth month of intrauterine life, but occasionally one or both have remained in the inguinal canal or less frequently in the abdomen. Ordinarily, they descend in the next few weeks or months. The prepuce of the penis is usually adherent to the glans and does not separate for several months. In the female infant the labia majora are somewhat underdeveloped and do not lie in close proximity as in the older child, thereby making the labia minora appear relatively large. A hymenal tag is often present. The vagina contains a mucous discharge which may be slightly bloody during the first week.

Although the kidneys are not essential during fetal life, when the placenta is taking care of all waste excretion, they do assume functional form very early, and excretion begins about the seventh week. At the time of birth they are functioning quite efficiently. Urine is found in the bladder at the fourth month of fetal life, and the presence of albumin and urea in the amniotic fluid suggests that urine is voided by the fetus. Since urine is present in the bladder at birth the infant may void immediately after he is born, but emptying of the bladder may be delayed for 12 to 24 hours, and sometimes even longer.

The urinary output may be relatively low, and the voidings scanty during the first few days of life or until fluid intake has increased, unless the baby is edematous at birth. This edema fluid, which is excreted through the kidneys soon after birth, may make the first voidings large and frequent. Ordinarily, however, the ouput is low until the fluid intake increases, which will then increase both frequency and volume. The amount of urinary output is greater proportionately in the child than in the adult.

The total amount of urine voided per day is from 30 to 60 ml (1 to 2 oz) during the first two days of life; the amount then increases up to 200 to 225 ml (7 oz) at the end of one week and continues to increase up to 450 ml (15 oz) by the end of two months. The frequency of voiding increases from an average of 2 to 6 times per day during the first few days up to 10 to 15 times per day and even up to 30 times a day after the immediate postnatal period. This frequency decreases again when the child gains bladder control.

Specific gravity of the urine is quite high in the early days of life; after the first voiding, which may be clear and pale, the urine appears cloudy and quite highly colored due to the degree of concentration and its rather high urate and mucous content. After the fluid intake increases, the specific gravity drops, and the urine again becomes a pale yellow color. It is practically odorless during infancy. Due to an albuminous matrix, which is deposited in the kidney tubules during fetal life, albumin is present in the voided urine and may be considered physiologic during the first week. Uric acid excretion in the newborn is high; it may be deposited in crystal form in the albuminous matrix and produce infarcts. As these uric acid crystals are passed in the urine they may appear as red spots on the baby's diaper and are sometimes confused with blood in the urine.

Although the kidneys function quite adequately under normal conditions, at the time of birth they may be immature enough to make excretion of excessive amounts of water and electrolytes difficult; parenteral fluids must therefore be given with caution. A low fluid intake and the necessity of excreting considerable albumin and uric acid crystals may already have placed them under an increased strain in the immediate postnatal period. Development of good renal function is a gradual process, and the adequacy of the kidneys apparently increases with the age of the infant. Certain lobulations seen in the fetal kidney remain during the first year of life.

## THE NERVOUS SYSTEM

The nervous system of the newborn is not completely developed anatomically or physiologically and is characterized by immaturity. Most of the bodily functions are carried on by the midbrain and cord reflexes. The baby is born with a large brain, and all of the neurons are present at birth; but many of these must continue to mature for a number of months or years, and nerve fibers must continue to make new connections with one another. Because the nervous system is immature and cerebral influence is lacking, there are not many coordinated movements or specific actions; examples of immaturity are the poor control of heat-regulation activities and the irregularity of pulse and respiration as previously noted. Development takes place rapidly, however, and continues to progress. Certain behavior patterns, including those which regulate intrauterine movements, are present before the baby is born, but it is after birth that behavior becomes more coordinated and comes under the higher levels of control. Soon certain pathways which control the activity of various muscles are used, nerve fibers make new connections with one another, more complex behavior patterns develop, and the higher cerebral levels begin to function. Gradually coordinated movements, conditioned reflexes, habits, inhibitions, and discriminations develop. The newborn has a great capacity to learn.

**Reflexes.** The baby is born with certain reflexes which it is significant to note because they are evidences of normal development. Their presence or absence and the time at which they appear or disappear are indicative of progress. The manner in which they are used gives evidence of the functioning of the nervous system; for example, a weak or absent reflex may indicate the presence of a lesion in the central nervous system. Certain reflexes, which are evidences of immaturity, are normal only in the newborn infant. With progress in development of the nervous system these disappear in the first few months of extrauterine life.

The *Moro reflex,* or startle reflex, requires certain nerve tracts which are present at birth, unless there has been damage to either

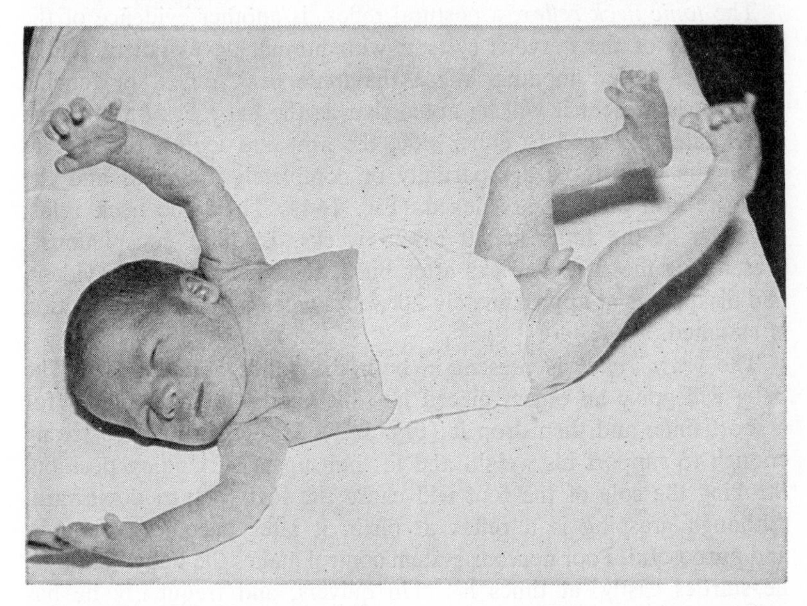

**Fig. 163.** The Moro reflex. With a sudden stimulus the infant brings his arms forward as in an embrace, draws up his legs, and often begins to cry. The response is symmetric in the normal infant. (Note the mottling of the skin which is probably due to chilliness.)

the central nervous system or the peripheral nerves. It demonstrates an awareness of equilibrium in the newborn infant. This reflex should be tested when the baby is lying quietly and is more easily elicited when he is undressed. With a sudden stimulus such as jarring the table on which he lies, quickly jerking his blanket, or a sudden change in position the baby draws up his legs, brings his arms forward as in an embrace position, and frequently begins to cry (Fig. 163). The movements should be symmetric; when one arm does not come forward the possibility of an injury to the arm or clavicle must be considered. If the Moro reflex is absent at birth but present on the following day, it may have been absent due to edema of the brain; the reflex returns when the edema subsides. If this reflex is present at birth, but absent soon thereafter, increasing edema of the brain or slow bleeding due to intracranial hemorrhage must be considered as possible causes. If brain injury has occurred during delivery the reflex is absent at birth and for the next several days; it will return, however, in three or four days if the damage is not too severe.

The *tonic neck reflex,* a postural reflex, is another evidence of the immaturity of the nervous system; with normal development it disappears in a few months. When the tonic neck reflex, or fencing position, is present it will be noted that as the baby lies on his back and rotates his head to either side, the arm and leg on the side to which the head faces are partially or completely extended and the opposite arm and leg are flexed (Fig. 164). The tonic neck reflex develops in the fetus at 20 to 28 weeks, is quite conspicuously present for the first 8 weeks after birth, then becomes less evident, and disappears at approximately 20 weeks when a symmetric position is assumed.

The *grasp reflex* is present in both the hands and the feet. The baby will grasp an object placed into his hands, hold on tightly for a short time, and then drop it (Fig. 165). His grasp may be strong enough to support his weight and lift him up to a standing position. Stroking the sole of the foot will cause the toes to turn downward. Although grasping is a reflex at birth, it later becomes voluntary and purposeful. Poor nervous system control makes the baby "jumpy"; he startles easily, at times his chin quivers, and frequently he has tremors of short duration of the arms and legs. He is able to turn his head from side to side easily, but prefers to keep it on one side or the other. He is able to raise his head from the prone but not the supine position. He will make crawling movements when placed on his abdomen and stepping movements when supported in an upright position (Figs. 166 A and B).

Reflexes in relation to obtaining food are also very active in the normal newborn. The *hunger* and *satiety reflexes* make him cry when he is hungry and know when he has had enough to eat. The *rooting reflex,* by which the baby searches for food, functions whenever the cheeks are touched with the hands, the mother's nipple, or any other object or when the baby smells milk; he immediately moves his head toward the source and opens his mouth in anticipation of food. The *sucking, swallowing,* and *gag reflexes,* which are responsible for getting food to the stomach, are all active in the full-term newborn

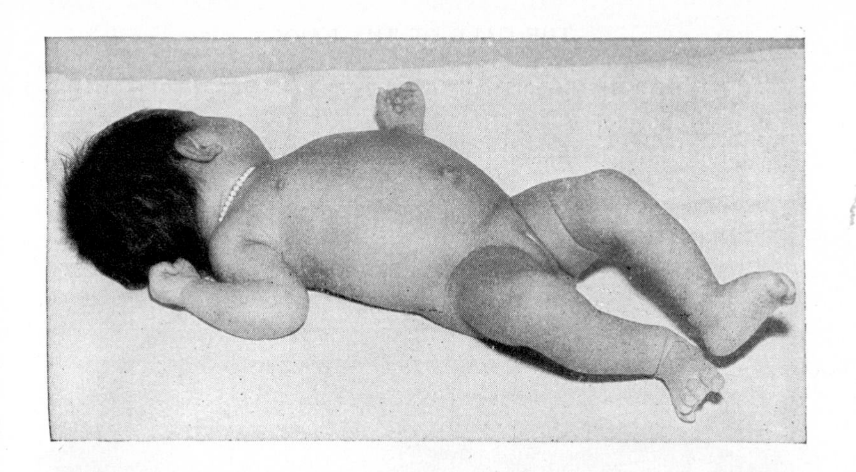

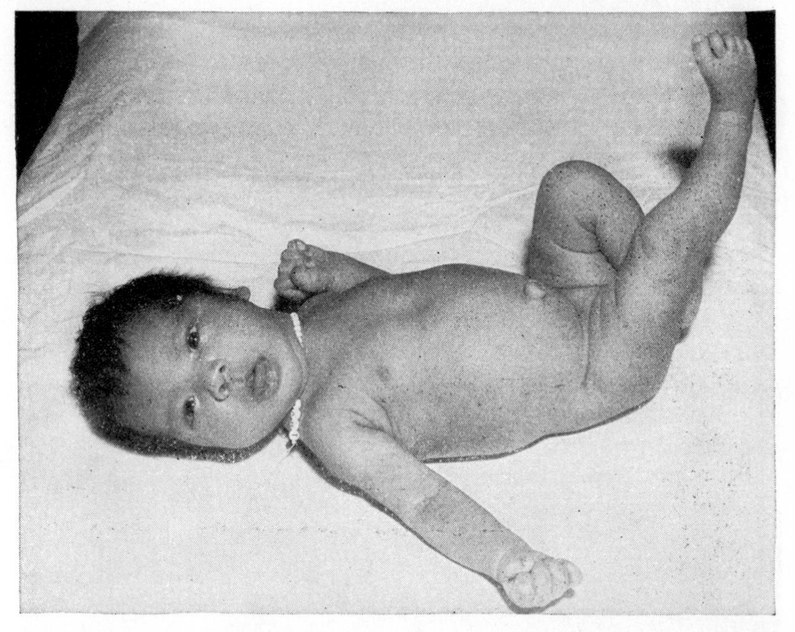

**Fig. 164.** The tonic neck reflex.

(*Top*) With the baby lying on her back and her head turned to the left side, the left arm and left leg are partially extended and the right arm and right leg are flexed.

(*Bottom*) As she turned her head to the right side, she extended her right arm and right leg and flexed the left arm and left leg.

infant, but may be absent in the premature baby. The sucking reflex is so well developed that the baby may suck his fist or thumb immediately after birth, and sucking movements are stimulated when-

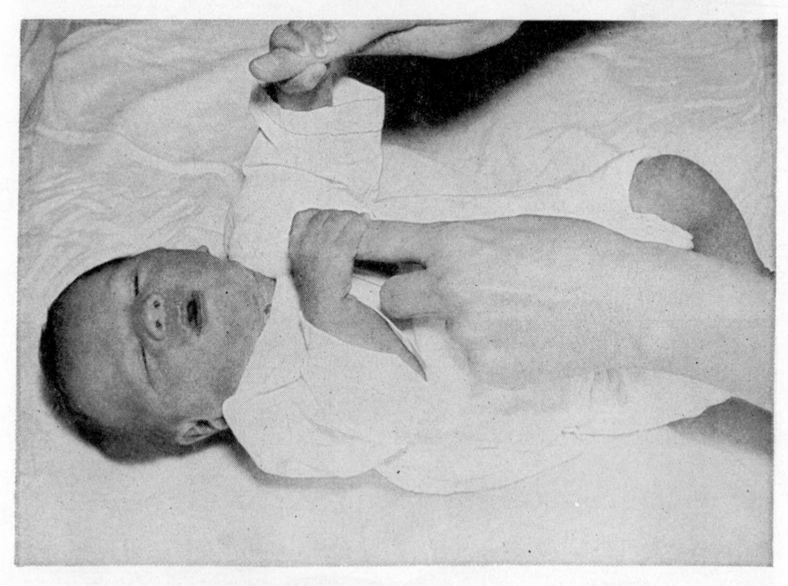

**Fig. 165.** The grasp reflex. The baby will grasp an object placed in his hands and hold on tightly for a short time.

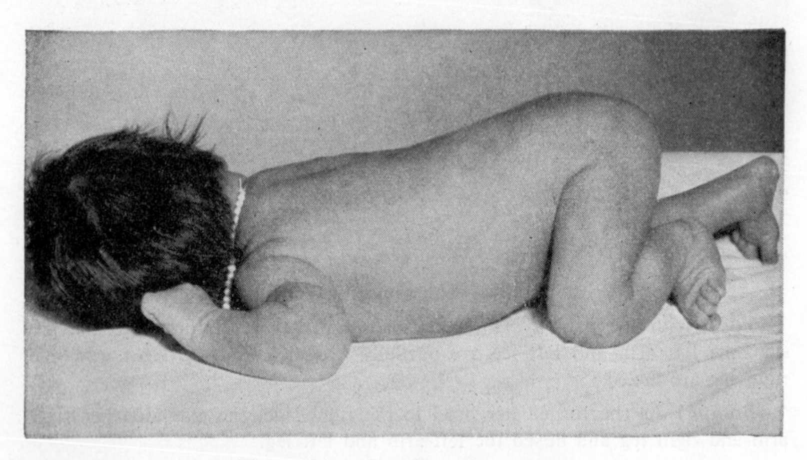

**Fig. 166A.** Crawling movements.

ever anything touches his lips. An absent or weak sucking reflex indicates immaturity, narcosis, or intracranial injury.

Many of the baby's actions are protective or defensive in nature. Others which may be mentioned are the ability to yawn, the ability to clear the respiratory tract by coughing and sneezing, to blink when the eyes are exposed to bright light, to shiver when cold, to resist restraint, thus demonstrating a muscle and joint sense, to withdraw from painful objects, and to cry when disturbed by pain or any other discomfort.

By the end of the neonatal period there is already evidence that nerve fibers have made new connections and that early behavior patterns are better developed. There is less choking and regurgitation, the breathing is more regular, the temperature more stable, the eyes begin to follow bright objects, there is more distinction between sleeping and waking periods, and the baby is less easily startled.

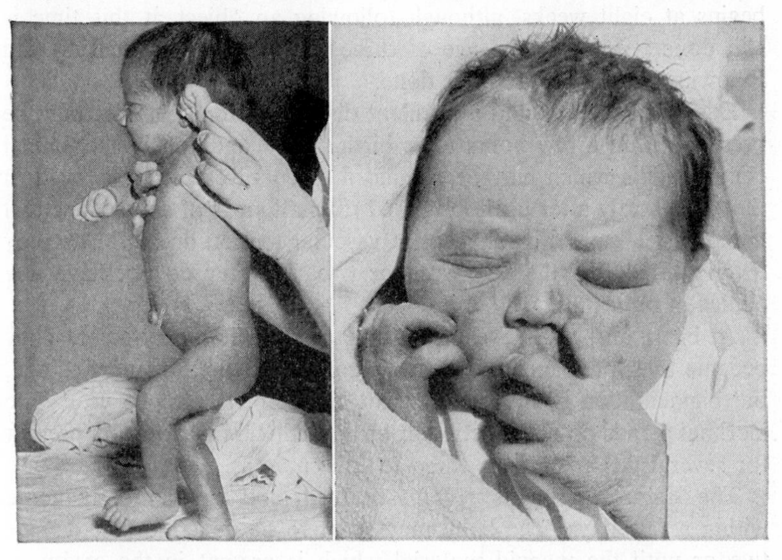

**Fig. 166B (left).** Stepping movements. The umbilical cord has separated and fallen off, but note that the skin of the abdomen had extended up on the umbilical cord a short distance and appears quite prominent.

**Fig. 167 (right).** Newborn infant—18 hours old. With the arms remaining flexed at the elbows and moving from the shoulders, the baby frequently scratches his face. This baby has edema and redness of the left eyelids, which is probably the result of trauma to the lids during instillation of silver nitrate and/or a chemical conjunctivitis.

## SPECIAL SENSES

**The Eyes.** The newborn baby keeps his eyes closed most of the time or when he opens them he frequently does so only half way. Vision except for distinguishing between light and dark is lacking, but the pupils react to light very readily. There is no doubt that light perception is present because the baby will close his eyes whenever he is in a bright light. Sight is not acute in this early period since both the retina and the nerves which transmit impulses to the brain develop more completely after birth. Focusing is not possible at birth, and movement of the eyes is uncoordinated for several months; a cross-eyed appearance is normal in the first few months of life during which time the nerves and muscles that control the focusing of the eyes develop enough to coordinate well. By the age of one month the eyes will begin to follow a bright object. Definite fixing begins at eight weeks, although following an object at this time is still done jerkily; by the age of three to four months focusing and following an object are well done.

Edema of the lids and a purulent discharge from the eyes may be present within a few hours after birth. This condition is a chemical conjunctivitis which may be produced when silver nitrate is used in the eyes shortly after birth (Fig. 167). Small areas of subconjunctival hemorrhage, caused by changes in vascular tension during birth, may be present during the first week or two, but they do not have any clinical significance.

At birth, all babies' eyes are a blue or slate blue-gray color. They become their permanent color at approximately three months of age, but pigmentation of the iris may not be complete for one year. The lacrimal glands do not function at birth, and tears may not be present for several weeks or even three to four months.

**The Ears.** Hearing is present at birth and is apparently acute within a few days. The baby may seem to be deaf the first day or two or until the mucoid material which is present in the cavity of the middle ear at birth has disappeared and the eustachian tubes are aerated. Not only is it known that the ear and the nerve tracts to the brain are anatomically complete at birth, but the presence of hearing is demonstrated by the startle reaction that the baby has to loud sounds.

**Taste and Smell.** The ability to smell seems to be quite acute in the newborn infant as demonstrated by his search for food when he smells milk. His ability to taste is also present at birth and is apparently quite well developed. He seems to be able to differentiate well between sweet and sour; most babies prefer sweet-tasting foods. The baby is apparently also well aware of the temperature of his food.

**Touch.** Although a baby feels pain and pressure, heat and cold, and hunger when his stomach is empty, his cutaneous sensitivity to touch, temperature, and pain is not developed as strongly as it will be later in life. The lips are very sensitive to touch, however, and sucking is stimulated immediately after anything touches them.

## THE UMBILICAL CORD

The cord begins to discolor and shrink soon after birth; within a few days the stump has shriveled and turned black, and a red line of demarcation has begun to appear at the juncture of the umbilical cord with the skin of the abdomen. This skin may extend just to the base of the cord or it may extend up onto the cord a short distance. By the sixth to tenth day the cord has atrophied to a dry black string; it then sloughs off and leaves a small granulating area which heals entirely in another week (Figs. 168, 169, and 170). The amount of granulation tissue is determined by the amount of Wharton's jelly that was present in the umbilical cord. Occasionally there is a delay in separation of the cord into the third week of life, but this is not significant if it appears dry and healthy.

The blood vessels at the base of the umbilical cord are sealed off by the formation of thrombi, but final obliteration does not occur until the end of the neonatal period when the thrombi organize and the vessels become fibrous cords. Until this anatomic closure has occurred the blood vessels are portals of entry to pathogenic organisms.

An umbilical hernia may develop, but strapping of the area cannot be done during this first month because of the danger of infection; it may not be necessary at all. If support to the umbilical area seems advisable during the first month, an abdominal band may be somewhat firmly applied during this period. The hernia frequently disappears during the baby's first year.

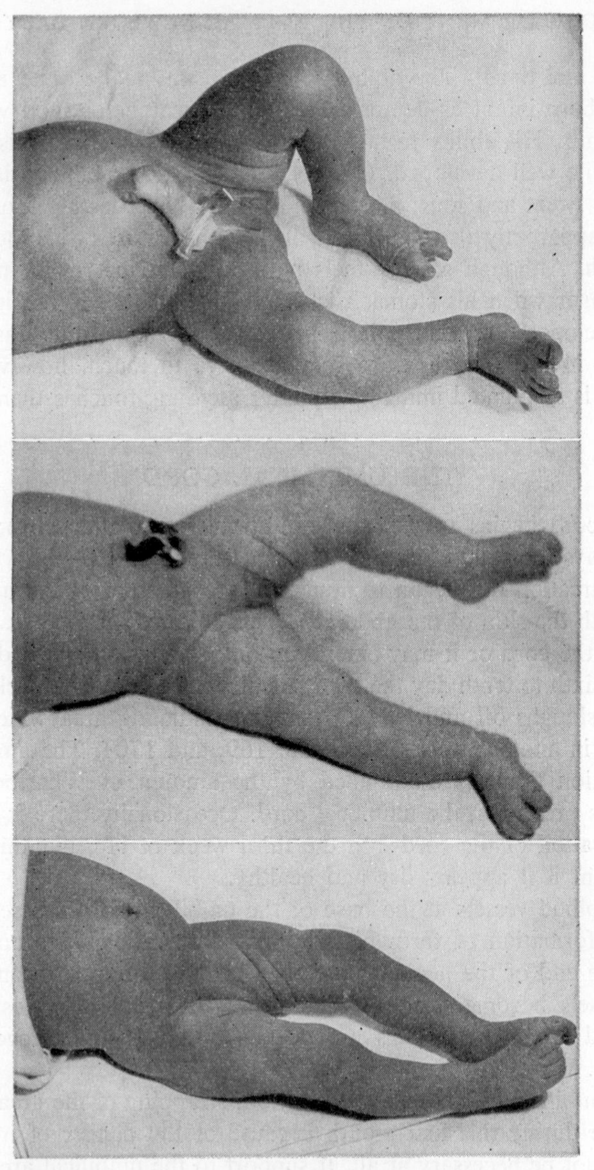

**Fig. 168.** (*Top*) Appearance of umbilical cord six hours after birth.

**Fig. 169.** (*Center*) Appearance of umbilical cord four days after birth.

**Fig. 170.** (*Bottom*) Appearance of umbilicus one day after separation of cord.

## SKIN

The skin which is a dark red or pinkish-red color shortly after birth changes to a pinker hue in a week or two. Pallor, especially if accompanied by pale lips and pale mucous membranes, is not normal. The hands and feet are often a slightly cyanotic color for the few hours after birth, during which oxygenation and circulation improve. A persistent blueness of the hands and feet or cyanosis of other parts of the body is suggestive of heart disease, pulmonary pathology, or birth injury. *Petechiae,* accompanied by bluish discoloration of the skin, may be present on the face for a day or two after delivery as a result of pressure during the process of birth. Edema and extravasation of blood into the tissues of the buttocks and genitalia are frequently seen following a breech delivery because of pressure changes in the area lying over the cervical opening, as well as bruising of the tissues as the breech is pushed through the birth canal (Fig. 171). Between the third and fourteenth day varying degrees of jaundice of the skin may be present.

A greasy, white, cheese-like material, known as *vernix caseosa,* which consists largely of secretion from the sebaceous glands plus epithelial cells and lanugo hair, covers the skin at birth. This material may be present as a very thin covering or as a thick layer; it is especially heavy in the folds and creases of the skin and between the labia. With the exception of that which is found in the creases, the vernix will be absorbed, rub off on the clothing, or dry and fall off within the first day; much of it disappears within 8 to 12 hours.

*Lanugo hair,* the downy covering which develops on the fetus at the sixteenth week and begins to disappear after the thirty-second week of intrauterine life, may still be present on certain parts of the body, especially over the shoulders, back, ear lobes, and forehead (Fig. 172). Most of the lanugo is lost during the first week of the neonatal period. The covering of the head varies from almost complete baldness to a growth of thick dark hair extending over the temples; this hair may later be lost and replaced by a new growth. Eyebrows and eyelashes are present, but may be thin and very light in appearance.

A good distribution of subcutaneous fat gives the skin a soft elastic texture. The epidermis comes off in flakes during the first two to three weeks, and peeling may be quite generalized. During this time the skin may be quite dry, and the presence of fissures at the

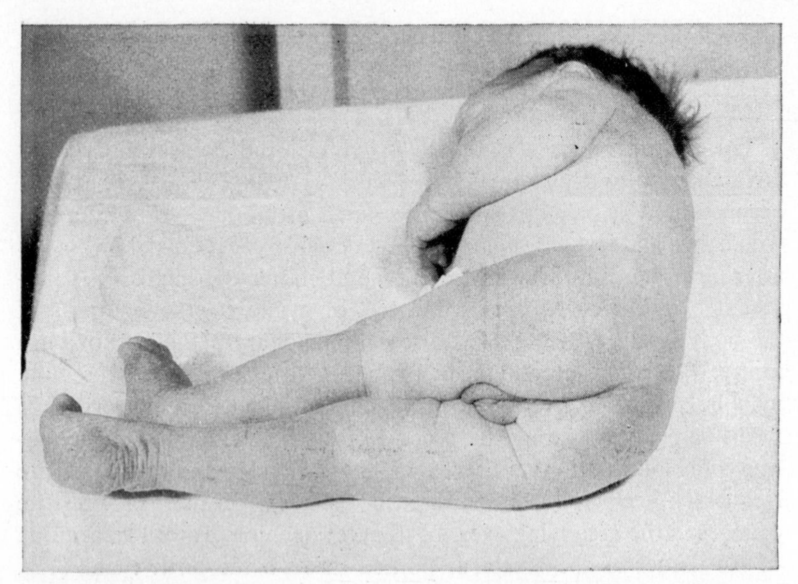

**Fig. 171.** Infant delivered by breech extraction—age 18 hours. The legs continue to assume the intrauterine position by remaining in extension, with the toes pointing toward the shoulders. There is edema and extravasation of blood into the tissues of the buttocks and genitalia. This is the result of pressure changes in the area which presents at the cervical opening during labor and bruising of the tissues as the breech is pushed through the birth canal.

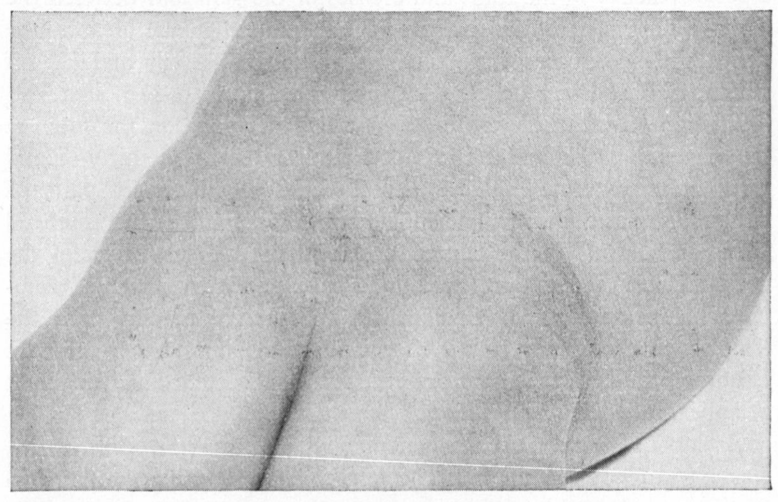

**Fig. 172.** Back covered with lanugo hair.

wrists and ankles is not uncommon (Fig. 173). Occasionally desquamation of the hands and feet is seen at birth.

The *sweat glands* do not function well during the neonatal period, and the baby does not perspire at all or does so very inadequately

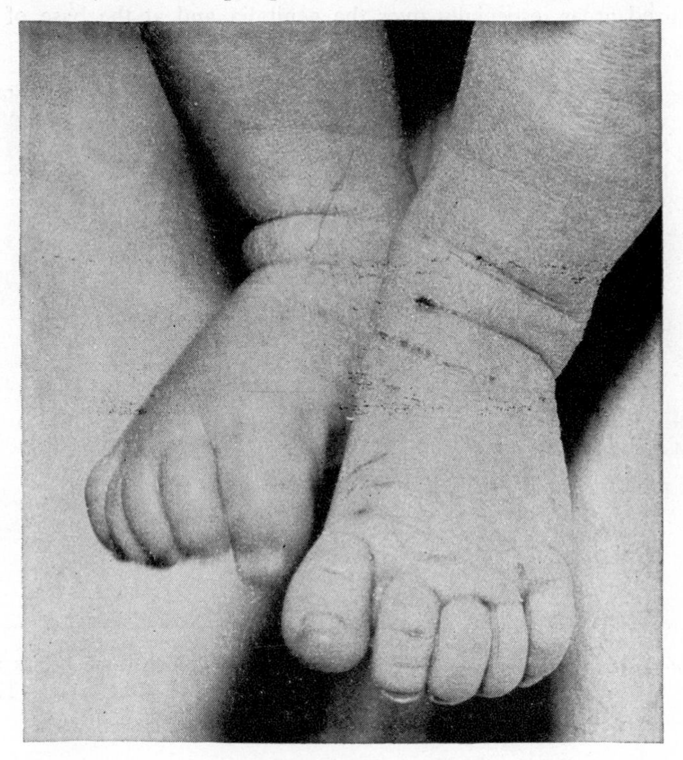

**Fig. 173.** Dryness and cracking of the skin which is often temporarily present in the newborn—this infant is 4 days old.

during the first few weeks. This is one of the factors responsible for the baby's inability to regulate his body temperature easily.

The fingernails are well developed and may even extend well beyond the tips of the fingers. The toenails are also well formed, but may appear embedded at the distal end.

Flat *hemangiomatous areas,* light red in appearance, may be present on the upper eyelids, between the eyebrows, on the upper lip, or at the nape of the neck; these eventually fade and disappear. *Papillomas* of the skin may be present; they are seen most frequently near or in front of an ear. Babies of Negro or Oriental parents and of parents from the Mediterranean countries may have bluish pigmented areas, known as *mongolian spots,* on the back or buttocks. Those of the dark-skinned races may have areas of dark pigmentation in certain localized areas, especially over the genitalia and at the base of the nails.

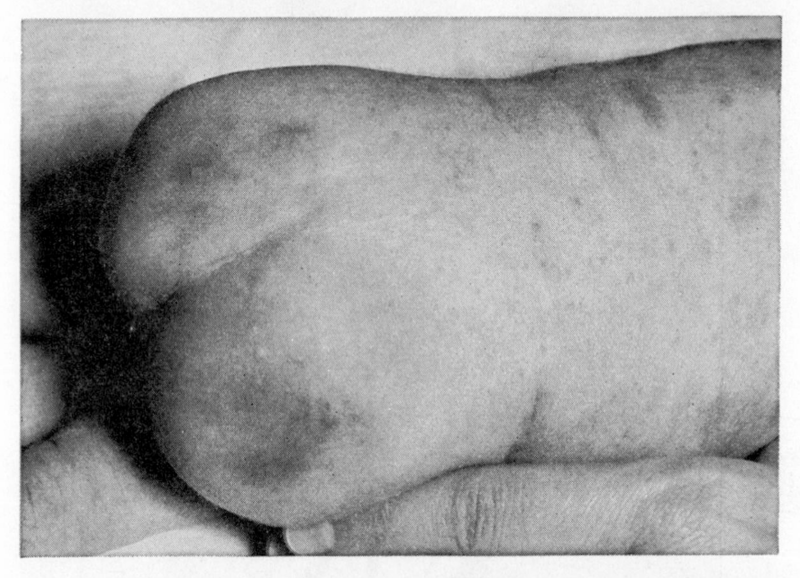

**Fig. 174.** Erythematous blotches. Hive-like areas which some babies may have following irritation from clothing or bathing or after crying. These appear and disappear at intervals during the first few days of life.

*Milia,* pin-point size white spots beneath the epidermis, may be seen over the nose and chin during the first one to two weeks. These spots are concretions of sebaceous material which has been retained in the ducts of the sebaceous glands.

The newborn infant's skin is very sensitive. Some babies have *erythematous blotches,* or hive-like areas, appearing and disappearing at intervals during the first few days of life, following irritation from clothing or bathing or after a period of crying (Fig. 174). The skin may become mottled due to chilling. Minor irritations easily produce nonspecific rashes and breaks in the skin. *Denuded areas* are seen following even minor, but frequent, irritation of one specific region. The active baby may rub some part of his body, mainly the nose, knees, or toes, against the crib covers during crying and break the skin enough to cause active bleeding. The skin of the buttocks is likewise irritated easily, and if the baby has frequent stools it may become quite raw and sore (see Chap. 22, p. 632).

## HORMONE REACTIONS

Changes such as breast hypertrophy, uterine bleeding, and vulvar or prostatic hypertrophy which occur in the genital organs of newborn infants are produced by maternal or placental hormones which have been transmitted through the placenta or occur as a reaction to their sudden removal. The moist congested external genitalia, hymenal tags of tissue, and vaginal discharge, at first watery and later a thick white mucoid material, are also a result of the endocrine substances which affect the genital organs. The maternal hormones present in the fetus and their subsequent withdrawal and exhaustion following birth are considered responsible for the hypertrophied vaginal epithelium, resembling the adult type, which is present at birth, and for the desquamation and mucosal changes with regression to an infantile type of tissue which takes place in two to three days. Within a week or two after birth the congestion of the genitalia has disappeared, and the vaginal discharge decreases.

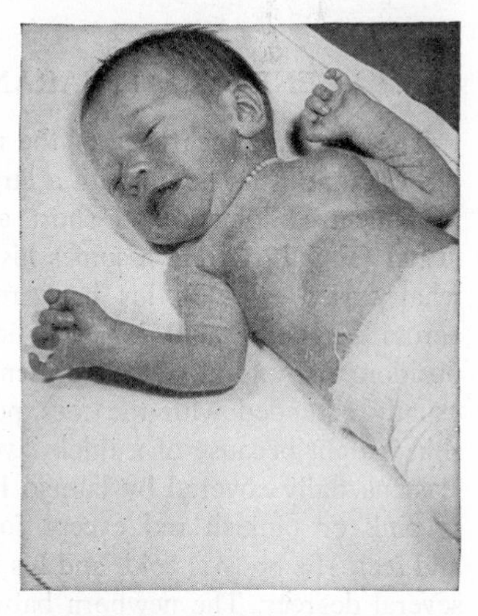

**Fig. 175.** Breast engorgement in the newborn infant. This may occur in infants of either sex during the first week of life.

Bleeding from the vagina, which occurs in some infants during the first neonatal week, is also caused by a temporary imbalance in the endocrine system which produces hyperemia of the pelvic organs and subsequent bleeding. This pseudomenstruation is considered physiologic, occurring because of the activity of the maternal hormones which have been transmitted to the baby in utero.

Another manifestation of the reactions which are produced by the maternal hormones is the breast enlargement, with swelling and tenseness, which occurs in babies of either sex during the first week of life (Fig. 175). A milky fluid, called witch's milk, may be secreted from the engorged breasts. The engorgement and secretion are much more pronounced in some babies than others. This also disappears in approximately one month.

## IMMUNITY

Antibodies to measles, smallpox, mumps, diphtheria, and probably to some of the other infectious diseases pass from the mother to the infant, through the placenta, providing the mother herself has an immunity to the disease. This passive immunity lasts for varying periods of time; to some infections the period of resistance may be very short, while to others it is active for four to eight months. There is very little or no immunity, however, to whooping cough or chickenpox. The newborn's capacity to form his own antibodies is not as well developed as it is a few months later in life; early immunization is therefore difficult.

## GENERAL APPEARANCE AND BEHAVIOR

The general appearance of the normal newborn immediately after birth is that of an infant with a large head, short neck, narrow chest, prominent abdomen, and short arms and legs which are sharply flexed (Fig. 176). He assumes his intrauterine position, lying somewhat curled up with his back rounded, his arms bent and lying across his chest, and his legs flexed on his abdomen unless the position was one of breech presentation, in which case the legs are usually extended with the toes pointing toward the shoulders. His skin is tight because of a thick layer of subcutaneous fat and it is at least partially covered by lanugo hair and vernix caseosa. His color is pink or pinkish red except for a slight cyanosis of the hands and feet. His body is cold, and his temperature has probably dropped several degrees. The newborn baby should be crying lustily immediately after birth and he usually draws up his arms and legs and clenches his fists during periods of crying. His Moro reflex should be complete, and his grasp reflex strong. He may begin to suck his thumb or his fist almost immediately after he is born.

The baby's appearance and behavior at the time of birth are affected to some extent by the duration of the labor, the type of delivery, and the amount of analgesia the mother has received during labor and delivery. His head may show very little to a considerable amount of molding with overlapping of the cranial bones, a caput succedaneum may be present, and there may be an asymmetry of the face due to pressure from intrauterine position. Edema and ecchymosis of the presenting part are sometimes observed. The baby may be quiet but alert, may cry readily following minor stimulation, may be irritable and easily startled, or he may be sleepy and listless.

The **cry** of the newborn infant should be loud and vigorous and should follow even mild stimulation. When it does not start with

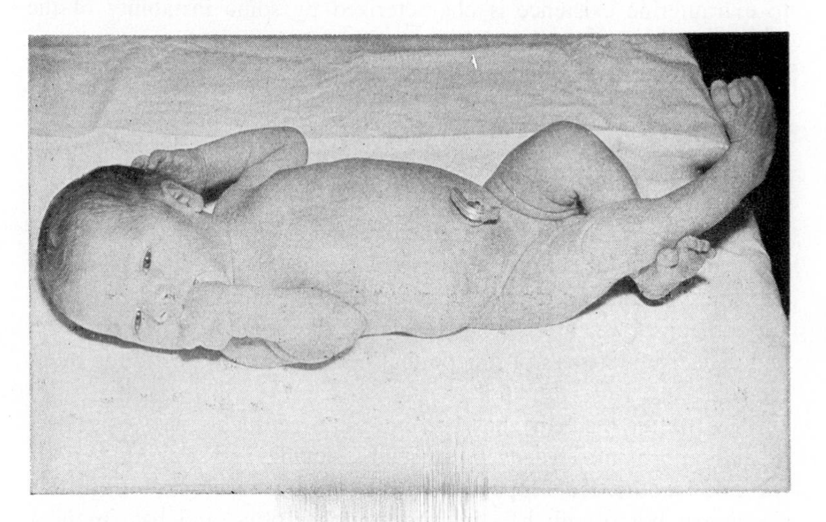

**Fig. 176.** The newborn infant—two days old. The head is large, the eyes are crossed, and lanugo hair is present on the forehead and in front of the ears. The abdomen is prominent and very relaxed, the pelvis is small, and the neck, arms, and legs are relatively short. The arms are flexed at the elbows with the hands near the face. The fist is clenched, and attempts are being made to suck the hand. The umbilical cord is clamped and drying. The legs are abducted, flexed, and bowed so that the soles of the feet nearly face each other. The skin on the feet is dry and wrinkled. The baby appears alert and has good muscle tone.

stimulation or is weak or whining or poorly maintained, an abnormal condition caused by atelectasis, cerebral injury, immaturity, or the effect of narcotics must be suspected. A grunting cry or a moaning respiration may indicate respiratory distress or some degree of cerebral injury. The baby normally cries lustily whenever he is hungry or uncomfortable.

**Good muscle tone** is present in the normal newborn (Fig. 176). Although his head and back need support when he is picked up, a sensation of good tone should be conveyed; a limpness or relaxation with little or no resistance when an attempt is made to restrain him or change his position is not a normal reaction and may mean that the baby is suffering from shock, narcosis, or intracranial injury.

**General Reaction.** During the first few days the baby recovers from the shock of birth. The period of transition from intrauterine to extrauterine existence is characterized by some instability of the various systems. This instability shows itself in many ways; tremors and quiverings, gagging, choking, poor sucking, regurgitation, irregular pulse and respiration, and hyperactivity during sleep, even awakening every few minutes, may be included in these manifestations.

Within a few days to a week the effects of birth and sudden change of environment have largely been overcome. Molding of the head has receded; edema of the presenting part has disappeared; the face has become symmetrical; temperature regulation is improved; the appetite is good; birth weight is being regained; the respiratory, circulatory, and digestive systems are functioning better; and the posture is more relaxed.

**Sleep.** After the baby has become adjusted to his new existence, he has approximately seven to eight sleeping and waking periods within 24 hours. He sleeps about 20 hours out of every 24, but this sleeping is not sound; he stirs and stretches often and has frequent periods of waking up momentarily. He startles easily, even in his sleep. When he does awaken he will not lie contentedly, but is fussy due to discomfort from hunger or from a wet diaper. He cries hard, waving his hands and feet vigorously, but he will become quiet, at least for a short time, when he is picked up.

The young baby continues to prefer a rather flexed position; even in sleep this is not relaxed. He usually sleeps with his hands near his head or chin. If he is on his back when awake he takes the tonic neck reflex position. Whenever he moves his arms about they remain flexed at the elbows and move from the shoulders. This brings his hands near his face which he frequently scratches or where he may stick his fingers in his eyes which, fortunately, are usually closed (Fig. 167). At the end of the neonatal period this flexion is much less noticeable, but it is not until later in infancy that the arms move at the elbows. The fists are kept clenched for the first eight weeks. Control over muscle movements always begins at the proximal and moves to the distal parts.

When the baby is in the prone position he will pick his head up momentarily and rotate it from side to side. He can also move along a short distance with a crawling motion. When he is held against the shoulder he will attempt to, and can, hold his head up for a moment, but the neck muscles are not strong enough to maintain this position and his head soon drops back. When in the supine position he turns his head to either side, preferring one side more than the other, however.

**Hunger.** At varying intervals the baby will show signs of hunger by becoming restless, crying fretfully, moving his head about in search of food, and sucking on his fingers, clothing, or anything he finds near his mouth. The time at which he first desires food depends somewhat upon his size, the type of labor and delivery, and the amount of analgesia his mother received. He may show signs of hunger immediately after he is born or he may have little or no desire for food for 24 to 48 hours. He usually falls asleep immediately after he is fed, but may stay awake and cry for a short time before he sleeps. After a feeding period he should sleep quietly from one to several hours, only to awaken again when uncomfortable because of hunger or a wet diaper.

The normal newborn will have good color, good muscle tone, cry lustily, sleep 20 hours a day, awake only when hungry or uncomfortable, eat well, and gain weight steadily.

## BIBLIOGRAPHY AND STUDENT REFERENCES

Adams, Margaret M.: "Appraisal of a Newborn Infant," *Am. J. Nursing,* **55**:1336–37, (Nov.) 1955.

Aldrich, C. Anderson, and Aldrich, Mary M.: *Babies Are Human Beings,* 2nd ed. The Macmillan Company, New York, 1954.

Bookmiller, Mae M., and Bowen, George L.: *Textbook of Obstetrics and Obstetric Nursing,* 2nd ed. W. B. Saunders Co., Philadelphia, 1954.

Davis, M. Edward, and Sheckler, Catherine E.: *DeLee's Obstetrics for Nurses,* 15th ed. W. B. Saunders Co., Philadelphia, 1951.

Dunham, Ethel: *Premature Infants,* 2nd ed. Paul C. Hoeber, Inc., New York, 1955.

Eastman, Nicholson J.: *Williams Obstetrics,* 11th ed. Appleton-Century-Crofts, Inc., New York, 1956.

Gesell, Arnold: *The Embryology of Behavior.* Harper & Brothers, New York, 1945.

Gesell, Arnold, and Ilg, Frances L.: *Infant and Child in the Culture of Today.* Harper & Brothers, New York, 1943.

Greenhill, J. P. (ed.): *Obstetrics,* 11th ed. W. B. Saunders Co., Philadelphia, 1955.

Holt, L. Emmett, Jr., and McIntosh, Rustin: *Holt Pediatrics,* 12th ed. Appleton-Century-Crofts, Inc., New York, 1953.

Jeans, Philip C.; Wright F. Howell; and Blake, Florence G.: *Essentials of Pediatrics,* 5th ed. J. B. Lippincott Co., Philadelphia, 1954.

Lyon, Robert A., and Wallinger, Elgie M.: *Mitchell's Pediatrics and Pediatric Nursing,* 4th ed. W. B. Saunders Co., Philadelphia, 1954.

Nelson, Waldo E. (ed.): *Textbook of Pediatrics,* 6th ed. W. B. Saunders Co., Philadelphia, 1954.

Parmelee, Arthur H.: *Management of the Newborn.* The Year Book Publishers, Inc., Chicago, 1952.

Sanford, Heyworth N., and Grulee, Clifford G.: "The Newborn," in McQuarrie, Irvine (ed.): *Brennemann's Practice of Pediatrics,* Vol. I. W. F. Prior Co., Inc., Hagerstown, Maryland, 1948, Chap. 42.

Smith, Clement A.: *The Physiology of the Newborn Infant,* 2nd ed. Charles C Thomas, Publisher, Springfield, Ill., 1951.

———: "The Valley of the Shadow of Birth," *A.M.A. Am. J. Dis. Child.,* **82**:171–201, (Aug.) 1951.

———: "The Newborn Patient," *Pediatrics,* **16**:254–63, (Aug.) 1955.

Woodward, H. L.; Gardner, B.; Bryant, R. D.; and Overland, Anna E.: *Obstetric Management and Nursing,* 5th ed. F. A. Davis Co., Philadelphia, 1955.

Zabriskie, Louise, and Eastman, Nicholson J.: *Nurses Handbook of Obstetrics,* 9th ed. J. B. Lippincott Co., Philadelphia, 1952.

*Chapter 22*

# Nursing Care of the Newborn Baby

A great improvement in maternal and infant care during the last two decades has reduced the infant mortality rate considerably during the past 15 to 20 years (Fig. 177), but in spite of this improvement, the first month of life remains hazardous for the infant and has a higher death rate than any of the remaining months. Infant mortality is highest on the first day of life, particularly during the first hour; after this it decreases day by day and month by month (Fig. 177). Deaths on the first day account for more than one-third of the total deaths in the first year; more than two-thirds of the total occur during the first four weeks of life. That the neonatal month is a very dangerous period of life is evident from statistics of infant mortality that are arranged according to age. Although the mortality rate in the neonatal period has been reduced during the past twenty years, the decrease during this period has been much slower than that of the post-neonatal months. More progress has been made in the control of diseases that cause death in later infancy than in the control of abnormal conditions before or at the time of birth. Immaturity is the chief cause of death in the neonatal period; congenital malformations, injury at birth, and asphyxia and atelectasis are other important causes. Medical supervision of the prenatal period is an important factor in the reduction of the infant mortality rate since the condition of the newborn is influenced considerably by the health

[*Text continued on p. 620.*]

INFANT MORTALITY RATES BY DETAILED AGE, RACE, AND SEX: UNITED STATES, 1940 AND 1952

(Exclusive of fetal deaths. Rates per 1,000 live births in each specified group)

| AGE AND YEAR | ALL RACES | | | WHITE | | | NONWHITE | | |
|---|---|---|---|---|---|---|---|---|---|
| | Total | Male | Female | Total | Male | Female | Total | Male | Female |
| **1952** | | | | | | | | | |
| UNDER 1 YEAR | 28.4 | 31.8 | 24.9 | 25.5 | 28.7 | 22.1 | 47.0 | 52.3 | 41.7 |
| Under 1 day | 9.7 | 11.0 | 8.4 | 9.2 | 10.4 | 8.0 | 12.8 | 14.3 | 11.2 |
| Under 1 hour | 2.0 | 2.1 | 1.8 | 1.9 | 2.0 | 1.8 | 2.5 | 2.8 | 2.2 |
| 1–23 hours | 7.7 | 8.8 | 6.6 | 7.4 | 8.4 | 6.2 | 10.2 | 11.5 | 9.0 |
| 1 day | 3.0 | 3.5 | 2.5 | 2.9 | 3.4 | 2.4 | 3.8 | 4.5 | 3.1 |
| 2 days | 2.1 | 2.4 | 1.7 | 2.0 | 2.4 | 1.6 | 2.5 | 2.9 | 2.1 |
| 3 days | 1.1 | 1.2 | 0.9 | 1.0 | 1.2 | 0.8 | 1.5 | 1.7 | 1.2 |
| 4 days | 0.6 | 0.7 | 0.5 | 0.5 | 0.6 | 0.4 | 1.0 | 1.1 | 0.9 |
| 5 days | 0.5 | 0.5 | 0.4 | 0.4 | 0.5 | 0.4 | 0.8 | 0.9 | 0.7 |
| 6 days | 0.3 | 0.4 | 0.3 | 0.3 | 0.3 | 0.3 | 0.6 | 0.7 | 0.6 |
| 7–13 days | 1.3 | 1.4 | 1.2 | 1.1 | 1.2 | 1.0 | 2.3 | 2.6 | 2.1 |
| 14–20 days | 0.7 | 0.8 | 0.7 | 0.6 | 0.7 | 0.6 | 1.5 | 1.6 | 1.4 |
| 21–27 days | 0.5 | 0.6 | 0.5 | 0.4 | 0.5 | 0.4 | 1.2 | 1.3 | 1.1 |
| Under 28 days | 19.8 | 22.5 | 17.0 | 18.5 | 21.1 | 15.8 | 28.0 | 31.6 | 24.4 |
| 28–59 days | 1.8 | 2.0 | 1.6 | 1.5 | 1.7 | 1.3 | 3.9 | 4.4 | 3.4 |
| 2 months | 1.4 | 1.6 | 1.2 | 1.1 | 1.3 | 1.0 | 3.1 | 3.3 | 2.8 |
| 3 months | 1.1 | 1.2 | 1.0 | 0.9 | 1.0 | 0.8 | 2.5 | 2.7 | 2.3 |
| 4 months | 0.9 | 1.0 | 0.9 | 0.7 | 0.8 | 0.7 | 2.0 | 2.2 | 1.9 |
| 5 months | 0.8 | 0.8 | 0.7 | 0.6 | 0.6 | 0.6 | 1.8 | 1.8 | 1.7 |
| 6 months | 0.6 | 0.7 | 0.6 | 0.5 | 0.5 | 0.5 | 1.5 | 1.7 | 1.3 |
| 7 months | 0.5 | 0.5 | 0.5 | 0.4 | 0.4 | 0.4 | 1.2 | 1.2 | 1.1 |
| 8 months | 0.5 | 0.5 | 0.4 | 0.4 | 0.4 | 0.4 | 1.0 | 1.1 | 0.8 |
| 9 months | 0.4 | 0.4 | 0.4 | 0.3 | 0.3 | 0.3 | 0.8 | 0.9 | 0.8 |
| 10 months | 0.3 | 0.3 | 0.3 | 0.3 | 0.3 | 0.2 | 0.6 | 0.7 | 0.6 |
| 11 months | 0.3 | 0.3 | 0.3 | 0.3 | 0.3 | 0.2 | 0.6 | 0.7 | 0.5 |

| AGE AND YEAR | ALL RACES | | | WHITE | | | NONWHITE | | |
|---|---|---|---|---|---|---|---|---|---|
| | Total | Male | Female | Total | Male | Female | Total | Male | Female |
| **1940** | | | | | | | | | |
| UNDER 1 YEAR | 47.0 | 52.5 | 41.3 | 43.2 | 48.3 | 37.8 | 73.8 | 82.2 | 65.2 |
| Under 1 day | 13.9 | 15.7 | 12.1 | 13.6 | 15.3 | 11.8 | 16.0 | 18.1 | 13.9 |
| Under 1 hour | ... | ... | ... | ... | ... | ... | ... | ... | ... |
| 1–23 hours | ... | ... | ... | ... | ... | ... | ... | ... | ... |
| 1 day | 3.5 | 4.1 | 2.9 | 3.4 | 3.9 | 2.8 | 4.7 | 5.1 | 4.2 |
| 2 days | 2.2 | 2.7 | 1.8 | 2.1 | 2.5 | 1.7 | 3.3 | 3.9 | 2.7 |
| 3 days | | | | | | | | | |
| 4 days | | | | | | | | | |
| 5 days | 3.6 | 4.2 | 3.0 | 3.3 | 3.8 | 2.8 | 5.7 | 6.8 | 4.6 |
| 6 days | | | | | | | | | |
| 7–13 days | 2.4 | 2.7 | 2.2 | 2.1 | 2.4 | 1.9 | 4.6 | 5.1 | 4.0 |
| 14–20 days | 1.6 | 1.7 | 1.5 | 1.4 | 1.5 | 1.3 | 2.9 | 3.1 | 2.8 |
| 21–27 days | 1.4 | 1.6 | 1.2 | 1.3 | 1.4 | 1.1 | 2.5 | 2.7 | 2.2 |
| Under 28 days | 28.8 | 32.6 | 24.7 | 27.2 | 30.9 | 23.3 | 39.7 | 44.9 | 34.5 |
| 28–59 days | 3.5 | 4.0 | 3.0 | 3.1 | 3.5 | 2.6 | 6.3 | 7.2 | 5.5 |
| 2 months | 2.9 | 3.1 | 2.6 | 2.6 | 2.8 | 2.3 | 5.0 | 5.5 | 4.5 |
| 3 months | 2.4 | 2.5 | 2.2 | 2.1 | 2.2 | 1.9 | 4.5 | 4.6 | 4.3 |
| 4 months | 1.9 | 2.1 | 1.8 | 1.7 | 1.8 | 1.6 | 3.6 | 4.1 | 3.1 |
| 5 months | 1.6 | 1.7 | 1.5 | 1.4 | 1.5 | 1.3 | 3.1 | 3.3 | 3.0 |
| 6 months | 1.4 | 1.4 | 1.3 | 1.2 | 1.3 | 1.1 | 2.7 | 2.8 | 2.7 |
| 7 months | 1.2 | 1.3 | 1.0 | 1.0 | 1.1 | 0.9 | 2.2 | 2.7 | 1.8 |
| 8 months | 1.0 | 1.2 | 0.9 | 0.9 | 1.0 | 0.8 | 2.1 | 2.4 | 1.8 |
| 9 months | 0.9 | 0.9 | 0.8 | 0.8 | 0.8 | 0.7 | 1.8 | 1.8 | 1.7 |
| 10 months | 0.8 | 0.9 | 0.7 | 0.7 | 0.8 | 0.6 | 1.4 | 1.5 | 1.2 |
| 11 months | 0.7 | 0.8 | 0.7 | 0.7 | 0.7 | 0.6 | 1.3 | 1.4 | 1.2 |

**Fig. 177.** Infant mortality rates by detailed age, race, and sex: United States, 1940 and 1952. (U.S. Department of Health, Education, and Welfare. National Office of Vital Statistics, Washington, D. C.)

of the mother, especially by her nutritional status and the presence or absence of constitutional disease. Care and supervision of the expectant mother will prevent many of the antenatal conditions which are unfavorable to good physical development of the fetus.

The nurse has an important share of the responsibility in the prevention of some of these antenatal conditions by helping and encouraging the expectant mother to seek care and supervision during her pregnancy. She can also help in reducing the mortality rate by giving expert nursing care during the crucial first month of life. By good nursing care of the premature baby she can increase his chances of survival, and by her knowledge of the physiology and needs of the normal newborn, by close observation for signs of complications, and by prevention of infection through the use of careful technics, she can help keep the well baby well.

In addition to the care she herself gives the baby, she has a responsibility for continued good care by teaching the parents. She must help them gain an understanding of the baby's needs, acquire some skill in his care, and develop confidence in themselves by giving them an opportunity to care for him under her supervision and guidance.

In caring for the newborn baby and in guiding his parents, the nurse must be concerned, however, not only with providing expert physical care, important as this may be, but also with developing attitudes which will help the parents satisfy the baby's needs for love and security and help him make a happy and satisfactory adjustment to life.

Just as the physical condition of the newborn infant is influenced by good prenatal care, so provision for his emotional health can begin before he is born. Giving consideration to the mother's emotional needs as well as her physical condition during the prenatal period is an important factor in the development of a healthy happy attitude toward the coming baby. The father's attitudes must also be considered very important, especially insofar as they affect his wife and the baby. To provide a healthy environment for the child, a happy relationship between the parents and the infant must be maintained.

The prenatal period is an ideal time to orient prospective parents to the psychologic care of their baby and to teach them about the normal development and the basic needs of infants. It is also an opportune time in which to interest the mother in the physiologic and psychologic value of breast feeding.

By providing close parent-child relationships soon after birth, especially through the use of the rooming-in plan, and by encouraging parents to show the baby love and affection through fondling him, rocking him, and attending to his cries, a good beginning is made toward the development of sound mental health. During the rooming-in period the parents can learn to recognize the baby's needs and to adjust their care of him to these needs. In general, very satisfactory relationships can be started between baby and parents during this time.

## THE FIRST DAY OF LIFE

Some of the care the baby receives immediately after birth, especially the establishment of respirations, clamping and dressing of the umbilical cord, care of the eyes, and identification has been described in Chapter 12. This immediate care is usually given in the delivery room; the baby is then wrapped in a warm blanket and placed in a warmed crib and transported to the nursery. There he is examined closely, dressed in warm clothing, which usually consists of shirt, diaper, gown, and blanket, shown to his parents, placed into a warmed crib, and carefully observed for both normal and abnormal reactions.

Since the greatest hazard postnatally is in the first few hours of life, the nurse must watch the newborn baby very closely during this early period in which he is making drastic adjustments to his environment. His breathing, color, and general behavior must be closely observed. Respiratory distress may develop at any moment due to choking caused by mucus which the baby spits up or by vomiting of maternal discharges swallowed at the time of birth. To aid in clearing the air passages of mucus the baby is placed on his side with the head of the crib lowered several inches during the first 24 hours of life; he may, however, have periods of choking in spite of this position due to an excessive amount of mucus and may need extra assistance in clearing the respiratory tract. Lowering his head, stroking his neck in the direction of the mouth, and firmly patting his back, methods discussed in Chapter 12, may all be used to help him clear his air passages. The nurse should know how and when to use an aspirator (Figs. 102 and 103), and should have one available near the crib of the newborn at all times. Oxygen should also be available, and, in the absence of a doctor at the time that respiratory distress occurs, the nurse must make a decision to administer oxygen if she believes that it is indicated and whenever there is any sign of respiratory disturbance, however mild or temporary it may seem.

Inspection of the umbilical dressing for bleeding from the cord and immediate clamping or retying in case of bleeding are also an important duty of the nurse during the first 24 hours of life.

During this first day it is necessary to check the body temperature frequently to determine the amount of external heat necessary and to discover when the baby can maintain his temperature adequately in the normal nursery environment.

Observations should also be made during this early period for reactions expected in the newborn infant which indicate normal behavior. The frequency and kind of cry should be observed. The normal cry is lusty and spontaneous at birth and continues or occurs at frequent intervals while the baby is being handled during the immediate care after birth. It should occur spontaneously at intervals after he is placed in his crib and especially when handled for care and observation. If the baby seems sleepy for the first few hours after birth, it may be necessary to stimulate him to cry at approximately hourly intervals to force deeper respiratory movements. Besides observing the respirations and the color of the skin, it is important to check the Moro reflex, to note the general body tone, alertness, a desire to suck which the baby demonstrates by attempting to suck on his fingers, or on any object that comes near his mouth, and his ability to nurse. The first bowel movement and first voiding, both of which may occur in the delivery room, should be noted and recorded as evidences that the intestinal and urinary systems are functioning.

## BODY TEMPERATURE

The full-term newborn baby's temperature always drops immediately after birth and returns to normal spontaneously within approximately eight hours. To prevent undue chilling and to assist the baby in regaining his normal temperature quickly, it is wise to protect him with adequate clothing and with external heat. He should be wrapped in a warm blanket immediately after birth and placed in a warmed crib or an explosion-proof incubator in the delivery room. Further care can be given while he is in the incubator. As soon as possible after birth, identification and eye treatment should be done, and the baby moved to the nursery where he can be dressed in dry clothes, since the blanket in which he was wrapped at birth becomes wet with the amniotic fluid which is on his skin. After he has been dressed in warm clothes and wrapped in a blanket he may be shown to the parents again, although this may have been done on the way to the nursery, and then placed in his crib. Except in very hot weather, when clothes alone may furnish sufficient warmth, he should have external heat applied for a few hours. This heat may be supplied by hot-water bottles placed on the outside of the crib covers; great care must be taken that the heavy bags are not placed so near the chest as to interfere with respiratory movements. To avoid burning the baby's sensitive skin, precautions must be taken that the temperature of the water is not above 51.7° C (125° F), that the bag is encased in flannel covers or wrapped in a towel, and is carefully checked for leakage. Since the hot-water bottles may be dangerous, cool rapidly, and need refilling frequently, a more satisfactory and more constant temperature can be maintained by placing the baby in an incubator, heated to approximately 26.7° C (80° F), for somewhere between 4 to 12 hours. This method makes it necessary to check the baby's body temperature every one to two hours because it may respond very readily to environmental temperature and the baby may become too warm. It may be necessary to reduce the incubator temperature in one to two hours. After the body temperature has returned to normal, external heat is not necessary for the average newborn baby.

The incubator is particularly satisfactory for the baby who is light in weight or the one who has been delivered with difficulty; in either of these instances the body temperature may take a longer period of time to return to normal or may be unstable for a day or two after birth.

After the first few hours the amount of clothing the baby needs will depend upon the weather and his ability to maintain a normal body temperature. In the hospital, where the body temperature is usually taken once or twice daily, the nurse can use this temperature reading as a guide in making a decision in dressing the baby, but frequent temperature readings are not recommended at home and the mother must use other methods. Since the natural tendency is to dress the baby too warmly, the nurse must remember this and explain to the mother that a baby's hands and feet are normally cool and that any effort which is made to put enough clothing on him to keep his hands and feet warm will probably result in overdressing. Observing the color of the face, which will show flushing if the baby is too warm, and have a pale and bluish appearance if too cool, and the feel of the arms, legs, and neck help to determine the amount of clothes the baby needs. He may be fussy if he is either too hot or too cold.

Since a baby cannot compensate for variations in external temperatures very well it becomes necessary to use good judgment in adjusting the amount of clothing to the temperature changes during the day. When the atmospheric temperature is 32.2° C (90° F) it is usually necessary to remove all of the baby's clothing with the exception of the diaper; great care must be taken, however, to put more clothing on him as soon as the temperature drops. It becomes just as important to remove clothing when the baby has been dressed warmly in the morning and the outside temperature becomes hot during the day. With the small baby, under 2700 gm (6 lb), who has a more unstable temperature-regulating mechanism than a larger baby, it may be necessary for the mother to check the body temperature for a few days after she takes him home to determine the amount of clothing he needs.

The newborn baby's temperature is taken (rectally or axillary) at least every four hours until stabilized and then once or twice daily unless the baby's condition requires more frequent checking. This helps to determine how well he is maintaining his own body temperature and is a check for fever, which may be due to dehydration or other causes, during the early days of postnatal adjustment. There should be a separate thermometer for each baby. Frequent insertion of a thermometer into the rectum may be injurious to the rectal mucosa, and many doctors recommend that the temperature be taken in the axilla, since such a method, if done properly, is sufficiently dependable.*

When the mother is taught how to bathe and care for her baby she should be given an opportunity to take his temperature. She should understand, however, that this is not a part of the daily care

* Axillary readings, if taken properly by holding the thermometer in place and pressing the baby's arm gently but firmly against his chest for 1½ minutes, are satisfactory and preferable when the temperature must be taken often.

at home, but that she is learning this procedure only to use when she believes that the temperature is not normal.

## WEIGHT

The baby's weight is always taken and recorded at birth and is usually checked daily for the first week or two of life. In a fairly warm nursery the average newborn may be weighed completely undressed without undue exposure, but if the baby is small, under 2270 gm (5 lb), it may be necessary to protect him against temperature changes by weighing him with his clothes on or while he is wrapped in a blanket. To obtain an exact reading, the weight of the clothing or blanket is ascertained separately and deducted from the total weight. The nurse should compare the day's weight with the birth weight and that of the day before; she must report to the doctor any great loss during the first few days of life as well as a stationary weight or a very slow gain after the first week. These weights are recorded on the baby's hospital record each day; they may be charted on a graph (Fig. 189A and Chart VII).

The mother should be taught how to weigh her baby before she leaves the hospital and warned of the danger of the baby falling off the scales while he is active and kicking. By placing one end of the scales (the end toward which the baby's head will be placed) near but not against a wall and watching him carefully during the weighing instead of concentrating completely on balancing the scales she will avoid any accident. Since there are daily fluctuations in the weight or times at which a plateau is reached instead of a steady consistent daily gain, it is well to recommend to the mother that she weigh her baby only once a week. Thus she is relieved of worry on the days on which the weight is stationary, but she can expect a gain of 210 to 240 gm (7 to 8 oz) each week, with 150 gm (5 oz) being the minimum gain and 360 gm (12 oz) the maximum. When her baby's weight does not fall within this range she should notify the doctor.

## POSITION

During the first 24 hours of life the baby is placed in a position which will facilitate drainage of mucus from the respiratory tract.

To keep his head at a lower level than the rest of his body, the foot end of his crib or mattress must be elevated to a 15- or 20-deg angle, and to further facilitate drainage he is placed on his side with a change of position from one side to the other every two to three hours.

The position which the baby assumes during the early weeks of life affects the shape of his head. When he maintains the same position constantly or takes a certain one frequently, deformities develop because his bones are soft and are not able to resist pressure. If he lies on the back of his head too much it becomes flattened and if he is on one side more than the other his face becomes asymmetrical. His position must be watched because he likes to turn his head toward the side, seems to prefer one side more than the other, and likes especially to turn toward a light if it is not too bright. To protect the shape of his head, it therefore becomes necessary to change his position frequently. When the infant is too young to change his own position it is a good plan to alternate the side on which he is placed after each time he is picked up or fed. When he lies on his side he has a tendency to roll slightly backward; the prone position is therefore best, but it is not entirely safe unless the baby is in a crib and on a firm, flat mattress. The bassinet is not as safe a place to put the baby on his abdomen as is a crib because he can move considerably and can crawl snugly up into a corner where he might feel trapped or actually be trapped. Since it is important, however, to have him become accustomed to sleeping on his abdomen early in his life, he can be conditioned to the prone position by being placed on his abdomen during a time of day in which he can be watched closely. It is wise to begin using a crib immediately after arriving home or to change from bassinet to crib as soon as possible.

A baby's head must be given considerable support when he is picked up because the muscles of his head and neck are not strong enough for him to hold it up. To keep his head from falling back the individual picking him up must place one hand, with fingers spread, under his head and shoulders while the other hand supports the lower part of his body either by firmly grasping his legs or by placing the hand under the buttocks (Fig. 180). To give him a feeling of security he should be held firmly whenever he is picked up or moved.

## CARE OF THE UMBILICAL CORD

Care of the umbilical cord immediately after the birth of the baby has been described in Chapter 12. To avoid serious hemorrhage it must be observed closely during the next 24 hours for any evidence of bleeding; inspection may be necessary every one-half to one hour until it appears quite evident that bleeding will not occur. The danger of bleeding is greatest when the cord contains a large amount of Wharton's jelly which shrinks and leaves a previously tight ligature or clamp loose. In some instances bleeding does not occur even when the ligature is loose because a blood clot has formed at the end of the cord stump. This clot may become loosened, however, with manipulation or the movements of the baby which may cause pulling on the umbilical dressing, and bleeding may then occur. The nurse will usually find that the quickest way to stop bleeding from the cord is to apply a sterile hemostatic forceps. This should be placed as far away from the abdominal wall as possible allowing for adequate room to apply another ligature, especially if the forceps should in some way injure the cord itself and make hemostasis at this point impossible. After the bleeding has been controlled, the nurse or doctor can apply another ligature or clamp and dressing, using aseptic technic.

In the daily care of the umbilical area, it is important that asepsis be maintained until healing is complete. Until then, any of the pyogenic bacteria can produce an infection which may extend to the peritoneum, the liver, or into the blood stream. Many doctors believe that a cord dressing is not necessary or even desirable, but others believe that its use is necessary to protect the baby from infection and that it serves as a constant reminder to everyone caring for the baby of the need of keeping the umbilical area clean. Some hospitals apply a cord dressing for only the first 24 hours. When a cord dressing is used continuously the original dressing is applied in the delivery room and is left on the cord for 24 to 48 hours or until the cord has begun to dry unless the dressing becomes soiled and must be changed sooner.

Daily care consists of wiping the stump and the area around the umbilicus with 60 per cent alcohol. When a dressing is used a sterile dry gauze dressing or gauze saturated with 60 per cent alcohol, which has a drying effect and hastens healing, is applied. If the dressing should become soiled, however, it must be changed more than once daily; sometimes it slides out of position and the umbilical area is exposed and at other times it becomes wet with urine, especially if the diaper is applied too high. After the cord drops off, the granulating area is cared for in the same manner as the cord until the area is completely healed. This takes approximately one week. The nurse applying the dressing must be very careful to wash her hands immediately before the procedure and use every precaution to avoid contamination. She should note any signs of infection and report these to the doctor immediately. There should be no odor or moistness of the cord while it is mummifying. If it is moist, which is indicative of a mild infection, or if there is a moist granulating area at the base of the cord with a slightly mucoid or purulent discharge, the doctor usually recommends the application of alcohol dressings at more frequent intervals or the application of an ointment containing an antibiotic after the area has been cleaned with alcohol.

Before the baby leaves the hospital the mother must be given full instructions in regard to the care of the umbilicus. If the cord is still on she must be told that it will soon be found loose, that there will probably be a small amount of bloody discharge from the navel for a few days, but that the navel should appear more healed every day. She should be instructed not to give the baby a tub bath or to allow the navel to get wet until the scab has come off and the area is completely healed. The mother should be instructed in the method of applying the dressing if used and in the precaution she must take to keep the area clean. It is advisable that she apply the dressing, under the nurse's guidance, before she leaves the hospital. This will help her to learn the technic and also to overcome the anxiety she may have of the care of the umbilical cord.

**Abdominal Bands.** An abdominal band is used mainly to hold the umbilical cord dressing in place. It should be applied with firm even pressure, but not too snugly, and held in place with ties or safety pins. It frequently needs adjusting or changing when the diaper is changed. It must always be loosened before a feeding to allow the stomach to expand.

Ordinarily the abdominal band is not necessary after the umbilicus has healed or if a dressing is not used, but sometimes the doctor recommends the use of a band for several weeks, for support when the navel has a tendency to bulge with crying.

Ready-made bands may be purchased, but they can easily be made at home by cutting a strip of flannel or muslin 4 to 5 in. wide and 18 to 20 in. long. Strips of stockinet material cut at least 6 in. wide, because they become narrower on stretching, are frequently used in the hospital, and the mother can be advised to make similar ones at home if she has a piece of ribbed material which she can cut with the ribbing running the width of the band. This allows for extra stretching of the band when necessary.

## CARE OF THE SKIN

The care of the skin of the newborn infant has changed from time to time over the years and varies from one hospital to another at the present time. One of three methods—the "dry" technic, the oil bath, or the soap and water bath—may be used or a combination of any of these methods is sometimes chosen. The present consensus of opinion seems to be that the less handling the skin receives, the less the irritation, and consequently the less the danger of infection. Rubbing to remove the vernix caseosa, some soaps, some oils, and rubbing with washcloths and towels may traumatize the skin and allow bacteria to enter. Skin irritations will occur in some infants regardless of the method of skin care, but those handled the least are less susceptible.

The so-called "dry" technic means that neither water nor oil is used on the baby's skin for 7 to 10 days. As soon as possible after birth the blood on the face and scalp is washed away with cotton balls or a soft washcloth dipped into warm water, and the baby is dressed in his warm clothing. No attempt is made to wash or wipe off the vernix caseosa. To avoid undue chilling it is quite possible to dress the baby in his warm clothes first and then wash the blood from his face and scalp. If the body is still a little moist from amniotic fluid or from a wet receiving blanket, patting it dry with a soft cloth or diaper will keep his clothes from getting moist and thus becoming cool and clammy.

The vernix acts as a vanishing cream and has either rubbed into the skin or off onto the clothes within 12 to 24 hours. It will remain for a longer time, however, in the creases and folds of skin where a heavy deposit may be found. These areas instead of being protected may become irritated if vernix is left indefinitely, and it should therefore be removed in 24 to 48 hours.

This technic of skin care does not eliminate daily morning care.

The only aspect omitted is the soap and water or oil. Careful inspection of the condition of the skin and of the eyes, nose, mouth, ears, umbilicus, and genitalia must be done as thoroughly as any observation made during the more traditional bath. Special care must be taken to inspect the creases behind the ears, around the neck, in the axillae, and in the groins for skin irritation. The skin may become very dry and peel in large flakes after a few days, and dry cracks may appear around the wrists and ankles (Fig. 173). These have no significance except insofar as they cause the mother concern, and the nurse must be prepared to explain that this is only a temporary condition of the skin which does no harm and that after a few days of bathing and oiling the flakiness and the cracks will disappear. It is important for the nurse to note and report to the doctor moist irritated areas, pustules, or water blisters which may be impetigo and therefore may need special attention.

Even with the dry technic it will be necessary to use some water on the baby's skin, but the amount is minimal. The face is washed with clear warm water and a soft washcloth to remove regurgitated formula or mucus. A cotton ball may be used for washing, but special care must be taken to moisten the cotton ball completely to prevent cotton wisps from getting into the eyes and nose where they would produce irritation. For this reason it is necessary to use a soft towel rather than a cotton ball for drying the face. The vernix that remains in the axillae may be spread as a cream to other parts of the body for the first day or two; after that the axillae should be wiped with a wet cloth during the daily morning care unless the skin in that area is dry. The groins and buttocks must be washed with warm water each time the diaper is changed. It may even be necessary to use some bland soap to wash the buttocks and the crease between the buttocks if water alone does not clean the stool off sufficiently. Some doctors recommend using oil for the diaper area, but others are definitely opposed to the use of any oil during the hospital stay because they believe a moist skin is more susceptible to infection than one that is kept completely dry.

After a thorough inspection of the skin, the morning care is completed by weighing the baby, taking his temperature, changing the gauze on the umbilical cord, and dressing him in clean clothes. Fingernails and toenails may need trimming if they extend beyond the ends of the fingers and toes.

If the vernix is not to be left on the skin until it rubs off it is removed with soap and water or oil, either immediately after birth or in approximately 12 hours, at which time the baby has usually regained a normal temperature.

When an oil bath is given, a warmed nonirritating oil is applied freely to all areas of the skin with the fingers, and the excess is wiped off with a soft cloth. Mineral oil, olive oil, cottonseed oil, or a commercial baby oil may be used. The commercial baby oil may be mineral oil or a mixture of mineral and vegetable oil; it is usually perfumed and may have a chemical added to keep it from becoming rancid. Care must be taken to avoid contamination of the stock container. The oil bath may be used daily or less often; it is most frequently advocated in cold weather. It may be used from the beginning or started after 7 to 10 days of dry technic and then it may or may not be alternated with the soap and water bath. As with other technics of daily care, it is important to inspect all areas of the body very closely for irritation or infection, and the face and buttocks will need to be washed with water before the application of oil.

The first soap and water bath may be given immediately after birth to remove vernix, it may not be given until the baby has recovered from the shock of birth and regained a normal temperature, or it may not be given for a week. To avoid getting the umbilical cord wet it is usually given as a sponge bath by soaping and washing a small area of the body at a time, or it may be done by soaping the entire body at once and then rinsing; the procedure depending somewhat upon the size of the baby and the season of the year. A complete tub bath should not be used until the umbilical cord has been off for at least one day. A bland nonirritating soap should be used; some doctors definitely specify the use of a superfatted soap, which is the least drying to the skin. This bath may or may not be followed by oil. Some doctors recommend the use of oil following the soap and water bath at home, but do not wish to use it in the hospital where the danger of impetigo, and its spread to other babies, is greatest. They prefer to keep the skin dry throughout the hospital stay.

Talcum powder is usually not necessary following the bath, but is sometimes used for esthetic reasons. It is ordinarily not used in the hospital, although mothers like to use it at home. The mother should be adequately instructed in its use. She should be warned against dusting it freely over the baby because there is danger that the baby may inhale it; she should also be cautioned to avoid an accumulation of the powder in the folds of skin where it will become moist, cake, and produce irritation. Zinc stearate powder, which is very irritating to the lungs, should never be used.

Some infants are susceptible to skin irritation regardless of the kind of care given. These infants may develop a heat rash, especially in the neck region and in the groins, if they become too warm for even a short period of time. Occasionally pin-point- or pinhead-sized erythematous papules or vesicular lesions develop. Treatment of skin irritations consists of washing the affected area with soap and water, applying talcum powder frequently but in small amounts, and using less clothing on the infant. Sometimes calamine lotion, which has the same drying effect that powder has, but stays on the skin better without caking, is applied to the rash. A baby may develop *intertrigo,* which is a chafing, where two moist surfaces rub together, especially in the creases of the neck, in the axillae, and in the groins. These areas must be washed and kept as dry as possible. Abrasions may occur on the heels, toes, or knees from kicking or rubbing against the sheets. Further irritation is prevented, and healing takes place if the areas are bandaged. The buttocks may become reddened and raw due to irritation from stools. When this occurs, the diaper must be changed frequently, and the stool and urine washed off carefully. The use of an ointment such as petroleum jelly, zinc oxide, or one of several commercial preparations, such as Vitamin A and D Ointment or methylbenzethonium (Diaparene), helps keep the stool off the raw area and aids in the healing process. Exposure to the air, which is accomplished by leaving the baby with his diaper placed under him but not pinned on, is beneficial in healing. Heat from an ordinary electric-light bulb, obtained by placing a tall lamp over the crib, is also effective and helps somewhat in keeping the exposed baby warm (Fig. 178). It is important that he lie in a prone position for this treatment. Great care must be taken, of course, to avoid any possibility of the lamp falling, and it must be kept far enough away to prevent a burned skin. Treatment can be alternated by exposing the buttocks to the air while the baby is asleep and applying an ointment when he must be picked up to be fed. As explained in Chapter 21, the baby's skin is very sensitive and frequently shows signs of minor irritations which have no significance, but the nurse must always be alert for any evidence of skin infection.

**Bath Demonstration.** Regardless of the method of skin care in the hospital the new mother should be given an opportunity to give her baby a soap and water bath before she takes him home. Although

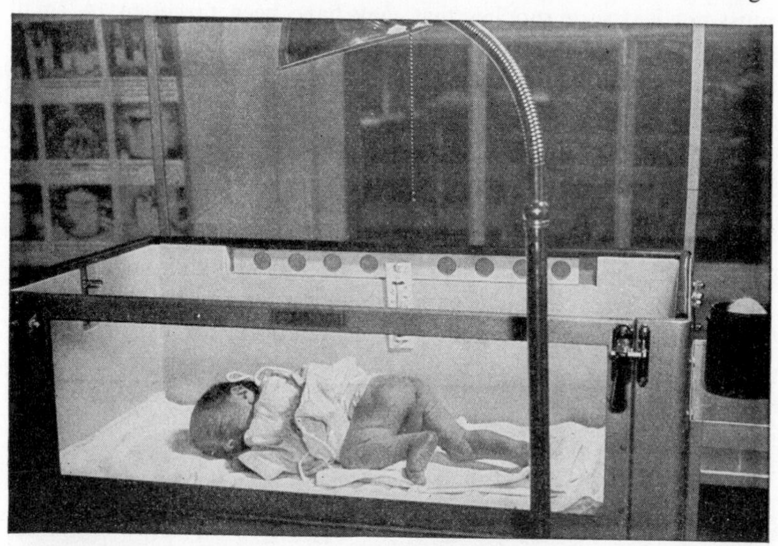

**Fig. 178.** The baby with sore buttocks may be left with his diaper unpinned in order to expose the irritated skin to the air. Heat from an ordinary electric-light bulb, 40 to 60 watt, obtained by placing a tall lamp over the crib, is also effective in healing and aids in keeping the exposed baby warm. During this treatment the baby should be placed on his abdomen.

the doctor may recommend that her baby have oil baths with only an infrequent soap and water bath, it is well for her to learn the procedure. If she can give the soap and water bath with confidence, she will be able to give the oil bath easily. Because the student nurse and the mother can read complete descriptions of the tub bath in infant care pamphlets and read about many of the "do's and don't's" listed there, only an incomplete description will follow. Other parts of this chapter also give suggestions for teaching the mother, and the nurse should be able to apply these as necessary in her daily contact with the mother.

A room should be selected which is not drafty and which can be heated to between 23.9° to 26.7° C (75° to 80° F) for the baby's bath. This bath is usually given before a feeding, frequently before the morning feeding, but can be given at any time of day. In hot weather it may be necessary to give two or three baths a day to keep the baby comfortable. All equipment must be assembled and conveniently located since the baby must never be left alone; the mother must not leave for supplies that may have been forgotten. A small enamel tub, a dishpan, or a folding rubber tub which has legs long enough to bring it to a convenient height and has a canvas top that can be used as a work table is usually selected for the bath. The baby's face is washed first using only warm water; next the scalp is soaped and rinsed. The mother should be shown how to place her left arm under the baby's body with his head resting on her hand and his buttocks held securely between her hip and elbow. In this position his head can be held over the tub and thoroughly rinsed (Fig. 179). To avoid undue exposure, unless the day is hot, this much of the procedure can be done without removing the baby's clothes.

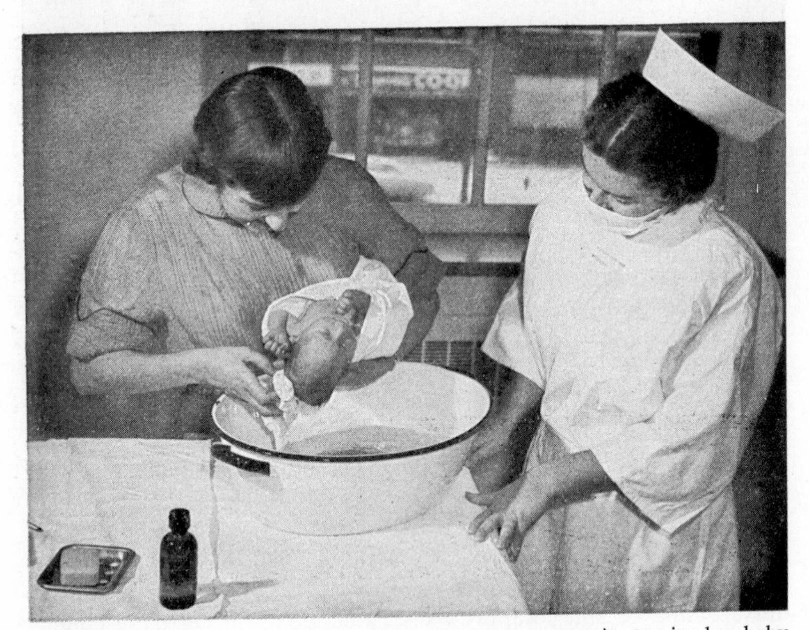

**Fig. 179.** The new mother should be given an opportunity to give her baby a bath, with the nurse's help and guidance. Holding the baby on her left arm and holding his buttocks securely between her hip and elbow, the mother can support his head with her left hand while she washes it with her right hand.

The diaper is removed next, and, if there is stool, the diaper area is washed with a separate cloth or cotton ball. If the mother needs experience in taking the baby's temperature it may be done at this time. The baby is now ready to have the rest of his clothing removed and to be weighed. It is usually advisable to weigh the baby before his skin is damp from the bath. The mother may need to learn how to balance and read the scales, and she must be shown how to pick up the baby and place him on the scales (Fig. 180). Finally the rest of the baby's body is soaped and thoroughly rinsed. If the navel has not healed the rinsing must be done with the washcloth used as in a sponge bath, but when this is necessary it is a good plan to have the mother practice placing her baby into a tub filled with only 1 in.

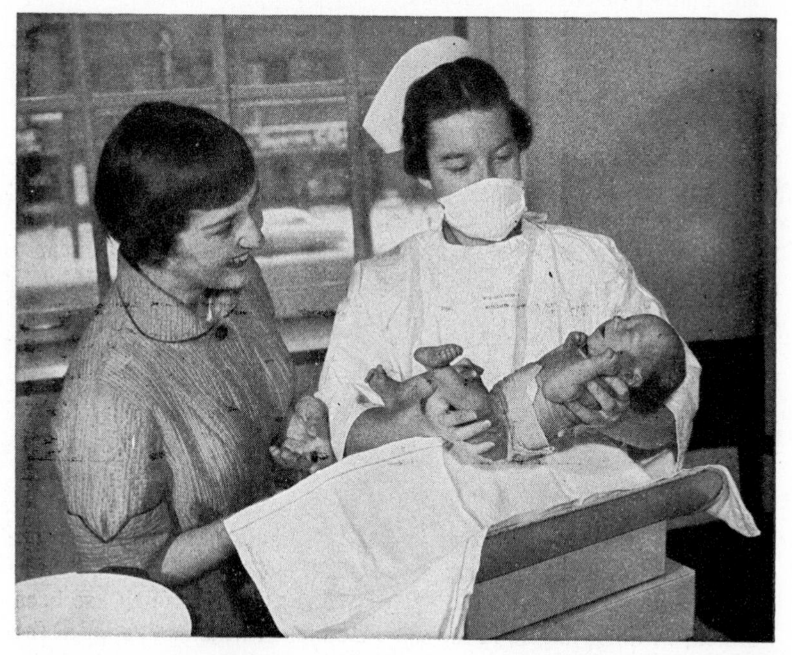

**Fig. 180.** Weighing the baby. The scales is balanced with a towel on the pan to keep the baby from becoming chilled from the cold metal surface. The nurse demonstrates a good method of supporting a baby whenever he is picked up. One hand with fingers spread supports his head and shoulders while the other hand supports the lower part of his body by firmly grasping his legs or buttocks. The nurse will let the infant's buttocks rest on the pan and then gently release his shoulders and head.

of water to learn the proper technic of holding him. She should place her left arm under the baby's head and shoulders and grasp his left arm firmly with her left hand; with her right hand she can grasp his ankles. She now has a firm grip and can lower him into the tub gently and place him in a sitting position. After the baby is in the tub, the mother can release her ankle grasp; this leaves her right hand free to rinse him. At this early age, the baby will not wish to play in the tub and he should be taken out again quickly, patted dry, and dressed in his clean clothes. Particular attention must be given to thorough washing and drying in all the skin folds and creases, especially around the neck and in the axillae and groins. Bath time provides an excellent opportunity to warn the mother against any manipulation of engorged breasts.

During the bath the mother can learn to test the temperature of the water with her elbow by testing it at the same time that the nurse does or by using a bath thermometer. The temperature of the water should be between 36.7° and 37.8° C (98° and 100° F). The very important habit of closing all safety pins and putting them out of reach should now be started. Some time during the bath procedure the mother should be reminded of the importance of selecting a firm table on which to place the bath tub, the danger of placing it near a stove or fire, and the danger of adding hot water after the baby is in the tub.

The baby usually thoroughly enjoys his bath by the age of four weeks. However, if he is afraid of the tub he should not be forced into it until he gradually overcomes his fear, a fear which may have started by having his bath water too hot or too cold, or having it splashed onto him too suddenly. He may react negatively to his bath because he is not being held firmly enough while in the tub.

If oil is being recommended for the daily bath at home, the nurse can explain to the mother that she should wash the face and buttocks with warm water first and that she can apply the oil, which has been warmed, with her fingers in the same manner in which she applied the soap with her hands. (The mother can be told that the oil is easily warmed by placing the bottle in a small saucepan to which warm water has been added.) The excess oil is wiped off in much the same manner as if the skin were being dried with a towel following a water bath.

## SPECIAL ORGANS

**Eyes.** A baby's eyes do not require daily care other than the removal of accumulated secretions in the corners of the eyes using a soft washcloth and clean water. They should not be irrigated unless there is a conjunctival discharge. Boric acid had for many years been a favorite irrigating solution, but the clinical experience of many doctors has resulted in a general disapproval of the use of boric acid for any care that is given an infant, not only because of some danger of absorption, but also because of the more serious danger of boric acid poisoning if the solution is mistakenly used for drinking water. Boric acid solution and crystals should never be used in the nursery, and the mother should be warned against their use in the home. Whenever it is necessary to irrigate the eyes, a physiologic salt solution may be used; the mother can be given instructions in how to prepare this at home.

**Nose and Ears.** The nose and ears should be cleaned externally only. The baby may sneeze and secrete mucus because of lint and dust and may develop some noisy breathing due to mucus, but no attempt should be made to clean the nose internally. Mucus may be removed if it is well down in the nostrils and can be wiped away easily by using a twisted piece of cotton which has been moistened with water or oil and the excess solution squeezed out. Dried mucus must not be worked out of the nose with an applicator. It is never advisable to introduce any object into any body orifice.

**Mouth.** The mouth should not be washed; there is great danger of injuring the tissue and predisposing to an infection. If the baby's mouth seems dry, he should be offered a bottle of sterile water between feedings.

**Genitalia.** The vulva should be cleaned by gentle washing with soap and water; special care must be taken to separate the labia in order to remove secretion which may collect between the labia minora and majora. At birth there is a heavy layer of vernix caseosa between the labia which may be washed away over a period of several days. It is impossible to remove all of the vernix at one time unless the area is washed vigorously and it is therefore a better practice to remove a little of it each day by gently washing between the labia at bath time and whenever the buttocks are cleaned following a stool.

This vernix should however be completely washed away by the time the baby is discharged from the hospital to relieve the mother of the worry of removing it. The mother must be given explicit instructions at the time she is learning to bathe the baby to wash between the labia each day (Fig. 181). During instructions regarding the care

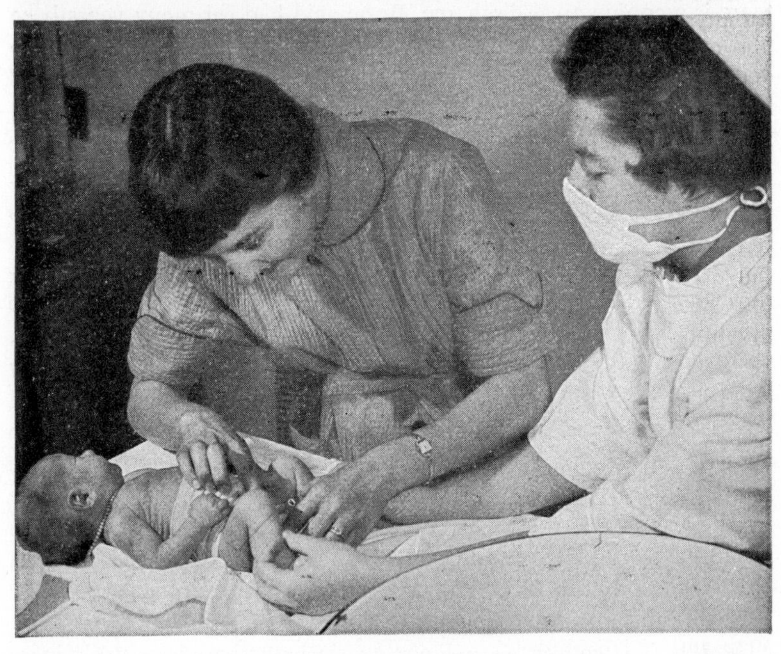

**Fig. 181.** Every mother needs instruction on how to clean the genitalia of her infant.

of the vulva, she should also learn of the importance of washing from the front backward, both at bath time and when she is wiping stool from the genital area. She should be instructed to use a different area of the washcloth for each downward stroke to avoid contamination of the vagina from the anal region.

In the male, if a circumcision is not performed, the foreskin must be retracted each day and the glans cleaned. *Smegma,* a cheese-like material, collects under the foreskin, and, with bacteria added, it will produce an irritation. After the first week of life the foreskin may be retracted daily; this should be done gently and only as far as it will go easily. The smegma is washed from the exposed portion of the glans or wiped with oil. Some doctors recommend postponing retraction of the foreskin for several months since an adherent foreskin at birth may separate with further development; it is then much easier to retract. The skin must be pulled back into its normal posi-

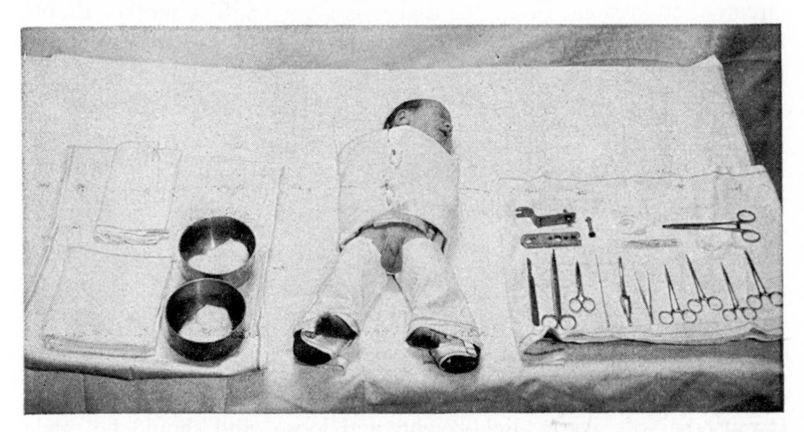

**Fig. 182.** Baby restrained on Y board for circumcision. Sterile tray contains cotton balls and solutions for cleaning the area and towels for draping. Tray with sterile instruments is placed in a convenient position.

tion, over the glans, within a few seconds, because its tightness will reduce circulation in the penis, cause edema, and finally make it impossible to draw it forward. A *paraphimosis* would then develop. The mother may find it quite difficult to retract the foreskin in the early weeks of life, when it is still quite adherent, and the doctor may prefer that this procedure be postponed for several months. If the doctor recommends that retraction of the foreskin be started early, the mother should be instructed how to retract it a little more each day, if possible, but without causing the baby pain.

A *circumcision,* which is the surgical removal of the foreskin of the penis, is frequently performed on the newborn baby (Fig. 182). It makes cleaning the area much easier and is important in the prevention of disturbances such as inflammation of the prepuce and glans with consequent dysuria later in life. It is often done between the sixth and eighth day of life, an age at which the baby has recovered from physiologic hypoprothrombinemia, if at this time he is in good physical condition and his coagulation and bleeding time of blood are within normal limits. If this procedure is done before the sixth day it may be necessary to administer vitamin K preoperatively.

Following a circumcision the nurse must watch for postoperative bleeding. An ointment, frequently petroleum jelly, is applied to the circumcised area each time the diaper is changed. The mother should be instructed to continue this care at home until the operative area has healed to the extent that the diaper will not adhere to it. It may be necessary to regularly retract the foreskin that remains following a circumcision, after danger of bleeding is past, in order to prevent adhesions to the glans during the healing process. If adhesions do form, the doctor will separate them later with a sterile probe or small forceps.

## CLOTHES

The baby's clothing should be suitable to the climate, the season, the temperature of the room, and the size and condition of the baby. It must be soft, warm, lightweight, and loose, and should be made of a material which is easily washed. A baby does not like to be dressed and undressed; it is therefore advisable to make the clothes very simple with a large enough neck to slip over the head easily and with large armholes. Clothes that open all the way down the back are easy to put on and take off. Since wool is sometimes irritating, a cotton material is preferable for the clothes worn next to the skin. Wool blankets give the most warmth, however, with the least weight.

A shirt, band, diaper, and gown usually make up the maximum amount of clothing worn in the hospital; the minimum may consist of only a band and a diaper. The baby may or may not be wrapped snugly in a lightweight cotton blanket. If he is cool, this amount of extra wrapping helps to keep him warm. It is believed that some babies feel more secure and sleep better when wrapped in a blanket; no doubt others prefer less covers. The baby's reactions may give a clue as to which he prefers.

Crib covers depend somewhat upon the temperature in the nursery. During cool weather the baby needs covers over him while he is asleep. A lightweight blanket folded twice and placed inside a pillowcase makes an excellent crib cover of the proper size for the bassinet. This arrangement supplies several layers of covering that may be handled in one piece. If the room temperature is quite warm a blanket or a pillowcase alone are adequate; in hot weather covers are not necessary and may even be undesirable at certain times of the day.

The baby is usually wrapped in a lightweight cotton blanket when he is picked up to be fed. He needs this protection even on hot days when he wears only a diaper because he may get cool while being carried through the corridor to his mother's room.

The mother usually has all of her baby's clothes before she enters the hospital, but if the nurse is asked for advice as to the proper amount she can recommend a minimal supply because the baby outgrows his clothes very rapidly. Laundry facilities will, of course, also have to be considered in determining the amount. Three to four shirts and bands are usually considered adequate; four to six gowns may be needed. The subject of long- or short-sleeved shirts is controversial. Some believe that if the baby needs a shirt at all he needs his arms well covered; on the other hand the short sleeves are usually long enough to reach well down on the baby's short arms. Three to 5 doz diapers are usually sufficient if the laundry is done at home; if a diaper service, which many laundries offer, is to be used, they either furnish the diapers or specify the exact number the mother must supply. Two to three blankets, one of wool, which furnishes warmth with the minimum amount of weight and bulk, and a sweater or two are usually enough additional clothing at home and for outdoor wear.

The diapers should be made of a soft, absorbent, lightweight material which is easy to wash and dry. Those made of a fine-meshed, gauze-like material probably meet these requirements best, but are also the most expensive; mothers sometimes prefer to use a cotton bird's-eye cloth or sometimes a flannel material. Diapers may be made in 27-in. squares or in an oblong shape measuring 20 by 40 in. Diapers used in the hospital nursery may be quite small because they are always put on small babies, but the mother must consider getting a large size which will fit the baby for as long as he wears diapers. There are various methods of folding a diaper. Whenever possible it should be folded so that there is an extra thickness in one area; this is usually in a center panel. It is frequently suggested that the extra thickness of the diaper should be in front on the boy and in back on the girl. It would seem that the position in which the baby sleeps would determine the place for the extra padding; if the girl is lying on her abdomen she may need the extra thickness in front also. The diaper must be put on snugly but should not be applied tightly enough to hamper the baby's movements. It is important for the mother to keep her hand between the diaper and the baby while she is pinning it.

Waterproof pants, over the diaper to protect other clothing and bedding, should be worn only on special occasions. The diaper must be changed more frequently than is normally necessary when worn under the rubber pants because it gets wetter and warmer and bacteria accumulate faster. Rubber pants should not fit too snugly around the waist or legs and they should have air holes to allow for some evaporation. Knit woolen pants are a good substitute for the rubber kind because they allow for a certain amount of evaporation. When pants are not absolutely necessary for protection it is best to place another diaper or a quilted cotton pad under the buttocks to absorb the extra moisture and to allow for some air between the baby's diaper and the rubber bed sheet under the linen sheet.

A change of diaper before and after a feeding is sufficient for the average baby, but some are uncomfortable from a wet diaper and wake up and cry between feeding times. Others may need more frequent changing because of an irritation of the skin in the diaper area. Diapers should be placed in a covered container immediately after removal; in the home they may be put to soak in a covered pail of cold water. If soiled with stool the diapers should be rinsed. In the hospital provision is made for rinsing of diapers in a flush sink outside of the nursery; in the home this rinsing is often done in the toilet.

The diapers need more attention than any of the other clothing because a *diaper rash,* consisting of a diffuse redness of the buttocks and possibly blisters and pustules and an irritation of the urethral orifice in the circumcised baby, may develop from what is known as an ammoniacal diaper. Bacteria from the stool decompose the urea in the urine and liberate free ammonia which causes this ammonia dermatitis. Some commercial antiseptic solutions used for diaper rinses have a marked bactericidal action and are useful in controlling the bacterial growth if directions are carefully followed, but boiling of the diapers is a safe and very satisfactory means of killing the organisms. Three minutes of boiling is sufficient time to destroy these bacteria; with a large pan full of diapers, however, it may be necessary to boil them 15 minutes to get the heat to those in the middle of the pan. A long-handled wooden spoon may be needed to keep the diapers under the water level. (The container and spoon should be used for diapers only.) If the ammonia rash is severe it may be necessary to boil all the other clothes that become wet with urine, since ordinary washing does not destroy these bacteria. An ammonia dermatitis is ordinarily not a problem in the hospital; besides a very adequate laundering many hospitals autoclave all the clothes used in the newborn nursery.

Everyone seems to find many uses for diapers; they often serve as sheets, or towels, or bibs. If the diapers have not been boiled it is not wise to use them for any area of the body other than the buttocks.

**Bed.** The baby's bed may be a bassinet or a large basket at first, but he soon outgrows this and may, therefore, be placed in a crib from the very beginning at home. If he does occupy a basket or bassinet it should be large enough to give him some room to move about and it should always have square corners to allow him adequate room to breathe in case he moves up to the corner of his bed. When a crib is chosen, care must be taken that the bars are close together. Whenever possible the crib should be placed in a room where the baby can be alone. It must be kept in a part of the room where he will not be in a draft. A bassinet should not be kept on the floor, which is more apt to be drafty.

The crib mattress must be firm so that the baby's head does not sink down into it. A pillow should never be used as a substitute for a mattress because a pillow is too soft; several thicknesses of a cotton pad or blanket are firmer and may be used quite satisfactorily. It is never advisable to place a pillow under the baby's head, and loose towels or diapers should not be left around the head end of the crib. A rubber or waterproof sheet is always necessary to protect the mattress from becoming wet or soiled.

## PSYCHOLOGIC CARE

It is generally agreed that the newborn baby responds emotionally to many stimuli and that the manner in which his needs are met and the experiences of his early childhood help to determine his adult behavior. He becomes uncomfortable from hunger, a wet diaper, and extremes of temperature; he jumps when he hears a loud noise and objects to being restrained; and he is pleased and comforted with rocking, patting, soft words, warmth, and being allowed to suck. The attitude with which he is picked up, held, cuddled, smiled at, and talked to begins to make impressions upon him from the time of birth. He needs loving care to feel safe and secure and to develop a sense of belonging. Nurses and parents should therefore be urged to pick him up when he cries, smile at him, talk to him, rock him, play with him, and hold him while he is fed. An early close parent-child relationship in the newborn period in which the parents can care for his needs as they arise is most easily accomplished by rooming-in. Parents must be given adequate explanation and assistance in the care of their baby to help them to overcome their worry and anxiety, and they should be urged to follow their natural impulses in his care. The developing needs of the child are usually good guides in determining this care.

Early indulgence does not mean that the baby will develop into a spoiled child or that he will place too many demands on his parents later. If he is cared for when he is distressed he will be happy without attention while he is comfortable. He will have to adapt to waiting some of the time, but satisfaction in infancy, which gives him an early sense of security, will help him to learn to wait and to accept restrictions more easily later in life.

A baby usually sleeps interruptedly for periods of two to four hours, awaking frequently to move, yawn, and open his eyes momentarily, but he will awaken and cry when distressed. He cries because he needs attention; it is his only means of letting someone know that he is uncomfortable. The person taking care of him must determine the cause of his distress and comfort him when he is fussy. Hunger is the most common cause of crying, although some babies may cry for a few minutes after a feeding, before they fall asleep. He may be uncomfortable because of a wet diaper, abdominal distress, an unpleasant temperature, close restraint, or he may be fussy because he needs to be held. Some babies do not mind a wet diaper while others are quite uncomfortable when they are wet. If the crying baby is not hungry or wet he may need to be picked up and patted for an air bubble, he may need more or less covers or a change of position, or he may need to be held and talked to for a few minutes. Short periods of crying do no harm; in fact, they may even be good exercise, but if the crying continues for more than 10 to 15 minutes after the baby has been given attention he may need something else;

perhaps he needs to be held and played with longer. It is sometimes very difficult to determine the baby's needs when he cries frequently or for long periods.

Nurses in the newborn nursery should meet the babies' needs as much as possible with the self-regulating feeding schedule, frequent changing of wet diapers, change of position, and close check on environmental temperature. Even when the baby is not rooming-in, the mother can assist in his care if the nurse takes the baby to her to be fed or for her to hold and play with when other methods of quieting him do not meet his needs.

Babies react so differently in the amount they protest to discomfort and in their response to handling that all care must be adapted to the individual child. The phlegmatic infant is neither readily awakened nor easily disturbed by noise or handling while the hypertonic infant is wakeful and fussy and responds to minimal stimulation. Some make their demands much stronger than others, cry harder and more frequently, and offer more resistance to restraint. They may even make it more difficult to change their clothes because they are very tense and do not allow their arms and legs to be straightened. All babies derive a great deal of pleasure from sucking and usually stop crying by being allowed to suck; many times they will soothe themselves by sucking their fingers when they do not receive immediate attention. Some babies need much more sucking than others, more than they get from the nursing periods, and they will suck any part of their hand—thumb, fingers, or knuckles—that they get to their mouth in order to take care of their need.

## FEEDING

The newborn baby may either be breast or artificially fed. Breast milk, which is the ideal and natural food for the young baby, should be given during the first months of life whenever possible. Nursing should be encouraged, when there is no contraindication, not only for its food value but also for the emotional benefits both mother and baby derive from breast feeding. (See Chap. 17.) The close relationship which is established between the mother and her baby may help to make later relationships easy and natural.

If the mother is unable to nurse her baby, he must be held while he is being fed his bottle. "Propping" a bottle is dangerous because the baby may choke and aspirate milk; there is also the possibility that he may suck in air that will cause distention and therefore discomfort. Aside from these very important reasons for holding the baby's bottle he gets more enjoyment from eating when he is held. He needs the closeness and cuddling that accompanies a feeding. The food which quiets his hunger pains, the feeling of being held, and the mother's pleasant manner during his feeding all make eating enjoyable, and although his hunger will cease even when he receives his bottle lying down, he does not get as much satisfaction from it as if he receives this feeding in a more comforting manner. Complete pleasure and satisfaction in eating may help to make adjustments to other situations easier.

The method and technic of breast feeding have been discussed in Chapter 17. For purposes of review and comparison of the similarity of technic of breast and bottle feedings, a few points will again be mentioned. Feedings may be withheld for 4 to 12 hours and sometimes for 24 hours to allow the mother and baby to recover from the shock of birth and to give the baby an opportunity to spit up mucus with which he is frequently troubled during the first 12 to 24 hours of life.* Since the main purpose of starting breast feeding early is to stimulate the breasts, bottle feedings are usually withheld the longer period. Feedings offered on a self-regulating schedule are most satisfying to the baby; he knows when he wants to eat. Hunger usually wakes him, and he begins to cry when he gets contractions of the stomach which produce pain; food stops the contractions, and he gets a pleasant sensation of pain relief. If food is supplied whenever the baby is hungry, so that he experiences this pleasant sensation of relief, he will develop a good appetite. The baby may be sleepy and may not wish to eat frequently, or in amounts that seem adequate, during the early days of life; he should not be prodded or patted too firmly in an effort to awaken him and to make him eat more than he wishes. Even when he appears to be hungry he may dawdle during the first few days; feedings should be attempted with patience and calmness. The breast-fed baby can be placed with his cheek near the mother's breast so that he can find the nipple when he begins to

* Some doctors prefer to have the baby that is to be breast-fed put to breast just as soon as possible following birth if the mother's and baby's condition permits.

root; if fed with the bottle he should be allowed to feel the nipple with his lips, take it and let go of it several times if he wishes, until he finally starts sucking well. Since the baby knows when he has had enough to eat he will stop when he is satisfied and should not be forced to take more than he is eager to take from either the breast or bottle; forcing the feedings will make them unpleasant.

With the bottle, as with the breast feeding, the baby should, therefore, be hungry and ready to eat; he should be made dry and comfortable, and the mother should be pleasant and unhurried. The bottle of formula, which has been stored in a refrigerator, is placed in a pan of warm water until it has become warmed to the temperature to which the baby is accustomed. Since the baby's palate is very sensitive to temperature changes he may like his formula the same temperature each time; otherwise the temperature is relatively unimportant unless the formula is too hot or too cold. In a hospital, bottles must always be warmed in a nursery warming pan or preferably a thermostatically controlled bottle warmer, and not in a lavatory sink where they may become contaminated. The holes in the nipple should be of such a size that the milk drops freely when the bottle is inverted, but does not flow out. As the baby is sucking, air bubbles should be seen going up into the bottle regularly. It should take him from 5 to 20 minutes to obtain his feeding. If the holes are too small, the baby may become so tired that he cannot finish his bottle; if too large, he may take his feeding so quickly that he does not have his desire to suck satisfied.

While the baby is in the hospital the mother should be allowed and urged to feed him during the daytime hours so that she can become accustomed to his reactions and way of eating (Fig. 183). For the sake of the mother's rest the night feedings are given in the nursery with the nurse always holding the baby during his feeding (Fig. 184). The mother should be instructed to hold her baby in a semireclining position while he is eating in order to keep the air which he swallows at the top of the stomach contents. To prevent having the baby swallow even more air than he ordinarily does while sucking, the bottle must be tilted enough to keep the nipple filled with milk at all times.

The mother should understand that the amount of formula (or breast milk) which the baby wishes may increase each day for a week or more, but that he will not take exactly the same amount from

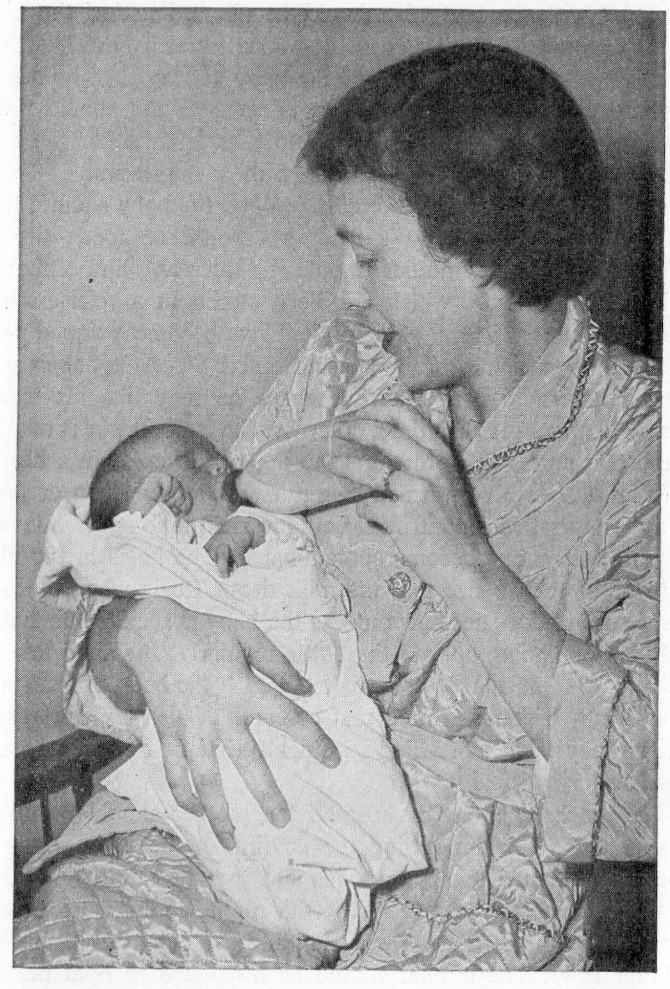

**Fig. 183.** A mother giving the baby his bottle feeding. The artificially fed baby should be held for his feeding since it is the only safe way to feed him to prevent choking and aspiration of milk. The baby also needs the closeness and cuddling that accompanies the feeding while he is being held. Mothers enjoy being given the opportunity to bottle-feed their babies in the hospital.

his bottle at each feeding. When he ordinarily takes 4 oz at a time he may stop after only 2 oz at some feedings; the bottle should not

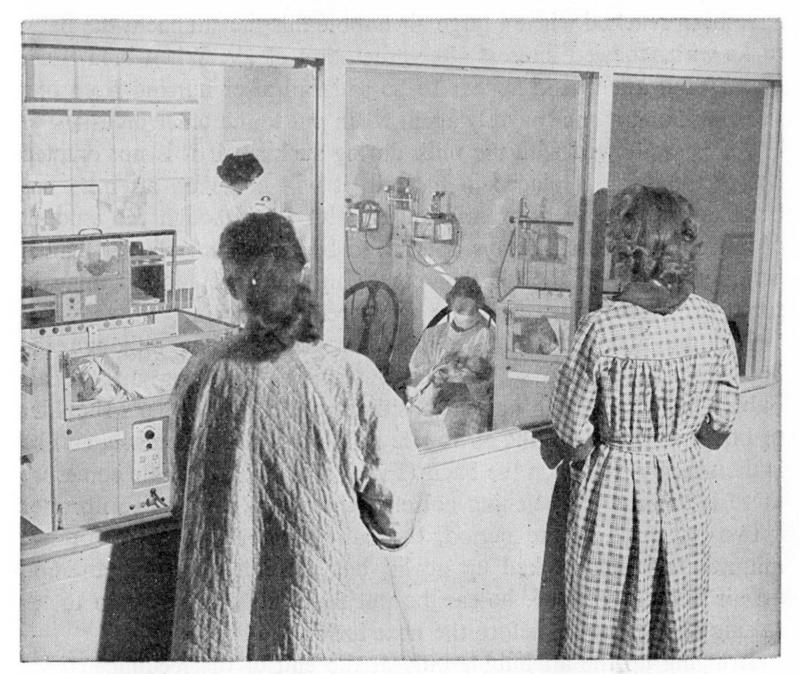

**Fig. 184.** Nursery at University Hospitals, Madison, Wisconsin.
If the nursery shades are up at all times, the mothers take advantage of the opportunity to watch their infants. Many of their learnings are incidental, gained by watching the nurses as they care for the infants. This picture also demonstrates the policy of holding infants for bottle feedings. It is hoped that this picture also makes it apparent that each infant has a complete unit for his care, thus eliminating the common work table.

be jiggled to try to get him to take more. It is also important for her to learn that caloric needs and gastric capacity vary greatly in infants of the same size and age and that her baby may not need the same amount that another baby born at the same time takes. The question frequently asked, "How much should my baby be eating now?" gives the nurse an excellent opportunity to explain the importance of allowing the baby to determine his needs.

When the infant's stomach is full, sucking becomes intermittent and slower and he gradually falls asleep. The nipple may be taken away for a few minutes and then offered again to determine whether he was satisfied or had become tired. Sometimes satiety seems to have been reached when a large air bubble fills the stomach; the baby sucks with renewed interest after eructation of air. When breast-fed, he may fall asleep and appear to be satisfied after nursing from one side, but he may suck eagerly again when put to the other breast.

Air is swallowed with the milk during sucking; if it is not eructed before the baby is placed in his crib it will come up after he has been put down and bring milk along with it. Although the amount of milk thus vomited always appears to be many times larger than it actually is, due to the air that comes up with the food, it may in some instances be necessary to feed the baby again.

A baby may not eructate air after each feeding although the bottle-fed baby does so in most instances. To bring up the air bubble he is held in an upright position against the mother's shoulder or body, which allows the air to rise to the top of the stomach, and he is then gently patted on the back (Fig. 147). As the bubble comes up there is definitely a belching noise. If the air has not come up after a two- to three-minute period, the baby can be put down for five minutes and then picked up again; but if, after a second attempt, no air bubble is heard, he can be put to bed. It is then wise to try raising an air bubble before the next feeding is begun.

Bringing up the air bubble only at the end of the feeding may be sufficient, especially with the breast-fed baby, but if it is known that a baby swallows considerable air and ordinarily vomits before he finishes a feeding it may be necessary to stop once or twice during the feeding to make an attempt to raise the bubble. If he seems satisfied with only a small amount of his feeding, his stomach may be filled with an air bubble and raising it may allow him to eat more.

The mother must be adequately instructed in raising the air bubble when she feeds her baby, but she must also be reassured that the spitting-up of milk, and some vomiting after a feeding, is normal in the newborn and not always due to inadequate raising of the bubble. She must also be reassured that vomiting will decrease as the baby gets older and that it becomes significant only if it continues. Adequate bubbling, gentle handling after a feeding, and avoiding placing the baby's head lower than the rest of his body when he is put to bed all help to decrease regurgitation. Since the amount of food vomited is frequently less than it appears, the mother does not need to be concerned that the baby is not receiving an adequate amount of food unless he does not continue to gain weight. Persistent vomiting, of course, may have a serious underlying cause and may also result in a decrease in body fluids. The mother also needs to be reassured that hiccuping is common after a feeding and is not significant. When the baby has hiccups an attempt can be made once again to raise an air bubble, but further treatment is not necessary to try to stop hiccups; they will soon disappear.

## ARTIFICIAL FEEDING

Although breast milk is the ideal food for the newborn baby it may become necessary to use an artificial feeding when the mother is not able or does not wish to breast-feed her baby. Artificial feedings are much easier, safer, and simpler at present than they have been in the past. Since cow's milk is the most common substitute for breast milk a comparison of the constituents of cow's milk and human milk may be valuable in understanding the necessity for the modification of cow's milk when it is used in infant formulas.

A comparison of human and cow's milk shows:

| | Human Milk | Cow's Milk |
|---|---|---|
| Water and solid content | Same in both; 87 to 87.5 per cent being water | |
| Calories | Same in both; 20 calories per ounce | |
| Protein | 1 to 1.5 per cent; 60 per cent of this is lactalbumin, and 40 per cent is casein | 3.5 per cent; 15 per cent of this is lactalbumin, and 85 per cent is casein |
| Carbohydrate (in form of lactose) | 6.5 to 7.0 per cent | 4.5 per cent |
| Fat(s) | Variable from time to time, but both have approximately 3.5 per cent. Differs qualitatively | |
| | Contains more olein which is more readily absorbed | Contains more volatile fatty acids which are irritating to the gastric mucosa |

| | Human Milk | Cow's Milk |
|---|---|---|
| Fat(s) | Digestion of fat easy | Digestion of fat sometimes difficult |
| Minerals | 0.15 to 0.25 per cent | 0.7 to 0.75 per cent. Contains more of all the minerals except iron and copper |
| | Iron content is low in both of these milks | |
| Vitamins | Varies with maternal intake; vitamin content of cow's milk may also vary with cow's intake | |
| Vitamin A | Relatively large amount in both milks | |
| Vitamin B | Probably adequate in both milks | |
| Vitamin C | More is found in human milk | |
| Thiamine | Higher content in cow's milk | |
| Riboflavin | Higher content in cow's milk | |
| Vitamin D | Relatively small amount in both milks | |
| Digestion | Cow's milk has a higher buffer content and can therefore absorb much more gastric acid than breast milk before it reaches the acidity necessary for digestion. The large amount of casein in cow's milk makes large tough curds in the stomach as compared to the fine, easily broken-down curds of breast milk | |

The curd in cow's milk is altered, made smaller, and less tough by boiling, by pasteurization, by homogenization, by the addition of acid or alkali, and by the heat necessary for making evaporated milk; this change in the curd is due largely to an alteration in the casein, but also is in part due to the homogenization of fat.

Formulas are made with milk, water, and sugar. The kind of milk used may depend somewhat upon its availability and upon individual preferences, but it should never be used raw because of its high bacterial count and the large tough curd that is produced by raw milk. Even pasteurized milk should be boiled. Evaporated milk is very frequently used. Many sugars are used satisfactorily. Lactose, which is the natural milk sugar, has no advantage over the other kinds and may even be less well tolerated. It may cause more flatulence because of its greater degree of fermentation. Cane sugar is easily obtained, is well tolerated by the normal baby, but is sweeter than all of the other sugars. Combinations of maltose and dextrins are commonly used; they digest and absorb more slowly than some of the other preparations. Corn syrup is also used quite frequently. Many of the sugars contain 120 calories per ounce.

Although the infant is to be fed on a self-regulating schedule as to frequency and amount, it is necessary to begin with a formula which fulfills the nutritional requirements for his size and age. Alterations can then be made as the individual infant needs a change for adequate growth and for satisfaction of hunger. Caloric and fluid requirements must therefore be considered in the construction of a formula, remembering that the full-term infant needs 110 to 120 calories per kilogram (50 to 55 calories per pound) of body weight and 130 to 200 ml of fluid per kilogram (2 to 3 oz per pound) of body weight in a 24-hour period.

There are a few basic rules which may be applied in determining the proportions of milk, water, and sugar to be used in formulas suitable for newborn infants of various weights. First, it must be remembered that the baby needs from 1.5 to 2 oz of whole milk or ¾ to 1 oz of evaporated milk per pound of body weight in a 24-hour period except that this requirement may be less during the first two weeks of life. Protein requirements are fulfilled by 1.5 oz of whole milk, but appetite may not be satisfied. To determine the total amount of fluid necessary in a formula the infant's fluid requirement for a 24-hour period is calculated. Since most or all of the newborn infant's fluid intake is formula, the milk is diluted with water up to the amount which will fulfill this total fluid requirement. (A dilution of approximately three-fifths parts of milk to two-fifths parts of water is the average concentration of formula used for the normal newborn; it does not need to be weaker than this and can often be tolerated somewhat stronger.)

Sugar is usually added to the milk mixture to bring the sugar content of the formula close to 7 per cent, which is the approximate amount of sugar found in breast milk. To determine the amount of sugar to be added, the following rule may be used: $\frac{1}{10}$ oz of sugar per pound of body weight. Frequently less than this amount of sugar is used in formulas and sometimes none is added.

It is well to remember that the number of tablespoons of sugar per ounce varies considerably with the various kinds of sugars. If a tablespoon is to be used in measuring the sugar it is very important to know the number of tablespoons per ounce of the particular kind of sugar to be used.*

Applying the above rules, a 24-hour supply of a cow's-milk formula which will fulfill the needs of an infant whose weight in 3600 gm (8 lb) would be calculated as follows:

| | | |
|---|---|---|
| Total fluid requirement is approximately 3 oz for each pound of body weight | =24 oz | |
| Total whole milk requirement is approximately 2 oz for each pound of body weight (16 oz of milk x 20 cal per oz) | =16 oz | =320 cal |
| Amount of water to be added to the milk to make a total of 24 oz of formula | = 8 oz | |
| Sugar in amount of $\frac{1}{10}$ oz per lb of body weight (8 lb) | =0.8 oz (⅘ oz) | = 96 cal |
| Total | 24 oz fluid | 416 cal |

Therefore the formula prepared may read as follows:

| | | |
|---|---|---|
| Whole boiled milk | =16 | oz |
| Water | = 8 | oz |
| Cane sugar | = 1½ | tbsp |

This might be divided into eight bottles with each bottle containing 3 oz or six bottles containing 4 oz, depending upon the amount the infant ordinarily takes at a feeding.

Since this formula furnished 416 cal, an infant weighing 3600 gm (8 lb) receives 114 cal per kilogram (52 cal per pound) in a 24-hour period if he takes all of the formula during that time.

Besides fulfilling fluid and caloric needs, this formula will fulfill the infant's protein, carbohydrate, and fat requirements.

An evaporated-milk formula is frequently used in the feeding of the newborn baby. It is easily available, relatively inexpensive, and is very easy to prepare. In addition to these advantages it is more easily tolerated by the infant than whole milk because of the small curd which is produced in the stomach and because its buffer value is changed so that it takes less acid, in that the process of evaporation so alters the casein that the curd in the stomach is quite similar to that of breast milk. Its easy digestibility makes it possible to give a higher concentration of evaporated-milk formula than would be possible

* Cane sugar —2 tbsp per ounce
Dextri-Maltose—4 tbsp per ounce
Dexin —6 tbsp per ounce
Corn syrup—2 tbsp per ounce

with whole milk; caloric intake could thus be increased above the normal if this should become necessary. Each fluid ounce of evaporated milk contains 44 calories.

The same rules that apply to whole-milk formula can be applied to evaporated milk by remembering that this milk has been evaporated down to approximately one-half of the original volume of whole milk. Thus only ¾ to 1 oz of milk is used per pound of body weight; it is never necessary to dilute evaporated milk with more than two times its volume. Therefore, 8 oz of evaporated milk diluted with 16 oz of water is not too strong for the newborn infant. Sugar added to this formula should, however, be less than that used in a whole-milk formula; ½ oz of sugar being used in place of the ⅘ oz. Sugar is not tolerated in the amount the rule calls for during the first six weeks of life. A 24-hour supply of an evaporated-milk formula which will fulfill the needs of an infant whose weight is 3600 gm (8 lb) would be calculated as follows:

| | | |
|---|---|---|
| Total fluid requirement is approximately 3 oz for each pound of body weight | =24 oz | |
| Total evaporated milk requirement is approximately 1 oz for each pound of body weight | = 8 oz | |
| (8 oz of evaporated milk x 44 cal per oz) | | =352 cal |
| Amount of water to be added to the milk to make a total of 24 oz of formula | =16 oz | |
| Sugar (a smaller amount than the rule states) | =½ oz | = 60 cal |
| Total | 24 oz fluid | 412 cal |

Therefore the formula prepared may read as follows:

| | |
|---|---|
| Evaporated milk | = 8 oz |
| Water | =16 oz |
| Dextri-Maltose | = 2 tbsp |

This may be divided into eight bottles with each bottle containing 3 oz or six bottles containing 4 oz, depending upon the amount the baby ordinarily takes at a feeding.

Since this formula furnishes 412 cal, an infant weighing 3600 gm (8 lb) receives 113 cal per kilogram (51.5 cal per pound) in a 24-hour period if he takes all of the formula during that time.

Whole milk has a tendency to cause constipation, while evaporated milk tends to produce loose stools; with a large amount of sugar in the formula the stools would become too loose. The baby can, however, tolerate more than 1 oz of evaporated milk per pound of body weight; if he is hungry, more than the average amount can be satisfactorily given. A 7.5- or 8-lb baby may even need 10 oz of milk to satisfy his hunger. Evaporated-milk formula is sometimes given without sugar, but the caloric intake may then not be sufficient to satisfy the baby's hunger. The amount of sugar needed should be determined by the character of the baby's stools. In general, the more concentrated the formula, the less the amount of sugar that is tolerated. If a newborn infant develops loose stools during the time he is being fed an evaporated-milk formula containing sugar, it becomes necessary to reduce the amount of sugar in the formula or to eliminate it entirely.

During the first few days of life it is most important to supply the infant with an adequate fluid intake; after this, more consideration must be given to the caloric intake. Both of the above formulas will fulfill the fluid and caloric requirements of the newborn baby.

Proprietary infant foods, which are of approximately the same composition as breast milk and which usually require only the addition of water for preparation, are used by some physicians in place of the whole-milk or evaporated-milk formula. With the consultation of her physician, a mother who is breast-feeding her baby often uses a selected proprietary infant food for the single artificial feeding which she finds is occasionally necessary or convenient to give in place of a breast feeding.

As the infant grows older and reaches a weight of approximately 4500 gm (10 lb) he usually gives evidence of being dissatisfied with the proportion of the original formula. Alterations are then made which will supply the needs for growth and will satisfy hunger. The baby will continue to need 2 oz of milk per pound of body weight, but a more concentrated formula becomes necessary. At this time less water may be added to the milk since some of the infant's total fluid intake is furnished by orange juice and other foods and by water taken between feedings. The rule for determining the amount of sugar is continued until 1.5 oz of sugar is reached; the amount of sugar added to a day's feeding should not exceed 1.5 oz and sometimes not more than 1 oz is added.

## FORMULA PREPARATION

Proper preparation and sterilization of infant formulas are of the utmost importance in the prevention of digestive upsets. These procedures should be carried out in a section of the hospital removed, insofar as possible, from traffic of hospital personnel and visitors and in an area where there is no danger of contamination from sick infants. The cleaning of bottles and equipment should always be separated from the actual mixing of the formula by a partition between the unit that is used for cleaning of utensils and bottles and the one that is used for the preparation and sterilization of the feedings; or, when this is impossible, by arranging for a separate time at which these procedures are performed.

All equipment in the formula room must be constructed so that it can be washed easily and should be kept in a scrupulously clean condition. Mops and cleaning equipment must be reserved for formula room only. Dry dusting is prohibited. Personnel in the formula room should have a pre-employment physical examination and periodic checkup examinations at stated intervals thereafter. Gowns should be worn in the formula room and caps to cover the hair. Employees must be educated to the importance of reporting early signs of illness. Assignment to duties outside of the formula room should never be with sick patients.

In the preparation of formulas great care should be taken that the ingredients are accurately measured and that the bottles of formulas are carefully labeled. All formula used for infant feedings should be prepared in a manner which is bacteriologically safe. For many years it was prepared by means of a sterile technic, a method which is still used, but is recommended only for those special formulas that are curdled by heat. Terminal heating of all formulas that will tolerate the degree of heat necessary for this process is the accepted technic for a bacteriologically safe formula and serves as a means of eliminating one source of infection in the nursery. Terminal heating is a process by which the entire formula unit, consisting of a bottle filled with the milk mixture, nippled and capped, is exposed to a degree of heat which will destroy bacteria but will not cause nutritive or physical damage to the formula. Theoretically, the aseptic technic is safe, but there is always danger of breaks in technic which can result in high bacterial counts and contamination by pathogenic organisms; terminal heating reduces the danger of error, and is often an easier method of preparation.

With the *aspetic technic* all equipment for preparation of formula and the bottles, nipples, and nipple caps are washed in soap and water, rinsed, and sterilized by boiling for 10 minutes or autoclaving for

10 minutes at a temperature of 110° C (230° F). The work table is scrubbed and covered with sterile draping sheets. Ingredient containers are washed with soap and water. Water to be used in mixing the formula is sterilized by boiling. When a whole-milk formula is made the milk as well as the water must be boiled; this is also true of pasteurized milk. The person making the formula prepares the hands by careful scrubbing and wears a sterile gown, a cap to completely cover the hair, and a face mask. Sterile gloves may be worn. After careful preparation of equipment and of the person making the formula, the milk, water, and sugar are mixed.

For making an evaporated-milk formula the required amount of water is poured into a graduated pitcher; the syrup or sugar is measured, added, and stirred until dissolved; and milk is added up to the required amount. The ingredients are then well mixed, and the formula is poured through a sterile funnel into sterile bottles and covered with sterilized nipples and bottle caps. All equipment is handled with sterile forceps during the entire procedure. After the bottles of formula have been cooled they are stored in the refrigerator until needed. In preparation of a whole-milk formula the required amount of water is put into a pan and brought to the boiling point; the milk is measured and added; and the milk and water mixture is boiled for three minutes. Since some fluid evaporates during boiling, enough sterile water is added to bring the total amount of fluid back to the original amount. The sugar is then added to the milk and water mixture, and after the ingredients are well mixed the formula is poured through a sterile funnel into sterile bottles and covered with sterile nipples and bottle caps. As in the preparation of an evaporated-milk formula all equipment is handled with sterile forceps and the formula is stored in a refrigerator after it has been cooled.

For the preparation of formula to be *terminally heated* it is not necessary to presterilize the ingredients, utensils, or bottles, but extreme care in cleanliness of equipment and technic is essential. All utensils, bottles, and nipples must be thoroughly cleaned and inspected. Bottles which are used daily without thorough cleaning will collect a milk film in which heat-resistant organisms, that survive terminal heating, may build up and produce a contaminated formula. The extra precaution of presterilization of bottles and equipment before formula preparation may be taken but is not necessary and does not eliminate the danger of contamination by heat-resistant organisms. Nipples, however, should be boiled, even when the terminal heating method is used, because, due to their shape and texture they are more difficult to clean.

The use of a detergent for cleaning formula bottles and equipment is far superior to a soap which combines with milk casein to form a gummy substance that is difficult to remove from the surface of bottles, nipples, and utensils.

Adequate cleaning of the bottles and nipples is a particularly important part of the thorough cleaning of equipment and also the most difficult. For good results the bottles, nipples, and caps should be rinsed under cold running water immediately after use and then submerged in cold water to loosen milk solids and coagulated protein. After a period of soaking they should be washed in a warm detergent solution with the aid of a hand or mechanically operated brush that reaches to the bottom of the bottle so that all particles of formula adhering to the glass can be removed. Next they are rinsed in hot running water until all detergent is removed and finally inspected in a good light to be certain that they are clean. Following this they should be inverted in a rack to drain. Nipples and bottle caps should be cleaned in the same manner. A small brush may be used to reach the ball of the nipple or it may be inverted for thorough cleaning. Nipples are then boiled for five minutes fully submerged in water by wrapping them in a towel or several thicknesses of gauze. All feeding equipment from the suspect or isolation nursery should be boiled before it is returned to the formula room.

As in the preparation of formula under aseptic precautions the person mixing the ingredients must prepare her hands by scrubbing and should wear a clean cap and gown. The work table should be washed and the ingredient cans cleaned with soap and water. The formula is mixed in clean utensils, the required amount is poured into clean nursery bottles, nipples and caps are applied, and the bottles are placed into racks ready for terminal heating.

Terminal heating is performed by either a nonpressure or a pressure method. In the nonpressure method the formula is heated at a temperature of 100° C (212° F) for 25 minutes with flowing steam or with boiling water and steam in a water bath. It takes approximately 15-minutes' exposure to the steam, or to the boiling water and steam, before the formula itself approaches 100° C (212° F). During the total 25 minutes, the formula itself is therefore at a temperature very close to boiling (98.3° to 99.4° C [209° to 211° F]) for 10 minutes; this amount of heating kills all pathogenic bacteria, but does not destroy spore formers.

Pressure heating is carried out in an autoclave where steam is under pressure and temperatures higher than boiling are reached; the temperature of the steam increases as the pressure in the autoclave is increased. It is recommended that formula be heated at 110°C (230° F) (7-lb pressure) for 10 minutes; this will produce within the formula a temperature of 110° C (230° F) for 6 to 8 minutes depending upon the length of time required for the autoclave to reach the proper temperature.

The pressure method has the advantage of producing a higher percentage of sterile formula because some kinds of spores are killed by the degree of heat that is reached, but there is also a disadvantage in the danger of overheating the formula and thereby causing some physical damage in the form of caramelization or curdling and nutritive damage which results in a partial loss of ascorbic acid, thiamine, and lysine.

Sterility in every bottle of milk cannot be assured by terminal heating since the degree to which heat can be applied without damaging the milk is limited. Nonpathogenic heat-resistant bacteria may occasionally survive. Although each bottle of formula may not be sterile the bacterial count of these nonpathogenic organisms is low enough to make the formula bacteriologically safe.

To keep the remaining organisms, although nonpathogenic, from increasing due to a prolonged incubation period the formula must be cooled quickly and must be adequately stored. Temperatures in the range of 54.4° C (130° F) down to 10° C (50° F) are most favorable for proliferation of these organisms, and unless this period of cooling is reduced to a minimum the bacterial count may increase considerably. Formula may be cooled by immersion in cool circulating water or by allowing it to air-cool. Water cooling is quicker but is difficult when high pressure heating has been used and it may introduce the danger of contamination. Air cooling at room temperature for approximately one hour is more practical and safer. Final cooling is accomplished in the refrigerator, which should be adequately large to store all of the formula and have a cooling capacity which will maintain a temperature of 4.4° C (40° F) to 7.2° C (45° F). The formula may be placed in the refrigerator almost immediately upon removal from the autoclave if a heavy-duty refrigeration unit is available.

Nipple caps are essential to terminal heating and will keep the nipple surface bacteriologically safe for at least 24 hours. To allow for escape of air and circulation of steam during the heating process and to prevent complete dislodging of the caps they must not fit snugly at the shoulder of the nipple during sterilization, but should be pressed down firmly immediately after sterilization. These caps should never be removed until the baby is fed.

Changing of nipples in the nursery because of plugging or too rapid a flow is accompanied by great danger of contamination and should never be permitted. Whenever a nipple cannot be used, another bottle of formula should be substituted. A scum, which sometimes forms on the formula, may clog the holes in the nipples and leads to the practice of changing them. This plugging can be prevented by using a nipple with a crucial incision (cross-cut).

Nipple openings may be made either by puncturing holes or by making the crucial incision (Fig. 185). When the holes are made by puncturing, several openings are best since there is less chance of complete plugging when there are more than one. These openings are usually made by burning small holes into the rubber with the point of a fine needle, the eye of which has been pushed into a cork to make for ease in handling. The point of the needle is heated to a red heat over a flame and quickly plunged through the end of the nipple. The size of the holes can be tested by inverting the formula bottle and observing the speed of the drops.

The crucial incision consists of two 4-mm incisions made at right angles in the form of a cross. This opening has a valve-like action which opens as the infant sucks and closes as the pressure from the baby's mouth is released. The opening cannot be tested by inverting the bottle to observe the speed of the drops, but must rather be done before sterilization by milking the nipple on an inverted bottle of fluid. Nipples with crucial incisions may be purchased ready-cut, but if they cannot be obtained the opening can be made with a razor blade, sharp knife, or pointed scissors. The opening must be made very carefully because with one that is too large the baby receives a stream of milk too great to handle and with an opening which is too small the nipple plugs or a partial vacuum may be created in the bottle.

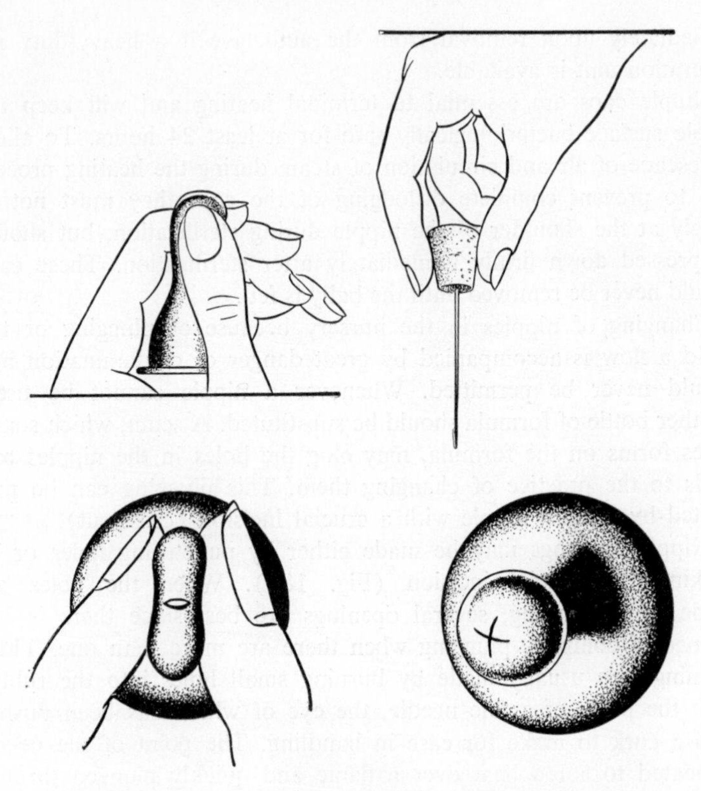

**Fig. 185.** Two types of nipple holes.

(*Top*) Two or three small holes are burned into the rubber with the point of a fine needle which is heated over a flame and quickly plunged through the end of the nipple. Pushing the eye of the needle into a cork makes for ease in handling.

(*Bottom*) The crucial incision (cross-cut). Two 4-mm incisions are made in the form of a cross. (Courtesy of Pet Milk Company, St. Louis, Mo.)

While mothers are in the hospital they should be taught how to make a baby's formula by being given the recipe, a set of instructions, and a demonstration of the procedure (Fig. 186). They may be instructed in either the aseptic technic or the terminal heating method or both; many show great interest in the terminal heating procedure which is safer and can easily be carried out in the home

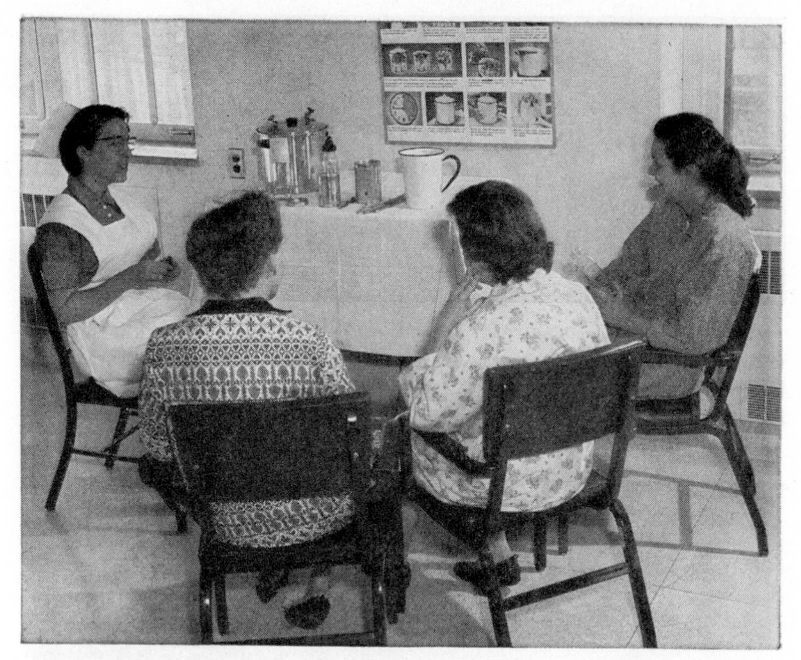

**Fig. 186.** A student nurse talking about formula preparation informally with a group of mothers.

by using boiling water and steam in the water-bath method (Fig. 187). Teaching by hospital personnel can be supplemented with booklets from evaporated-milk companies showing in pictures, step by step, how to prepare formula by either method.

## WATER

Fluid requirement is high during infancy. Ability to survive is greatly reduced by an inadequate fluid intake; the infant reacts more quickly than the adult to a lack of water. The daily need ranges from 130 to 200 ml of fluid per kilogram of body weight (2 to 3 oz per pound). This need is very great in hot weather and may increase to over 200 ml per kilogram of body weight (3 oz per pound) when the temperature is high. The normal baby will ordinarily fulfill his own requirement if enough fluid—formula, orange juice, and water

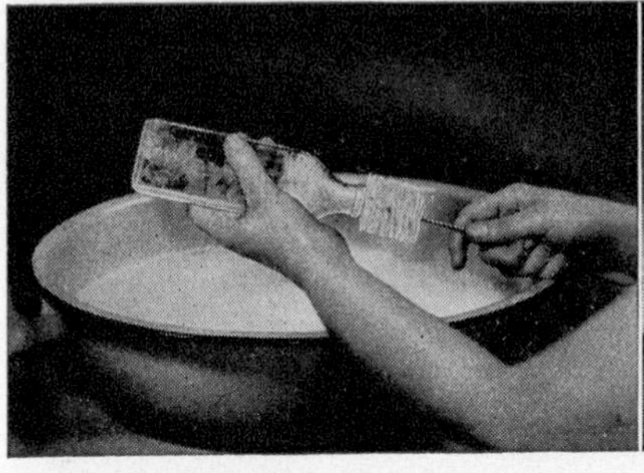

(1) Wash all utensils in hot soapy water or detergent. Scrub bottles with bottle brush. Rinse in hot clear water. Let drain.

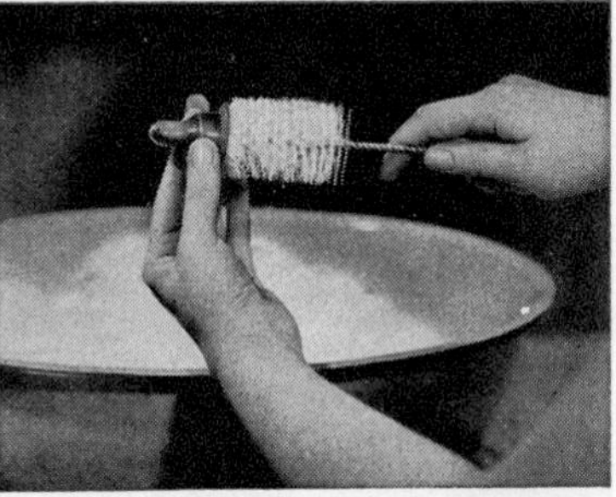

(2) Scrub nipples thoroughly—inside and out—with bottle brush. Rinse with hot clear water.

**(Fig. 187, pp. 664–68; Courtesy of Pet Milk Company)**

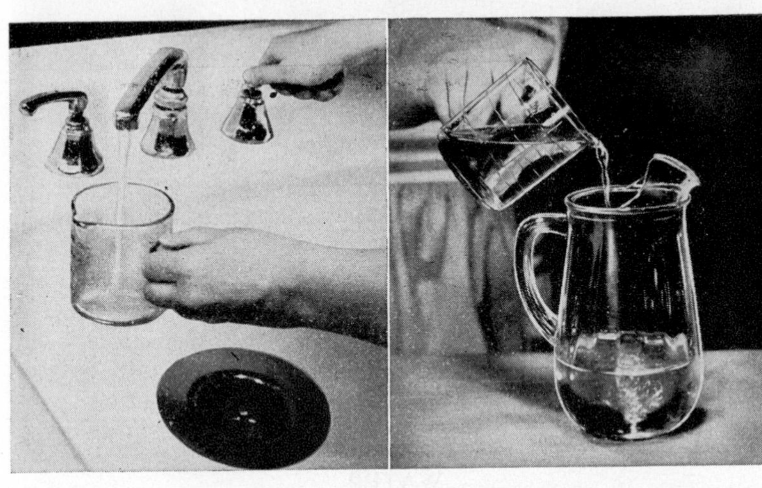

(3) Measure required amount of warm water from tap.

(4) Pour water into pitcher or quart jar.

between feedings—is offered. Water must be given frequently if the formula intake is inadequate because of poor appetite or poor sucking in the early days of life, if body fluids are lost due to heat, or if the baby has a fever. It may be necessary to offer water between all feedings when the need is great.

If it should suddenly become necessary to place an entirely breast-fed baby on artificial feedings, he may refuse to suck from a rubber

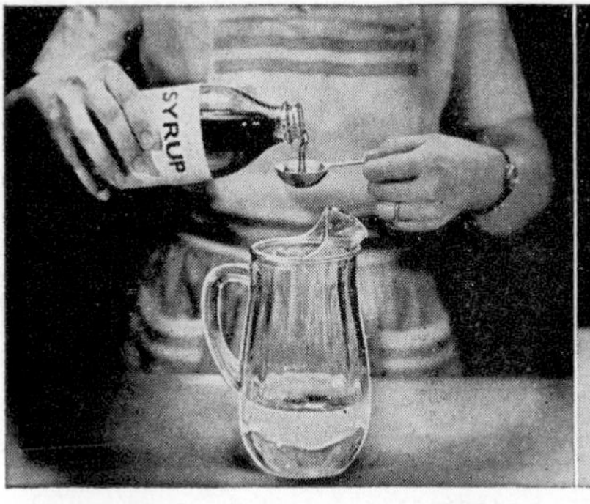


(5) Measure required amount of syrup or sugar in measuring tablespoon. If you use syrup, pour from bottle into spoon.

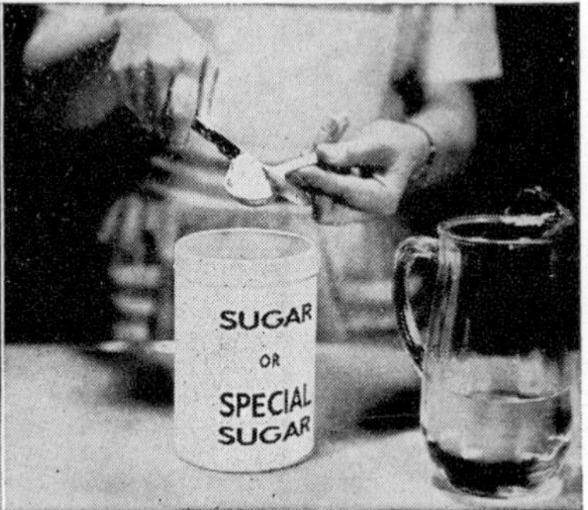


(6) If sugar, level off spoon with back of table knife. Add to water in pitcher. Stir with long-handled spoon until dissolved.

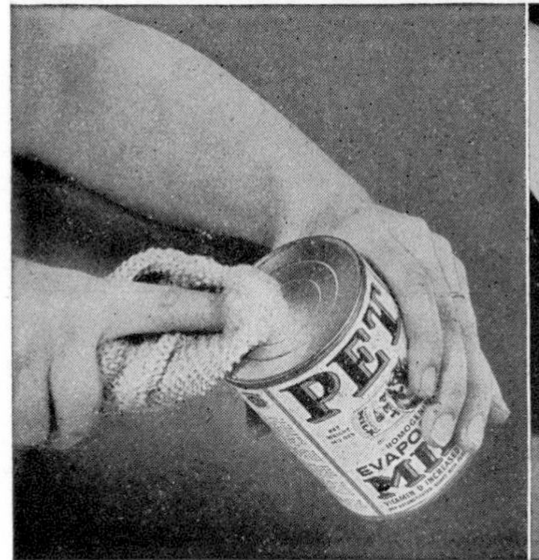

(7) Scrub top of can with soapsuds. Rinse in hot tap water. Punch two holes in top of can. (Open fresh can daily.)

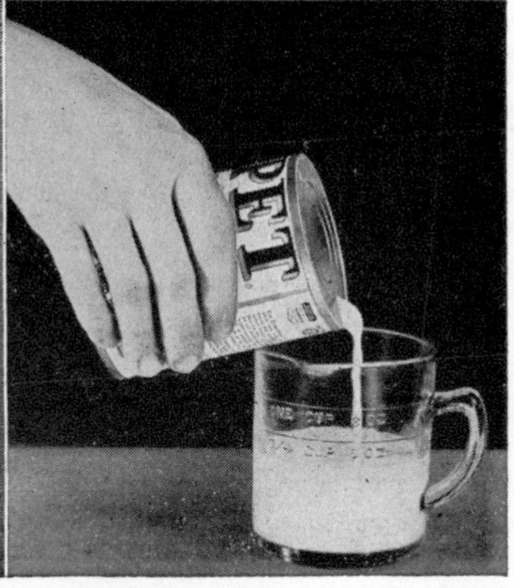

(8) Measure required amount of milk into measuring cup.

nipple unless he is accustomed to taking water from a bottle. Sterile water should, therefore, be offered once or twice daily for educational reasons when the baby otherwise has no need for fluid above that which is obtained from milk. Drinking water from a bottle also helps him learn to accept fluids other than milk from a rubber nipple.

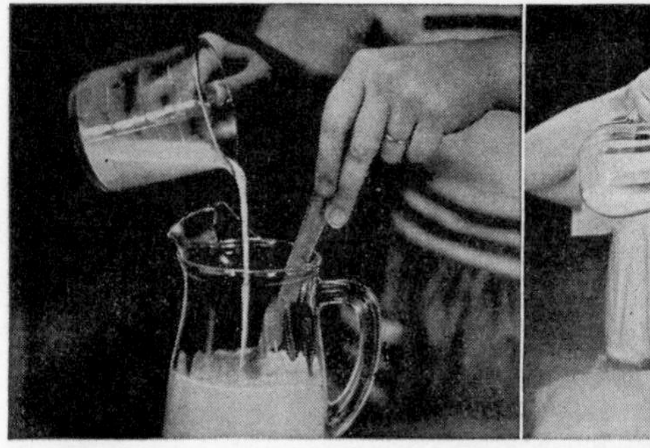

(9) Pour milk into water-sugar mixture and stir with long-handled spoon.

(10) Use funnel to pour correct amount of formula into bottles. (A bottle of water to drink may be sterilized with formula.)

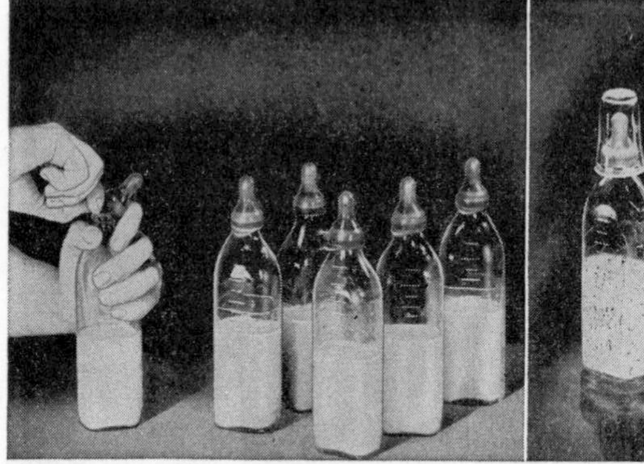

(11) Put nipples on bottles. (Boil new nipples five minutes before using for the first time.)

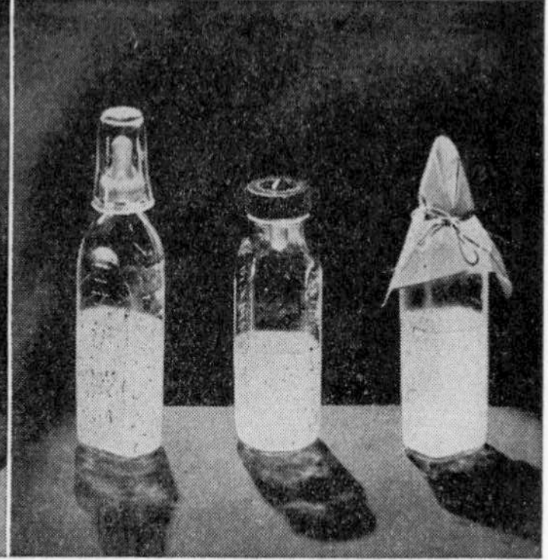

(12) Place nipple covers over nipples in one of three ways shown. Be sure covers or screw caps are loose. Brown paper covers should be fastened with string or rubber bands.

## VITAMINS

Rapid growth makes the infant's vitamin requirements high; they must be given early and in adequate amounts for proper development of rapidly growing bones and tissues. The quantity of the various vitamins that are present in milk will vary to some extent with maternal intake. The amount of vitamin A is relatively large, how-

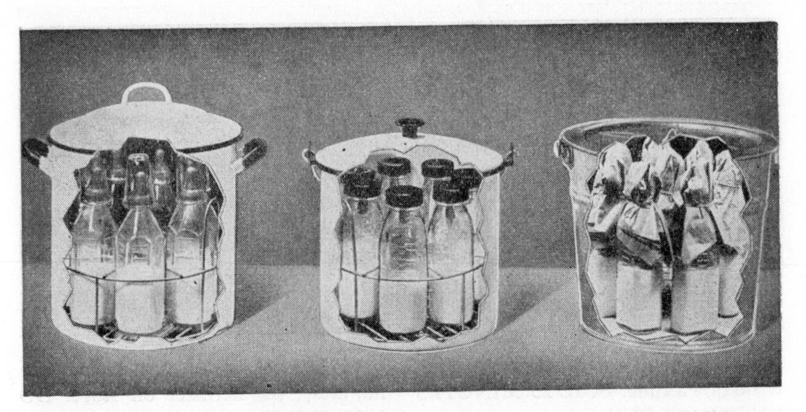

(13) Any one of three types of sterilizers shown, or deep pan with lid, may be used.

(a) Tall sterilizer with rack for bottles.

(b) Standard height sterilizer for screw cap bottles.

(c) Pail with washcloth in bottom, handle removed, and tight fitting lid.

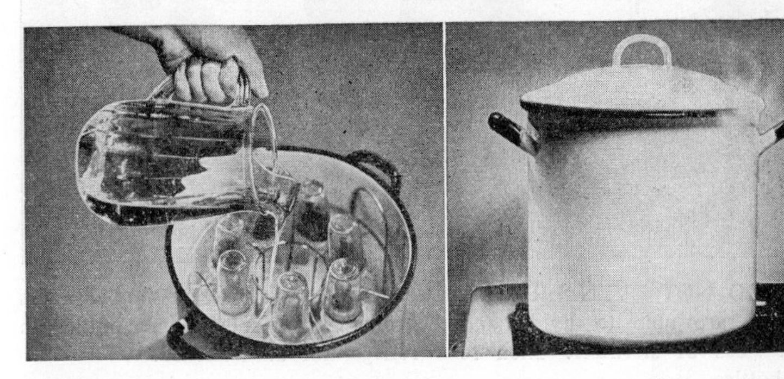

(14) Place rack or washcloth in sterilizer. Stand bottles of formula on it. Pour in 2 in. of water.

(15) Cover sterilizer and place on stove. Turn on heat.

ever, in both breast milk and cow's milk and may be sufficient to supply the baby's needs; the vitamin B content is adequate until the baby takes other foods. The C vitamin is found in human milk in a quantity which is sufficient for the infant providing the mother's diet is adequate, but cow's milk is low in this vitamin at all times, even when the milk is raw. Heat used to modify this milk for the

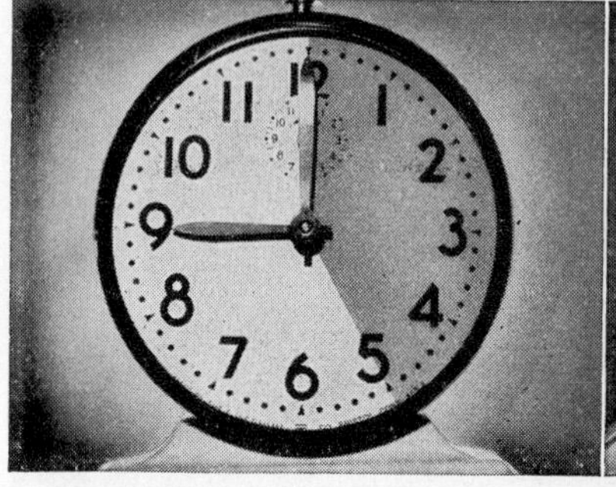

(16) When water starts to boil, write down time. BOIL 25 MINUTES BY THE CLOCK.

(17) After water has boiled "25 minutes," set sterilizer off stove. DO NOT REMOVE LID.

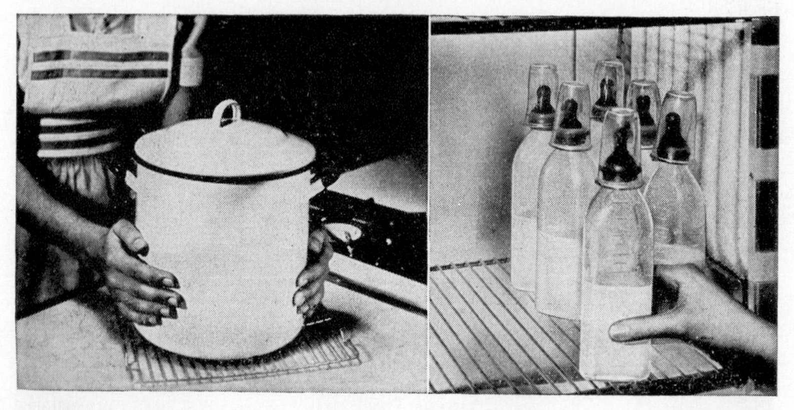

(18) DO NOT EVEN LIFT LID until you are able to hold hands against sides of sterilizer. Then remove bottles.

(19) Press or screw nipple covers firmly over nipples. Place bottles in refrigerator until needed.

**Fig. 187.** Preparation of formula by the terminal heating method. (Reprinted from a Pet Milk Company publication, "Your Baby's Formula.")

baby destroys part of this vitamin that is present, bringing the total amount even lower and making the addition of ascorbic acid necessary whenever artificial feedings are given. Vitamin D must be given as a supplement to both breast milk and cow's milk since the amount present in either is inadequate for the baby's needs.

Ascorbic acid, being water soluble, may be added directly to a bottle of formula or, if it is prescribed for a baby who is entirely breast-fed, it may be put into a small amount of water and given from a 4-oz bottle. Ascorbic acid is given in a concentrated form, in dosages of 25 to 50 mg daily, beginning at the seventh to tenth day of life and is continued until the time at which the baby is taking approximately 2 oz of undiluted orange juice daily. Orange juice is usually begun at the age of four to six weeks, and although the breast-fed baby receives an adequate amount of vitamin C it is given to him at this age also to accustom him to taking it. To prevent loss of vitamin C, orange juice should not be squeezed and strained until shortly before it is given to the baby, or if used from a can as either canned or frozen juice it must be kept refrigerated after the can has been opened. A fresh can should be used each day. Orange juice can be obtained in small cans, especially for infants. Orange juice is started in small amounts, approximately 1 tsp twice daily, and is increased by 1 tsp every day or two until 2½ to 3 oz are given. It is diluted with two to three parts of boiled water at first, then with equal parts of water, and finally, as the water is decreased even more, the orange juice is given undiluted.

The antirachitic vitamin should be started at the age of 10 to 14 days. Although 400 units of vitamin D per day are adequate for most babies, from 800 to 2000 units are frequently given to ensure a good margin of safety. Since vitamin D can be obtained from sources which also have a high vitamin A content it is better to give a preparation containing both vitamins A and D than to use one that supplies vitamin D alone. These vitamins may be given in the form of a concentrated fish liver oil, the preparations ordinarily containing around 200 units of vitamin D per drop. The usual dosage of 10 drops daily thus assures an adequate amount of vitamins A and D. When these vitamins are given in the form of an oil they will not mix with milk and must be administered by dropping the oil directly on the back of the baby's tongue. If these vitamins are given in a water-soluble mixture, which is commonly used, they may be dropped on the back of the baby's tongue or given in the formula or a small amount of water.

The administration of vitamin D is not quite as important in the summer as it is in the winter providing the baby receives a great deal of sunshine. If the amount of sunshine received is questionable, however, as when the baby is in the shade most of the time or when the atmosphere is smoky, it is best to continue with the regular dose. A small amount is usually given throughout the summer in any case, to keep the baby accustomed to taking it.

A number of water-soluble vitamin preparations containing vitamins A, B, C, and D are available and are used in this combined form in many instances instead of being administered separately.

Vitamin K is frequently administered shortly after birth to prevent a low prothrombin level of the blood which would otherwise normally occur in the infant between the second and fifth postnatal day. Some doctors recommend its administration to all infants; others use it mainly for the baby born following a difficult labor or delivery or the one showing a tendency to bleed. To the normal infant it is given as one dose of 1 to 2 mg, intramuscularly, very soon after birth. This dose may be repeated on the following day or two in instances where maintenance of a high prothrombin level seems indicated.

## URINE AND STOOLS

As has been previously mentioned it is important that the nurse make a record of the first voiding and stool, since they furnish good evidence that the urinary and intestinal systems are functioning; they are important observations in making an appraisal of the newborn infant. The baby may void at the time of birth or this function may be delayed for 12 to 24 hours, but the nurse must watch for and carefully record the first time. Following this the number of voidings daily are recorded on the baby's chart and if the amount seems scantier or larger than average a comment should also be made of this observation. Highly colored urine due to concentration, evidence of uric acid crystals, or observation of abnormal conditions, such as blood, should be charted and reported to the doctor. The quantity and frequency of the voidings will assist the doctor in determining the amount of fluid intake that he wishes the baby to have. Efforts may be made to increase the fluid intake when the voidings are scanty and infrequent and when uric acid crystals are present on the diaper. On the other hand, if the first voidings occur frequently and are large in amount, because of tissue edema at birth, fluids may be withheld from one to several days or until the edema has decreased or disappeared.

In charting the stools the nurse notes the frequency and describes the color and consistency. Some of the descriptive terms used are greenish brown, brownish yellow, greenish yellow, pale yellow, formed, semiformed, pasty, semiliquid, and liquid. The normal stools are frequently curdy, may contain some mucus, and occasionally may contain a minute amount of blood. It is important for the nurse to consider the day of life and the kind of feeding the baby is taking in order to judge the normalcy of the color and consistency of the stools. Greenish-yellow curdy stools containing some mucus are normal in the young infant, and the stools may be loose during the first week or two of life if the baby is ingesting a large quantity of milk. Diarrhea must be considered, however, if the stools are watery.

The baby may have from four to eight stools daily at first, possibly a small stool after each feeding; these become more infrequent later. The mother should be told the number and kind of stools she can expect her baby to have and must be advised to report watery stools to the doctor.

## PREVENTION OF INFECTION

The prevention of infection is an important part of the planning for nursery care and is the individual responsibility of everyone concerned with the care of the newborn baby. Perhaps the first and foremost precaution is thorough hand washing whenever the baby is handled. An antiseptic detergent or a soap or detergent containing hexachlorophene is considered superior to soap for nursery hand washing. Doctors, nurses, auxiliary workers, and mothers should wash their hands with soap and running water every time the baby is cared for or before clean nursery equipment is handled. It is especially important that the hands be washed carefully before the baby is fed or the upper part of his body is handled after a diaper has been changed. Jewelry should not be worn by the nursery staff. The mother, during her stay in the hospital, can be taught the importance of washing her hands before handling her baby and after changing his diaper if she is told of the reasons for this precaution and reminded to wash her hands before she feeds him.

One essential preventive measure against the acquiring of infection from nursery personnel is a pre-employment and annual physical examination of the nursing and auxiliary staff. All personnel must also fully understand the importance of not entering the nursery when they develop any signs of an upper respiratory infection, a diarrhea or other gastrointestinal upset, skin rashes, or any other infection, and the necessity of remaining away from the nursery for a long enough period of time to have fully recovered from any such disease. Any similar signs of infection in the mother must be given special attention. If the mother's infection is discovered before the baby has been exposed, it is best to keep him away from her. If he has already had contact, the baby can be isolated from his mother and from the other babies. Unless the mother's condition contraindicates nursing, her breasts can be pumped to maintain her milk supply. This milk may be sterilized and fed to the baby or it may be discarded until the mother recovers from her infection. As a safeguard against infection from an outside source, visitors should never be allowed in the nursery or in the room when the mother is feeding her baby; children should be excluded from the obstetric unit.

To prevent spread of infection from one baby to another the nurse must observe all babies closely for evidence of infection. Any baby having a fever; frequent and loose stools; a discharge from the umbilical area, the eyes, or the vagina; skin lesions; respiratory disease; or any other signs of infection should be removed from the nursery immediately.

To protect the baby from contact with uniforms, a gown, which should be changed several times daily, is worn in the nursery and masks may be worn to prevent droplet infection. Masks become wet from the breath and to be effective must be changed every one-half hour. Everyone should realize that handling or adjusting of the mask means contamination of the hands and necessitates washing them. Mothers are sometimes asked to wear a mask if they have had a recent cold; they must then have very careful instruction in the proper use of the mask.*

The best possible physical facilities to make nursery care easy will help prevent spread of infection. It is recommended that the bassinets be well spaced, with at least 2 ft between the cribs, and that the aisles be 3 ft in width. Equipment should be simple enough

* It may at times be advisable for the mother to wear a mask at home, while caring for her baby and preparing the formula, if she has a cold. For this purpose she can purchase masks or she may tie a soft cloth over her mouth and nose. She must be given proper instructions in their use and be told to use a clean one each time she wears a mask.

to be easily cleaned. Dry dusting is prohibited in the nursery. Common bathing and dressing tables should not be used. Soiled diapers are less of a source of contamination if they are placed in containers with foot-control covers and if they are never rinsed in the nursery. Two containers for diapers are advisable; one for diapers wet with urine and one for diapers soiled with stool. If possible, all infant laundry and supplies should be autoclaved. Every obstetric unit should have a suspect or observation nursery, where babies can be placed for observation when there is a question of infection, such as unexplained fever, loose stools, suspicious skin lesions, or infection in the mother which may be transferred to the infant. There should also be an isolation unit which is completely separated from the regular nursery and cared for by a separate staff. Here babies with diarrhea, impetigo, respiratory infection, or other types of infection are cared for. Babies born outside of the hospital should not be admitted to the newborn nursery; these babies are cared for in the suspect nursery. The nurse should be authorized to transfer a baby suspected of illness to the observation nursery until the doctor arrives to examine the infant.

Since increased traffic raises the bacterial count, nursery units small enough for one nurse to care for alone or with the assistance of one auxiliary worker are best. The American Academy of Pediatrics' Committee on the Newborn recommends that at least two hours and preferably three hours of nursing care be given to each baby in a 24-hour period. This requires one nurse at all hours of the day for every 12 babies and preferably for every 8 babies. Auxiliary workers in the nursery may give some of this care. They should be chosen for their ability, interest, and sense of responsibility and should be given good instruction and supervised experience.

## ROOM TEMPERATURE

Ideally the temperature of the hospital nursery is thermostatically controlled, kept between 22.2° to 23.9° C (72° to 75° F), and the relative humidity is maintained between 30 to 50 per cent. Keeping the humidity high, especially in the wintertime, if the source of heat is a radiator, is practically impossible, and whenever a baby particularly needs an environment in which the temperature and humidity can be specially controlled it may be necessary to place him in an air-conditioned incubator. When the nursery is not air-conditioned there may be a problem of keeping it cool enough on certain days in the summer; frequently one of the easiest ways of keeping the babies from becoming too warm is to remove their clothing during the hottest part of the day. It may be necessary to maintain good circulation of air on hot days by means of electric fans which, of course, must be so placed that air is not blown directly on the babies. The floor is a very satisfactory area for the fans if they are placed where the nursery personnel is protected from any danger of coming too near them.

It is usually necessary to advise the mother in regard to the proper temperature for the baby's room in the home, and, as with the clothing, it is difficult to tell someone just how warm it should be kept; the general tendency is to overheat the room. It is well to remember that the new baby who lies covered up in his crib will usually be quite comfortable in a cool room. Ordinarily the instructions concerning the temperature of the baby's room are to keep it from 20° to 22.2° C (68° to 72° F) during the day, if the baby is well covered, and to allow the temperature to drop to 18.3° C (65° F) at night until he weighs 3600 gm (8 lb), following which the night temperature may drop to 15.6° C (60° F). The room thermometer should be placed on an inside wall at the level of the crib and not near a source of heat.

Babies, because of their poorly developed sweat glands, are more easily distressed by heat than adults and are often very irritable and exhausted on warm days. During excessively hot weather the baby should have the coolest best-ventilated room available. Adjusting shades and awnings to keep the hot sun out and keeping the air in circulation by means of an electric fan, which, of course, must be adjusted in such a manner that the current of air is not directed toward the baby, may help to keep the room comfortable. Offering drinking water whenever the baby is awake and giving two or three cool sponge baths per day also help to reduce the baby's discomfort.

## FRESH AIR AND SUNSHINE

The baby has great need for an abundance of sunlight and fresh air to increase his resistance, improve his appetite and aid digestion, and to improve his color. In general, the more the baby is in the sunshine and the more fresh air he has while indoors, the better his physical condition.

While in the hospital the baby cannot be supplied with direct sunshine, but outside windows providing adequate sunlight and shades to control the amount are desirable. Circulation of air should also be provided. Ideally the hospital nursery is completely air-conditioned with temperature, humidity, and circulation of air controlled, but since the average nursery is not air-conditioned it is frequently necessary to depend upon windows and air ducts for fresh air. These must be opened in such a way that circulation of air can be obtained without a draft around the bassinets. If partitions are used in the nursery to provide individual units, better ventilation is obtained if these partitions do not reach to the ceiling.

The air of the room which the baby occupies at home should also be changing constantly in order that it may always be fresh, but the temperature should be equable and the baby protected from drafts. During cold weather it is important to place the baby's crib away from the window and to protect him from direct currents of cold air by the use of a window board in the window or a screen in front of it. In hot weather, circulation of air does not present as much of a problem except that the coolest room in which it is possible to have good circulation of air without a draft should be selected.

Direct sunshine is a valuable source of vitamin D, which is essential to the utilization of calcium and phosphorus by the body. Although a sufficient amount of vitamin D is not obtained from this source alone in the Frigid and Temperate zones, nor on cloudy days or in smoky areas, which do not allow for adequate exposure to the ultraviolet rays, sunshine should be provided whenever possible. There are also days in which it may be too hot to leave the baby out in the sun. It is best, therefore, to give an additional amount of vitamin D, in the form of special preparations, to most babies.

In spite of the need of giving vitamin D, it is important to put the baby outside early in life for all the beneficial effects he can obtain from both sunshine and fresh air. Extremes of heat and cold and dampness should be avoided, but the mother can and must be assured that he will tolerate being outside very well whenever the weather is not extreme and that he will benefit greatly from this outside environment.

The normal newborn baby can usually be placed outside for two to three hours a day as soon as he leaves the hospital. A baby weighing between 2950 to 4500 gm (6½ to 10 lb) may be out if the temperature is 15.6° C (60° F) or above, and some doctors say that he may even be outdoors anytime that the temperature does not go below 0° C (32° F) providing that he is well wrapped, that the day is not windy, and that the air is not damp and chilly. After he weighs 4500 gm (10 lb) he may be placed outdoors to sleep for two hours in the morning and two hours in the afternoon whenever the temperature is above 0° C (32° F); some doctors recommend that when he reaches this weight he may even be out anytime that the temperature does not drop below —9.4° C (15° F), providing he can be placed in a sunny protected area which will actually be much warmer than the temperature record for the day would indicate. The best time to place the baby outdoors in the wintertime is in the middle of the day, usually between the late morning and early afternoon feeding.

In hot weather the newborn baby may be outside more hours than in the winter; the middle of the day is frequently too warm, however, and it may be better to keep him in as cool a room as possible during this time. When sleeping outside in hot weather the baby should be kept in the shade, since even here he will get fairly good exposure to ultraviolet rays if the day is hot and sunny. In an attempt to expose the baby's skin to sunlight great care must be taken to avoid a sunburn which may be produced by even a few minutes of too much exposure. Excessive exposure, even after tanning of the skin has taken place, is dangerous.

## RECORDS

A daily record sheet kept in the nursery, on which to write observations at the time they are made, is very helpful to the doctor and all nursery personnel. Each hospital staff needs to decide on the type of record sheet they wish to use and on the kind of information they want to have on it, but there are several things which nearly all record sheets have in common (Fig. 188). The baby's day of life, birth weight, and yesterday's weight are usually written on this sheet; when today's weight is recorded it is possible to tell at a glance whether or not it compares favorably with the past weights. The time and amount of feedings are usually recorded; this makes it possible to check very easily how frequently and how much the baby has eaten during the day and how long since the last feeding was taken. This record also shows if the amount of breast milk is increasing as the days post partum increase and whether the baby can be expected to get enough breast milk at each nursing or if a bottle of formula should be offered. When a baby is crying, the information on the chart may guide the nurse in deciding whether hunger or some other discomfort may be the reason for the cry. The record will show the kind and number of stools the baby has had during the day; if he has a stool which is liquid or in some other way seems abnormal, it is possible for the person recording it on the daily sheet to notice immediately how many and what kind of stools he has had previously and to decide if it is necessary to be concerned about the present one.

The daily record sheets are usually not permanent records; the nurse must transfer information from them to the baby's permanent chart (Fig. 189A). Charting at spaced intervals takes less time than it would to go to the baby's chart at frequent intervals to do the charting. The daily sheet may have information of several babies on it and therefore makes for ease in checking on their general condition very readily. Another advantage of the daily record sheet is that auxiliary workers record their observations on this sheet, which they would ordinarily not do on the permanent chart. Whenever there is a need to check back on the food intake, the weight, or the output record of previous days this information can be found on the baby's permanent record or chart, which will contain the observations made each day since birth.

## BIRTH REGISTRATION

Registration of birth is of the utmost importance to the baby. It is the duty of the physician, midwife, nurse, or other attendant at the birth to register, with the local registrar, the name of the child, the date of birth, the place of birth, names of the parents, and any other information that is required. The proper blanks for registration of births may be obtained from the state board of health. All information should be accurately reported and legibly written. These records

[*Text continued on p. 680.*]

**UNIVERSITY OF WISCONSIN**
**UNIVERSITY HOSPITALS**

**NURSERY RECORD**

| Room | Name | Day of Life | Birth Weight | Yester-day's Weight | Today's Weight | Output | A.M. Temp. | Cord | Skin | Eyes | Mouth | Water | |
|---|---|---|---|---|---|---|---|---|---|---|---|---|---|
| | | | | | | | | | | | | | Time |
| | | | | | | | | | | | | | Output |
| | | | | | | | | | | | | | Weight |
| | | | | | | | | | | | | | Br. Milk |
| | | | | | | | | | | | | | Comp. |
| | | | | | | | | | | | | | Time |
| | | | | | | | | | | | | | Output |
| | | | | | | | | | | | | | Weight |
| | | | | | | | | | | | | | Br. Milk |
| | | | | | | | | | | | | | Comp. |
| | | | | | | | | | | | | | Time |
| | | | | | | | | | | | | | Output |
| | | | | | | | | | | | | | Weight |
| | | | | | | | | | | | | | Br. Milk |
| | | | | | | | | | | | | | Comp. |
| | | | | | | | | | | | | | Time |
| | | | | | | | | | | | | | Output |
| | | | | | | | | | | | | | Weight |
| | | | | | | | | | | | | | Br. Milk |
| | | | | | | | | | | | | | Comp. |
| | | | | | | | | | | | | | Time |
| | | | | | | | | | | | | | Output |
| | | | | | | | | | | | | | Weight |
| | | | | | | | | | | | | | Br. Milk |
| | | | | | | | | | | | | | Comp. |
| | | | | | | | | | | | | | Time |
| | | | | | | | | | | | | | Output |
| | | | | | | | | | | | | | Weight |
| | | | | | | | | | | | | | Br. Milk |
| | | | | | | | | | | | | | Comp. |
| | | | | | | | | | | | | | Time |
| | | | | | | | | | | | | | Output |
| | | | | | | | | | | | | | Weight |
| | | | | | | | | | | | | | Br. Milk |
| | | | | | | | | | | | | | Comp. |
| | | | | | | | | | | | | | Time |
| | | | | | | | | | | | | | Output |
| | | | | | | | | | | | | | Weight |
| | | | | | | | | | | | | | Br. Milk |

**Fig. 188.** Nursery record (University Hospitals, Madison, Wisconsin). A daily record sheet which is kept in the nursery. It has pertinent information concerning each baby and space in which to write observations at the time at which they are made. This up-to-date information is helpful to the doctors

DATE ________________ 19____

| FEEDINGS | | | | | | | | Feeding Orders | Medicines and Treatments | Pediatrician |
|---|---|---|---|---|---|---|---|---|---|---|
| | | | | | P.M. Temp. | | | | | |
| | | | | | | | | | | |
| | | | | | | | | | | |
| | | | | | | | | | | |
| | | | | | | | | | | |
| | | | | | | | | | | |
| | | | | | | | | | | |
| | | | | | | | | | | |
| | | | | | | | | | | |

and all nursery personnel. This is not a permanent record, but it serves the purpose of providing a place to record observations until they can be transferred to the baby's permanent record.

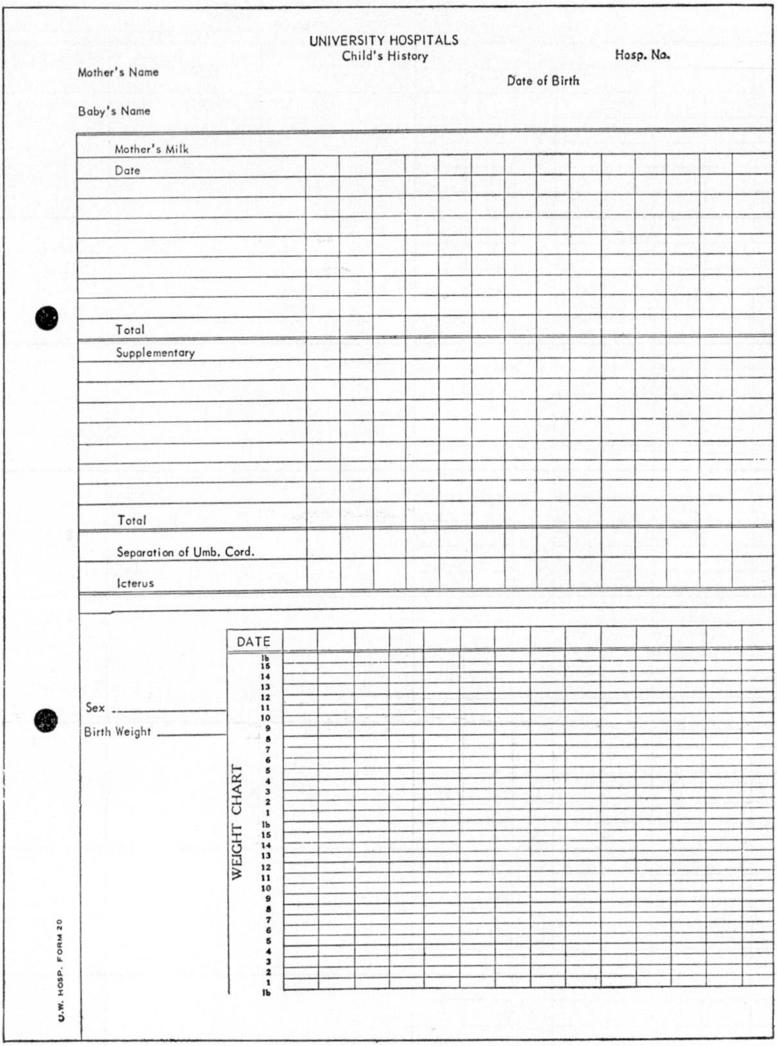

UNIVERSITY HOSPITALS
Child's History

Hosp. No.

Mother's Name

Date of Birth

Baby's Name

Mother's Milk

Date

Total

Supplementary

Total

Separation of Umb. Cord.

Icterus

DATE

WEIGHT CHART

lb 15 14 13 12 11 10 9 8 7 6 5 4 3 2 1 lb 15 14 13 12 11 10 9 8 7 6 5 4 3 2 1 lb

Sex

Birth Weight

U.W. HOSP. FORM 20

**Fig. 189A.** A sheet for the baby's permanent chart. (University Hospitals, Madison, Wisconsin.)

are permanently filed with the state Bureau of Vital Statistics; a photographic copy of the birth certificate or some other form of notification of the registration is sent to the parents.

EXAMINATION AT BIRTH

PROGRESS NOTES

BLOOD STUDIES

DISCHARGE EXAMINATION AND SUMMARY

Ant. Font. Sag. Suture & Post. Font.

Measurements: Head Crown-Rump

Chest Length

Abdomen

Umbilical cord off on th day. Umbilical Cicatrix

Circumcised on th day. Result

Eyes

Mouth

Skin

Birthmarks

Heart Femoral Pulses

Feedings

Date of Discharge Examined by Dr.

**Fig. 189B.** Back of a sheet for the baby's permanent chart, illustrated in Fig. 189A. The doctor records his observations on this sheet. (University Hospitals, Madison, Wisconsin.)

A birth certificate is necessary for a number of reasons and must be retained throughout life. The following list of reasons is partial, but demonstrates the importance of this document: to prove place of birth; to prove parentage and legal dependency; to prove age for entrance to school, for right to vote, for right to marry, for social security; to prove right to inheritance of property; to obtain a passport; and for other legal purposes.

The parents should understand their responsibility for receiving a photographic copy of the birth certificate, or a notice of registration, as absolute proof that their baby's birth has been registered.

## TEACHING PARENTS

Helping the parents of a new baby gain confidence in themselves and develop a feeling of security is one of the many valuable services the obstetric nurse can give her patients. She has an excellent opportunity to help them gain an understanding of their baby and develop attitudes which will be of inestimable value later on. The nurse can also help the mother become skillful in the handling of her infant by providing opportunities for her to give the actual physical care her baby requires. The mother can learn to make decisions as to the baby's needs with the nurse's help and guidance at first and finally by herself. It is important to make her feel that she has good judgment in planning his care so that she will have confidence in herself at home.

The nurse herself must have a good understanding of the needs of newborn babies; she must know how the doctor advises his patients so that she can correlate her teaching with his instructions, and she must familiarize herself with the equipment and procedures that would be suitable for care in the home in order to make all teaching adaptable to the home situation. She should be able to do her teaching with ease and must not allow the parents to sense a feeling of haste and pressure. A knowledge of what is taught in the prenatal classes and what the public health nurses do in the home will help her correlate the teaching she does in the hospital with that which has been done before the patient comes to the hospital and which will be given after she leaves.

The more infant care that is given at the bedside and that the mother herself can perform, under supervision, the more the mother has an opportunity to learn about her baby. Rooming together of mother and baby is, of course, as near to an ideal situation as the hospital can provide. Besides learning how to bathe and dress the baby, procedures that always seem complicated and terrifying, there is much more for the mother to learn which will be equally or more valuable to her. Among these may be included learning to turn the baby; to support his head; to determine what his cry means; to determine when he is hungry; to learn how to make, store, and warm formula; how to get up the air bubble after nursing; to learn the number and type of stools that are normal; that regurgitation, sneezing, and hiccuping are normal; how to judge the amount of clothing and proper room temperature; to learn the value of cuddling and rocking the baby; and many other things. If the parents learn that an absolutely rigid procedure need never be followed, but that several similar methods will accomplish the same purpose, they may find it easier to transfer their learning to their home situation. The mother may wish or may be asked if she would like to keep a record of the baby's behavior so that she can see what pattern her baby follows for sleeping, waking, and eating and so that she can learn which reactions are normal and which may need to be reported to the doctor. A record of this kind, kept by the mother whose baby is rooming-in, can be used by the nurse to transfer to the baby's chart information that should be recorded on the hospital record.

Whenever it is impossible to give individual instruction to mothers, group teaching saves time and proves very valuable. This may be a good method for those mothers who have other children or have developed skill in handling infants, but would like to have some demonstrations and review. A demonstration of giving a bath and of preparing formula can easily be given to a group of women at one time, and a discussion of some of the normal characteristics of the new baby and the psychologic aspects of his care can also be given to a group. The pediatrician may wish to conduct this discussion. The mothers who do not have the advantages of a rooming-in arrangement and feel they need to develop some skill in handling their babies before they take them home will gain some security by being given an opportunity to bathe their babies once or twice before they leave the hospital.

Providing the mothers with infant care books or pamphlets from a nursing unit library and giving them information on how to obtain pamphlets from their state Bureau of Maternal and Child Health or from the United States Children's Bureau constitute a valuable supplement to individual teaching.

## DISCHARGE FROM THE HOSPITAL

Even after the mother has had adequate instructions and has had practice in the care of her baby during her hospital stay, it becomes necessary to adapt this learning to the care of the baby at home. Referral to a public health nursing agency, so that one or more follow-up visits by a public health nurse can be made to the home, will make this adjustment easier and will assure continued nursing supervision for as long as necessary. The public health nurse can assist the mother in applying her learning in the hospital to the care of her baby at home and can help her to solve problems that arise in the home which the mother herself could not have anticipated earlier.

In some instances, where financial aid is needed, where the mother needs extra help to care for her family, or where more adequate food, clothing, or housing is necessary, it is important to refer the parents to a family service agency before discharge from the hospital. A check on the health of other members of the family, especially if someone has a communicable disease, may necessitate further planning before discharge.

If the baby will not remain under the medical supervision of the doctor in the hospital after he is discharged, continuous medical care can be assured by referral to the family physician or to a community agency maintaining a well-baby clinic.

### BIBLIOGRAPHY AND STUDENT REFERENCES

Addams, Ruth, and Scott, Ruth B.: "The Unbroken Circle," *Am. J. Nursing,* **51**:181–82, (Mar.) 1951.

Aldrich, C. Anderson: "The Role of Gratification in Early Development," *J. Pediat.,* **15**:578–82, (Oct.) 1939.

———: "Neonatal Crying, A Study of Its Incidence, Causes and Control," *Hospitals,* **20**:68–78, (Apr.) 1946.

———: "High Lights on the Psychology of Infancy," *Ment. Hyg.,* **30**:590–96, (Oct.) 1946.

Aldrich, C. Anderson, and Aldrich, Mary M.: *Babies Are Human Beings,* 2nd ed. The Macmillan Company, New York, 1954.

Aldrich, C. Anderson; Norval, Mildred A.; Knop, Catharine; and Venegas, Francisco: "The Crying of Newly Born Babies," *J. Pediat.*, **28**:665–70, (June) 1946.

American Academy of Pediatrics: *Standards and Recommendations for Hospital Care of Newborn Infants—Full-term and Premature.* The Academy, Evanston, Ill., 1954.

American Hospital Association: *Manual—Procedures and Layout for the Infant Formula Room.* The Association, Chicago, Ill., 1949.

Bakwin, Harry: "The Emotional Status at Birth," *Am. J. Dis. Child.*, **74**:373–76, (Sept.) 1947.

———: "Psychologic Implications of Early Child Care," *Am. J. Nursing,* **51**:7–10, (Jan.) 1951.

Beane, Geneva F.: "The Prevention of Impetigo," *Am. J. Nursing,* **36**:1207–10, (Dec.) 1936.

Benson, Reuel A.; Slobody, Lawrence B.; Lillick, Lois; Maffia, Anthony; and Sullivan, Norbert: "The Treatment of Ammonia Dermatitis with Diaparene," *J. Pediat.*, **34**:49–51, (Jan.) 1949.

Blake, Florence G.: *The Child, His Parents and the Nurse.* J. B. Lippincott Co., Philadelphia, 1954.

Bookmiller, Mae M., and Bowen, George L.: *Textbook of Obstetrics and Obstetric Nursing,* 2nd ed. W. B. Saunders Co., Philadelphia, 1954.

Carithers, Hugh A.: "Mother-Pediatrician Relationship in the Neonatal Period," *J. Pediat.,* **38**:659–60, (May) 1951.

Carney, Ruth: "A Parent Teaching Program," *Am. J. Nursing,* **51**:187–89, (Mar.) 1951.

Clifford, Martha L.: "Well Babies and Hot Weather," *Am. J. Nursing,* **50**:459–60, (Aug.) 1950.

Davidson, William D.: "A Brief History of Infant Feeding," *J. Pediat.*, **43**:74–87, (July) 1953.

Davis, M. Edward, and Sheckler, Catherine E.: *DeLee's Obstetrics for Nurses,* 15th ed. W. B. Saunders Co., Philadelphia, 1951.

Eastman, Nicholson J.: *Williams Obstetrics,* 11th ed. Appleton-Century-Crofts, Inc., New York, 1956.

Faust, Otto A.: "There Is Always More to Learn about Children," *The Child,* **13**:170–73, (May) 1949.

Finley, R. D.; Smith, F. R.; and Louder, E. A.: "Terminal Heating of Infant Formula. II. Bacteriological Investigation of High-Pressure Technique," *J. Am. Dietet. A.*, **24**:760–63, (Sept.) 1948.

Frank, Lawrence K.: "The Newborn as a Young Mammal with Organic Capacities, Needs and Feelings," *Psychosom. Med.*, **7**:169–73, (May) 1945.

Grayson, Robert, and Cranch, Gene S.: "Care of the Foreskin," *Am. J. Nursing,* **56**:75–76, (Jan.) 1956.

Greenhill, J. P. (ed.): *Obstetrics,* 11th ed. W. B. Saunders Co., Philadelphia, 1955.

Haddy, Theresa, and Adams, Forrest: "Factors of Importance in Breast Milk," *J. Pediat.*, **40**:243–53, (Feb.) 1952.

Hayt, Emanuel: "Circumcision Rites and Rights," *Mod. Hosp.,* **74**:73–74, (Feb.) 1950.

Heineman, H. E. O.; Huey, Grace; O'Connell, Elizabeth; and Campbell, Ann J.: "Converting to Terminal Formula Heating," *Am. J. Nursing,* **51**:605–6, (Oct.) 1951.

Hodson, A. Z.: "Terminal Heating of Infant Formula. III. Retention of Heat-Labile Nutrients," *J. Am. Dietet. A.,* **25**:119–22, (Feb.) 1949.

Holt, L. Emmett, Jr., and McIntosh, Rustin: *Holt Pediatrics,* 12th ed. Appleton-Century-Crofts, Inc., New York, 1953.

Huffman, Helen C.: "What the Birth Record Means for a Child," *The Child,* **11**:202–4, (June) 1947.

Illingworth, R. S.: "Crying in Infants and Children," *Brit. M. J.,* **1955, 1:** 75–78, (Jan. 8) 1955.

Jackson, Edith B.: "Should Mother and Baby Room Together?" *Am. J. Nursing,* **46**:17–19, (Jan.) 1946.

Jackson, Robert L.: "Feeding Healthy Infants," *Am. J. Nursing,* **55**:1076–79, (Sept.) 1955.

Jeans, Philip C.; Wright, F. Howell; and Blake, Florence G.: *Essentials of Pediatrics,* 5th ed. J. B. Lippincott Co., Philadelphia, 1954.

Latham, Helen C.: "How Does Your Nursery Rate?" *Mod. Hosp.,* **81**:79–82, (Sept.) 1953, and **81**:81–82, (Oct.) 1953.

Levine, Milton I.: "A Modern Concept of Breast Feeding," *J. Pediat.,* **38**:472–75, (Apr.) 1951.

Levine, Milton I., and Bell, Anita I.: "The Treatment of 'Colic' in Infancy by Use of the Pacifier," *J. Pediat.,* **37**:750–55, (Nov.) 1950.

Lyons, Robert A., and Wallinger, Elgie M.: *Mitchell's Pediatrics and Pediatric Nursing,* 4th ed. W. B. Saunders Co., Philadelphia, 1954.

MacDonald, Mary: "Nursing Observation of the Infant," *Pub. Health Nursing,* **38**:615–20, (Nov.) 1946.

Metropolitan Life Insurance Company: "The Hazardous First Month of Life," *Statist. Bull. Metrop. Life Insur. Co.,* **33**:1–4, (Feb.) 1952.

Murray, Marjorie F.: "Doctor Should Be Mother's Guide, Philosopher, and Friend," *The Child,* **13**:122–24, (Feb.) 1949.

Nelson, Waldo E. (ed.): *Textbook of Pediatrics,* 6th ed. W. B. Saunders Co., Philadelphia, 1954.

Norval, Mildred A.: "Sucking Response of Newly Born Babies at Breast," *Am. J. Dis. Child.,* **71**:41–44, (Jan.) 1946.

Parmelee, Arthur H.: *Management of the Newborn.* The Year Book Publishers, Inc., Chicago, 1952.

Peck, Elizabeth: "A Rooming-In Program," *Am. J. Nursing,* **51**:184–86, (Mar.) 1951.

Peto, Marjorie: "The Normal Newborn Infant," *Am. J. Nursing,* **52**:1353–55, (Nov.) 1952.

Powers, Grover F.: "Infant Feeding, Historical Background and Modern Practice," *J.A.M.A.,* **105**:753–61, (Sept. 7) 1935.

Ribble, Margaret A.: *The Rights of Infants.* Columbia University Press, New York, 1943.

Richmond, Julius B.: "Health Supervision of Infants and Young Children," *Am. J. Nursing,* **52**:1460–63, (Dec.) 1952.

Sanford, Heyworth N., and Grulee, Clifford G.: "The Newborn," in McQuarrie, Irvine (ed.): *Brennemann's Practice of Pediatrics,* Vol. I. W. F. Prior Co., Inc., Hagerstown, Maryland, 1948, Chap. 42.

Senn, Milton J. E.: "After the Midcentury White House Conference—What?" *The Child,* **15**:81–86, (Dec.) 1950.

Shea, Nilda; Klatskin, Ethelyn; and Jackson, Edith B.: "Home Adjustment of Rooming-in and Non-Rooming-in Mothers," *Am. J. Nursing,* **52**:65–67, (Jan.) 1952.

Smith, F. R.; Finley, R. D.; Wright, H. J.; and Louder, E. A.: "Terminal Heating of Infant Formula. I. Bacteriological Investigation of Low-Pressure Technique," *J. Am. Dietet. A.,* **24**:755–59, (Sept.) 1948.

Smith, L. Howard: "The Prevention of Impetigo," *Am. J. Nursing,* **36**:1206, (Dec.) 1936.

Spock, Benjamin: *The Common Sense Book of Baby and Child Care.* Duell, Sloan, and Pearce, New York, 1946.

———: "Common Behavior Disturbances in the First Two Years of Life," *J.A.M.A.,* **136**:811–13, (Mar. 20) 1948.

Stevenson, Stuart S.: "The Adequacy of Artificial Feeding in Infancy," *J. Pediat.,* **31**:616–30, (Dec.) 1947.

Stone, Samuel, and Bakwin, Harry: "Breast Feeding," *J. Pediat.,* **33**:660–66, (Nov.) 1948.

Tenney, H. Kent, Jr.: *Let's Talk about Your Baby.* The University of Minnesota Press, Minneapolis, 1947.

U.S. Department of Health, Education, and Welfare: *Infant Care,* Publication No. 8. U.S. Government Printing Office, Washington, D.C., 1955.

Weinfeld, Gustave F.: "Self-Demand Feeding and Indulgence in Early Infancy," *J. Pediat.,* **31**:203–6, (Aug.) 1947.

Wessel, Morris A.; Cobb, John C.; Jackson, Edith B.; Harris, George S. Jr.; and Detwiler, Ann C.: "Paroxysmal Fussing in Infancy, Sometimes Called 'Colic,'" *Pediatrics,* **14**:421–35, (Nov.) 1954.

Woodward, H. L.; Gardner, B.; Bryant, R. D.; and Overland, Anna E.: *Obstetric Management and Nursing,* 5th ed. F. A. Davis Co., Philadelphia, 1955.

Zabriskie, Louise, and Eastman, Nicholson J.: *Nurses Handbook of Obstetrics,* 9th ed. J. B. Lippincott Co., Philadelphia, 1952.

# Chapter 23

# The Premature Infant: Characteristics and Nursing Care

A premature baby is one born before full-term gestation, or any time before the thirty-seventh week of pregnancy is reached. The twenty-eighth week has long been considered the borderline of viability, but babies apparently younger have survived. Weight and length have seemed the best criteria of age because it is sometimes impossible to know the number of weeks of gestation, and occasionally even a supposedly full-term baby shows the deficiences of a premature; weight, which is the easiest to measure, is the most frequently used criterion of prematurity. A premature infant is defined as any liveborn infant with a weight of 2500 gm (5 lb, 8 oz) or less at birth. Any baby whose weight is 2500 gm or less should, therefore, receive premature care regardless of the estimated period of gestation.

**Cause and Prevention.** Adequate prenatal care, started early and continued throughout pregnancy, is a very important factor in the prevention of premature births. The mother is in this way kept in the best-possible health, and abnormal conditions can be detected and treated as soon as they arise. Treatment of disorders in the mother and improvement of her health by adequate nutrition and improvement of hygiene will help bring her and her baby to the end of pregnancy in the best-possible condition. Adequate nutrition is considered a very important factor in the prevention of premature birth.

Premature labor occurs without known cause in a fairly large number of cases. In others—such as multiple pregnancy, premature rupture of the membranes, placenta previa, and hydramnios—no preventive measures are known. Hospitalization of the mother, however, does increase the infant's chance of survival.

Known causes in which prevention may be possible by early diagnosis and adequate treatment include the toxemias of pregnancy, syphilis, chronic diseases (such as diabetes, tuberculosis, cardiovascular renal disease), acute infectious diseases, genital tract abnormalities, overfatigue, inadequate diet, or trauma. Syphilis is not the important cause of premature delivery that it was some years ago because of earlier and better prenatal care. Some premature births caused by genital tract abnormalities can be prevented by preconceptional examination and treatment. Some of the fetal abnormalities, another factor in premature deliveries, may possibly be prevented by adequate prenatal diet and by advising the mother to avoid exposure to the virus infections.

Premature induction of labor is sometimes necessary because of maternal complications, but should be performed as late as the mother's health will permit to give the infant the longest possible intrauterine existence. The pregnancy can in some of these cases be prolonged by hospitalization of the patient which may improve or slow the progress of the disease.

**Incidence and Cause of Deaths.** The incidence of premature births varies widely, ranging from 4 to 12 per cent of the total births in different countries. Although the mortality rate of these infants has decreased during the past two decades, prematurity is still the leading cause of infant deaths. Most deaths of immature infants occur during the first month of life, with the first day being the most critical period. Nearly one-third of all infant deaths in the first year of life and nearly one-half of those in the first month of life are attributed to premature birth. The mortality rate is inversely proportional to the birth weight; infants weighing less than 1500 gm (3¼ lb), measuring less than 37.5 cm (15 in.), and born close to 28-weeks' gestation have a high mortality rate.

Determining the exact cause of death is often difficult, and in a large proportion of cases no specific factor will be found. There are, however, some conditions which are the principal causes of death. Many infants whose birth weight is very low are too immature to survive, their death being due to immaturity alone.

Many of the fatalities during the first day of life are associated with the respiratory tract. The central nervous system and the lungs are immature, and atelectasis, periods of apnea, and cyanosis are very common.

Intracranial hemorrhage is another common cause of death. With

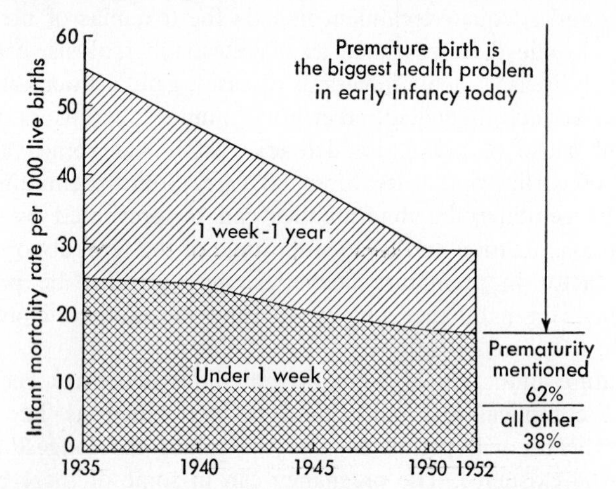


**Fig. 190.** Reduction in infant mortality. While the infant mortality rate has dropped sharply since 1935, deaths among babies in their first week of life have not decreased to any appreciable extent. (Kirkwood, Samuel B.: "Twenty Years of Maternal Care," *Children* **2**:136, 1955.)

all the structures of the body very inadequate, the premature baby cannot resist the forces of labor and delivery well and is therefore very susceptible to birth injury. Because of the fragile capillaries and the prolonged prothrombin time only slight trauma may cause damage. The possibility of a premature baby being expelled from the birth canal rapidly and the more frequent breech presentations in a premature labor can easily cause intracranial injury, since both conditions are traumatic. If the membranes have ruptured prematurely, as they frequently do in a premature labor, and if the head is the presenting part, it has much pressure exerted on it during labor and delivery. Asphyxia, by causing venous congestion in the brain, may also cause intracranial hemorrhage.

Death may also be due to infection, to which the premature baby is very susceptible and for which it has very little resistance. Upper respiratory tract infections and epidemic diarrhea of the newborn are followed by a very high mortality rate.

Defective renal function and poor water and acid-base metabolism may lead to acidosis or edema and death.

Other less frequent causes could be mentioned but those listed above are the most common. With all organs poorly developed it is not surprising that the mortality rate is very high, and it is quite apparent that the premature baby requires expert medical and nursing care from the moment of birth.

## CHARACTERISTICS AT BIRTH

The premature baby weighs 2500 gm (5 lb, 8 oz) or less and measures less than 46 cm (18½ in.). The head is round and relatively large. Growth of the head is rapid in fetal life, as compared to the rest of the body, especially in the earlier months, and it is therefore large in relation to the body when the baby is born. There is a disproportion between the circumference of the head and the thorax; the younger the baby, the greater this disproportion. The neck and extremities are short, and the trunk is broad and long. The eyes are prominent, and the tongue is large. The ears are soft and flabby and hug the scalp. The thoracic cage is less rigid than that of the full-term infant; the abdomen is round and full, and hernias are common. The mammary glands are small, do not become engorged, and do not secrete milk. The genitalia are small.

The skin is thin, through which the blood vessels can readily be seen; it is delicate, loose, and wrinkled, and lanugo hair is prominent. Physiologic jaundice is present in all premature babies in a few days after birth, and it lasts longer than in the full-term infant. Fingernails and toenails are soft, but contrary to popular belief extend to the ends of the digits. There is very little subcutaneous fat; this is true even when the infant is born fairly close to the full gestation period, because fat is deposited rapidly in the last month of intrauterine life (Figs. 191 A and B).

Respirations are irregular in rate and volume, and the baby is susceptible to atelectasis, attacks of cyanosis, and periods of apnea. There is a tendency to snuffles due to mucus in the nose and large adenoids which fill the nasopharynx. Body temperature is subnormal and markedly unstable.

The infant is inactive, and the cry is feeble, whiny, and monotonous. Gag, swallowing, and sucking reflexes are weak or absent.

The infant has a lowered tolerance of the alimentary tract with a tendency to vomiting and diarrhea; abdominal distention is more

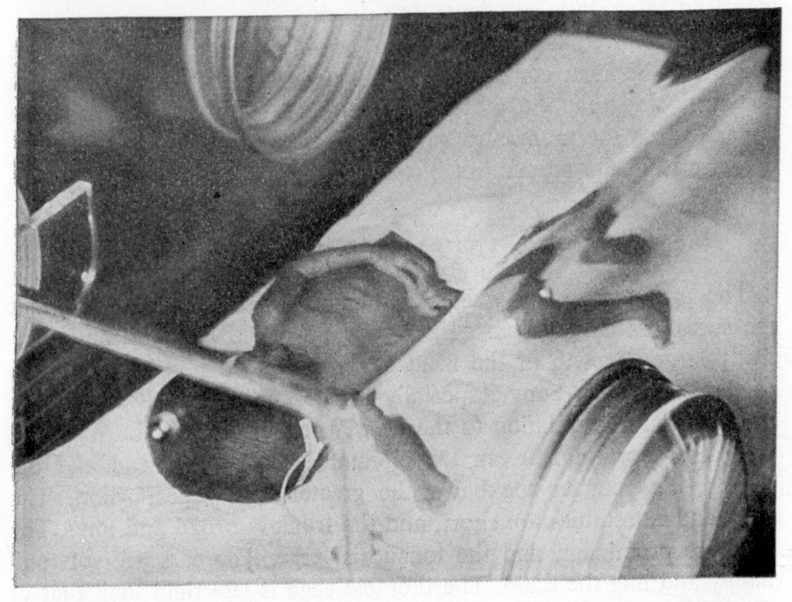

**Fig. 191A.** A premature infant 23 days old, weighing 874 gm (1 lb, 14 oz). Note the paucity of subcutaneous fat. (Distortions in the picture are a result of the curving glass of the incubator. It was considered unwise to open the incubator for the purpose of photography.)

common than in the full-term baby. The stools tend to be infrequent due to hypomotility of the intestinal tract; they can be loose and frequent due to lowered food tolerance, but may be so infrequent that they dry out and become constipated. The premature infant loses a larger amount of weight relatively than does the full-term baby and he does not regain it as quickly as the normal infant.

Impairment of renal function and a poor water and acid-base metabolism may cause edema or dehydration and acidosis. A heightened capillary fragility increases the tendency to hemorrhage, and defective hematopoiesis causes anemia.

Hepatic immaturity with bilirubinemia, hypoglycemia, hypoprothrombinemia, and hypoproteinemia is common. Deficient placental transmission causes poor antenatal storage of minerals and vitamins, immune substances, and maternal hormones and thus may be the cause of rickets, anemia, and/or infection. The premature infant also has an incompletely developed enzyme system. Congenital malformations are believed to be more common in the premature baby.

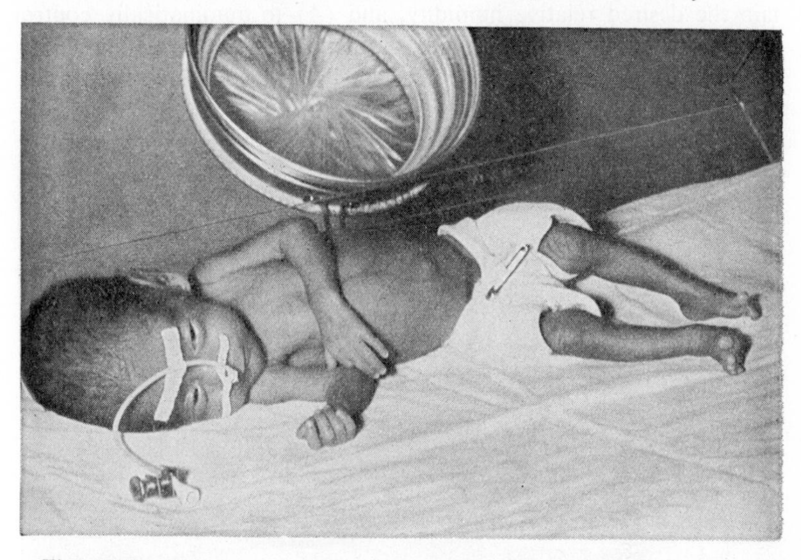

**Fig. 191B.** The same premature baby three weeks later. Note the large head as compared to the rest of the body. Blood vessels are visible through the thin skin of the abdomen. A polyethylene tube is in place for feedings.

## MEDICAL AND NURSING CARE

The care the nurse gives the premature infant is a very important factor in the prognosis. She must be keenly interested in his care, must be conscientious in attending to all of his special needs, understand his physiologic differences from the full-term infant, and be alert to very minor changes in his behavior, which may be a warning sign of impending danger. No care given the premature baby can take the place of the intelligence and interest of a nurse well trained in his special needs.

### INCUBATORS

Incubators are considered essential for the care of small premature infants—under 1500 gm (3¼ lb)—and are desirable for the larger premature—over 2000 gm (4½ lb). The ideal incubator provides the baby with an optimum environment at all times; in such an incubator it is possible (1) to accurately regulate the environmental temperature, (2) to maintain a desirable oxygen concentration, (3) to maintain the desired relative humidity, and (4) to automatically control circulation of air. Several types of incubators are available (Figs. 192 and 193). They may be completely air-conditioned with auto-

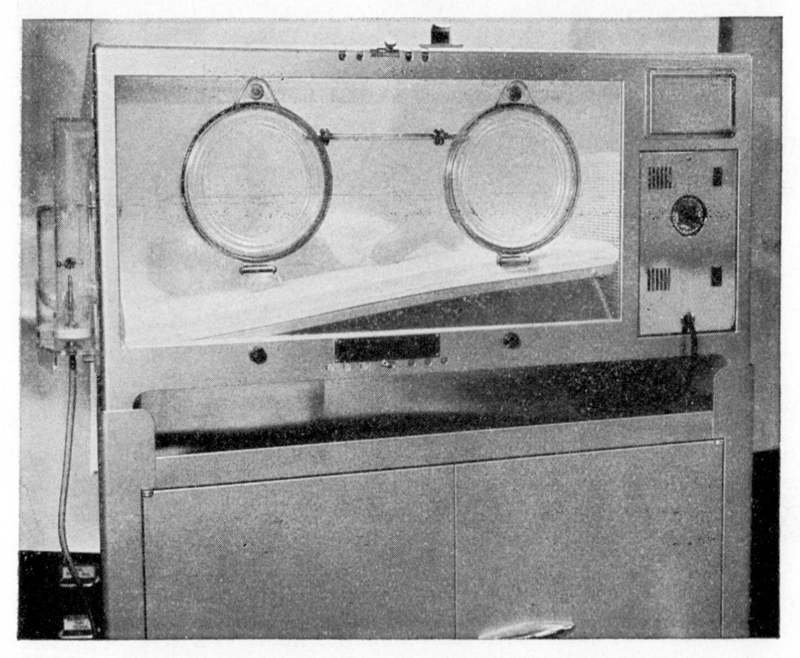

**Fig. 192.** Armstrong De Luxe H-H (hand-hole) baby incubator. (Courtesy of The Gordon Armstrong Company, Inc., Cleveland, Ohio.)

matic control of temperature, humidity, and circulation of air or they may be partially air-conditioned with automatic control of temperature and humidity, but not of the circulation of air. In still others only the temperature is automatically controlled. In some incubators there is provision for increasing the humidity to 100 per cent with the use of a vaporizer which produces a mist (pp. 770–71). Some are so constructed that they can be cooled in hot weather as well as heated in cool weather. All incubators should be free of fire and electrical hazards.

The nurse may occasionally find herself in a situation where an incubator is temporarily not available for the care of a premature baby. In such an instance hot-water bottles used in the crib, and changed in rotation, will help keep the body warm, and a partial cover over the crib will reduce the loss of heat. Precautions must be taken that the water is not over 51.7° C (125° F), that the bags are en-

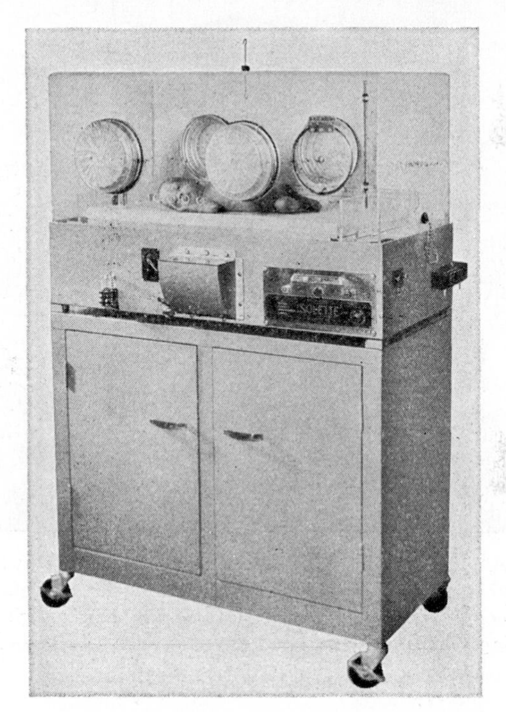

**Fig. 193.** Isolette infant incubator. (Courtesy of Air-Shields, Inc., Hatboro, Pennsylvania.)

cased in flannel covers or wrapped in a towel, and that they are carefully checked for leakage. Even with these precautions they must always be placed outside the baby's wrapping blankets. Portable incubators, for transporting a baby from home to hospital or from one hospital to another, are available. These may be heated with electricity (the cord is plugged into the socket of the dashboard light of a car) or with hot-water bottles.

Incubators may be constructed so that an ideal environment can be maintained at all times or so that they may maintain an even environment except when the crib is opened for purposes of giving the baby care. In the former, all care given the baby is conducted through entry ports (Fig. 194); the incubator thus remains closed

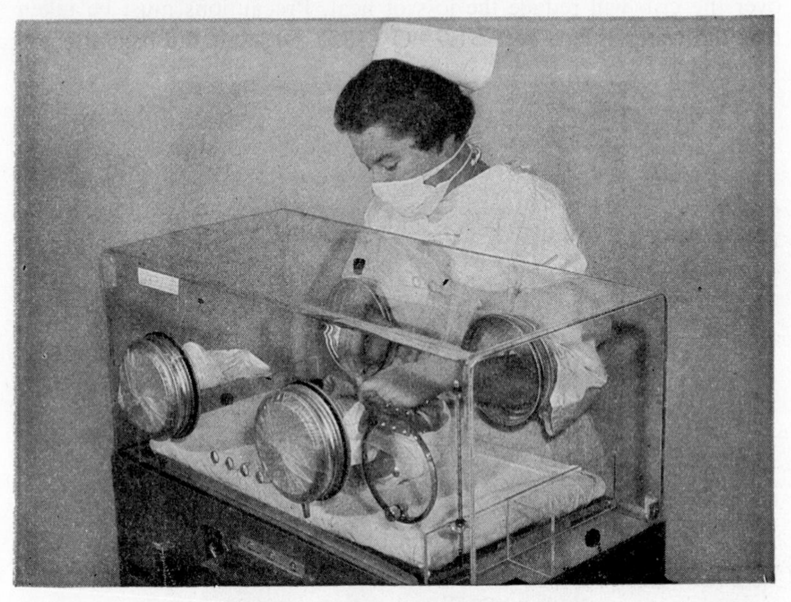

**Fig. 194.** A nurse demonstrating the use of the entry ports in the incubator. It is seldom necessary to raise the hood while caring for the infant; therefore, atmospheric conditions remain constant, and the baby is protected from droplet infection. The transparent hood provides ready observation of physical changes in the infant.

at all times, and the environment remains constant. This type also serves to protect the baby from droplet infection. If an incubator must be opened while medical and nursing care are given, the environment changes during the time that it is open. The very immature infant is cared for best in a unit that is completely air-conditioned and that can be kept closed during medical and nursing care. The larger premature infant does not necessarily need a completely air-conditioned incubator; he can be cared for quite adequately in a unit in which the temperature and the humidity can be controlled or even in one in which temperature only can be controlled.

There are great variations in the different types of incubators in regards to control of oxygen concentration, temperature, and humidity. In some incubators the temperature changes much faster than in others when the thermostat is moved; in some the percentage of oxygen is much different at the same rate of flow than it is in another. It is very important that the nurse understand this and that she knows approximately what changes to anticipate, but most of all that she has an awareness of the fact that there are variations so that she will check the environmental conditions very carefully until they are quite well stabilized at the desired point. After this, careful checking at regular intervals is, of course, still necessary.

Air-conditioned nurseries are ideal for the care of premature infants. (This is also true for the normal newborn.) Babies that are not placed in air-conditioned incubators will benefit from the environment of an air-conditioned nursery. The desired atmospheric conditions may be much easier to maintain in an air-conditioned incubator when the incubator is located in an air-conditioned nursery.

## ESTABLISHMENT AND MAINTENANCE OF RESPIRATION

Respirations are more frequently delayed and need stimulation in premature babies than in full-term infants. This delay may be due to a number of factors, including the immaturity of the lungs and the central nervous system; abnormal conditions in the mother which may have brought about premature labor, such as premature separation of the placenta or toxemia; the greater danger of intracranial injury to the fragile tissues; and the effects of analgesia and anesthesia administered to the mother. To prevent this last-mentioned difficulty the administration of pain-relieving drugs, especially to the woman in premature labor, should be kept at a minimum.

Whenever possible a doctor and a nurse should be ready in the delivery room to give their undivided attention to the premature baby. As for all deliveries, equipment to establish respirations and administer oxygen should be available. A catheter attached to a mucous trap or a rubber ear bulb must be ready to remove mucus and fluid from the respiratory tract (Figs. 102 and 103). The administration of oxygen may be necessary immediately. In establishing respirations, described on pages 327–32 and 763–67, special emphasis must be placed on keeping the infant warm throughout the procedure, and all efforts must be very gentle to prevent injury to the delicate issues or rupture of alveoli.

Oxygen was formerly administered to all premature infants for prophylactic reasons even in the absence of clinical evidence of need. Since an association between blindness in premature infants and high concentrations and prolonged use of oxygen has been noted and studied, oxygen is used much more cautiously. It is now believed that oxygen should be administered only in the presence of respiratory difficulty and cyanosis. If oxygen therapy is started at birth, the general trend at present is to discontinue it as soon as possible. Oxygen may not be necessary for more than a few hours or perhaps even less than one hour. The National Society for the Prevention of Blindness recommends: "Discontinue oxygen as soon as possible. Less than an hour's therapy is often sufficient. Prolonged therapy even at presumably safe concentrations (below 40%) has been associated with cicatricial retrolental fibroplasia. Discontinue oxygen at least once every 8 hours unless the infant is cyanotic while in oxygen." * If the baby does not become cyanotic when the oxygen is discontinued, its therapy is then not resumed unless cyanosis reappears later. When oxygen is administered to the premature infant its concentration should be kept below 40 per cent, unless a definite improvement in respiratory distress is evident in a higher concentration. Nurses need a standing order from the doctor that they may temporarily increase oxygen concentration above 40 per cent when the infant's condition definitely appears to warrant such an increase. When respiratory distress is such that the need for higher oxygen concentration seems indicated, the nurse must always notify the doctor as soon as possible. Maintaining a desired oxygen concentration is difficult without proper equipment. Methods by which the oxygen percentage can be controlled to a certain extent are: (1) the rate of oxygen flow to maintain the percentage at certain levels is often recommended by manufacturers of incubators; (2) oxygen may be used from tanks which contain 40 per cent oxygen and 60 per cent nitrogen; (3) the oxygen concentration is controlled by the use of a mixing device which dilutes 100 per cent oxygen to 40 per cent by delivering an air-oxygen mixture to the incubator. Although these methods help to regulate the percentage of oxygen that is administered there may be unpredictable variations. The use

* Lanman, Jonathan T., and McLaughlin, Ada: "Prevent Retrolental Fibroplasia in Premature Infants with Oxygen Control," National Society for the Prevention of Blindness, New York.

of an *oxygen analyzer* to measure the concentration each time that oxygen is used for short periods or at least every three hours when it is used over long periods is very important for accurate control of the amount of oxygen administered. The nurse has a great responsibility to measure the oxygen and administer it accurately according to the doctor's order.

Oxygen may be administered with a funnel placed close to the infant's mouth and nose for temporary treatment. For prolonged use it is given in an incubator which serves as an oxygen chamber or with an oxygen hood that can be placed over the top of the bassinet. Whenever oxygen is administered the relative humidity in the incubator or the oxygen hood should be increased to at least 65 per cent. If the humidity cannot, for some reason, be increased the oxygen should be bubbled through water. Although this does not provide adequate humidity it does help to moisten the gas somewhat and may reduce the irritating effect that dry oxygen has upon mucous membranes.

Premature babies are often placed in a supersaturated atmosphere for the first day or two of life as a prophylactic treatment against respiratory tract complications (pp. 770–71). If this treatment is used when oxygen is not necessary, compressed air can be used instead of oxygen to operate the nebulizer or vaporizer that is used to produce the mist in the incubator.

The premature baby's respirations are often rapid, shallow, and irregular with periods of apnea, but these signs are not necessarily indications for the administration of oxygen. An increasing respiratory rate may be evidence of distress; the respirations must be counted and recorded every one to two hours at first. Movements of the intercostal muscles and the diaphragm are weak, and varying degrees of atelectasis exist. It takes from two to three weeks for the premature baby's lungs to become fully expanded. Respiratory difficulties often occur because of the immaturity of the respiratory system and of the central nervous system, the weakness of the muscles used in respiration, the weak thoracic cage, and the absence or weakness of the gag and cough reflexes. These conditions predispose to aspiration pneumonia.

It is apparent that the nurse must watch the premature infant very closely during at least the first 24 hours of life for evidence of respiratory distress. More premature babies die during this period than at any other time, the main cause being respiratory failure. The nurse should have a catheter with mucous trap or a rubber ear syringe available in the nursery to remove mucus (gently) if it accumulates. The baby's head is often kept dependent by putting him in a Trendelenburg position for the first 24 hours to aid in the drainage of secretions from the air passages. His position must be changed approximately every two hours. The nurse must try to re-establish breathing if it stops. Sometimes a change of position or cutaneous stimulation is all that is necessary to re-establish breathing; at other times artificial respiration, done gently, may be required. If the baby has a moaning respiration, an indication of distress—central nervous system damage, a large area of atelectasis, or hyaline membrane disease *—he must be watched very closely. Stimulating the baby that is lethargic to cry occasionally may aid in lung expansion, but it must be done very gently to prevent injury or exhaustion and is contraindicated if there is any evidence of intracranial hemorrhage.

The baby who has survived the first 24 hours with very little or no respiratory distress is usually considered to be in fairly good condition, but the nurse must continue to observe him for evidence of cyanosis which may be precipitated by very minor disturbances. Occasionally cyanosis may even occur after several weeks of life. These episodes can be caused by such factors as exposure to cold, overfeeding, rapid feeding, abdominal distention, or fatigue. If cyanosis occurs while the baby is being fed, the feeding must be discontinued. Intermittent attacks of cyanosis, which should be considered serious, may be caused by congenital atelectasis, hyaline membrane disease, cerebral damage, heart disease, or infection, although the infection may not manifest itself by other signs. Continuous cyanosis is very serious and is a poor prognostic sign; it is probably due to extensive areas of atelectasis or hyaline membrane disease, severe cerebral damage, or serious heart disease.

## MAINTENANCE OF BODY TEMPERATURE

The premature baby has an unstable body temperature and is very susceptible to environmental conditions. His temperature tends to be subnormal and it is very easily lowered in a relatively cool environment because he has poor central nervous system control over his

* See Chapter 24, page 770, for a discussion of hyaline membrane disease.

heat-regulating mechanism; heat is readily lost due to a relatively large skin surface which allows for more radiation than that of the full-term infant's, and the premature has poor insulation because of a small amount of subcutaneous fat. Added to these factors are his inability to produce heat well because of his relative inactivity and his low-caloric intake during the first few days of life. On the other hand, he may develop hyperthermia if his environmental temperature is too high; this is due to the poor central nervous system control over heat regulation and because the sweat glands of a premature are poorly developed, making it difficult to lose heat by perspiration.

Keeping the body temperature of the premature baby constant until he has matured enough to maintain a stable, normal temperature in an environment normally provided for full-term infants is an essential part of the nursing care. Because he reacts so readily to environment it is, therefore, the nurse's duty to determine the best environmental temperature for the individual baby and to change it as his needs change, always remembering to keep his body temperature constant. It is impossible to know at birth what his environmental needs will be, and the nurse can decide this only by careful and frequent checking of his body temperature. She should remember that there will be a sudden change at birth from the carefully controlled intrauterine existence, and she must be prepared to conserve his body heat from the moment of birth. When a premature delivery is imminent, the delivery room should be warmed to a temperature close to 23.9° C (75° F), the incubator or a crib must be preheated, and a sterile warmed blanket made available to place on the delivery table in which to receive the baby as soon as he is born. He should be wrapped in the warm blanket immediately after delivery, even before the umbilical cord is cut. As soon as the cord is severed he can be placed on a table warmed with a heat lamp or in an incubator for further care. If resuscitation is necessary great care must be taken to keep him warm during this procedure. Tying the umbilical cord, eye treatment, and identification can all be done after he has been placed in the incubator. Some of these procedures, especially the eye treatment and identification, may even be postponed until the baby has been changed from the blanket which has become wet with amniotic fluid and blood into a clean dry blanket that has been preheated.

The weight of the baby should always be taken while he is wrapped in a blanket, which is later weighed or has previously been weighed, so that the weight of the blanket can be subtracted from the total weight. By this method an accurate birth weight can be obtained without chilling the infant, since even a few minutes of exposure will lower his temperature considerably.

In transporting the infant from the delivery room to the nursery, care must also be taken that he is kept warm. If possible, the incubator he will occupy should be taken to the delivery room to receive him; if this is not practical it is best to move him in another heated crib.

Even with the utmost care the baby's temperature is usually lowered to somewhere between 33.3° C (92° F) and 34.4° C (94° F), rectally, shortly after birth and it should gradually be raised to nearer a more normal level. During the first 24 hours after birth, or perhaps longer, the nurse must take the baby's body temperature every one to two hours either rectally or in the axilla, until she learns his ideal environmental temperature.* The incubator temperature must be adjusted as necessary (by raising or lowering the thermostat or turning electric heating units on or off) to keep the baby's temperature between 35.6° C (96° F) and 36.7° C (98° F) for the larger prematures and between 34.4° C (94° F) and 35.6° C (96° F) for the smaller ones. Many premature babies, especially the very immature, seem to progress better when the body temperature remains rather low for several days or longer. The body temperature should not vary more than 1.1° C (2.0° F) during any day. Both the body temperature and the crib temperature should be recorded each time they are read. If the baby's temperature is quite unstable and drops or rises more than desired, a gradual adjustment of the incubator temperature is necessary. The baby cannot tolerate sudden changes well, and a gradual, rather than sudden, raising or lowering of his body temperature is best. If the crib has been overheated he must be given very close attention while the temperature is being lowered because he may become very distressed from the heat. During hot weather it may be necessary to be more concerned with lowering the body temperature than with raising it after the initial adjustment in the period immediately after birth has been made. With the pre-

* Axillary readings, if taken properly by holding the thermometer in place and pressing the baby's arm gently but firmly against his chest for 1½ minutes, are satisfactory and preferable when the temperature must be taken often.

mature baby's tendency toward a subnormal temperature this is usually accomplished by reducing the incubator temperature or turning it off completely. It may, however, become necessary to remove some of his clothing.

It is obvious from what has been said that the temperature at which the incubator must be kept will be dependent entirely upon the baby's body temperature, but the following schedule may serve as somewhat of a guide: a weight of 1360 gm (3 lb) or less requires an incubator temperature of approximately 32.2° C (90° F); between 1360 gm (3 lb) and 1800 gm (4 lb) a temperature of 29.4° C (85° F); between 1800 gm (4 lb) and 2270 gm (5 lb) 26.7° C (80° F); and if the baby's weight is over 2270 gm (5 lb) an environmental temperature of 23.9° C (75° F) may be sufficient. With these temperatures the relative humidity should be increased to somewhere between 55 and 65 per cent; it should be at least 65 per cent for infants weighing under 1800 gm (4 lb).

The baby's temperature may fluctuate a great deal for two to three days and then gradually become more stable; the earlier it is stabilized the better the prognosis. Great fluctuations with an even environmental temperature indicate a great degree of immaturity. Hypothermia; hyperthermia, which may be accompanied by acidosis; and great fluctuations in temperature, either due to a great degree of immaturity or poor regulation of external heat, are very difficult for the baby to tolerate and may cause death.

As soon as the baby's temperature becomes quite stable, a check every three to four hours may be adequate. As he gets older and his temperature is less unstable he should gradually be changed to a normal nursery environment. He may still need extra clothing or need to be wrapped in an extra blanket after he is discharged to his home to supply additional warmth in a room which is perhaps not as warm as the nursery, but by this time he should be adjusted fairly well to living in a normal environment.

### HUMIDITY

From what has previously been said it is evident that the ideal relative humidity of the premature infant's environment, at least during the early days of life, is approximately 65 per cent. The humidity should be at least 65 per cent for infants receiving oxygen and for infants under 1800 gm (4 lb). Studies have shown that the baby's general progress and ability to maintain a stable body temperature are lessened when the humidity is 30 per cent or lower. An optimum humidity can only be maintained in an incubator in which the humidity can be increased and controlled or in an air-conditioned nursery. It is necessary for the nurse to keep careful check on the incubator humidifying device in order to maintain an adequate water level since this water evaporates rapidly when the humidity in the incubator is maintained at a high level. As the premature infant matures he can gradually be changed to an ordinary room environment.

If an air-conditioned nursery and/or an incubator with increased humidity are not available it is practically impossible to maintain a relatively high humidity when the nursery is heated in cold weather. If humidity pans have been placed next to radiators they should be filled regularly in order to keep the air as moist as possible.

### PREVENTION OF EXPOSURE AND FATIGUE

If the nurse will remember that two of her objectives as she gives the baby daily care are to prevent exposure and fatigue, she will know what she must do in regards to clothing, skin care, and the general handling of the infant.

**Clothing.** The blanket into which the baby has been received on the delivery table is usually damp with amniotic fluid and blood, and it is necessary to transfer him into a dry warmed blanket as soon as respirations are established and the umbilical cord is dressed. The eye treatment may even be done after this transfer has been made. It is at the time of this change of blanket that the weight can be obtained with a minimum of exposure. The baby may be weighed in the soiled blanket, which is weighed later, and its weight subtracted from the total weight.

The amount of clothing the baby will need will depend entirely upon the facilities available for his care. If he is placed in an incubator that does not need to be opened to give nursing care, the environmental temperature will remain constant and he will need no clothing other than a diaper. (This type of incubator makes close observation of his condition easy since his breathing and his color can readily be observed when he is not clothed.) If the baby is to be cared for in a bassinet or an incubator which must be opened for care he should be well clothed to keep him insulated and prevent loss of body heat. These clothes must be soft and lightweight and should be autoclaved to prevent infection. A fairly practical arrangement is to dress him in a shirt and a diaper, and to wrap him in a blanket. The diaper of necessity should be small and not too bulky, and if the baby is very small, pads of cotton placed against the genital region may be used instead of a diaper.

**Skin Care.** Skin care usually consists of the "dry" technic, described on pages 629–30. This care must be reduced to a minimum if the baby is very immature.

A daily weight may be obtained if the baby can be weighed without being removed from the incubator; some incubators make this provision. If the baby is in an incubator which must be opened for care he ordinarily has his clothes changed and his weight taken only every second or third day in order to prevent heat loss and exposure. The skin and umbilicus should, however, be inspected daily, but the shirt need not be removed for this inspection. On every second or third day he is taken out of the incubator, only long enough to be weighed. This weight should be taken while he has all of his clothes on; he is then put back in the crib to be changed. To have an accurate record of his weight the soiled clothes, which have been removed, are then weighed and their weight is subtracted from the total weight. Because of this infrequent change of clothing the baby's blanket should be well protected with an extra diaper or pad under his buttocks which can be changed whenever wet or soiled.

As the baby gets older, weighing between 2000 and 2270 gm (4½ and 5 lb), and as his temperature becomes stabilized, he may have his clothes changed daily. A change to the care of the normal newborn must be a gradual process and must depend entirely upon his progress. This change should, however, be complete a few days before his discharge from the hospital.

**Handling of the Baby.** The premature baby becomes exhausted very easily in the early days of life; to avoid undue handling his examinations, feedings, and treatments, as well as his general care, should be done without removing him from the incubator. An infant suspected of having intracranial injury must be handled just as infrequently as it is possible and with the utmost gentleness to prevent stimulation of bleeding. In these cases feedings may be withheld longer than usual.

To allow the baby to rest for fairly long intervals and to prevent frequent environmental temperature changes, several short procedures in his care should be performed at one time. For example, the temperature can be taken at the same time the diaper is changed. On the days his weight is to be taken, plans can be made to weigh him, change his clothes, and feed him in close succession. If, however, this much handling seems too exhausting or if it is necessary to do additional treatments, it is best to space them in such a manner that the baby does not become exhausted by a long period of manipulation. The nurse must observe each infant closely and use judgment in determining the frequency and the amount of handling he can tolerate without tiring.

**Position.** The premature infant must be kept on his side to prevent aspiration of formula in case regurgitation occurs. He should be changed from one side to the other each time that he is handled to protect the shape of his head, which is very easily molded. It is not safe to place him on his abdomen unless he is constantly observed because he is unable to pull his head off the anterior chest wall and turn it from side to side as the full-term infant is able to do. The premature baby is not placed on his abdomen to sleep except when he can be watched closely until he reaches a weight of 3175 to 3400 gm (7 to 7½ lb).

## NUTRITION

Feeding of the premature baby is made difficult by the lowered tolerance of the alimentary tract, the weakness or absence of the sucking and swallowing reflexes, the tendency to vomit and develop abdominal distention, and the incomplete development of the digestive enzyme system. The more immature the infant is, the more difficult the feeding problem. In addition, the baby must take and absorb large amounts of food because of his low antenatal storage and his need to grow rapidly.

**Beginning Feedings.** All fluid is withheld from the premature baby for at least the first 12 hours of life. The present tendency is to wait a longer period of time than formerly before the administration of fluids; some doctors even wait two to three days before they give feedings, especially with the less vigorous infant. If the baby is very small or appears to become dehydrated he can be given parenteral fluids during this period, care being taken not to administer large amounts of physiologic salt solution, which may cause edema. The larger infants can usually be fed safely at the age of 24 hours. This interval of rest before feedings are started gives the infant time to adjust to extrauterine life and gives him an opportunity to recover from respiratory difficulties that are easily increased with feedings. There is little danger of dehydration by withholding feedings because many premature babies have excess fluid in their tissues, water accounting for a larger part of their body weight than that of the full-term infant, but if dehydration does develop it can readily be overcome by the use of parenteral fluids.

**Meeting the Food and Fluid Requirements.** Proper food and fluid are of utmost importance in feeding the premature. In the calculation of the infant's milk mixture the total volume of fluid to be given and the caloric needs for the baby's age and size must be considered. Up to the fourth or fifth day the caloric intake is of little concern, but considerable attention must be given to supplying an adequate fluid intake; after this early period the concentration of the feeding can be increased to ensure an adequate caloric intake. By using half-strength breast milk or standard formula * to fulfill the fluid requirement, it is possible to supply some calories and to evaluate the infant's ability to handle food as well as fluid.

It is well to remember that although a full-term infant needs one-sixth of his body weight to cover his fluid requirements (2 to 3 oz per pound of body weight), he does not take this amount for the first four to six days of life. Similarly the premature infant will not be able to take one-sixth of his body weight, which is the ideal fluid intake for any infant, during the first few days.

To make certain that the baby is getting fluid in an adequate amount, but not in too large a quantity for him to tolerate, a schedule can be figured whereby he is given fluid equaling one-twentieth of his body weight on the second day, one-tenth to one-eleventh on the third day, and one-eighth on the fourth day. Then the total amount can be continued at one-eighth of his body weight with an increase in the strength of the formula each day to ensure an adequate caloric intake. By the tenth day he is usually ready to take one-sixth of his body weight in fluid. This means one-sixth of his actual body weight

* The term "standard formula" when used in this section means a formula which furnishes 20 calories per ounce.

in ounces on the day on which his requirements are calculated. His schedule is frequently planned in such a way that he is given approximately 4 ml at the first feeding, 6 ml at the second, 8 to 10 ml at the third, and increasing the amount by 2 ml every second or third feeding depending, of course, upon his ability to tolerate the amount offered. For the very small infant it may be necessary to make the initial feeding as low as 2 ml and to slowly increase the amount by 2 ml only every third or fourth feeding. The large premature infant may tolerate 6 to 8 or even 10 ml for an initial feeding, and the rate of increase can be quite rapid, even up to 4- or 5-ml increase per feeding. These feedings are ordinarily given on a three-hour day-and-night schedule, but sometimes feedings are given every two hours at the beginning, later at three-hour intervals, and still later at four-hour intervals. There are such great variations in premature infants in the tolerance of food, especially in the first few days of life, that all feeding schedules must be individualized.

Using the above figures for calculating a premature baby's food and fluid needs, the following example shows how a feeding schedule could be planned for a baby weighing about 1600 gm (3½ lb).

INFANT WHOSE BODY WEIGHT IS 3½ lb = 56 oz

| | FIRST DAY | SECOND DAY | THIRD DAY | FOURTH DAY | FIFTH DAY |
|---|---|---|---|---|---|
| 2 A.M. | 0 | 4 ml | 16 ml | 24 ml | 26 ml |
| 5 A.M. | 0 | 6 | 16 | 24 | 26 |
| 8 A.M. | 0 | 10 | 18 | 24 | 26 |
| 11 A.M. | 0 | 10 | 18 | 24 | 26 |
| 2 P.M. | 0 | 12 | 20 | 26 | 26 |
| 5 P.M. | 0 | 12 | 20 | 26 | 26 |
| 8 P.M. | 0 | 14 | 22 | 26 | 26 |
| 11 P.M. | 0 | 14 | 22 | 26 | 26 |
| Total | | 82 | 152 ml | 200 ml | 208 ml |
| | No food or fluid | 1/20 of 56 oz = 2.8 oz (84 ml) | 1/11 of 56 oz = 5 oz (150 ml) | 1/8 of 56 oz = 7 oz (210 ml) | 1/8 of 56 oz = 7 oz (210 ml) |

Second to fourth day—Breast milk or standard formula is diluted with equal parts of sterile water.
Fifth day—Dilution of breast milk or standard formula is changed to three-fourths milk and one-fourth water.
Sixth or seventh day—The caloric intake is increased by offering full-strength breast milk or standard formula. The total intake is continued at one-eighth of the body weight until the tenth day.
Tenth day—The amount of feeding offered is increased up to one-sixth of the body weight.

When a schedule such as this is set up for an infant the nurse adheres to it if the baby does not show distress by attacks of cyanosis, by regurgitation or vomiting, or by signs of abdominal distention. The nurse must always use her judgment in discontinuing a feeding before the entire amount is given or in omitting a feeding entirely if the baby has any signs of distress. Subsequent feedings are rescheduled after the physician has evaluated the infant's condition.

A small premature infant may be given a 5 per cent glucose in water solution on the first day of feeding. This infant will progress to half-strength breast milk or formula according to his ability to handle small amounts of fluid. When breast milk is being used it may be possible to give it full strength by the third or fourth day of feedings rather than on the fifth or sixth day. If the infant weighs more than 2000 gm (4½ lb) and appears robust, full-strength breast milk may be used. The heavier, robust premature can handle standard formula without dilution earlier than the less mature infant. Within two weeks the infant's ability to handle food will be understood, and his feeding schedule will be stabilized so that increases can be made daily or even at longer intervals.

At the age of 10 to 14 days the premature baby may need a caloric intake above the requirements of the full-term infant for satisfactory weight gain. Some doctors believe that 110 to 120 calories per kilogram of body weight (50 to 55 calories per pound)—which is the requirement of the full-term infant—are adequate; others recommend increasing the calories to between 120 and 130 per kilogram (55 to 60 calories per pound) for adequate weight gain; still others recommend that the caloric intake be increased to 135 to 140 calories per kilogram (62 to 64 calories per pound). To supply such a caloric intake it is necessary to feed the baby a quantity amounting to near one-fifth of his body weight, using either breast milk or a formula which furnishes 20 calories per ounce.

Each baby's feeding must, of course, be individualized to his tolerance. Because of the respiratory embarrassment to which the baby is subject with overfeeding and the tendency to abdominal distention and diarrhea, he is fed the minimum amount of food on which he can gain weight satisfactorily rather than the maximum amount that he wishes or can take.

**Formula.** The premature infant requires a diet high in protein, calcium, and phosphorus because of his low storage of these elements at birth and his needs for rapid growth. The baby born before full term is reached has a poor supply of calcium and phosphorus because one-fourth or more of the calcium and a somewhat lesser amount of the phosphorus are stored during the last eight weeks of intrauterine life. Protein requirements are higher than those of the full-term baby, and the daily intake recommended is 4.4 to 6.0 gm per kilogram of body weight for those babies weighing less than 2000 gm (4½ lb) and 4.4 to 5.0 gm per kilogram if the weight is over 2000 gm. Some doctors believe that cow's milk meets the special needs of the premature infant better than human milk because of its higher protein, calcium, and phosphorus content. The premature baby does not, however, metabolize the protein in cow's milk as well as the protein in breast milk unless an increased amount of vitamin C is added to aid in this metabolism.

The premature baby tends to have difficulty in fat absorption, and those who recommend the use of cow's milk believe that another of its advantages over human milk is the ease with which the fat content can be reduced by the use of skimmed milk. Carbohydrate is quite well tolerated, and when cow's milk is used for feeding sugar is added up to the content of human milk or even increased above this amount to compensate for the calories lost by the removal of fat.

While some doctors advocate the use of cow's milk in the feeding of premature babies, especially the very small ones, others believe that human milk is tolerated better and is still to be considered the ideal food for all infants. They believe that, if necessary, breast milk can be modified to meet the requirements of the premature by the addition of skimmed milk or calcium caseinate.

Another recommendation for feeding premature infants is the use of a skimmed cow's milk formula for the very small babies because they gain weight rapidly when fed this formula. It is felt by many that as the baby matures human milk is as satisfactory as cow's milk and that for this reason as well as for psychologic reasons the mother's lactation should be maintained so that the infant may eventually nurse at the breast.

Included among recommended feedings for premature infants then are: unmodified breast milk; breast milk fortified with protein in the form of skimmed milk, calcium caseinate, or other commercial protein preparations; a skimmed-milk formula which decreases the fat content; formulas made of proprietary preparations which have a lowered fat content and an increased protein, vitamin, and mineral content; or an evaporated-milk formula which is quite easily tolerated by most infants because of the small soft curds it forms.

**Minerals and Vitamins.** The baby fed on a modified cow's milk mixture does not require extra minerals because of the high-calcium and high-phosphorus content of cow's milk, but there is some evidence that supplements may be necessary when human milk is used. When calcium caseinate or skimmed milk is added to breast milk the protein, calcium, and phosphorus content of the feeding mixture is adequately increased. Calcium caseinate is particularly valuable as a supplement if the baby has a tendency toward loose stools.

The premature infant's need for vitamins is high because of low antenatal storage and the great demands made by rapid growth. Information as to the vitamin requirements of the premature is not complete, but the necessity of prophylactic administration is recognized. The baby will not obtain enough vitamins in his milk, and, therefore, the entire daily requirement is given in the form of supplements.

*Vitamins A and D.* Vitamin D deficiency is manifested by rickets and associated with tetany. Because of the importance of this vitamin in increasing calcium retention it should be started even earlier in the premature than in the full-term infant, and the minimum daily requirement is believed to be greater. The premature is highly susceptible to rickets, sometimes even when vitamin D is administered, and large doses are started at one week of age. It is recommended that 800 to 1000 I.U. of vitamin D be given daily and if any signs of rickets should appear that this dosage be increased up to 6000 I.U. per day. In the small, weak premature there is danger of aspiration of the fish liver oils, resulting in lipoid pneumonia. It is therefore considered advisable to use a concentrate of vitamins A and D in a preparation which is miscible in milk or water.

Vitamin A must also be supplemented early. Due to faulty fat absorption this vitamin may not be absorbed very efficiently, and if the baby is fed a formula with a reduced fat content the amount of this vitamin obtained from the milk is greatly decreased. Vitamin A is usually administered with vitamin D, and if the requirement for vitamin D is met the infant will receive an adequate amount of vitamin A also. Recommended dosage is 5000 to 10,000 I.U. daily. Absorption of vitamin A is greatly increased when it is given in a nonoil menstruum.

*Vitamin B.* The daily prophylactic requirement for vitamin B complex has not been established, but it is usually administered in combination with other vitamins. This group is not stored well in the body, and the amount of milk taken by the baby is probably too small to contain protective amounts.

*Vitamin C.* The feedings should always be supplemented with vitamin C even when human milk is used because the amount of milk taken is small; if it has been boiled, a process which destroys much of the vitamin, even less is obtained. When a high-protein formula is fed, the need for vitamin C is increased because of its importance in protein metabolism. The administration of vitamin C is begun during the first few days of life; the dosage is gradually increased over a few days until 50 to 100 mg are given daily. This vitamin is administered in the concentrated form, as ascorbic acid, mixed in milk or water, and given with the feedings.

*Vitamin K.* This vitamin is important in prothrombin formation and therefore in blood coagulation. It is administered at birth because the prothrombin value decreases in all infants during the first few days of life, thus increasing the blood clotting time. It is particularly valuable in the premature because of the tendency toward hemorrhage in these infants. Vitamin K is given intramuscularly in a dose of 1.0 to 2.4 mg soon after the baby is born and may be repeated once daily for several days if there is any evidence of hemorrhage or suspicion of intracranial injury. The physiologic drop in the prothrombin level of the blood during the first few days of life can be prevented by the administration of vitamin K.

**Method of Feeding.** Premature babies are fed by indwelling nasogastric tube, gavage, medicine dropper, Breck feeder (Fig. 195), or bottle depending upon their size and vitality, ability to suck, and tendency to cyanosis. The only safe way to feed a baby weighing 2000 gm (4½ lb) or less is to start with gavage; when it is ascertained that he can suck well a change can be made to a Breck feeder and finally to bottle feedings. If a baby is small he may need gavage

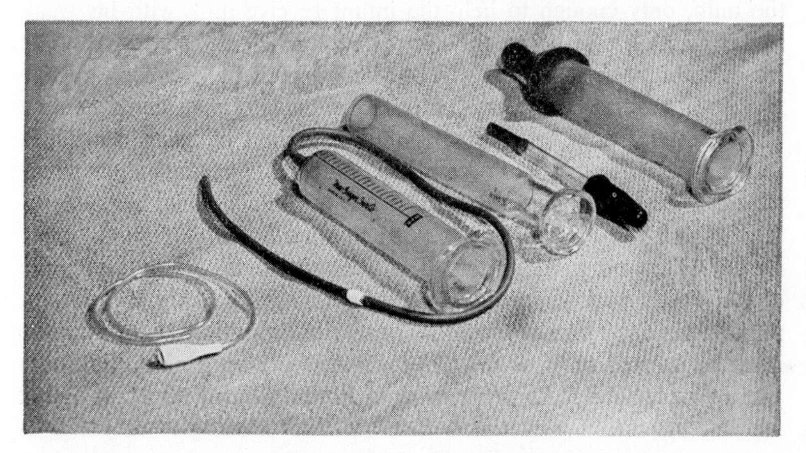

**Fig. 195.** Examples of equipment used for feeding premature infants. *From left to right:* Polyvinyl feeding tube No. 5 French, 37.5 cm (15 in.) long. A 20-ml syringe with a No. 8 or No. 10 French catheter. The catheter is marked for the distance of insertion for an individual infant.

A medicine dropper with a rubber tip.

The barrel of a 20-ml syringe with nipple attached—to be used as an open Breck feeder (without a rubber bulb).

feedings for a long period of time, this method being continued until he shows signs of sucking ability. It is believed that the baby's sucking and swallowing ability develop simultaneously and that he must, therefore, not be started on a Breck or medicine-dropper feeding until he shows signs of sucking well on the gavage tube. Putting milk into the infant's mouth, which he is unable to swallow, is a very dangerous procedure. An important observation for the nurse to make while feeding the baby is noting his ability to suck on the gavage tube. When he does this quite vigorously he is ready to be offered *Breck feedings,* at first only once a day to prevent tiring. As he becomes strong enough to take the Breck feeding well, one or two Breck feedings can be added each day until he is completely changed over to this method. Some doctors object to the use of a Breck feeder because of the danger of forcing food into the baby's mouth. There is, however, no danger if the Breck feeder is used skillfully and started only after the baby shows that he has the ability to suck and swallow.

In using the Breck feeder, the nurse applies gentle pressure on the bulb, only enough to help the infant receive milk with his weak sucking action and never enough to force milk into his mouth. The infant's ability to suck well will be strengthened by practice, and the nurse will regulate the flow of milk to see that it comes easily enough to prevent fatigue. Another satisfactory method of using the Breck feeder is to leave the bulb off entirely, allowing the baby to suck from it just as he would from a bottle. It has advantages over bottle feedings in that the baby does not need to suck as hard from the open feeder where no partial vacuum is created as there may be in the closed bottle and where atmospheric pressure can help the flow of milk as the baby sucks. When the rubber bulb is used, slight pressure must be exerted on it or the baby will be working against a vacuum just as he would if he were using a bottle. During the first Breck feeding the infant may tire before the total feeding is taken. It is not wise to finish the feeding by gavage at this time because he may regurgitate as the tube is inserted. The feeding is halted when fatigue is observed, and the next feeding is given by gavage.

Those who object to a Breck feeder prefer the use of a specially prepared *medicine dropper*. A ¾-in. piece of rubber tubing is attached firmly to the end of a dropper so that it extends ¼ in. beyond the glass tip to prevent injury to the mouth. The tip of the dropper is placed well back on the infant's tongue. As the milk is released it should be directed toward the side of the mouth and pressure should be exerted on the back of the tongue with the dropper tip to stimulate swallowing. This method, if used too early, is as dangerous as the Breck feeder because it may deliver fluid to the back of the baby's mouth which he is unable to swallow. The mouth must be inspected after each dropperful of milk is given to make certain that the milk has been swallowed. The medicine-dropper technic is frequently unsatisfactory; by the time it can be employed safely the quantity of feeding may be so large that it is a slow and tiring method.

The usual procedure then is to feed all premature babies weighing below 2000 to 2270 gm (4½ to 5 lb) by indwelling nasogastric tube or by gavage until they show ability to suck well and then gradually replacing one or two gavage feedings with Breck or medicine-dropper feedings each day as the baby can tolerate them without tiring. After all feedings are given by one of these methods, a gradual change is made to a bottle.

If the baby weighs around 2270 gm (5 lb) at birth and appears vigorous, a nipple may be placed in his mouth to determine his sucking ability. If he can suck vigorously he may be fed by a Breck feeder or medicine dropper from the beginning and changed to bottle feedings more quickly. A premature baby should not be breast-fed for the first few days of life even when he appears very robust because breast feeding always requires considerable effort from the small young baby.

If the mother has an adequate supply of breast milk (which has been maintained by pumping her breasts), when the premature infant reaches a weight of 2270 gm (5 lb), and if he can suck vigorously he may be allowed to nurse. One or two bottle feedings may be replaced with breast feedings each day. At first the time allowed at the breast should be limited to five minutes for each feeding to prevent tiring the baby. Nursing gives the mother an opportunity to handle her baby and become better acquainted with him since she has been deprived of this opportunity earlier by his specialized care. If she does not have breast milk she should be encouraged at this time to visit him daily and to give him his bottle feeding once a day.

To avoid undue exposure the baby must at first be left in his crib for his feedings, but the upper part of his body should be raised and supported in a semiupright position while he is fed. This position is maintained by elevating the head of the incubator mattress, if it is adjustable, to approximately a 30-deg angle, or by support to the head and shoulders with the nurse's hand. When the baby is strong enough to maintain his temperature well he should be wrapped in an extra blanket and held during his feedings. With feedings by all methods except gavage the baby should be bubbled midway in the feeding and again at the end of the feeding. Bubbling may not be necessary when the very weak baby, unable to suck, is fed by gavage, but should always be done at the end of a feeding as soon as he begins to suck on the tube, at which time he will swallow air. The baby who is not being removed from the incubator for feedings may be bubbled by being held in a sitting position while he is supported with the nurse's hands. To prevent regurgitation, and possibly aspiration, of milk following a feeding the nurse must handle the baby very gently and place him on his side after feedings. The right side is preferred since in this position the cardiac opening of the stomach is up. This position allows further air bubbles in the stomach to rise upward and helps to prevent regurgitation. If the baby is placed on his right side after each feeding he should be turned to the left side midway between feeding times to ensure adequate change of position. If the head of the bassinet has been raised it is advisable to allow it to remain elevated at approximately a 30-deg angle for 30 minutes after feedings, as a further safeguard against regurgitation.

*Gavage Feeding.* A gavage feeding is given through a catheter passed into the esophagus to just above the cardiac end of the stomach. Formula is poured through the glass barrel of a syringe which is attached to the catheter. The size of the catheter is somewhat determined by the size of the infant. For the very small baby a No. 8 French catheter is best, while for the baby weighing approximately 1500 gm (3¼ lb) a No. 10 catheter is more satisfactory. The distance to which the catheter should be passed is also determined by the size of the infant; each baby should, therefore, have its individual catheter. The distance from the bridge of the baby's nose to the tip of the ensiform cartilage of the sternum is measured, and the catheter is marked at this point with a narrow strip of adhesive tape (Fig. 196). When the catheter is boiled the adhesive tape comes loose, but it leaves a mark and is therefore satisfactory. Two more marks may be made 2 and 4 cm (.8 to 1.6 in.) above the first one for further guidance in passing the catheter.

To prepare for the feeding the catheter, after it has been measured, and the glass barrel of a syringe are sterilized, and the breast milk or formula is warmed. The baby is prepared for his feeding by changing his diaper so that he will be comfortable, and, to avoid handling after feeding, his temperature is taken if it should be checked at this time. If he has gastric distention he may be supported in a sitting position for a moment, and an attempt made to raise the air bubble. He is then placed on his back on a flat surface with his head in a straight line and on a level with his body, and the catheter is passed through the mouth into the esophagus until the first mark is even with the baby's lips (Fig. 197). The catheter is usually passed without difficulty because it does not enter the larynx and there is little or no gagging or retching because of weakness or absence of reflexes. If the catheter does not enter the esophagus it will turn upon itself and come out of the mouth. A lubricant should not be used on the catheter because oil may drop into the pharynx.

When the catheter is passed to the first mark it is just above the

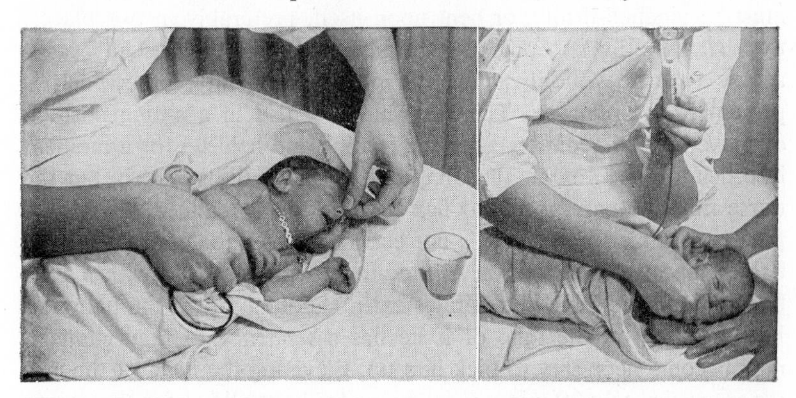

**Fig. 196 (left).** Measuring the distance from the bridge of nose to the tip of the ensiform cartilage in order to determine the exact length of gavage tube to be inserted. The gavage tube is marked at this time.

**Fig. 197 (right).** The tube, with the mark at the infant's lips, is held between the nurse's thumb and forefinger while her other fingers are in firm contact with the infant's chin. This assures the nurse that the tube will remain in the same position in the esophagus throughout the feeding. If the infant is active, it is advisable for a second person to hold the infant's hands and head.

cardiac opening of the stomach and is in the best position for the feeding. At this distance it does not stimulate the reflex at the cardiac opening and does not irritate the gastric mucosa. If gastric distention is present, which could not be relieved by bubbling the baby before the catheter was passed, it becomes necessary to insert the catheter to the second or third mark so that it enters the stomach and allows the gas to escape. As soon as the stomach is entered the gas can be heard coming through the tube. The catheter may be left in the stomach for the feeding or may be pulled out to the first mark on the tube so that its eye again rests in the esophagus.

After the catheter has been inserted the nurse should wait a few moments to assure herself that it is not causing the baby distress. Then an accurately measured amount of the feeding is poured into the glass barrel of the syringe, which has been attached to the catheter, and the barrel is elevated to a level at which the formula will flow freely, but not rapidly. The time required for all of the feeding to be given is ordinarily from three to five minutes.

Proper withdrawal of the catheter is very important. The tube must be pinched firmly, or bent upon itself, preferably in two places, to prevent spilling of milk into the pharynx. The baby usually gasps as the tube is withdrawn and he may aspirate any food which is present in the pharynx. The baby may be held in a sitting position or picked up immediately after the feeding and held up for a moment in order to raise any air that may be present in the stomach, but the nurse must be careful not to flex his body in a manner which puts pressure on his stomach. It is not customary to bubble all premature babies, because they get very little air into the stomach with a tube feeding, and bubbling necessitates extra handling, but if the baby has been sucking on the tube or if he has a tendency to regurgitate, it may become necessary to pick him up. Elevating the head of the crib for approximately 30 minutes following feedings allows for the escape of an air bubble. The baby is gently placed on his side after feedings, preferably the right side, and changed to the left side midway between feedings.

*Indwelling Nasogastric Tube Feeding.* This is a gavage feeding in which a plastic tube is passed through the nostril into the stomach and left in place from one feeding to another (Fig. 191B). This method is often considered preferable to the method in which a tube is introduced into the esophagus at each feeding time since the very small baby can be fed frequently without the trauma and the fatigue that may accompany frequent insertion of a gastric tube. With this method nurses are relieved of the responsibility of inserting a tube each time a feeding is done. Complications which may be encountered are a purulent rhinitis due to irritation from the tube and possibly some irritation of the esophagus or gastric mucosa.

A polyethylene tube of approximately 30 cm (12 in.) length and 0.965 mm outside diameter has commonly been used for this procedure. Recently a polyvinyl-type plastic tube, No. 5 French, has been recommended on the basis of this material being softer and more pliable, and thus lessening the danger of trauma to the mucous membrane during its passage into the stomach. The end of a polyethylene tube is rather sharp and rough, and several methods for blunting the tip have been advocated. The gastric end of the polyvinyl tube is closed and smooth, with openings along the side near the end; therefore, it does not present much of a problem of irritation from the tip.

Before the tube is inserted it is measured and marked with a small piece of adhesive tape at the approximate distance at which it will enter the stomach. The doctor inserts the tube through the nostril until the marker is reached. To make certain that the catheter has not entered the trachea a stethoscope may be placed over the region of the stomach while a small amount of air is injected into the tube with a syringe; this air can be heard to bubble in the stomach. If the tube has entered the trachea the baby is apt to show signs of respiratory distress. The tube is secured to the baby's face with adhesive tape; it is necessary to secure it quite firmly since the baby may hook his fingers around the tube and pull it out. If the skin of the face shows signs of irritation from the adhesive tape it may be protected with an application of tincture of benzoin.

The baby is placed on his right side before the feeding is begun, and the head of the mattress, if it is adjustable, is elevated to approximately a 30-deg angle. The desired amount of feeding is *slowly* injected through the nasal tube with a 20-ml syringe. The syringe is attached to an adaptor on the end of the nasal tube; if there is no adaptor a No. 22- or 20-gauge needle is attached to the syringe and inserted into the tube. After the feeding has been introduced, 1 to 2 ml of sterile water are injected to clear the tube of milk. The tube may be kept closed between feedings with a small clamp or with a rounded toothpick inserted into the end of the tube, or it may be left open between feedings to allow for escape of air from the stomach. To prevent spillage of milk through the tube it is necessary to keep the open end of the tube raised above the level of the baby for approximately one-half hour after each feeding; this is done by placing the open end on a folded towel, and it must even then be closely observed. If the tube is kept clamped between feedings, it should be opened for a few minutes before each feeding is given; this allows for escape of air, which may be present in the stomach, before the feeding is introduced.

The nasogastric tube is changed every three to four days, with the new tube being introduced into the opposite nostril. The baby may be given a rest without a tube for two to three hours if it is removed immediately after one feeding and reinserted just before the next feeding on the day on which it is to be changed.

## PSYCHOLOGIC CARE

The premature baby, because of his physiologic handicaps, cannot be given the same consideration of his emotional needs during his early days of life that the full-term infant receives. He is isolated in his incubator, must remain in the hospital a long period of time, and cannot demonstrate a demand for food as the full-term baby can. The special care he must be given deprives him of being held, of rooming-in with his mother, of breast feeding, and self-demand schedule, but as soon as his condition warrants he may be placed in a regular bassinet and be held by the nurse for his feedings. It may also be possible to allow him to have a self-demand feeding schedule when he is old enough to indicate his needs.

The later emotional life of the baby is greatly dependent upon the reactions of the mother. Separation from her baby gives her anxiety over his condition. Being unable to hold him, unable to nurse him for several weeks, if at all, seeing him in the incubator receiving special care, and leaving him in the hospital when she goes home—all add to giving her a feeling of inadequacy. To overcome some of the effects of the enforced separation from her baby, the mother should be allowed to see him as soon after birth as this can be arranged by permitting her to observe him through the nursery window. She should be given the opportunity to observe his care often during her hospital stay (Fig. 184). Before she goes home she should have a demonstration in the care of the full-term infant and be assured that she can handle her baby as a normal baby when he is ready to go home. The mother's breasts may be pumped to stimulate and maintain her milk supply so that she will be able to nurse the baby when he becomes strong enough. Arrangements can ordinarily be made for her to pump her breasts at home. She can send the milk to the hospital for the baby's use. She should be encouraged to visit the baby frequently after she leaves the hospital and allowed to hold him when he is strong enough, feed him as soon as she can safely do so, and bathe him before he leaves the hospital so that she will have confidence in the care she gives him at home. Both parents often come for observation and learning experience.

## PREVENTION OF INFECTION

After the baby has survived the first two or three days of life he may succumb to infection unless he is very carefully protected. The immaturity of the baby's organs and a deficiency of immune substances give him a high susceptibility to disease and a very low resistance. Birth has taken place before protective antibodies are transferred from the mother to the baby, and his capacity to produce immune substances is impaired.

Precautions which are important in any nursery, discussed in Chapter 22, must be strictly observed. Traffic in and out of the nursery should be reduced to a minimum, being limited to the personnel actually caring for these infants. Small nurseries make the observation of these precautions easier. Ideally, premature babies are kept in a nursery especially designed for their care, and each baby is isolated in his unit, but where this is not possible he must be protected in the regular newborn nursery. It is important that the personnel be free of any type of upper respiratory tract infection, skin infection, and gastrointestinal symptoms and that persons caring for premature babies have not recently taken care of an infectious patient. Any member of the staff who has had an infection must be excluded from the nursery until several days have elapsed after signs of infection disappear. A gown, and often a mask, should be worn in the nursery. Individual technic for each baby with thorough hand washing between the handling of each infant is essential. When babies are admitted that have been born outside of the hospital they should be carefully isolated until it is ascertained that they are free of infection.

Upper respiratory tract infections are common in the premature, and every precaution possible should be taken to prevent contamination by contact or by aspiration of food. The immaturity of the lungs, the presence of asphyxia, and the low neonatal immunity all contribute to the baby's susceptibility to respiratory infections.

The skin is another highly susceptible area. It is thin and easily traumatized; even a slight break allows organisms to enter and produce infection. Trauma and unnecessary handling can be reduced by the omission of baths and oiling. The skin must be inspected for lesions daily, but only the face and buttocks are washed or oiled, leaving all other areas dry. This method of care has the added advantage of minimizing exposure and temperature change. The autoclaving of all clothing and supplies taken into the nursery also affords protection against skin diseases.

Epidemic diarrhea, an acute condition characterized by loose watery stools, vomiting, weight loss, and listlessness, which has a high mortality rate in the normal newborn, is particularly fatal to the premature and must therefore be carefully guarded against.

Clinical manifestations of infection are variable; they may have an abrupt onset with fever and constitutional signs or be so minimal that they are easily missed unless everyone caring for the baby is very alert to all minor changes in his condition. The nurse must be observant of an increase in the respiratory rate or more frequent attacks of cyanosis, which may be the only signs of an infection located anywhere in the body. The respiratory system of the premature is always easily disturbed, but such a disturbance becomes more pronounced when an infection is present, and death may occur with no apparent signs or symptoms other than a change in respirations.

## COMMON PHYSIOLOGIC DISTURBANCES

**Anemia.** Soon after birth all newborn infants develop a neonatal physiologic anemia from which they recover spontaneously. There are some immature cells present in the blood of the infant at birth, more in the premature than in the full-term baby, and the erythrocyte count and the hemoglobin level are high. A physiologic decrease takes place with a gradual reduction in erythrocytes and hemoglobin. A low level is reached by the eighth to twelfth week of life after which there is a rise until a normal level is attained at seven to eight months of age. This is a normal process for all infants, but is more pronounced and more persistent in the premature, especially in the very small baby. This destruction of red blood cells produces bilirubinemia, which causes the physiologic jaundice seen early in life. Recovery from neonatal anemia is spontaneous, but if the erythrocyte count and hemoglobin level become quite low, treatment may improve the baby's general condition, hasten his progress, and give protection against infection. Iron administered during the neonatal period does not prevent this anemia of prematurity. Its severity may be decreased by a delay in severing the umbilical cord at the time of birth until pulsation has ceased, thereby giving the baby a higher erythrocyte and hemoglobin level to begin with, which may keep it from becoming too low. Administration of properly typed and crossmatched blood, 10 ml per pound of body weight, is often considered the best treatment; one transfusion is usually sufficient, but two or three may occasionally be necessary.

In the second or third month the premature develops an iron deficiency anemia which is associated with the immaturity of the hematopoietic system, low storage of iron before birth, rapid growth, and poor absorption and utilization of iron. An illness will increase the degree of anemia. Although iron does not prevent the neonatal type of anemia, the iron deficiency type can be prevented or modified by prophylactic administration of iron. Iron may be started in six to eight weeks after birth or even at four weeks of age if the baby can tolerate it, in the hope that he can store it for later use. Its administration is not delayed beyond the age of three months.

Although anemia must be diagnosed by an examination of the blood, the nurse should note any pallor of the skin and mucous membranes as she makes her daily observations and report these to the doctor. When the baby is receiving iron she should watch for signs of intolerance; gastrointestinal upsets and diarrhea occur most commonly.

**Acidosis.** Premature babies tend to have an acidosis in early life which is physiologic and from which recovery is spontaneous; in the later neonatal period acidosis may be associated with infection, especially diarrhea, and improper feedings. To prevent this condition the infant should be observed carefully for signs of dehydration, edema, or infection, and treatment should be instituted early. The nurse must watch the baby carefully for any signs which may indicate the presence of acidosis. A premature baby does not show the continuous rapid breathing seen in adults or older children with this condition; he may have some hyperpnea, but this change cannot be relied upon. She must, therefore, watch and report to the doctor other signs associated with this metabolic disturbance, such as a change in the ability to suck, failure to gain weight, evidence of dehydration or edema, an anxious expression, signs of fatigue, sluggishness, or restlessness. Laboratory findings of a reduced carbon dioxide combining power of the blood plasma confirm the diagnosis.

Acidosis, especially when associated with diarrhea, requires very careful and individualized treatment. For its correction 1/6 molar sodium lactate solution is used parenterally; glucose solution is given to provide calories, and blood transfusions are used to sustain the red cell and plasma volume. In the presence of dehydration, water and electrolytes must be replaced and the needs for daily maintenance provided. Great care is taken, however, to keep the salt intake at a minimum because too much physiologic salt solution can easily produce edema, a condition which may occur spontaneously during the neonatal period. Acidosis may recur after it has been corrected, and close observation of the infant must be continued.

**Edema.** Edema may occur spontaneously in the early neonatal period, probably due to some metabolic disturbance which is associated with a relatively high water content of the body and the inability of the kidneys to excrete salt easily. If it becomes necessary to give parenteral fluids to the infant, the amount of physiologic salt solution used must be carefully regulated and kept at a minimum to avoid exaggerating any tendency toward edema. Since these babies have excess water in their tissues at birth they are seldom given fluids during the first 24 hours of life. Sometimes fluids may be withheld for two to three days without evidence of dehydration. Withholding oral fluids for the first one to three days of life gives the baby time to recover from respiratory disturbances and to adjust to extrauterine existence before he has the added exertion that the feedings entail.

**Rickets.** Rickets tends to develop earlier, to progress to a more severe stage, and to be more difficult to prevent in the premature baby than in the full-term infant. This is due to many factors, among which are low antenatal storage of calcium, rapid growth, which increases the calcium requirement, inefficient utilization of calcium and phosphorus from food, and poor fat absorption which affects absorption of vitamin D. Clinical signs are insidious in onset and may not appear for three to four months. *Craniotabes* is frequently the first sign of the disease. Because of this special susceptibility, antirachitic treatment is usually started in the first week of life by the administration of vitamin D in adequate doses in a safe, absorbable form. The premature baby has a tendency to develop rickets even with the administration of vitamin D, and if any evidence of the disease appears it becomes necessary to increase the dosage above the prophylactic amount.

**Retrolental Fibroplasia.** Retrolental fibroplasia is a disease of the premature characterized by a deposition of fibrous tissue behind the lens of the eye which produces a severe loss of vision or complete blindness. This disease is most apt to develop in the baby that weighs 1800 gm (4 lb) or less at birth. The greater the prematurity, the higher the incidence. It is the leading cause of blindness in children today.

The disease is not present at birth. At about four weeks of age the retinal vessels dilate and become engorged and tortuous, the retina becomes edematous, and bands arise from areas of proliferative retinitis and extend into the vitreous; this is followed by retinal detachment. A retrolental membrane then forms by fusion of the vitreous bands and folds of detached retina; this appears as an opaque tissue or grayish membrane behind the lens. The disease produces destructive lesions in the eye; the growth of the eye is arrested, the cornea remains small, the anterior chamber is shallow, and adhesions form between the iris and the lens and between the iris and the cornea. All vision, and usually light perception, is lost. The membrane is ordinarily complete by the age of four months, and the reaction becomes inactive. Occasionally development is arrested when only a partial membrane is formed, allowing for partial vision. Both eyes are ordinarily affected, but the membrane may be complete in one eye and partial in the other.

Since this comparatively new disease of premature infants (first reported in 1942 and now apparently decreasing) has been studied, many efforts have been made to determine its cause and method of prevention. The most recent of these studies have shown that there is apparently a relationship between irreversible changes in the eye and the administration of oxygen for a prolonged period of time and in a high concentration. It is now believed by many that retrolental fibroplasia can be almost entirely eliminated by the controlled use of oxygen. This means that oxygen should be used only when indicated by clinical evidence of need, for the shortest period of time possible, and in a concentration below 40 per cent.

## THE NURSE'S DAILY RECORD

Daily observations which the nurse should make and record have been discussed in detail previously, but are briefly summarized here.

Observation of the functioning of the respiratory system should include a record of the respiratory rate at one- to two-hour intervals at first, and a record of any change in the character of respirations, and of cyanosis. The temperature must be recorded hourly at first, with a change to every three hours and finally twice daily as the baby matures. The skin should be observed each time the baby is given care—feedings, change of diaper, change of position—for signs of infection, for degree of jaundice, or evidence of pallor. Muscular twitchings or convulsions may indicate intracranial injury, infection, hypoxemia, tetany, or gastrointestinal disturbance. Close observation should be made of any change of respiratory rate, fever, diarrhea, or other signs of infection. An anxious expression, fatigue, dehydration, or change in ability to suck may indicate acidosis. A record of the way in which the baby takes his feedings, how and when he sucks, his hunger or satisfaction after feedings, any vomiting or abdominal distention, and the character of the stools all help the doctor decide when to change the amount or strength of formula and the method of feeding. All of these observations are so important that the value of having a well-qualified nurse present in the nursery at all times is quite apparent.

## FUTURE DEVELOPMENT

Average development, both mental and physical, can be expected of the premature baby if his development at birth is normal for his intrauterine age and if he has no congenital abnormalities or has not had certain neonatal complications which may leave a permanent effect in any infant. Some allowance must be made, however, for delay in development during the first few years of life. The premature baby is somewhat retarded in growth, both weight and length, during the first two to five years of age, and the smaller the weight at birth the greater the delay; but given good care he will develop at the same rate as the full-term infant after approximately four years of age. Prematurity in itself does not affect mental development, especially if the time of conception rather than the date of birth is used in calculating the baby's age.

## DISCHARGE FROM THE HOSPITAL

The premature baby is usually ready for discharge from the hospital at a weight of 2270 to 2500 gm (5 to 5½ lb). This depends largely upon the baby's vitality, the intelligence and cooperation of the parents, and the physical condition of the home. The baby must be able to maintain his temperature in an average environment and be able to eat well from a bottle or the breast. He usually attains an adequate weight and stage of development for discharge from the hospital at approximately the time he was due to be born. To determine his physical status a complete examination should again be done and a complete blood count obtained before he is sent home.

Before the baby leaves the hospital the mother must learn to feed, bathe, and care for him and be encouraged to handle him as a normal child. If her lactation has been maintained the infant should be taught to nurse. It is important to learn the social, economic, and physical status of the family and to have a public health nurse visit the home to check on housing arrangements, illness in the family, or any other condition which would be hazardous to the baby, and to help the parents make final arrangements for his care. She must know if the parents are physically and financially able to care for him. It is a good plan to provide the public health nurse with specific recommendations for the individual baby. She should arrange to visit the home the day after discharge to assist the mother with the actual care of the baby and as often thereafter as the mother needs help. Specific plans for follow-up supervision of the baby by a physician and a public health agency are important.

## GENERAL CONSIDERATIONS

It is a well-recognized fact that the premature infant's chances of life are greatly increased by good hospital care. Since the first 24 hours are especially hazardous, careful plans must be made for handling the baby expertly at birth. The delivery room and nursery should, of course, always be ready for emergency care with equipment for resuscitation and the conservation of body heat, but when a patient is known to be in premature labor it is possible to make additional plans and thereby avoid loss of time in instituting prompt treatment. The pediatrician and nursery staff should be notified of the impending birth, and plans can be made for extra personnel in the delivery room to give special attention to the baby. The nurse can be of great assistance in giving the infant proper care by heating an incubator in advance, by checking that adequate oxygen and resuscitation equipment is available, and by having all supplies in readiness to care for the baby quickly, thereby taking a minimum amount of time to get him into an ideal environment. This infant may need the undivided attention of a doctor and a nurse in the delivery room and constant observation after he is moved into the nursery.

A separate nursery with a temperature maintained between 23.9° to 26.7° C (75° and 80° F) and air-conditioned if possible should be provided unless fewer than four premature babies are cared for at any one time, as in a small maternity department. In these hospitals, space must be made available in the newborn nursery with the provision of incubators for premature babies. Separate nurseries should always be provided for babies born outside of the hospital and for those suspected of having an infection.

The American Academy of Pediatrics recommends that every premature baby should be under the continuous care of a qualified pediatrician and that the nursing staff be under the supervision of a graduate nurse who has had postgraduate training or satisfactory clinical experience in the care of premature infants. Auxiliary workers in the premature nursery must be selected with great care and must demonstrate ability to understand aseptic technic and a willingness to follow instructions explicitly. Their duties should be limited to care that is not highly specialized. The nurse should care for the small prematures and those with complications; the auxiliary worker may assist with the care given the larger infants.

Five to six hours of nursing care for a 24-hour period is the average requirement for a premature baby. This means that one nurse must be on duty at all times for every four to five infants. If the baby is cared for in the regular newborn nursery, added personnel must be provided with the admission of a premature baby. To give expert care and make necessary observations it is important for a graduate nurse with special training to be present in the nursery at all times.

Improvements can be made in the care given premature infants by arranging periodic conferences of the medical, nursing, public health, and social service personnel in order to discuss policies and procedures.

Premature babies born outside of the hospital have less chance of survival, but many of these can be saved by making provisions for transfer to a premature center as quickly as possible. If facilities are not adequate to care for the premature baby where he is born, which may be either in the home or in the hospital, it is important to meet the immediate needs of the baby—to establish respirations and apply external heat—and then make arrangements for transfer to an institution where adequate equipment and qualified personnel are available. It was once considered difficult to move these babies to better facilities, but this is being done very satisfactorily in some cities at the present time. Transportation must be made in an ambulance equipped with a heated incubator, oxygen, and suction apparatus and staffed with a nurse trained in the care of premature infants.

## COMMUNITY RESPONSIBILITY

Premature care is a public health problem. The Children's Bureau has encouraged state health departments to set up plans for the care of the premature. Practically all states have some such plan. Their programs range from those on a small scale which lend incubators where necessary or train a few nurses in the special care of the premature to large state-wide programs which give complete care. This may include provision for special training of doctors and nurses, development of hospital standards, provision of medical and nursing consultation service, loan of incubators, transportation of prematures to hospitals, establishment of premature centers, and payment of hospital care. Saving lives means making increased efforts to prevent premature births, spreading knowledge of and making facilities available for the special care needed by these infants, and continuing research in regard to the problems of prematurity. Much emphasis is being placed on the prevention of maternal complications and on provision of expert care during pregnancy and labor, especially where complications exist. These programs should be administered by a health-department unit which is closely related to the maternity care section and should include home follow-up care. Most of these programs are assisted by grant-in-aid funds under the Social Security Act.

Public and private welfare agencies and nursing organizations may be called upon to assist the parents in preparation for the baby and in follow-up care. These parents frequently need considerable help from the public health nurse and in some cases from a medical social worker. The family may be overwhelmed by the responsibility of a small baby and unduly anxious over its future. They frequently worry about the details of his special care and over his physical and emotional development. Added to this is concern over finances because of the long period of hospitalization. The medical social worker can evaluate the emotional and social problems that arise with the birth of a premature infant. By her contacts with the family she learns their relationship to one another and their attitude toward the baby. Help in understanding that this infant can be handled as a normal child and avoidance of an overly protective attitude are especially important when there are other children in the family. Jealousy over the new baby can be minimized by treating him casually in the presence of his brothers and sisters.

Information obtained by the public health nurse and the medical social worker regarding the financial and physical setup of the home will help the doctor decide upon the best time for discharging the baby from the hospital. By their contact with the family in well-baby clinics and in home follow-up care they can guide the family in the proper utilization of help from community agencies. Their interpretation to these agencies of the home situation will be very valuable in determining the best method of providing the necessary aid. The care of the premature baby is expensive due to the long hospitalization period, and it is often necessary to assist the family through state and local funds when they are unable to pay for all of the baby's care.

## BIBLIOGRAPHY AND STUDENT REFERENCES

Allen, Elaine: "The Premature Is an Individual," *J. Am. M. Women's A.*, **8**: 327–30, (Oct.) 1953.

American Academy of Pediatrics: *Standards and Recommendations for Hospital Care of Newborn Infants—Full-term and Premature.* The Academy, Evanston, Ill., 1954.

Blake, Florence G.: *The Child, His Parents and the Nurse.* J. B. Lippincott Co., Philadelphia, 1954.

Clarke, Erma E.: "The Premature Infant Goes Home," *Am. J. Nursing,* **52**:882, (July) 1952.

Cohig, Ruth, and Mason, Helen: "Medical Social Work and the Premature Baby," *The Child,* **14**:157–58, (Apr.) 1950.

Dancis, Joseph, and Cardullo, Hugo: "Incubator Care of the Premature Infant," *Pediatrics,* **6**:432–40, (Sept.) 1950.

Denton, Robert: "Continuous Nebulization Therapy: A Technique for the Treatment of Abnormal Respiration in the Newborn Premature Infant," *Pediat. Clin. North America,* **1**:625–38, (Aug.) 1954.

Dimaggio, Gellestrina, and Gelinas, Marguerite: "Parents Learn about Their Premature Baby," *The Child,* **17**:106–8, (Mar.) 1953.

Dunham, Ethel: *Premature Infants,* 2nd ed. Paul B. Hoeber, Inc., New York, 1955.

Gesell, Arnold: "Behavior Aspects of the Care of the Premature Infant," *J. Pediat.,* **29**:210–12, (Aug.) 1946.

Gordon, Harry: "Feeding of Premature Infants," *Am. J. Dis. Child.,* **73**:713–18, (June) 1947.

Green, Doris M.: "Caring for the Premature Baby," *Am. J. Nursing,* **50**:458–59, (Aug.) 1950.

Greene, Doris M., and Zetzsche, Louise: "Premies Are Human Beings Too!" *Pub. Health Nursing,* **44**:253–55, (May) 1952.

Guy, Loren P.; Lanman, Jonathan T.; and Dancis, Joseph: "The Possibility of Total Elimination of Retrolental Fibroplasia by Oxygen Restriction," *Pediatrics,* **17**:247–49, (Feb.) 1956.

Hess, Julius H.: "Prevention and Control of Infections," *Am. J. Dis. Child.,* **73**:696–705, (June) 1947.

———: "The Premature Infant," in McQuarrie, Irvine (ed.): *Brennemann's Practice of Pediatrics,* Vol. I. W. F. Prior Co., Inc., Hagerstown, Md., 1948, Chap. 43.

Hess, Julius H., and Lundeen, Evelyn: *The Premature Infant,* 2nd ed. J. B. Lippincott Co., Philadelphia, 1949.

Jeans, Philip C.; Wright, F. Howell; and Blake, Florence G.: *Essentials of Pediatrics,* 5th ed. J. B. Lippincott Co., Philadelphia, 1954.

Koenig, Hedweg: "What Happens to Prematures," *Am. J. Pub. Health,* **40**:802–7, (July) 1950.

Lanman, Jonathan T.; Guy, Loren P.; and Dancis, Joseph: "Retrolental Fibroplasia and Oxygen Therapy," *J.A.M.A.,* **155**:223–26, (May 15) 1954.

Lanman, Jonathan T., and McLaughlin, Ada: "Prevent Retrolental Fibroplasia in Premature Infants with Oxygen Control," National Society for the Prevention of Blindness, New York.

Lesser, Arthur J.: "Premature Birth Is a Public-Health Problem," *The Child,* **14**:146–49, (Apr.) 1950.

Losty, Margaret A.; Orlofsky, Irene; and Wallace, Helen M.: "A Transport Service for Premature Babies," *Am. J. Nursing,* **50**:10–12, (Jan.) 1950.

Lundeen, Evelyn C.: "Prematures Present Special Problems. Basic Factors in Nursing Care," *Mod. Hosp.,* **82**:60–65, (Apr.) 1954.

Lyon, Robert A., and Wallinger, Elgie M.: *Mitchell's Pediatrics and Pediatric Nursing,* 4th ed. W. B. Saunders Co., Philadelphia, 1954.

Marquis, Henrietta: "When a Premature Baby Is Born," *The Child,* **14**:150–51, (Apr.) 1950.

Maternity Center Association: "Preventing Prematurity," *Briefs,* **14**:12–13, (June) 1950.

Nelson, Waldo E. (ed.): *Textbook of Pediatrics,* 6th ed. W. B. Saunders Co., Philadelphia, 1954.

Owens, William C., and Owens, Ella U.: "Retrolental Fibroplasia," *Am. J. Pub. Health,* **40**:405–8, (Apr.) 1950.

Parke, Priscilla C.: "Naso-Gastric Tube Feeding for Premature Infants," *Am. J. Nursing,* **51**:517, (Aug.) 1951.

Prugh, Dane G.: "Emotional Problems of the Premature Infant's Parents," *Nursing Outlook,* **1**:461–64, (Aug.) 1953.

Reese, Algernon B., and Blodi, Frederick C.: "Retrolental Fibroplasia," *Am. J. Ophth.,* **34**:1–24, (Jan.) 1951.

Royce, Stephen; Tepper, Clifford; Watson, William; and Day, Richard: "Indwelling Polyethylene Nasogastric Tube for Feeding Premature Infants," *Pediatrics,* **8**:79–81, (July) 1951.

Sanford, Heyworth N.; Root, J. Harold; and Graham, R. H.: "The Premature Infant," *Pediatrics,* **8**:431–34, (Aug.) 1951.

Taylor, E. Stewart: "The Prevention of Deaths from Prematurity," *Pub. Health Nursing,* **42**:280–81, (May) 1950.

U.S. Department of Health, Education, and Welfare: *Infant Care,* Publication No. 8. U.S. Government Printing Office, Washington, D.C., 1955.

Wagner, Edward A.; Koch, Carl A.; and Jones, Daniel V.: "An Improved Indwelling Tube for Feeding Premature Infants," *J. Pediat.,* **45**:200–201, (Aug.) 1954.

Wallace, Helen M., and Losty, Margaret A.: "The Premature Infant's Parents," *Am. J. Nursing,* **53**:68–69, (Jan.) 1953.

Wisconsin State Board of Health, Bureau of Maternal and Child Health: *Care of the Immature Infant. Basic Principles and Recommendations.* The Board of Health, Wisconsin, 1954.

*Chapter 24*

# Abnormalities and Diseases of the Newborn Infant—Medical Aspects and Nursing Care

The nurse who cares for the newborn infant must have a knowledge of those abnormalities and diseases which are peculiar to the newborn period or which originate before or at the time of birth. The nurse, because of her close contact with the newborn infant, is in a position to make valuable observations on the functioning of the various systems, on any deviations from normal behavior, and on the appearance of early signs and symptoms of disease. She should be able to recognize early manifestations of abnormalities or disease and have a good understanding of their significance. An early report to the doctor of any deviation from normal makes early treatment possible. Early treatment often has a profound effect on future development and may be essential for survival.

## CONGENITAL ANOMALIES

Any part of the body may be congenitally malformed to a small or large degree. These abnormalities may consist of such a minor deviation from normal that function is only very slightly impaired or not at all; they may be disrupting to varying degrees; or they may be so severe as to require a major surgical procedure for correction or even be incompatible with life. Congenital anomalies are a frequent cause of death just as anomalies of the embryo are a common cause of loss of life in early intrauterine existence. The extent of the total abnormalities which could occur is not known because structural defects of the embryo are often a cause of abortion. Of those abnormal fetuses which do survive to term many are unable to adjust to extrauterine existence and die soon after birth. Congenital anomalies are the fourth most frequent cause of deaths in the neonatal period; only prematurity and certain diseases of early infancy (mainly birth injuries and postnatal asphyxia and atelectasis) are more often the cause of loss of life in this period. Little is known about the actual causes of congenital defects, but it is evident that certain circumstances favor the development of abnormalities. Anomalies may be genetically determined or they may be influenced by environmental factors. Some of the conditions which may produce an adverse environment for the developing embryo are certain maternal diseases, of which rubella (German measles) is one of the most dangerous, maternal irradiation in therapeutic doses during pregnancy, possibly dietary deficiencies in the mother, and diseases of the area of implantation. Maternal diabetes increases the risk of congenital defects. An abnormal circumstance during the first two or three months of intrauterine life may have considerable effect on the fetus and lead to arrests in development; the part of the body that is growing and differentiating most rapidly at the time of the abnormal condition may be affected. Several anomalies may be present in the same individual.

The chance of preventing congenital anomalies increases with increased knowledge of causes. Adequate early prenatal care to ensure good health, an adequate diet, and protection insofar as possible against virus diseases, especially rubella, in the early months of pregnancy are all valuable in the prevention of an adverse environment for the fetus.

Diagnosis of developmental defects can sometimes be made before or during labor. Hydramnios is frequently associated with a congenital anomaly. An x-ray taken late in pregnancy may reveal an abnormality. Dystocia during labor may be due to an anomaly, and a diagnosis can sometimes be made at this time; congenital hydrocephalus may cause an obstructed labor. Many defects, however, are not apparent until after birth and may even then not be discovered easily. They may be obscure enough not to appear until they interfere with normal growth and development. Sudden death in the neonatal period may be due to congenital malformations of the heart, lungs, gastrointestinal system, or brain. Some deaths are not preventable because of the extent of the malformations, but others may be prevented by immediate treatment. A thorough examination of the newborn infant and close observation of the functioning of the various systems for characteristic clinical manifestations of internal defects of the body will be valuable in early detection and treatment of abnormalities. The nurse can be very helpful in making these observations.

## CENTRAL NERVOUS SYSTEM

Congenital malformations of the brain and spinal cord vary greatly in their location and in the extent of involvement.

**Anencephalus** is a condition in which the forebrain is malformed and deficient. A considerable portion of the cerebral hemispheres (and the cranium and scalp which lie over them) is lacking. This condition is not compatible with life.

**Hydrocephalus,** which is an accumulation of fluid in the intracranial cavity due to some interference in the flow or absorption of cerebrospinal fluid, may be caused by a congenital malformation. It is often associated with spina bifida. Evidences of hydrocephalus are an abnormally large head size, tense bulging fontanels, separation of skull sutures, a rapid increase in head size, vomiting, and convulsions. It may be necessary to rule out, by lumbar puncture and examination of the spinal fluid, increased pressure due to intracranial hemorrhage. Surgical treatment of congenital hydrocephalus is rarely successful.

**Spina bifida** is a developmental defect in the closure of the bony spinal canal, frequently in the lumbar region. The spinal cord membranes may remain in the canal or may protrude through the defect. Neurologic disability may or may not be present depending upon the extent of the anomaly. A meningocele, in which the meninges only protrude, is not as serious as a myelomeningocele in which nerve fibers are also present in the sac. Surgical correction of this condition may be possible. There is a chance that the protruding sac may break and become infected; meningitis would then follow.

**Mongolism** is a condition in which mentality is severely retarded and developmental defects of other tissues are present. Some of the physical characteristics are a small skull, eyes wide set and with a lateral upward slope, protruding tongue, short nose with a flat bridge, mobile relaxed joints, poor muscle tone, and often cardiac malformations. The cause is unknown. This condition must be differentiated from cretinism. Some of the signs of mongolism become more obvious with age, and diagnosis cannot be made easily at birth or not at all until later.

## CIRCULATORY SYSTEM

**Congenital heart disease** causes more deaths in the first year of life than any other congenital defect. Many infants with gross malformations die in the first few months of life; some die very soon after birth, others during infancy, and some live for several years. Defects may, however, be of a less serious nature; some individuals develop symptoms late in life, and others live quite normally and without symptoms through a normal life span.

Many and complex types of malformations involving the heart and/or the great vessels may be found. The heart goes through a very complicated developmental process in fetal life, and a disturbance at any one of the series of changes may result in a congenital anomaly. Some of the common defects are a patent ductus arteriosus in which the communication between the aorta and pulmonary artery persists; a patent foramen ovale in which the communication between the right and left atria continues; defects between the ventricles; an underdeveloped pulmonary artery, or a stenosis of the pulmonary valve; a constriction of the aorta; and transposition of the great vessels. Various combinations of these defects may exist. Some defects are functional and disappear within a few months, some remain but do not require treatment and do not produce a handicap, some require surgery to support life, and some are so marked that they are incompatible with life. Congenital heart lesions may be accompanied by anomalies in other parts of the body.

Signs and symptoms of heart disease may be absent in the infant, they may occur occasionally, or they may be constant in a mild or severe form. Signs and symptoms may occur because of a communication between the systemic and pulmonary circulation, which interferes with proper oxygenation of the blood, or because of an increased load placed on the heart when it is necessary to force blood through narrow passages or stenotic valves. Cyanosis is a common manifestation, but it may be absent or may not occur until later in life. Cyanosis is not present if the anomaly does not allow abnormal mixing of the arterial and venous blood. A blueness of the hands and feet is normal for a few hours after birth, but all other parts of the baby's body should be pink. A persistence of the cyanosis of the hands and feet after several hours, when oxygenation and circulation should be improved, is suggestive of heart disease, pulmonary pathology, or birth injury, and should be considered abnormal. A persistent heart murmur is another frequent sign of an abnormality. A precordial murmur in the early neonatal period may be due to delayed closure of one of the fetal openings and is, therefore, not significant unless it persists. Other signs of circulatory difficulty, such as rapid labored respirations and edema, may be present early or appear later. In some cases of heart disease the baby may not take his feedings well.

Diagnosis is made on the basis of clinical signs and their persistence and with the aid of fluoroscopic examinations and x-rays. When heart disease has been diagnosed other tests, such as electrocardiography and cardiac catheterization, may be necessary to determine the type and extent of the lesion. If the femoral arteries are palpated for pulsation at the time of the infant's physical examination, coarctation of the aorta may be detected before some of the other signs develop. Pulsations in the femoral arteries are decreased or absent in coarctation of the aorta because the circulation of the lower part of the body must, to a large extent, be carried on by a collateral circulation. If pulsation is absent further studies can then be carried out.

Cyanosis and rapid respirations can usually be relieved by the use of oxygen, and the nurse is justified in administering oxygen in the presence of cyanosis and rapid breathing until the doctor is consulted and leaves further orders. There is little else that can be done for the newborn infant. This oxygen is best administered by placing the baby in an incubator, flooding the incubator with oxygen, and then maintaining a concentration of 50 to 60 per cent, or possibly even higher if necessary to relieve signs of distress. As soon as the doctor is consulted he will order the percentage of oxygen that is desirable. If an incubator is not immediately available the oxygen can be temporarily given by running oxygen at 10 to 14 liters per minute through a rubber tube, or a tube with a funnel attached to the end, and placing this tube or funnel in front of the baby's mouth and nose.

Some congenital heart lesions are amenable to surgery in late infancy and early childhood; the condition may be corrected in some cases and improved in others by surgical procedures.

## GASTROINTESTINAL SYSTEM

**Tongue-tie** is a condition in which the vertical fold of mucous membrane (frenum) under the tongue, which is normally short and tight in the newborn, extends to the end or nearly to the end of the tongue. This may limit movement of the tongue, which is noticeable when the baby cries, but it usually does not interfere with sucking. Sometimes this fibrous band is nicked for a short distance with a sterile blunt scissors in order to free the end of the tongue, while in other instances no attempt is made to free it.

**Cleft lip (harelip)** and **cleft palate** are due to failure of the maxillary and palatal processes to close in early fetal life—between the sixth and tenth week. The cause is not known, but its occurrence may be seen in successive generations and in siblings. A cleft lip is a fissure in the upper lip to the side of the midline and may vary from a slight notch to a complete separation extending into the nostril. It may be unilateral or bilateral. A cleft palate is a fissure in the midline of the roof of the mouth; this fissure may be small or there may be complete separation involving both the soft and hard palate. These conditions may occur singly, or the two abnormalities may be seen together. Problems in the newborn nursery consist of finding the best method of feeding these babies, since sucking is often hampered, and of prevention of infection, to which these infants are very susceptible. The connection which exists between the mouth and nose in babies with a cleft palate permits some of the formula which is taken into the mouth to pass out through the nose. This connection between mouth and nose often contributes to respiratory infection. Feeding problems must be skillfully dealt with in order to have the baby in optimum physical condition for the surgery which is necessary to correct the defect. Soft nipples with large holes, which eliminate hard sucking, are often satisfactory for feedings, although it may be necessary to use a Breck feeder, a rubber-tipped medicine dropper, or an Asepto syringe with a rubber tip. A special nipple with a rubber flange which closes off the cleft is sometimes used. Occasionally gavage feedings must be given. Feedings must be slow enough to prevent choking. Holding the baby in an almost upright position may facilitate swallowing. Frequent bubbling during a feeding may be necessary since the infant often swallows considerable air. It is important to find the best method of feeding for each individual infant and to give the mother ample opportunity to learn how to feed her baby before he leaves the hospital.

Surgical correction of the defects is always necessary. The cleft lip is usually repaired shortly after birth, somewhere between the time birth weight has been regained and the age of three months has been reached, if the baby's condition otherwise is satisfactory (Fig. 198). The cleft palate is usually repaired between one and two years of age.

Since the development of the gastrointestinal tract is a very complicated process, malformations may occur anywhere else in the tract;

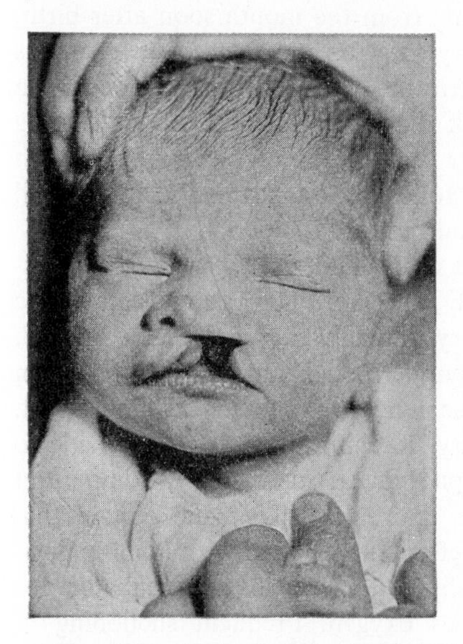

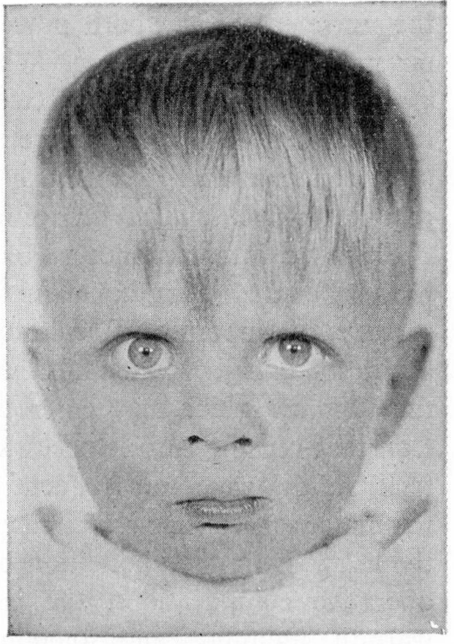

**Fig. 198.** *(Left)* Harelip. *(Right)* Harelip repair; this is a photograph of the infant *(left),* taken about two years after his operation which was performed at the age of 12 days. (Courtesy of Dr. William G. Heeks.) (West, John P.; Keller, Manelva W.; and Harmon, Elizabeth: *Nursing Care of the Surgical Patient,* 6th ed. The Macmillan Company, New York, 1957.)

these may be due to arrests in development in early fetal life or to a persistence of fetal structures. These anomalies may cause partial or complete obstruction depending upon whether stenosis or atresia is present. The anomalies of the intestinal tract may be single or multiple.

**Esophageal atresia** may take on different forms; both upper and lower segments of the esophagus may end in blind pouches or either one or both segments may be connected to the trachea by a fistulous tract. The commonest form of esophageal malformation is a *tracheo-esophageal fistula* in which the upper part of the esophagus ends in a blind pouch and the lower segment connects to the trachea.

When the infant is given his first feeding it is discovered that the baby has difficulty in taking food. He may take one or two swallows well and then cough and struggle; fluid returns through the mouth and nose, and cyanosis and respiratory distress follow. When this occurs it is important to discontinue the feeding immediately and suction the pharynx and the esophagus. The infant usually has an excessive amount of mucus flowing from the mouth soon after birth; the nurse in the newborn nursery may be the first to observe this constant, profuse drooling. When the above symptoms occur an esophageal anomaly is suspected; diagnosis is confirmed by finding that an attempt to pass a catheter through the esophagus meets with an obstruction and by an x-ray following an instillation of a small amount (only about 0.5 ml) of iodized oil (Lipiodol).

Since the infant cannot be fed orally and since he may have respiratory distress with this anomaly, an early diagnosis and immediate surgery are important. Respiratory difficulty may be caused by both aspiration of saliva which fills the upper pouch and by secretions from the stomach which may enter the lungs through the fistulous tract. Constant nursing care is necessary. Keeping the baby on his side to facilitate drainage and frequent pharyngeal suctioning are important to minimize aspiration of mucus and saliva. To make certain that the infant is in good condition before surgery and to minimize post-operative complications, the baby is placed in an incubator for warmth, humidity, and sometimes oxygen. Frequent suctioning of mucus and saliva is done, and chemotherapy and parenteral fluids are given.

The most common abnormality of the stomach is **hypertrophic pyloric stenosis,** which is due to hypertrophy of the musculature of the pylorus—chiefly of the circular muscles. This hypertrophy constricts the lumen of the pyloric opening and thus mechanically interferes with emptying of the stomach. This condition is much more common in the male than in the female.

Vomiting usually begins in the second or third week of life, occasionally even in the first week; it becomes more frequent and increasingly projectile. The baby vomits during or shortly after a feeding. Vomiting may occur with every feeding or only after every second or third feeding, but then food accumulated from the previous feedings also returns. It is important for the nurse or the mother who is feeding the infant to observe, record, and report the frequency and the amount of vomiting, the time in relation to the last feeding, the character of the vomiting (regurgitative or projectile), and the character of the emesis. The vomitus of the baby with pyloric stenosis does not contain bile or intestinal contents. Gastric peristaltic waves may be seen through the thin abdominal wall; they appear as definite characteristic waves which are most evident immediately after a feeding or just before vomiting. These waves begin at the left costal margin, pass transversely over the abdomen, and disappear in the region of the umbilicus. One, two, or three waves, appearing as long or as round globular contractions, may be visible. These are usually seen best from the right side with the eyes on a level with the abdomen and with a light, which is not too bright, coming from the left side. A tumorous mass may be palpable at the pylorus in the region of the umbilicus. As a result of the vomiting the infant does not obtain an adequate amount of food and fluid and thus becomes dehydrated, loses weight, and becomes constipated.

Surgical correction, by splitting the hypertrophied muscles of the pylorus, but without cutting the mucosa underneath, is almost always necessary in cases of pyloric stenosis. A differential diagnosis between hypertrophic pyloric stenosis and pylorospasm, a condition which can be controlled by an antispasmodic or a sedative must, however, be made before surgery is performed.

Some infants are hyperactive; they are easily disturbed and excited, sleep little, awaken easily, and seem very tense. These infants vomit frequently during the first few weeks of life; vomiting occurs suddenly and with considerable force. These infants are said to have *pylorospasm.* Slow, careful feeding; bubbling before, several times during, and after feeding; using a formula thickened with cereal;

refeeding if vomiting occurs soon after feeding; and treatment with an antispasmodic, such as atropine or an atropine derivative, or phenobarbital as sedation, or both simultaneously, usually control vomiting due to pylorospasm. Atropine is given in a small amount of water about 20 minutes before a feeding. The initial dose should be small to avoid a severe reaction in case of idiosyncrasy to the drug. The first dose may be 1 drop of a 1:1000 solution or, preferably, 10 drops of a 1:10,000 solution. The amount is gradually increased until the vomiting is controlled or until flushing of the skin occurs. The dosage is then maintained at that amount or one slightly smaller. Dosages above 3 or 4 drops of a 1:1000 solution are seldom given. Atropine is a toxic drug when an overdosage is given, and the tolerance dose varies greatly in different individuals. Flushing, which appears soon after the drug has been given and disappears after a short period of time, is a sign that tolerance has been reached. The nurse must watch for, record, and report flushing of the skin, dilatation of the pupils, and fever. Atropine in solution deteriorates rapidly, and the solution must be fresh every two weeks. When phenobarbital is used a 15-mg tablet (dissolved in water) may be given two or three times daily, or it may be administered in the form of an elixir which is given approximately 20 minutes before each feeding. Ten to 15 drops (2 to 3 mg) of the elixir may be given initially, and the dosage gradually increased to 30 to 40 drops (6 to 8 mg) if necessary. When vomiting is controlled the phenobarbital is again gradually decreased until it is completely eliminated. Whenever phenobarbital is used it is important to observe the baby for undue drowsiness and to decrease the dosage if this becomes evident.

**Intestinal obstruction** may be complete or partial and may be located at any level of the small or large intestine. It may be due to stenosis, or atresia, or absence of a portion of the intestine. Evidence appears early, in the first day or two of life, and consists of vomiting, abdominal distention, abnormal meconium which may be drier or lighter than normal, or absence of stools. The vomiting begins early and becomes more frequent and more severe. The character of the vomitus depends upon the level of the obstruction. It may consist of milk and thin fluid only; however, if the obstruction is below the ampulla of Vater it contains bile, and when the obstruction is as far down as the lower ileum or the colon, fecal material will be vomited.

Roentgenograms, even without contrast media, are valuable in diagnosis; there is a marked distention of the bowel above the obstruction. Barium is usually not given because of the danger of clogging the intestines.

Treatment of intestinal obstruction due to congenital malformations is by surgery, the success of which will depend upon the extent of the anomaly.

**Imperforate anus** may be caused by a persistent membrane over the anal opening with a normal anus just above the membrane or there may be complete absence of the anus with the rectal pouch ending some distance above. Direct inspection may reveal the defect; the nurse may discover the condition when she attempts to take the baby's temperature. A slight depression may be seen where the anal opening should be located. Meconium will not be passed, and the infant may strain, cry, and appear restless.

Surgery is necessary. An x-ray taken with the baby held head downward, thus allowing the gas in the intestinal tract to rise to the end of the blind pouch will help to determine how much of the rectum or anus is absent and whether perineal surgery will establish an opening or whether a colostomy must be done first, with plans to correct the rectal defect later.

Atresia or stenosis of the anus or rectum may be complicated by a fistulous connection with the genitourinary tract. Meconium or fecal material will be seen in the urine when a rectovesical fistula exists. With a fistula from the rectum to the urethra, more common in the male, meconium will be passed from the meatus of the urethra. In the female a rectovaginal fistula may be present.

**A diaphragmatic hernia,** which is a protrusion of the abdominal viscera, to varying degrees, into the thoracic cavity may be congenital, due to either an absence or a weakness of diaphragmatic tissue. Symptoms, which include respiratory distress, vomiting, and other evidences of intestinal obstruction, may be present at birth or appear later. Treatment is surgical. For severe types it is considered best to perform surgery in the first 48 hours of life since the intestines have not yet become distended and can be placed into the abdominal cavity more easily than they can be later.

**Biliary tract developmental abnormalities,** which obstruct the flow of bile into the intestinal tract, cause clay-colored or white stools, bile-stained urine, and early jaundice. The anomaly may or may not be amenable to surgery.

## GENITOURINARY SYSTEM

Malformations of the genitourinary tract are common; this is especially true in male infants. The development of the genitourinary system is a very complicated process, and any interruption in this development may result in a large variety of abnormalities. Many of these anomalies do not produce symptoms or disturb function at any time or at least not until sometime later in life—perhaps at a time of particular stress on the system. Among the anomalies found may be absence, aplasia, or duplication of the kidneys, ureters, or bladder; obstruction of ureters or urethra; and fistulas from the bladder and urethra to the rectum or vagina.

**Bilateral renal agenesis,** which is an absence of the kidneys and ureters, causes death within a few hours after birth. It is accompanied by characteristic facial features.

**Congenital cystic, or polycystic, kidneys** are the commonest of the kidney malformations. Many cysts, large or small, exist in one or both kidneys. They may not cause symptoms for several years and sometimes not until adult life. This condition will impair kidney function, but it may not be diagnosed until the cysts grow, replace kidney tissue, and thus diminish kidney function. It may, therefore, not be recognized during the neonatal period unless the kidneys are greatly enlarged or irregular.

**Exstrophy of the bladder** is a partial or complete exposure of the bladder mucosa through an opening in the abdomen. When complete, this defect is due to a failure of union of the abdominal wall, the anterior bladder wall, the symphysis pubis, and the urethra. The opening in the lower abdominal and anterior bladder wall exposes the posterior bladder wall and the ureters on the abdomen. The exposed area is a bright red color, has many folds, and is very sensitive. Urine is drained externally. Constant leakage of urine makes it impossible to keep the baby dry and is irritating to the surrounding skin. The exposed bladder wall must be covered with soft dressings to prevent irritation, the surrounding skin must be bathed frequently and protected by soothing ointments, and the dressings must be changed every one to two hours.

Treatment consists of ureteral transplants to the bowel and operative removal of the bladder if the exstrophy is complete. Plastic closure may be possible when the exstrophy is not complete. Other anomalies of the genitourinary tract and of the pelvic organs may also be present.

**Phimosis** is a narrowing of the preputial opening to a degree which makes it impossible to retract the foreskin. There is ordinarily no interference with urination, but the opening may be so small that straining is necessary during voiding and the stream of urine small. Difficulty in keeping the mucous membrane clean when the prepuce cannot be retracted may lead to inflammation of the prepuce and the glans, but symptoms may be absent. Treatment consists of stretching the prepuce with a forceps and forced retraction or performing a circumcision (pp. 639–40).

**Hypospadias** is an anomaly in which the urethra does not extend the entire length of the penis but rather opens on its lower surface somewhere behind the glans and in severe cases opens in the perineum. The tip of the penis is bent down. Treatment may not be necessary if the condition is not severe; in other cases a plastic operation may be performed. It is important to observe the urinary flow of these infants to make certain that the urethral opening is sufficiently large.

**A hydrocele,** which is an accumulation of fluid in the scrotum, making it a tense, fluctuating, translucent sac, may be congenital. Fluid may be present at birth or may accumulate later. Absorption of the fluid is usually spontaneous. A hydrocele may be accompanied by a hernia.

**Undescended testicles** make the scrotum appear small, or if only one testis is undescended there is a difference in size in the two sides of the scrotum. The testes develop in the abdomen and normally descend into the scrotum sometime during the last two months of fetal life. They may, however, remain in the inguinal canal, or even the abdominal cavity, for a longer period of time. Descent is usually spontaneous during the first few weeks of life or at any time up to the age of puberty. An undescended testicle may be associated with hernia.

## MUSCULOSKELETAL SYSTEM

Abnormal conditions of the musculoskeletal system may be caused by developmental defects and anomalies of bones and muscles or may be the result of an unusual fetal position in utero. Developmental defects may result in the absence of various muscles, absence of individual bones, supernumerary fingers or toes, union of fingers and toes due to either actual fusion of the bones or webbing of the skin only, and various other deformities.

As the fetus grows it becomes more and more confined in the uterine cavity, it does not move around as easily as earlier in its development, and it may finally maintain a certain posture, at least of some parts of the body. If this is an unusual position it may result in an asymmetrical development or a deformity. Severe molding of various areas of the body may be caused by such an unusual intrauterine position. When a certain part of the body is firmly pressed against another bony part, abnormalities, mild or severe, will result. Examples of molding due to pressure are abnormal positions of the feet, grooving due to pressure of the arms against the chest, and asymmetry of the face due to pressure of the chin against the shoulder or the chest. Developmental anomalies or position may cause shortening of muscles and result in contractural defects such as congenital clubfoot or torticollis.

The marked relaxation which characterizes the newborn period diminishes after one week, this being true especially of those muscles and joints which were stretched and strained by fetal position. They become restricted in motion. An example is resistance encountered to leg abduction in the potentially dislocated hip because the muscles splint an unstable hip joint. The joints and muscles that did not have strain in utero remain pliant for a longer period of time.

**Clubfoot** (talipes) is the result of an unequal pull of muscles producing a deformity in which the foot is turned at an abnormal angle. Intrauterine position or muscular imbalance is considered a possible cause. The condition is usually bilateral. Diagnosis is sometimes difficult because the foot of the newborn is often normally held in a position similar to clubfoot. Since muscular pull might increase the deformity as the muscles mature, corrective measures which change the direction of muscle pull are started early. The method of correction depends upon the severity of the condition. One form of treatment consists of passive overcorrection of the position of the foot at frequent intervals during the day. This manipulation may be started with the newborn infant before he leaves the hospital and continued at home. The nurses and the mother may be instructed to pull the foot as far as possible in the opposite direction and hold it in that position for a minute each time that the baby is handled (Fig. 199, *right*). During manipulation the leg must be supported

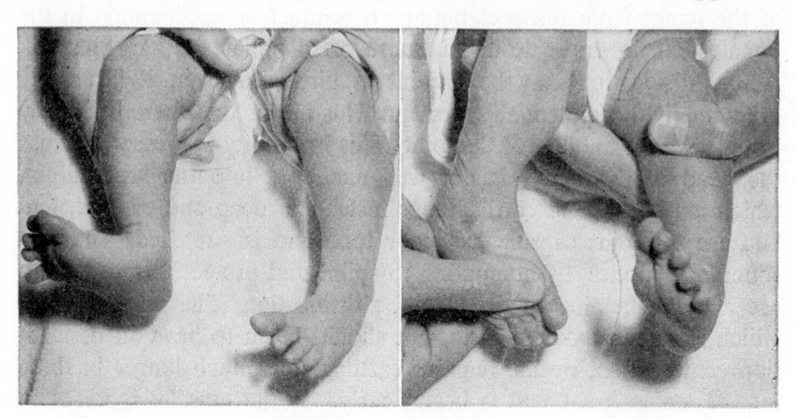

**Fig. 199.** *(Left)* Talipes calcaneovalgus; right foot—moderately resistant. *(Right)* Stretching of the foot downward and inward to overcome the resistance. The nurses were instructed to manipulate the foot in this manner three or four times each time the baby was picked up to be cared for, and the mother was instructed to continue this manipulation at home. If the resistance is not overcome by this treatment, casts will be applied.

under the calf and with the knee flexed in order to protect the lateral ligaments of the knee and the epiphysis of the tibia from strain, and the entire foot must be supported to avoid merely bending it in the middle. Bending the foot alone does not correct the shortened heel cord and may result in a rocker foot deformity. Plaster casts may be applied within a few days after birth; these are changed every one to three weeks to allow for growth of the foot and for further correction. Until the cast is thoroughly dry, care must be taken not to indent it with the fingers while handling the baby. It may be necessary to pick the baby up and hold him more than usual after application of the cast until he becomes accustomed to it. Following application of a cast the upper leg and the toes must be watched for signs of circulatory impairment. The toes should be warm and a normal pink color—not pale, dark red, or blue. There should be no signs of swelling as indicated by pressure of the edges of the cast against the thigh or the toes. A waterproof material applied to the edge of the cast at the thigh will help to keep it clean of urine and stool.

**Congenital dislocation of the hip** is a displacement of the head of the femur from the acetabulum. It is much more common in the female than in the male and is more often unilateral than bilateral. Actual dislocation may be present at birth; however, it is usually not actually, but potentially, present. This means that there is in most instances an instability of the joint. This instability is present because the head of the femur is not well anchored into the acetabulum, which is shallow and cartilaginous instead of deep and ossified, and because the joint capsule has poor tone and is stretched. The surrounding muscles, by attempting to splint and protect this soft joint, are actually helping to produce the dislocation. The femoral head which is cartilaginous at birth, but should begin to have an ossification center at six weeks, remains cartilaginous much longer in these infants, unless treatment is begun early. As the muscles increase in strength and finally as the baby stands, the femoral head is pulled and displaced more and more, the head and the socket are malformed, and the head of the femur is finally completely dislocated.

Early recognition of this condition from the standpoint of early treatment is very important to prevent an actual dislocation. At the first examination of the baby it may be difficult to recognize a potentially dislocated hip because of the great pliability of the joints of the newborn, but by the age of one month muscular splinting is evident. The thighs resist abduction. When the normal baby is placed on his back with the knees flexed, his hips and knees can be abducted until they nearly reach the examining table, but if a potential dislocation exists abduction of the affected leg is possible only to one-half of this distance. X-ray will reveal a persistence of fetal cartilage.

The nurse caring for a baby with a potential dislocation may find that she encounters some difficulty in moving one leg to the side when washing the groins or changing the diaper. This observation of an inability to abduct the leg completely should be reported to the doctor. The baby may also be observed to move this leg less than the unaffected one. Other early signs of congenital dislocation of the hip, such as apparent shortening of the affected leg, a higher gluteal and inguinal fold, and an additional transverse crease in the thigh may not be noticeable in the newborn period.

Early treatment, before the cartilaginous structures become malformed by pressure from muscle pull and weight bearing, is very important. Early treatment is directed toward maintaining the affected leg in complete abduction; the muscle pull then directs the femoral head into the acetabulum, and the pressure thus created stimulates ossification. A position of abduction may be achieved during the first two months by placing the baby in a prone position whenever he is put to bed and by keeping the legs flexed and abducted while in this position. The diaper can be pinned to the sheet in such a way that the legs are held in the desired position. The body weight helps to increase the degree of abduction. Another method of keeping the legs flexed and abducted is by the use of a Frejka splint, which consists of a square pillow placed against the infant's diaper and held snugly in place by suspenders or straps. The application of several diapers, in such a manner that there is a very heavy thickness in the center, is another method that may be used to keep the legs widely abducted. Extension of the leg should be avoided when handling the baby.

When treatment is not started early it becomes prolonged and a body cast may be necessary; when dislocation has actually occurred, surgery and a long period of treatment may be required. With early diagnosis and adequate treatment the baby may be able to walk normally at the average age.

**Congenital torticollis,** or wryneck, is characterized by an abnormal position of the head and a poorly functioning sternocleidomastoid muscle. The head is usually drawn downward on one side, the neck is shortened on the affected side, and the chin is rotated toward the opposite side. There may be a bony anomaly, but it is frequently due to muscular involvement resulting from a difficult delivery or an abnormal intrauterine position. Sometime between birth and ten days of life a boggy swelling is noticeable in the sternocleidomastoid muscle. This mass slowly increases in size for several weeks and then decreases and disappears. It may be quite tender at first. There may be no residual effect on the muscle or it may become short and noncontractile. If congenital torticollis is present without this swelling an x-ray may reveal a bony anomaly.

Since the deformity may be very mild or not noticeable at birth (becoming more apparent in several weeks), the nurse caring for a baby should notice any signs of limitation of movement of the head and neck and also be aware of any swelling in the muscle.

Treatment should be started early; it is directed toward restoring normal alignment of the head and neck. Manipulation by overextension and passive exercise is used, and the baby is positioned so that the head is bent to the side away from the contracture. If correction is not accomplished by manipulation and exercise alone, a cast or brace and sometimes surgery are necessary.

## THE SKIN

**Nevi** may be caused by a hyperplastic development of the blood and lymph vessels or of the epidermis and connective tissue. Nevi made up largely of blood vessels, known as *birthmarks,* are found on various parts of the body, and the nurse should observe the skin closely for any of these areas while she is caring for the baby. They may be flat or slightly raised, may range in color from a light red to a darker red, or to a blue-black color, and may or may not have a growth of hair. They may be variously described; some of the commonest names being a port wine mark, a strawberry mark, or a mole. Some lesions regress and disappear. Treatment varies considerably and may not be necessary at all. It must be individualized for the particular lesion.

## THE EYE

There are many congenital malformations of the eye, among them *congenital cataracts,* which may be caused by a rubella (German measles) infection in the mother in the first three months of pregnancy. This is an important time in the embryonic development of the eye, and the tissue may be particularly susceptible to the effects of the virus. The opacity of the lens is usually noticeable early if the eyes are observed as the baby opens them in a fairly good light.

## HELP FOR THE PARENTS

The parents of a child handicapped by a congenital anomaly have a problem with which it is very difficult to give them immediate help. Parents frequently blame themselves; they often have a deep feeling of guilt and self-accusation when their child has a congenital defect or a birth injury and either unconsciously assume or definitely express their feelings that they are at fault. They may believe an anomaly is caused by something they have done or something they have omitted to do during the prenatal period, and if they cannot think of a cause easily they may even search for one. They will quite naturally be very disappointed, and the baby's disability will sometimes, quite unconsciously, affect their behavior. Others find it difficult to accept the reality of the situation.

The doctor has the responsibility of informing the parents of the presence of a disability. Many believe that it is wise to tell the mother immediately after the birth of the baby and very frankly the kind and the extent of the anomaly present, at least insofar as it is possible to do so until further investigation is carried out. They believe that it is easier for the mother to accept an abnormal condition immediately than it is to have believed for even a short time that the baby is completely normal and then have her feel her disappointment more acutely. She will usually ask if the baby is normal almost immediately after delivery, and it is impossible to give a satisfactory answer unless she is told. If the abnormality is obvious it is necessary to tell her before she is shown the baby, and keeping him from her makes her suspicious that something is wrong. If information must, for some reason, be kept from the mother it is important that some member of the family be told without delay.

The nurse may find herself in a very difficult situation in meeting these parents. Although the doctor has explained the extent of the anomaly and the possibilities of treatment they will often want to talk about it further. The nurse, because of her close contact, is most commonly the person to whom they express some of their feelings, and many talk to the auxiliary workers. The nurse has therefore not only to make a decision of what she will say but also the problem of helping the auxiliary workers to understand. She must know what information has been given to the parents in regard to the extent of the anomaly and the possibility of corrective procedures. By demonstrating her acceptance of the baby, she will be able to help the parents gradually work through their first reactions to the anomaly and achieve acceptance of their baby.

Although the relationship between parents and a handicapped child can be, and frequently is, very healthy, a strain is always imposed. Parents, relatives, and friends must be helped to understand the problem and helped to accept the handicap on a realistic basis if possible. Much must be done to meet the social and emotional needs of these children, which are frequently more severe than the physical. Families must be helped in their adjustment since their reactions to the disability will greatly influence the child. Too much or too little should not be made of the handicap; it must be accepted as it is with allowances made for it as necessary but with no undue restriction of the child's activities. It is very important to give the child the feeling that he is genuinely loved and wanted in order to give him the security that he needs, but there is sometimes a tendency to give this child too much attention to make up for the difficulty; this overprotection may only serve to make him aware of his difference and make him overdependent. The newborn baby, of course, needs much love and attention, as any young baby does, but an attitude of overprotection may begin in this early period and may then be detrimental later in life. The parents may be helped to think in terms of how much their baby is like other children instead of how different he is.

Parents, therefore, need help not only in the medical care, but also in an understanding of and in assistance with their child's training, education, and social adjustment. Government services dealing with the problems of handicapped children were established by the Social Security Act of 1935 and its later amendments. The Children's Bureau of the Department of Health, Education, and Welfare has the responsibility of administering grants to states for crippled children's programs. Voluntary agencies are contributing to the care of the handicapped as well as tax-supported federal, state, and local agencies. All of these give both physical and psychologic care to handicapped children as well as counseling service for the parents.

## BIRTH INJURIES

Trauma during labor or delivery may involve any part of the newborn's body; some injuries produce only a temporary change while others cause permanent damage.

### SOFT-TISSUE INJURIES

Soft-tissue bruises usually occur in the presenting part of the fetus. Edema of the tissues and discolored areas due to an extravasation of blood into the tissues may develop in the part of the body that presents at the cervix and vaginal outlet at the time of delivery; this may be of the scalp in a vertex presentation (caput succedaneum and cephalhematoma), of the face in a face presentation, and of the genitalia, buttocks, and feet in a breech presentation (pp. 581–83 and 607–8). Reddened areas or abrasions are sometimes seen on the face and scalp due to bruising from the obstetric forceps. Most of these injuries are minor and the tissues return to normal in a few days, but they should be protected from further trauma while recovery is taking place. Petechial areas are sometimes seen on the face for a few days. Subconjunctival hemorrhages may be seen following spontaneous as well as instrumental deliveries; they are not serious and do not require treatment. Mothers will frequently observe this reddened area in the white portion of the baby's eye and inquire as to its significance. Occasionally an injury to one of the visceral organs, which is of serious consequence, occurs. Prognosis depends upon the site and amount of injury.

## INJURY TO BONES

Injury to bones occurs most frequently in the clavicle and the extremities; rarely of the skull, vertebrae, or ribs. The *clavicle* is the most common site of fracture; it is very susceptible to injury when delivery of the shoulders is difficult, but it may break during an apparently easy delivery. A fracture may be suspected if there is limitation of movement of an arm, if the Moro reflex is unilateral, and if there is spasm of the sternocleidomastoid muscle; these signs are, however, not always present. Crepitus may be felt on examination of the clavicle. A roentgenogram will confirm the diagnosis. Treatment usually consists of immobilization of the arm and shoulder on the affected side. This may be done by placing the arm against the chest wall with the hand lying across the chest and then, holding the arm quietly in place, wrapping a strip of stockinet material around the arm and chest. Complete immobilization is not always done, but the infant should then be handled carefully to prevent further trauma, and when the baby is picked up the shoulders should not be pressed toward the midline of the body. The arm on the affected side should not be put through a sleeve daily. When the arm is left out of the sleeve of the shirt and gown, the clothing helps to immobilize it somewhat. Healing takes place without deformity; a large callus forms within a week and then gradually absorbs. When a fracture is not suspected it may not be diagnosed until the callus is felt as a hard mass a week or more after birth.

A fracture of one of the extremities may occur if there is difficulty in delivery of an arm or leg. Spontaneous movement of the involved extremity is limited, and the Moro reflex is not symmetrical. These fractures heal rapidly; they heal without deformity when the extremity is immobilized in the corrected position.

### PERIPHERAL-NERVE INJURIES

Injury to peripheral nerves may sometimes occur during birth. The commonest of these injuries is to the *facial nerve*. Temporary paralysis of this nerve is usually due to pressure on the nerve during labor or pressure by a forceps blade during delivery. The affected side of the face is smooth, the eye may remain open, the corner of the mouth droops, and the forehead cannot be wrinkled. This condition is more obvious when the baby cries because the facial muscles on the affected side do not contract, and there is immobility of one side of the mouth; only the unaffected side of the face moves and the mouth is drawn to that side. There may be some difficulty in sucking during the first few days of life, but this is not always a problem. Treatment is not necessary, but if the eye does not close it must be protected from injury until it can close. If sucking is difficult for the first few days it may be necessary to feed the baby with a Breck feeder during this time. Prognosis is good. Improvement begins soon, and recovery is complete in a few weeks; sometimes this condition is quite transitory, and recovery is complete in a few days.

**Brachial palsy** is a partial or complete paralysis of certain muscles of the arm due to trauma to the nerve fibers of the brachial plexus. The brachial nerves may be injured by pressure, stretching, or actual severance. This injury may occur during delivery from the vertex position when traction is exerted on the head if delivery of the shoulders is difficult, or during delivery from a breech position if traction is made on the brachial plexus as an arm is stripped over the head or if tension is placed on the brachial plexus in making traction. The site of the injury determines which muscles are affected. The degree of paralysis, therefore, depends upon the amount of nerve involvement; the upper arm, the lower arm, or the whole arm may be paralyzed. The Erb-Duchenne (upper arm) paralysis in which the upper part of the plexus (the fifth and sixth cervical nerves) is injured is the most common type. The arm lies limp at the side; it is in a position of extension and is rotated inward; the forearm is in such a position that the palm of the hand faces downward and may even face outward. The baby cannot elevate or abduct the arm. The wrist and hand are normal. The Moro reflex is absent on the affected side. Pain seems to be present at first. The lower arm type of paralysis, which is rare, is seen when the nerves of the lower part of the plexus are injured; the hand and wrist are then paralyzed. The whole arm may be involved, and symptoms of both upper and lower arm type of paralysis are present. The nurse caring for the newborn should be aware of any abnormal arm position or diminished arm movements.

Treatment is directed toward restoring function in the involved muscles and preventing contractures in the unaffected ones. Treatment is started as soon after birth as the condition is noticed. At first treatment may consist of placing the baby in such a position that his arm is abducted and externally rotated and that the elbow is flexed. The arm is raised to shoulder height, and the elbow is flexed 90 deg. This position may be maintained in one of several ways. A strip of muslin, tied to the head of the crib, may be brought down and tied around the wrist to hold the arm up or the arm may be maintained in the desired position by placing it in a sling made of a folded towel which is pinned to the mattress. Another method of holding the arm up is to pin the sleeve of the baby's gown or shirt to the mattress or the top of the crib after the arm has been positioned. Later a splint may be used to hold the arm in the desired position, and massage and exercise may be given. In dressing the baby the arm should be supported at shoulder level. Clothing should be put on the affected arm first and taken off the affected arm last, and movement of the arm must be gentle.

Prognosis depends upon the amount of trauma. If this is slight due to edema or hemorrhage around the nerve fibers the condition will soon improve. If the nerves are not lacerated muscle power usually returns in a few months. Nerve laceration has a more serious prognosis.

## CENTRAL NERVOUS SYSTEM INJURY

Injury to the central nervous system is the most serious form of birth injury. *Intracranial hemorrhage,* which is the most severe form of injury, may be caused by trauma or hypoxia during birth or it may be due to a primary hemorrhagic disturbance of the newborn. The head may be traumatized in a prolonged hard labor, in a difficult delivery, by mechanical injury with the obstetric forceps, or in a precipitous labor and delivery. The shape of the fetal head changes during labor to fit the maternal pelvis; overlapping sutures and soft cranial bones make it possible for the head to accommodate to a pelvic canal of adequate size. Given time the head can usually make extreme adjustments; when compressed in one direction it will elongate in another. Excessive molding and overlapping of the cranial bones or sudden molding may, however, cause the meninges or sinuses to tear, with hemorrhage to a small or large degree the result. The differences in intrauterine and atmospheric pressure which produces caput succedaneum may at times affect the veins of the meninges and the brain in the same area. The short, apparently easy, labor and precipitous delivery are sometimes dangerous because blood vessels may break with the sudden changes in pressure.

Hypoxia prenatally, during delivery, or following birth (pp. 760--61) is sometimes a cause of brain injury. Common causes of hypoxia prenatally are placenta previa, premature separation of the placenta, and complications of pregnancy; among the paranatal causes are deep sedation or deep anesthesia and compression of the head as it passes through the birth canal. Ordinarily this compression is not harmful, but if changes in cerebral circulation are great and prolonged, a reduction in circulation and venous congestion may cause hypoxia which then predisposes to hemorrhage.

The premature infant is particularly susceptible to intracranial hemorrhage because the blood vessels in the premature are more easily broken than in the full-term infant, and the tendency to bleed is greater due to a prolonged prothrombin time. Premature rupture of the membranes, breech delivery, and short labor with precipitous delivery—conditions which cause more sudden changes in pressure—are more apt to occur in premature than in full-term birth.

Trauma to the brain may be slight and without hemorrhage, there may be edema only, or the bleeding may range from a minimal amount due to rupture of a few small vessels to a massive hemorrhage. Large hemorrhages are infrequent and usually fatal. Bleeding may occur from one or more of several sites; it may be subdural, subarachnoid, intraventricular, over the cerebellar area, or into the brain substance itself.

Signs and symptoms of intracranial injury are generalized and similar to those produced by several other conditions, one being atelectasis. Attacks of cyanosis, vomiting, listlessness, and poor sucking may be the only signs of cerebral irritation, but they may also be due to other causes, such as atelectasis, congenital heart disease, or diaphragmatic hernia. Included in the signs and symptoms of cerebral injury are irregular, difficult respirations; a pale, cold, clammy skin; cyanosis at intervals or continuously; an anxious expression, sometimes with the eyes open and staring; restlessness; failure to suck well; forceful vomiting; and a high-pitched cry. Localized muscular twitchings or generalized convulsions may occur a few hours after birth; the baby is flaccid at first and in 12 to 24 hours becomes spastic. The fontanels may be tense; the pupils may be of unequal size; Foote's sign, an adder-like, rhythmic protrusion of the tongue, may be present; the neck and spine may become rigid; and the infant may assume an opisthotonic position. Symptoms may be present immediately after birth or may be delayed for several days. With massive hemorrhage there may be practically no symptoms, but death may occur soon after birth, or there may be severe symptoms at or shortly after delivery. Where there is slight hemorrhage, due to rupture of small vessels, symptoms may develop gradually.

The difference in the signs and symptoms of cerebral irritation, cerebral edema, and intracranial hemorrhage is frequently only in the degree of severity and the length of time in which they are present. Slight trauma may give mild symptoms; the baby may be sleepy and listless and suck poorly during the first few days of life, but he usually recovers quickly and soon becomes alert, responds more readily, and begins to eat well. Cerebral edema is apt to give the same signs and symptoms as those of a mild hemorrhage, and it is frequently impossible to decide which is present. With edema the symptoms usually begin almost immediately after birth and as a rule they last only three to four days, after which improvement is rapid and recovery complete.

Observation of the Moro embrace reflex is important, and in cases of suspected intracranial injury it should be checked not only immediately after birth, but also on several succeeding days. Absence immediately after birth with a return in a few days is indicative of cerebral edema; the Moro reflex then returns because the edema has subsided. When hemorrhage has occurred the Moro reflex is usually present for 24 to 48 hours after birth, but then disappears and does not return until much later.

A spinal puncture, to test for increased pressure and for blood, is sometimes done as an aid in diagnosis, but interpretation of findings may be difficult since absence of these signs cannot exclude intracranial hemorrhage nor does the presence of blood confirm the diagnosis. The trauma of puncture may produce blood due to injury of a vessel of the spinal canal.

**Treatment** is largely directed toward keeping the baby quiet. Rest and a quiet environment are very essential in the prevention of prolonged bleeding or recurrence. The baby should not be handled more than is absolutely necessary until the acute stage has subsided. The usual nursery care of changing clothes, bathing, and weighing can be omitted for several days. Changing of diapers, taking of temperature, and other care that is essential can usually be done in the crib with a minimal amount of handling. The baby may need extra warmth, and body temperature will need to be checked to determine how much extra heat is necessary. Oxygen in a concentration of 30 to 40 per cent is often administered for several days whether or not cyanosis is visible. In cases of difficult delivery, the baby, regardless of size, may profit, during the first few days, from being given the same care a premature baby receives; he may be placed in an incubator where oxygen and external heat can easily be regulated. The head of the crib is usually elevated slightly; approximately at a 30-deg angle. If the baby's condition is questionable, the nurse should leave the head of the bed flat until she has orders from the doctor rather than lowering it, as is customary for drainage of mucus during the first few hours of life. Lowering of the head below the level of the body may increase bleeding if the baby has an intracranial injury.

Feedings are withheld for 48 hours or longer, and then easily digestible food such as breast milk is offered by a method that requires a minimum amount of exertion. A Breck feeder or rubber-tipped medicine dropper may at first be used; when it appears that the baby can suck easily the milk may be offered from a bottle. Breast feeding, because of the extra exertion for the baby, is not permitted until he is much improved, but breast milk, if it can be given by bottle, is an ideal food.

Vitamin K is ordered by some doctors for all babies after birth. When not used in this way it is often given prophylactically to a baby delivered with difficulty or as treatment when symptoms appear and for several days thereafter. Although hemorrhage is probably not due to a prothrombin deficiency, vitamin K may tend to control the amount of hemorrhage as it will prevent the physiologic drop in the prothrombin level of the blood which occurs in the early neonatal period.

Sedation is frequently given, especially if the infant is restless and hyperactive. Phenobarbital 8 mg (1/8 gr) is commonly used and may be repeated from two to four times daily depending upon the baby's response to its quieting effect.

Prognosis in cases of intracranial hemorrhage is guarded. Some of these babies are born dead and others may die after several days. In those that survive recovery is frequently complete, but there may be permanent cerebral damage. Sequelae may include convulsions, mental retardation, behavior problems, and spastic paralysis. Cerebral palsy is a common sequela when recovery is not complete. Congenital defects, as well as birth injuries, cause cerebral palsy, but an estimate of how large a factor this may be is impossible. Cerebral palsy may also be caused by other postnatal conditions such as asphyxia, erythroblastosis, head injury, encephalitis, and other infections, such as whooping cough or measles.

## THE RESPIRATORY SYSTEM

### ANOXIA *

Oxygen want is a great hazard to the fetus and the newborn baby. A deficiency of oxygen affects every tissue in the body and will pro-

* The term "anoxia" literally means "without oxygen," a condition that is incompatible with many forms of life; however, by common usage, anoxia is interpreted as a "shortage of oxygen in the blood."

Since this is a broad term, anoxia has been divided into four types, based on the underlying cause: (1) *anoxic* anoxia results from failure of ventilation; (2) *stagnant* anoxia is caused by a slowing of the circulation of blood; (3)

duce changes to a certain, and sometimes irreparable, degree depending upon the severity and duration of the anoxia and the susceptibility of the various tissues. It may cause temporary or permanent cerebral damage and is the cause of many neonatal deaths. Central nervous system symptoms may be due to the effect of the anoxia on the nerve tissue itself or due to its effect on blood vessels which lose tone and dilate and allow fluid and blood to escape, causing edema and even hemorrhage into the brain tissue. Anoxia may occur at any time during the baby's in utero existence, it may develop at any stage during labor and delivery, or it may not occur until after birth. It may be present at intervals or continuously and may be quite mild or very severe.

*Fetal anoxia,* which has occurred days or weeks before birth, is characterized by the presence of golden-yellow amniotic fluid and vernix caseosa at the time of birth and yellow staining of the baby's skin. These signs indicate that the baby may then also have respiratory difficulty at birth. Prenatal anoxia is usually due to an abnormal condition at the placental site caused by complications such as erythroblastosis fetalis, placenta previa, or premature separation of the placenta or it may be due to complications of pregnancy. Fetal anoxia may improve after birth if oxygen can be gotten to the tissues or it may have caused enough damage to interfere with normal functioning of the baby after birth.

*Anoxia during labor or delivery* usually manifests itself by a change in the fetal heart rate, either an acceleration or a slowing, by excessive fetal movements, and by the passage of meconium. Any condition that disturbs the normal functioning of the respiratory or circulatory system of the mother and thus interferes with an adequate oxygen supply to the placenta or any condition that disturbs adequate placental or umbilical cord circulation will interfere with the oxygen supply to the fetus. Anoxia during labor may be responsible for respiratory difficulty at birth.

---

*anemic* anoxia occurs when the hemoglobin level of the blood is low; and (4) *histotoxic* anoxia is the failure of tissue cells to utilize oxygen.

When an oxygen want exists in the newborn, it is usually an anoxic anoxia that results from inadequate oxygenation of the blood passing through the lungs because of depressed or delayed respiration.

The term "hypoxia" also means a "shortage of oxygen in the blood," and is used for an oxygen deficiency when the cause and/or degree have not been determined.

*Anoxia at birth or neonatal anoxia* is due either to a failure of the respiratory center to function or due to an interference with the normal functioning of the respiratory system. Pre-existing anoxia of the fetus may be the cause of initial respiratory failure at birth by having affected the respiratory center in such a way that its normal response to stimuli at the time of birth is diminished or the normal function of the respiratory center may be affected by trauma or maternal analgesia and anesthesia. Failure of the respiratory tract to function well may be due to mechanical obstruction or congenital defects of the respiratory or circulatory system. Neonatal anoxia may also occur when respirations that had already been established are interrupted. Included among causes of neonatal anoxia are (1) maternal analgesia and anesthesia which may produce narcosis, (2) antepartum bleeding, (3) toxemia of pregnancy, (4) long second stage of labor, (5) rapid labor, (6) trauma at birth with hemorrhage causing damage to the respiratory center, (7) prematurity, (8) compression of the umbilical cord, (9) obstruction of the air passages by mucus, blood, and amniotic fluid, (10) atelectasis, (11) congenital heart disease, and (12) malformations of the respiratory tract. Several factors may exist at any one time. Arterial oxygen saturation is approximately 50 per cent at birth and should increase up to 90 per cent or more within a few hours; any interference with this process may cause anoxia.

## ASPHYXIA NEONATORUM

This condition is a disturbance in the respiratory system which develops during or shortly after birth and results in anoxia; it is characterized by slow and irregular respiratory movements and cyanosis or by an absence of respiration. There may be initial respiratory failure or respiratory movements may be interrupted after they have been established. Any baby that does not breathe promptly after birth, or at least within the first 30 seconds, must be considered to be in danger of asphyxia. The chances of complications in the postnatal period are then increased.

Asphyxia may be present in any degree at birth. It may be mild with the baby having good color and good muscle tone and apnea for only a short time or it may be much more severe. It has frequently been divided into two stages depending upon the appearance of the child and has thus been designated as *asphyxia livida* and *asphyxia pallida.* A classification which is now more frequently used is one proposed by P. J. Flagg;* this denotes mild asphyxia as a stage of depression, moderate asphyxia as a stage of spasticity, and severe asphyxia as a stage of flaccidity. The stage of depression has milder manifestations and a better prognosis than the other two, but if anoxia is prolonged the asphyxia will progress into a more severe stage since the state of asphyxia does not remain stationary. The mild stage either improves rapidly or progresses to a more severe type.

In the *stage of depression* the respirations are slow and irregular; there is some cyanosis, either constant or recurring; the muscle tone is good; conjunctival and gag reflexes are present; the heart rate is normal or rapid; and there is resistance to movement of the head and extremities. In the *stage of spasticity* the respirations are irregular, shallow, gasping, and infrequent; cyanosis of mucous membranes is marked with blotching of skin and general pallor; muscle tone is diminished; the heart rate is rapid but may soon slow considerably; and the baby offers no resistance to movement, but will show some reflex action when resuscitation is attempted. When the infant is in the *flaccid stage* the respirations are absent or occur only at long intervals; the color is pale or gray; muscle tone is absent; the heartbeat is very poor; and reflex action is gone.

**Prevention.** Prophylactic measures are important in the prevention of asphyxia. Unless there are serious anomalies, almost all babies will breathe immediately if there have been no complications of pregnancy and labor and if analgesic drugs have not been given. There are many conditions that increase the incidence of asphyxia; among these are included prematurity, the toxemias, maternal disease such as diabetes, antepartum bleeding, abnormal presentations, long second stage of labor, operative deliveries, pressure on the umbilical cord, and analgesic drugs. A recognition of the causes of asphyxia and a careful evaluation of the individual patient as to the chances of fetal asphyxia make it possible to put forth every effort to eliminate or to reduce the danger of complications of pregnancy and labor and to determine the most suitable type of analgesia and management of delivery.

* Flagg, Paluel J.: *The Art of Anaesthesia,* 7th ed. J. B. Lippincott Co., Philadelphia, 1944.

Prevention is much more satisfactory than any treatment after asphyxia has occurred. Maintaining an adequate oxygen supply to the fetus before and during delivery and administering oxygen to a baby that does not breathe immediately and spontaneously at birth are important measures. Careful observation of the rate and rhythm of the fetal heart is the best method of recognizing an impending fetal asphyxia. There is an almost immediate change in the fetal heart rate with the development of anoxia. Other signs are excessive fetal movements and the passage of meconium. Oxygen administered to the mother when the fetus shows signs of anoxia may improve his condition by improving the oxygen saturation of the fetal blood. This may prevent respiratory depression at birth. Administration of oxygen to the mother may be very beneficial when the fetus is deprived of an adequate oxygen supply due to low concentration of oxygen in the anesthetic agent, obstruction in the maternal respiratory tract, respiratory depression due to drugs, a failing maternal circulatory system, placental separation, or pressure on the umbilical cord during contractions. If the cause of the intrauterine asphyxia cannot be corrected and if conditions are favorable for an operative procedure, immediate delivery of the baby may be advisable to prevent further danger from the effects of intrauterine asphyxia. Administration of oxygen to the mother while preparations are made for an operative delivery, during the delivery, and immediately after birth, before the umbilical cord is severed or stops pulsating, will help to supply the infant with oxygen.

**Treatment.** If the baby does not breathe, or breathes spontaneously but irregularly and feebly, or if he does not cry vigorously, prompt and sustained effort must be made to establish satisfactory respirations. Oxygen is absolutely essential in the treatment of asphyxia and must be available in the delivery room and the nursery at all times. It should be available for the first breath since this may get enough oxygen to the baby to help the respiratory center in the medulla function. If sufficient oxygen can be gotten to the tissues before irreversible damage has taken place, and this may occur any time between one to four minutes, there will be an improvement in the baby's condition so that the respiratory center will be able to function and spontaneous breathing may begin.

For these first breaths, oxygen can be administered with a mask or, if this interferes with other efforts at resuscitation, by means of a tube held in front of the mouth and nose with oxygen flowing at 15 to 20 liters per minute in order to increase the concentration of oxygen in the air surrounding the baby's head. After breathing is quite regular so that it is no longer necessary to make continuous effort to maintain respiratory movements the oxygen is administered most effectively in an incubator and is given at somewhere between 30 and 60 per cent, depending upon how well the baby breathes and the amount of oxygen necessary to relieve cyanosis. If a 50 to 60 per cent concentration is at first used, this is reduced to 30 to 40 per cent when the baby's condition improves, this reduction in concentration being particularly important with the premature infant.

An open airway is absolutely necessary for the beginning and maintenance of adequate respiration and this should be established before the infant breathes. If the simpler methods—postural drainage, wiping the mouth or suctioning with a rubber syringe, and milking the trachea—mentioned in Chapter 12 do not remove mucus, amniotic fluid, and other debris, then gentle and repeated aspiration of the mouth and oropharynx should be done before the first inspiration. This aspiration can be done with a rubber ear syringe inserted well back in the baby's mouth or with suction applied to a soft rubber catheter introduced into the back of the throat (Figs. 102 and 103). A catheter of soft rubber, size No. 14 or 16 French, attached to a DeLee mucous trap is very satisfactory. The opening of the catheter must be at the end or along the side very near the end. There must be no openings a little higher up since any efforts at suction on the catheter may only result in drawing air up through one or more of the openings that do not reach down to the level of the mucus. Suction is made on the glass trap as the catheter is placed as far back as possible into the baby's throat. The position of the catheter should be changed frequently during this procedure. Postural drainage can be used at the same time that the suctioning is done (Fig. 103). It is sometimes a little easier to get the catheter into a good position if the baby's head is allowed to drop slightly backward by elevating the shoulders than if he lies on a flat surface. The suctioning of mucus from the baby's mouth and throat with an ear syringe or a catheter is a procedure that the nurse can use at any time if more mucus accumulates after the respiratory passages have been cleared; this equipment should be readily available in the nursery. If obstruction with mucus is in the lower air passages a catheter, for aspiration of mucus, may be passed into the trachea either by direct visualization with a laryngoscope, of infant size, or with a finger guiding the catheter. Passing the catheter requires personnel skilled in performing the procedure. In cases of severe asphyxia the catheter which has been placed into the trachea may be left in place while oxygen is administered and while artificial respiration is carried out if necessary. With the catheter in place there is assurance of an open respiratory tract, and oxygen will reach the lungs more adequately. The tracheal catheter may be left in place until respiratory movements are well established. Oxygen should be administered in an incubator, and the baby must be observed very closely for need of further aspiration.

There are many ways of stimulating respirations. Sometimes after the air passages have been cleared skin stimulation is sufficient. Contact of the cool air in the delivery room with the skin furnishes some stimulation. The blowing of cold air over the baby has frequently been recommended, but this will chill the baby and the opinion of many is that the body heat should be conserved as much as possible. The skin may also be stimulated by rubbing the back, by gently spanking the buttocks, or by spanking the bottom of the feet.

When these simpler methods are inadequate in promoting normal respirations, artificial respiration becomes necessary. Direct inflation is sometimes employed by doing mouth-to-mouth breathing (Fig. 200). The baby's face is covered with two or three pieces of clean dry gauze, and the person giving the artificial respiration places his mouth over the baby's mouth and nose and breathes normally at the rate of 12 to 15 times per minute. If the baby's nose is not covered it must be held closed so that air will not come out through it. This procedure must be done gently, no more vigorously than normal breathing, so that the lungs are not injured. A small amount of chest movement is sufficient to indicate that the procedure is being done vigorously enough. Since air breathed into the baby's nose and mouth may enter either the stomach or lungs, the operator's hand should make slight pressure over the epigastrium to prevent the stomach from being filled by air. The elastic recoil of the baby's lungs will usually deflate them, but expiration will be favored by slight pressure on the baby's chest. Here again there is a difference of opinion, and the nurse will find that some doctors will disapprove of this method of resuscitation. Their reasons are that the pressure which is exerted may be so great as to rupture alveoli and that a

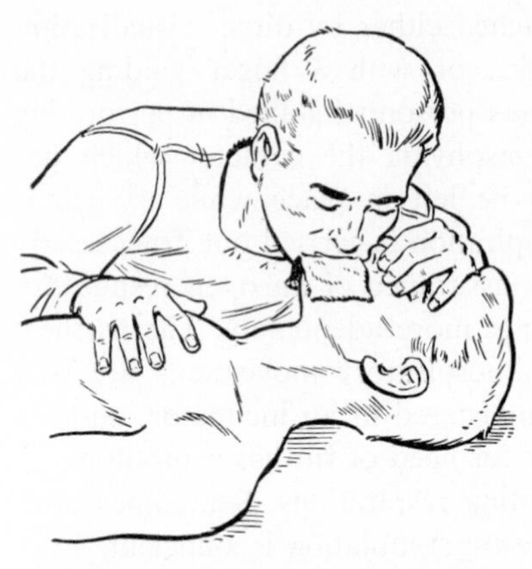

**Fig. 200.** With his left hand the operator holds the subject's nose closed while he blows into the mouth intermittently. A handkerchief or other light material prevents contamination. The operator's right hand rests lightly on the chest in order that he may appreciate when air is entering the lungs. (Waters, Ralph M.: "Simple Methods for Performing Artificial Respiration," *J.A.M.A.,* **123**:561 (Oct. 30), 1943.

*Note:* Resuscitation of the newborn is carried out in the same manner; however, it is important that the resuscitator's expirations are not too forceful.

respiratory infection may be communicated to the baby from the doctor or nurse. This method, however, is often very effective and is one that is always immediately available.

A mask and bag filled with oxygen can also be used for inflation of the lungs. Again pressure on the bag should be applied very gently; chest expansion must not be forced. If expiratory movements do not take place when pressure on the bag is released, they can be produced by applying pressure to the baby's chest. The movements of the chest should be watched during this procedure.

Artificial respiration can also be carried out by intermittent compression of the lower portion of the chest. With the fingers supporting the baby's back the lower anterior chest wall may be pressed down and in with the thumbs of one or both hands and then again released at the rate of 12 to 15 times per minute. Another method is to compress the chest from the sides with the thumb on one side of the chest and the fingers on the other side. All of this must be done gently in order to prevent injury.

Since it is very important to get an adequate oxygen supply to the baby's tissues as quickly as possible, oxygen should be administered by holding a tube, from which oxygen is flowing freely, in front of the baby's face while artificial respiration is carried out.

Respirators which supply oxygen and automatically carry out artificial respiration are not ordinarily necessary, and their use has not always proved to be entirely satisfactory. They may be of some value where the infant is under the effect of drugs and artificial respiration must be continued for some time. Usually a tracheal catheter must be left in place.

Regardless of the method of resuscitation it must never be carried out too vigorously. The baby is frequently already in shock, and vigorous treatment may be more harmful than beneficial.

Stimulants such as alpha-lobeline, caffeine sodium benzoate, pentylenetetrazol (Metrazol), and nikethamide (Coramine) are sometimes used if the baby remains asphyxiated after oxygen is given, but their value has remained questionable, and the difference between the therapeutic and toxic dose is quite narrow. When asphyxia is believed to be due to morphine or its derivatives which have been used for maternal analgesia, nalorphine (Nalline) 0.2 to 0.25 mg may counteract central nervous system depression.

Adequate warmth and gentle handling are very important during resuscitation. The baby should be kept warm by keeping him covered with warmed blankets or if prolonged efforts are necessary by carrying them out with the baby placed in a heated bassinet. Putting the baby in an incubator as soon as possible will help to supply warmth as well as oxygen.

After respirations have been established, the administration of oxygen should be continued for a period of a few hours or even 24 hours or longer depending upon the baby's color, the normalcy of breathing, and the general behavior of the infant. Even when the baby remains alert and cries spontaneously after he has once responded, oxygen may be administered for a few hours. The concentration of oxygen that is used following asphyxia may be anywhere from 30 to 60 per cent depending upon the color of the baby and the depth and rate of respirations. Whenever the higher concentration of oxygen is used at first, it is gradually reduced to below 40 per cent if the baby seems to do as well in a lower concentration. This is particularly important if the infant is immature. The body heat must be adequately maintained. Suction equipment should be available at all times, and the nurses should aspirate the mouth and oropharynx whenever mucus accumulates. It is advantageous to place the baby who has been asphyxiated in an incubator where the heat and oxygen can easily be regulated and where care similar to that given a premature baby can be provided. Feedings are usually withheld for a period of 24 hours or longer. The baby who has had asphyxia at birth may appear to be in fairly good condition after respirations have been established or he may continue to show evidence of severe respiratory distress for some time as characterized by labored respirations with periods of apnea, cyanosis, a feeble cry, poor or absent sucking reflex, limpness due to poor muscle tone, and petechial hemorrhages and areas of ecchymosis. When the baby has been narcotized as a result of deep maternal analgesia and anesthesia it may not only be difficult to initiate breathing, but the baby may continue to respond sluggishly even after he has cried. Frequent skin stimulation and change of position may be necessary until the effects of the anesthesia have worn off and respirations are normal. When recovery seems to have taken place following asphyxia the baby must be carefully watched for the next day or two for recurrence of respiratory difficulty. The nurse must realize that any baby, regardless of how good his condition seemed at birth, who later develops noisy breathing, shallow rapid respirations, more than average cyanosis of extremities, or periods of generalized cyanosis is having some respiratory disturbance and is in need of treatment.

## CONGENITAL ATELECTASIS

This condition may be described as an incomplete expansion of the lungs which persists for a longer than normal period of time postnatally. The lungs are atelectatic before birth; after birth they expand in a fairly systematic pattern. As expansion takes place it does so by an increase in the number of alveoli that are aerated rather than by an increase in the volume of each alveolus so that areas of atelectasis are present among areas of aerated lung tissue. Expansion is normally not complete for several days, but gaseous exchange is adequate during the early days of life in which this expansion is taking place. Atelectasis is closely associated with asphyxia or periods of apnea; when the infant does not breathe normally the expansion of the lungs does not progress at a normal rate.

Some atelectasis may be due to the natural cohesion of the moist surfaces. Surface tension is a large factor in the resistance of the lungs to aeration, but aspiration of fluid and debris and weak respiratory movements may contribute to inadequate lung expansion, this being true especially in cases where atelectasis is prolonged. Among the more common causes are obstruction of the bronchi with mucus and constituents of amniotic fluid, a poorly functioning respiratory center due to cerebral damage, immaturity of the respiratory tract as in the premature infant, and congestion and edema of the lungs.

Signs and symptoms of atelectasis depend upon the amount of involvement. A small degree of atelectasis may not present signs or symptoms, but large areas will give evidence of respiratory distress. A respiratory grunt which is loud enough to be heard throughout the nursery may be present. The respirations are rapid and shallow, and respiratory movements are almost entirely abdominal. Cyanosis may be continuous or intermittent; the baby's color improves with the administration of oxygen and stimulation to cry. Mucus, which is sometimes quite tenacious, may be present in the respiratory tract. The thorax may not expand well on one or both sides, and a retraction below the sternum and the lowest ribs may be noticeable. An x-ray will usually reveal the amount of unexpanded lung tissue.

**Prophylaxis** is directed toward preventing intrauterine hypoxia and asphyxia and aspiration of mucus postnatally.

**Treatment** consists largely of attempting to open the air passages, supplying oxygen, and avoiding extra exertion. When atelectasis is due to obstruction every effort should be made to open the airway. Immediate removal of any mucus and amniotic fluid present in the oral cavity and the oropharynx is important. Aspiration through a laryngoscope may be necessary, and even a bronchoscopic aspiration may occasionally be indicated when the lower air passages are obstructed. Removal of foreign material may bring immediate improvement. Postural drainage, obtained by elevation of the foot of the mattress at a 20- to 30-deg angle, and frequent aspiration of the upper air passages may be indicated for removal of mucus which may accumulate later. Since the amount of functioning lung tissue is diminished it is important to keep the baby in an atmosphere of 30 to 40 per cent oxygen concentration, or higher for a short period if the severity of the condition so indicates. This is usually administered in an incubator. The humidity of the atmosphere is increased to 100 per cent (pp. 700–771). A change of position every one to two hours is important to prevent further atelectasis due to hypostasis. Pulmonary expansion should be induced as much as possible; stimulating the baby to cry at hourly intervals is one effective means. Other treatment consists of maintaining an adequate body temperature, withholding feedings for 48 hours or longer, and administration of antibiotics to prevent infection.

Prognosis depends upon how well and how quickly the lungs become adequately expanded. If death occurs it is usually within 48 hours after birth. Infection may be a complicating factor. If there are any sequelae they are caused by the amount of damage due to hypoxia of the central nervous system.

### HYALINE MEMBRANE DISEASE

In this condition a material called a *hyaline membrane* lines the alveoli or plugs the alveolar ducts and interferes with gaseous exchange. Atelectasis is commonly associated with hyaline membrane disease, and is then called *resorption atelectasis,* because the lungs seem to have been relatively well expanded at first and then collapse again. The cause of the formation of this membrane is not known. Diagnosis is made on the basis of clinical signs and symptoms. Babies that are particularly susceptible to this complication are immature infants, those born by cesarean section, those born to mothers with diabetes and toxemias of pregnancy, and infants that have had intrauterine distress.

These babies develop respiratory distress shortly after birth or within a period of several hours. The respirations become rapid and grunting or moaning in character. This condition may soon improve again, or may remain the same for a period of time, but usually progresses to a severe stage. As the condition becomes severe, dyspnea develops, chest retraction is observed, and cyanosis appears. Respiratory distress may last two to four days and may cause death. If the infant survives, breathing becomes easier on about the third or fourth day, improvement is rapid, and recovery appears to be complete in five to seven days.

**Treatment** consists of placing the baby in an incubator in order to carefully control the environment—oxygen, humidity, and temperature. Oxygen is usually administered in a 30 to 40 per cent concentration unless it appears that a higher concentration improves the baby's condition. The atmosphere of the incubator is supersaturated with a mist of either water or a detergent such as an aqueous solution (Alevaire) that contains superinone, sodium bicarbonate, and glycerin. Supersaturation is obtained by the use of an atomizer or nebulizer through which the water or detergent is added to the atmosphere in the form of a cloud of very small or microscopic drops (Fig. 201). Postural drainage, obtained by elevation of the foot of the mattress at a 15- to 30-deg angle, is used. Mucus is aspirated from the mouth and oropharynx as it appears. The baby's position is changed frequently. Feedings are withheld for two to four days, usually during the entire period of respiratory distress. Antibiotics are administered to prevent respiratory infection.

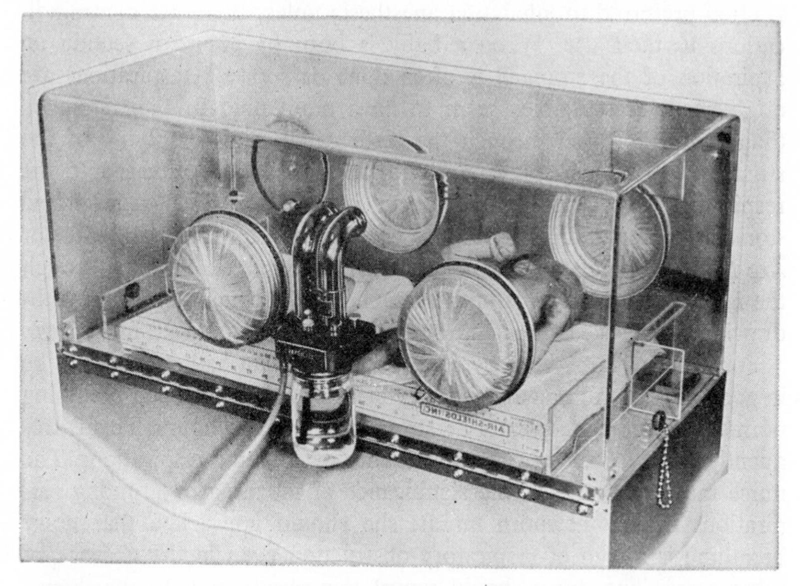

**Fig. 201.** The Vapojette supersaturation attachment on an Isolette infant incubator. (Courtesy of Air-Shields, Inc.; Hatboro, Pennsylvania.)

**Prevention.** Early and complete clearing of the respiratory tract by postural drainage and aspiration of the oropharynx is considered important. Although it is not known if supersaturation of the atmosphere has a specific effect, this treatment is often used prophylactically for immature infants, for babies delivered by cesarean section, for infants that had asphyxia at birth, and for babies that apparently had intrauterine distress as evidenced by meconium in the amniotic fluid. The baby is kept in this atmosphere until the danger of hyaline membrane formation is past or for a period of approximately 24 hours.

*Respiratory distress following birth by cesarean section* seems to be more common than following delivery through the birth canal; this appears to be true even when analgesic drugs and a general anesthetic have not been used. This difficulty may be caused by the complication which has necessitated delivery by cesarean section, but sometimes the asphyxia seems to be due to the method of delivery. Since asphyxia is more common in these infants every effort is made to reduce the danger of respiratory difficulty. Depressant drugs are not given to the mother before delivery of the baby, and a spinal or local anesthetic is often preferred to inhalation anesthesia unless there are contraindications to their use. When a baby is born by cesarean section an aspiration of the stomach is often done as soon as respirations are established; these babies seem to have more fluid in their stomach than those delivered through the birth canal. This emptying of the stomach will help to prevent aspiration of fluid and mucus into the respiratory tract which might occur in case the baby regurgitated stomach contents. This procedure can be done by passing a catheter size No. 14 French (No. 10 French for a premature infant) through the mouth and esophagus until it reaches the stomach and then withdrawing the gastric contents through the catheter with a 20-ml syringe.

Sometimes a baby born by cesarean section that had appeared to be in good condition immediately after birth and that has been breathing normally develops respiratory distress in one to two hours. This is frequently first suspected by the appearance of moaning respirations. The nurse must be aware of the significance of moaning or grunting respirations in any newborn infant; she should appreciate that noisy breathing is a sign of respiratory obstruction even in the absence of other signs. The nurse should report this observation to the doctor immediately in order to make early treatment possible.

## PROGNOSIS FOLLOWING RESPIRATORY DISTRESS

Prognosis depends upon the degree of asphyxia and the length of time that it existed. Delayed respirations may cause permanent damage to brain tissue, and the postnatal complications in the babies who have had asphyxia are greater than in those who have had no respiratory difficulty. Therefore, the incidence of atelectasis, respiratory infection, increased irritability, cerebral hemorrhage, and/or cerebral deficiency is greater.

The newborn infant can tolerate hypoxia to a greater degree than an older individual, but the longer the period of hypoxia, the greater are the chances of damage to the central nervous system. The brain cells may be able to survive several minutes without oxygen—four minutes have most frequently been cited as the maximum time that they can survive without some oxygen; sometimes the time is stated to be longer. It is important to remember, however, that even short periods of apnea may produce irreparable pathologic changes; irreversible changes may occur in less than one minute. The length of time that hypoxia can be tolerated after birth may be influenced by the amount of hypoxia the baby suffered in utero.

Certainly not all asphyxiated infants have nervous system manifestations, but the possibility must be considered. Damage may vary from a very mild degree which is quite inconspicuous to a severe degree resulting in convulsions, mental retardation, behavior problems, or cerebral palsy. Hypoxia may produce severe damage to much of the tissue or it may be partial and thus affect one area, leaving defects in either motor control or intellectual ability. Late effects of asphyxia may thus be manifested by defective physical, mental, nervous, or emotional development although there may be no evidence of permanent brain damage unless the asphyxia has been severe and prolonged.

## PNEUMONIA

Pneumonia may follow atelectasis; aspiration of amniotic fluid, meconium, or vaginal secretions during birth; aspiration of vomitus after birth; or it may be caused by a bacterial or virus infection. It may develop in utero or shortly after birth when labor is prolonged or when the membranes have ruptured early or be acquired after birth. Intrauterine asphyxia, difficult resuscitation, respiratory distress in the early neonatal period, and poor respiratory movements in the weak infant or the one with atelectasis or cerebral damage are predisposing factors.

This condition may involve different lobules rather than one lobe. Onset is insidious; clinical manifestations may be absent, or there may be some apparent respiratory distress, shallow breathing, and limited thoracic movement. The baby may have signs of a generalized infection with fever and listlessness, but fever may not be present. Diagnosis is by x-ray.

**Prevention** is important. If the membranes rupture early or labor is prolonged, prophylactic use of antibiotic drugs is usually instituted to prevent intrapartum infection of both the mother and the baby with infected amniotic fluid. Immediate aspiration of the upper respiratory tract, before the infant breathes, helps to prevent aspiration pneumonia. Infants with respiratory distress are given antibiotic therapy as a preventive measure against infection. Excluding all personnel with any signs of respiratory infection from the nursery reduces the chances of bacterial invasion.

**Treatment** consists largely of the administration of oxygen and antibiotics. Oxygen is given in a 30 to 50 per cent concentration, depending upon the degree of respiratory distress and cyanosis. Nutritional needs should be met, and adequate fluid intake should be maintained. If the baby does not suck well, feedings by Breck feeder or gavage may be necessary. Parenteral fluids may be indicated, depending upon ability to take fluids. The baby must be isolated to protect other infants in the nursery from infection.

## DISTURBANCES OF THE BLOOD

### HEMORRHAGIC DISEASE OF THE NEWBORN

This is a rare disease characterized by *spontaneous* and *prolonged bleeding,* either internally or externally, during the first week of life, especially between the second and fifth day. It is not associated with definite trauma or disease, but rather with the period of hypoprothrombinemia that is normal in newborn infants at this time of life; there is no proof, however, that this is entirely the cause of the disease. Bleeding occurs from various sites: (1) the skin, showing areas of ecchymosis, (2) the umbilical cord, (3) the conjunctiva or retina, (4) the nose, (5) the gastrointestinal tract as manifested by bleeding from the mouth, vomiting of blood, or melena neonatorum, (6) the lungs, (7) the genitourinary tract producing hematuria, or (8) the central nervous system. Bleeding may arise from several areas in the same baby. Onset is usually gradual, but may be abrupt. It may be started by minimal trauma, but is apt to be entirely spontaneous. Coagulation time is frequently, but not always excessively, prolonged.

**Prognosis** is good with immediate treatment. It depends upon the severity of the bleeding and its site; intracranial hemorrhage is more serious than bleeding from other areas, especially if these areas are external.

**Prophylactic** administration of vitamin K either to the mother during late pregnancy or labor or to the baby after birth prevents the normal physiologic drop in prothrombin level and may prevent hemorrhagic disease. Vitamin K is administered to all infants by some doctors; by others it is not given to all babies because of the rarity of the disease, but is administered to premature infants, who have a greater hemorrhagic tendency than full-term babies, and to those babies that have been delivered with difficulty and may be handicapped by trauma or asphyxia. Any surgery which can be postponed, such as circumcision, is more safely performed after one week of age. When surgery becomes necessary earlier, vitamin K is given preoperatively.

**Treatment** of active bleeding consists of the administration of vitamin K to increase the available prothrombin, repeated at intervals until the prothrombin level is normal, and blood transfusion of whole fresh blood (5 to 10 ml per pound of body weight) which will quickly raise the prothrombin level. Transfusions may be repeated if necessary to control bleeding or replace blood loss.

## ERYTHROBLASTOSIS FETALIS

This is a disease of the blood in late fetal or early neonatal life which occurs in infants in whom there is an incompatibility between the baby's and the mother's blood. In this disease there is maternal sensitization to antigens that are present in the fetal cells; the antibodies that are produced then pass back into the fetal circulation and there destroy red blood cells, sometimes to a severe degree. In order to compensate for the loss of cells this process is accompanied by an overdevelopment of the erythropoietic tissue in the bone marrow, the liver, and the spleen. Anemia and jaundice occur as a result of the erythrocyte destruction, and there are many nucleated red blood cells in the circulating blood due to hyperactivity of the blood-forming tissue.

**The Rh factor,** which is usually the *cause* of the incompatibility between the mother and infant, consists of several antigens which are found in red blood cells; it is similar to the factors *A, B,* and *O* that determine blood groups. Persons whose blood is agglutinated by anti-Rh serum are called Rh-positive; those whose blood is not agglutinated by this serum are called Rh-negative. About 85 per cent of the white population is Rh-positive; the other 15 per cent is therefore Rh-negative. There are fewer Rh-negative persons in the Negro population than among white people and still less in the Oriental race.

Landsteiner and Wiener discovered the Rh factor in 1940 in their work with the Rhesus monkey from which this factor takes its name. Although the signs, the familial tendency, and the hemolytic anemia of erythroblastosis had been known for many years and an understanding of the disease had increased from time to time, its exact etiology was not known until 1941 when Levine and his co-workers demonstrated an abnormal agglutinin in the blood serum of mothers who had erythroblastotic babies. This antibody agglutinated or clumped the red blood cells of the infant and the father; a factor was identified in their red blood cells which was absent in the mother's cells.

There are six common Rh antigens; these are called *C, c, D, d, E,* and *e.* Each of these antigens can stimulate the production of its particular antibody. These antigens are associated with three pairs of genes in the same chromosome. The chromosomes are found in pairs—one of each pair is derived from the mother and one from the father. Of that pair of chromosomes carrying the Rh genes one of the pair, therefore, carries those inherited from the mother, which may be a *C* or *c,* and a *D* or *d,* and an *E* or *e,* and the other one in the pair carries those inherited from the father which will also be a *C* or *c,* and a *D* or *d,* and an *E* or *e.* The chromosome does not carry both a *C* and *c,* a *D* and *d,* and an *E* or *e;* it must be either a large-letter or small-letter gene.

The kind of Rh genes that the chromosomes in an individual carry can be determined by laboratory tests with the use of anti-serum to the various antigens. Determination of the Rh genes present in the chromosomes of an individual is called *genotyping.* It is evident that there can be many combinations or Rh genotypes, but some of the commonest ones are *CDe/cde, CDe/CDe, cde/cde, CDe/cDE,* and *cDE/cde.*

Although it may at times be of clinical importance to know the genotype of a person, the majority of laboratory studies done on individuals are concerned only with whether a person is Rh-positive or Rh-negative. This is because the *D* antigen is responsible for most of the dangers due to Rh antigens. Clinically, therefore, the term Rh-positive is regarded to mean D-positive and Rh-negative to mean

D-negative. When the *D* gene is absent from a chromosome that chromosome has a *d* gene instead. The Rh-positive individual may have 2 *D* genes designated as *DD* in which case he is homozygous or one *D* and one *d* gene designated as *Dd* or heterozygous. Whenever there is one *D* gene present in a pair the individual is Rh-positive. If both genes in a pair of chromosomes are *dd* the person is said to be Rh-negative. As these genes are passed on to the offspring only one of a pair is inherited from each parent. If the father is *DD* (homozygous) all of the spermatozoa carry a *D* gene and all of his children will be Rh-positive. If he is *Dd* (heterozygous) half of the spermatozoa carry a *D* gene and half a *d;* a mating with an Rh-negative woman (*dd*) means that half of his children could be expected to be *Dd* (Rh-positive) and half *dd* (Rh-negative). (See Fig. 202.) The *C* and *c* and *E* and *e* genes are inherited in the same way; an ovum and a spermatozoan carry either a *C* or *c* and an *E* or *e*.

This Rh-positive factor or *D* antigen may stimulate in the Rh-negative person, the one who does not have the *D* antigen, the formation of antibodies which destroy Rh-positive (D-positive) red blood cells. This stimulation can occur when an Rh-negative (D-negative) person is transfused with Rh-positive (D-positive) blood or when red blood cells of an Rh-positive (D-positive) fetus pass through the placenta into the blood of an Rh-negative (D-negative) mother. Therefore, if the fetus is Rh-positive and some of its blood substances pass through the placental barrier into the circulation of a mother who is Rh-negative, she may produce antibodies to the fetal red cell antigens. The antibodies then pass back from the mother's blood into the fetal circulation and combine with its Rh-positive cells to destroy them.

The mating of an Rh-positive male with an Rh-negative female occurs about 14 times in 100, but the incidence of erythroblastosis is only approximately one in 200 births. Since immunization of the mother is slow, sensitization severe enough to cause the disease usually does not occur until after one or more pregnancies. Every pregnancy is not harmful. In some cases the fetus may be Rh-negative. Even when the fetus is Rh-positive the fetal blood substances are not always able to pass into the mother's circulation through the placenta which should be impervious to formed substances. If these substances do pass through to the mother she is not always able to produce antibodies. A first-born child is usually not affected unless the mother

MOTHER FATHER

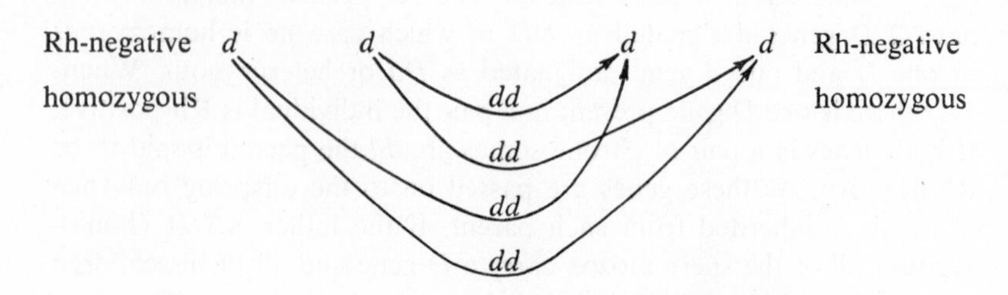


Illustrating a combination in which all of the ova and all of the spermatozoa carry a *d* gene. All of the children in this mating are therefore *dd* (Rh-negative).

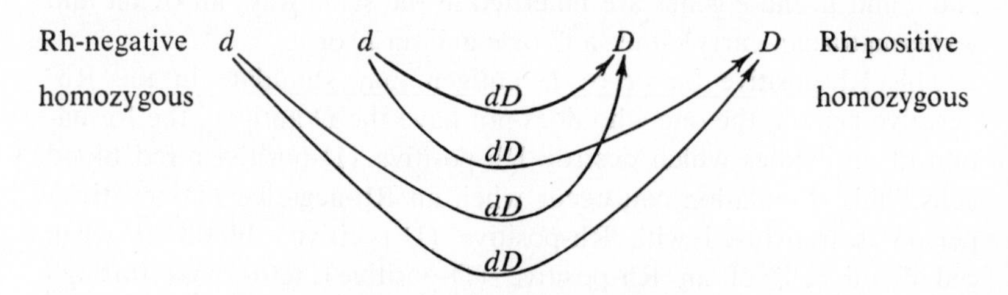


A combination in which all of the ova carry a *d* gene and all of the spermatozoa a *D* gene. All of the children in this mating are therefore *dD* (Rh-positive).

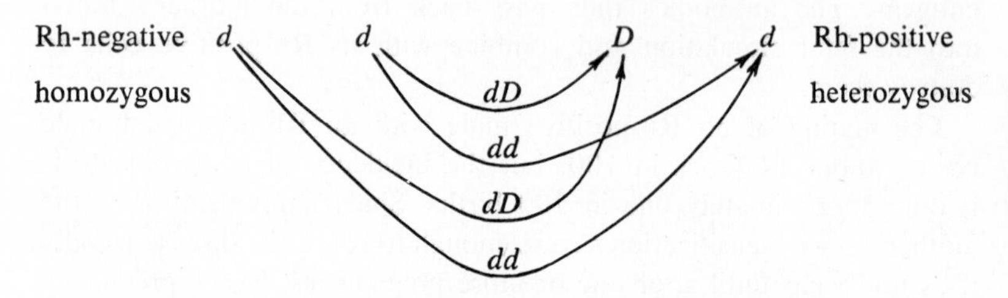


In this situation all of the ova carry a *d* gene, but half of the spermatozoa carry a *D* gene and half a *d*. In this mating half of the children can be expected to be *dd* (Rh-negative) and half *dD* (Rh-positive).

**Fig. 202.** Illustration of the inheritance of the Rh genes, *D* and *d*. The *C* and *c* and *E* and *e* genes are inherited in the same manner.

has been sensitized by a previous pregnancy which has ended in an abortion, by a transfusion with Rh-positive blood, or possibly by an intramuscular injection of blood at some time earlier in her life. (The administration of intramuscular blood was previously a form of treatment for some diseases of infancy.) Antibodies are certain to be present in the mother following a transfusion with Rh-positive blood because there is no doubt that these cells have entered the mother's blood stream as there may be concerning other routes. A subsequent pregnancy with an Rh-positive fetus is quite apt to result in an infant that has erythroblastosis fetalis. In the present day, transfusions are not done without checking for compatibility for the Rh factor as well as the blood group, but some Rh-negative women who have been transfused with Rh-positive blood had their transfusions before the Rh factor was discovered and before its ability to stimulate antibody production was known.

Whenever a mother has once developed a concentration of antibodies sufficient to have caused hemolysis in an infant, subsequent pregnancies with an Rh-positive fetus will cause hemolytic disease in that fetus because of the antibodies that are already present from a previous immunization and those that arise in response to further stimulation by the present pregnancy.

Although almost all cases of erythroblastosis fetalis are due to antibodies against the *D* antigen this disease is occasionally caused by antibodies to one of the other Rh antigens. Sometimes the disease is associated with an incompatibility between the mother and baby in the *A, B, O* blood groups in which case anti-A or anti-B antibodies may be produced in the mother and subsequently enter the infant's blood and there cause destruction of red blood cells. The mother in these cases may be Rh-positive and yet her baby develops the disease. Although the disease is not ordinarily anticipated in an infant born to an Rh-positive mother, all infants must be carefully observed for the appearance of jaundice in the first 24 to 36 hours of life because an incompatibility may exist between mother and baby due to a blood factor other than the *D* antigen. Erythroblastosis fetalis due to an *A* or *B* incompatibility is as apt to affect first-born as subsequent infants. Whenever jaundice appears early in life, laboratory studies are necessary to determine the severity of red blood cell destruction in the infant and to determine whether or not treatment is necessary. Laboratory studies on the infant's and the mother's blood which include blood grouping, genotyping, and antibody titration will determine whether or not an incompatibility exists and if so to which particular blood factor.

**Signs and Symptoms.** The classical signs of this disease are anemia, jaundice, and edema. In the individual baby any one of these signs may predominate. The disease may be present in a mild or severe form or in any degree between these two extremes. If all three of the major signs are present the disease is in its most severe form.

The clinical manifestations of the disease and the laboratory findings are largely due to hemolysis of red blood cells caused by the antibody-antigen reaction, the resultant end products of hemolysis, and the great increase that takes place in blood production and extramedullary erythropoiesis because of the hemolysis. Large numbers of *immature blood cells,* especially nucleated red cells, are found in the blood. The normal infant has from 200 to 2000 nucleated red blood cells per microliter of blood whereas the erythroblastotic infant has from 10,000 to 100,000 and even 500,000 nucleated erythrocytes per microliter of blood during the first 48 hours of life. This means more than 10 and usually from 25 to 200 nucleated red blood cells per 100 white blood cells. Normally the number of nucleated erythrocytes should not exceed 10 per 100 white blood cells at any time during the newborn period. The nucleated red blood cells in the erythroblastotic infant diminish and disappear within a few days after birth, but this finding does not mean an improvement in the condition.

*Anemia* is present at birth or it may develop any time during the newborn period. In mild untreated cases it may become pronounced in a week or two, and the baby begins to appear quite pale. The erythrocytes may, however, be destroyed so rapidly that even where there is only a slight suggestion of anemia at birth it may become quite evident within 12 hours and profound within a day or two. The erythrocytes may decrease as rapidly as a million cells per microliter per day. At birth or within a few days thereafter, the hemoglobin may range from 4 to 10 gm per 100 ml of blood (25 to 60 per cent) and the red blood cells from 1,000,000 to 3,000,000 cells per microliter. Whenever the hemoglobin level is less than 15 gm per 100 ml at birth and the red blood cell count less than 4,500,000 cells per microliter, the baby must be closely observed for severe anemia if treatment is not instituted immediately.

*Jaundice* is rarely seen at birth, but develops rapidly. It may appear within a few hours, or even within one hour, or sometime during the first day. It becomes increasingly severe and frequently masks the pallor of the anemia.

*Serum bilirubin* accumulates rapidly after birth, and figures as high as 50 and 60 mg per 100 ml of blood have been reported. (The bilirubin level at the height of physiologic jaundice does not rise above 5 or at the most 10 mg per 100 ml.) This high level of bilirubin in erythroblastosis fetalis is due to inability of the liver to clear the large amounts that result from the rapid destruction of the erythrocytes.

Jaundice may persist for several weeks in untreated cases, but if by treatment with blood replacement the serum bilirubin is not allowed to go over 20 mg per 100 ml of blood, jaundice will decrease rapidly after one to two days.

*Kernicterus,* or jaundice of the nuclear masses of the brain, may develop in the jaundiced baby between the second and sixth day of life. It is directly related to the severity of the jaundice. This is an unfavorable sign because most infants with this complication soon die or if they survive they frequently have brain damage which results in motor disability, mental retardation, and nervous manifestations. Clinical signs of kernicterus include severe jaundice, increasing lethargy, poor sucking, and loss of the Moro reflex. A rigidity, spasms, and an opisthotonic position are likely to develop. Respirations may be irregular and gasping, and death may be caused by pulmonary hemorrhage. Immaturity strongly predisposes to the development of kernicterus and is a contraindication to the early termination of pregnancy in an effort to avoid the effects of increasing antibodies in the mother's blood. Kernicterus is more common in the male than in the female infant. High maternal antibody titer prediposes to its development.

The *liver* and *spleen* become *enlarged* due to increased hematopoietic activity. They may be enlarged enough to be palpable at birth or may become palpable during the first week. Cardiac enlargement and murmurs may be present.

The *placenta* may be normal in size or it may be considerably enlarged. The *vernix caseosa* may be normal or it may have a golden-yellow color, and the amniotic fluid may be greenish yellow in appearance.

*Universal edema* (hydrops fetalis) may develop, but is usually found only in stillborn infants or in those that die within a few hours after birth (Fig. 203). The baby with hydrops fetalis is very waxy

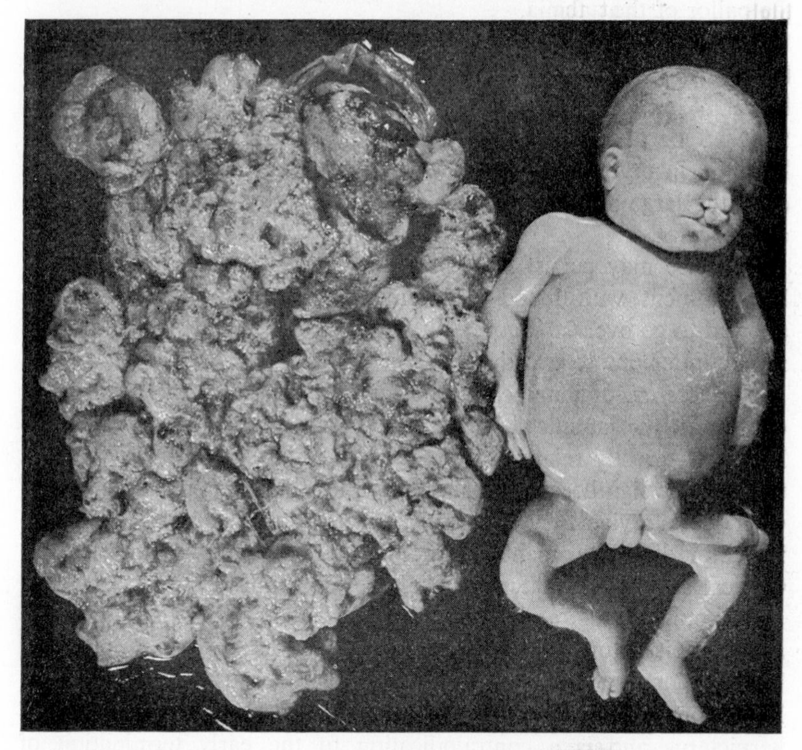

**Fig. 203.** A stillborn infant with hydrops type of erythroblastosis fetalis. The placenta is also markedly edematous and shows large prominent cotyledons. (Courtesy of Dr. Madeline J. Thornton.)

in appearance, has much fluid in all of its tissues, and has a very low hemoglobin level and red blood cell count.

**Course.** The disease may be so mild that there are no clinical signs of illness or it may result in such profound changes that death occurs in utero. Between these two extremes there are all degrees of illness. Many liveborn babies appear to be in good condition at birth, but rapidly become worse; this course must always be anticipated. Possible outcomes are (1) recovery with no clinical evidence of the disease, (2) recovery from a mild or severe anemia, (3) death from a severe anemia and edema, (4) development of kernicterus and recovery with or without central nervous system damage, (5) death due to kernicterus, or (6) stillbirth.

If the infant succumbs to a profound anemia, death usually occurs within the first 24 hours. This severe form of anemia, which is present at birth, is usually accompanied by a marked enlargement of the liver and spleen and by edema. If the baby survives this early period, the danger from anemia is lessened, but it is essential that the blood picture is watched carefully and treatment is adequate (pp. 786–88); the danger of the development of kernicterus is always present. Many of the deaths due to kernicterus and pulmonary hemorrhage occur between the second and sixth day of life, but some of these babies survive for part of the first year. More adequate treatment in recent years has done much to prevent kernicterus (pp. 786–87). Infants with hydrops fetalis are usually stillborn or they die soon after birth even when treatment is begun immediately.

**Prognosis.** In general, the chances of recovery for liveborn babies are good when treatment is adequate. After the first week prognosis is favorable, and there are no residual symptoms unless kernicterus has developed which may leave the baby with cerebral damage.

The first infant to be born after maternal sensitization can be demonstrated has a fairly good prognosis. When a sensitized mother has once had a child with the disease, any subsequent Rh-positive infants are in greater danger of having erythroblastosis with severe symptoms, and the chances of having a stillborn infant are greatly increased.

**Diagnosis.** The Rh type of all pregnant women should be determined at an early prenatal visit. If the woman is Rh-positive there is only a remote possibility of difficulty, and further studies are not indicated. If she is Rh-negative, her husband should also be typed, and if his blood is Rh-negative, there is no need to anticipate difficulty. Should he be Rh-positive the chances are still good that trouble will not be encountered, but the mother's blood should be examined both early and late in pregnancy for the presence of anti-Rh antibodies; whenever antibodies are found a titration should be made to determine the degree to which they are present.

In testing for antibodies it is necessary to check for both saline agglutinins and albumin agglutinins (blocking antibodies) since both may be present in the mother's blood. One kind, the saline agglutinins, produce clumping of cells when a physiologic saline solution is used for suspension of the cells that are used for the test. Albumin agglutinins (blocking antibodies) are another kind formed in the mother's blood; these are capable of combining with Rh-positive red blood cells to produce hemolysis, but they do not cause agglutination when the cells used for testing are suspended in a physiologic saline solution. Tests for albumin agglutinins must therefore be made with the red cells suspended in an albumin medium in which it is known that agglutination of cells will take place in the presence of these albumin, or blocking, antibodies. While albumin agglutinins will react only with an albumin suspension of red cells, the saline agglutinins will react with an albumin as well as a saline suspension of cells. Albumin agglutinins seem to appear in the blood later than saline agglutinins and seem to be indicative of a greater degree of immunization.

If there is a history of a preceding infant with the disease or if either saline or albumin agglutinins are found in the mother's blood, hemolytic disease can be anticipated unless the father is heterozygous and the baby to be born is Rh-negative. The detection of antibodies early in pregnancy, which indicates that sensitization had taken place before the present pregnancy, or the presence of high maternal titers, that is, large amounts of the antibody in the blood, are apt to lead to a severe form of the disease in the infant.

The mother pregnant with an erythroblastotic infant, especially with a severe type, frequently develops hydramnios and shows signs of toxemia early in her pregnancy.

When erythroblastosis is anticipated the baby must be carefully checked at the time of birth for all of the cardinal signs of the disease. Observation of the size and appearance of the placenta, the color of the vernix caseosa, and the color and general appearance of the infant is important. The liver and spleen should be palpated for an increase in size. It is necessary to collect blood specimens immediately, preferably from the umbilical cord (placental end), for determination of the Rh type, the Coombs test, the hemoglobin level, the erythrocyte count, and the nucleated red blood cell count.

A direct anti-human-globulin test (direct Coombs test) is very important in the diagnosis since it is positive when a baby has erythroblastosis due to an Rh-antigen incompatibility even in the absence of clinical evidence of the disease. The direct Coombs test is used to reveal the presence of maternal antibodies attached to the red blood cells of the baby. The red blood cells of an erythroblastotic baby may be coated with anti-Rh antibodies; these antibodies will cause hemolysis of the baby's cells, but may also interfere with the normal agglutinating activity of typing serum. The baby's cells are therefore not agglutinated with anti-Rh serum under ordinary methods of testing and thus appear to be Rh-negative. If the mother is known to have anti-Rh antibodies and the baby appears to be Rh-negative, it is necessary to exclude the possibility of a false Rh-negative reaction; this false reaction occurs when the maternal antibodies which have been absorbed on the surface of the baby's red blood cells interfere with the agglutination tests. A negative direct Coombs test excludes the presence of antibodies on the baby's red blood cells; a positive test indicates that antibodies are present on the surface of the cells. The Coombs test is not specific for anti-Rh antibodies, but in the newborn baby it can be assumed that the antibodies present are most likely antibodies to one of the Rh antigens. The diagnosis of erythroblastosis depends to a large extent upon demonstrating by the Coombs test that the baby's red blood cells are Rh-positive and are coated with anti-Rh antibodies unless the incompatibility is caused by the *A* and *B* group, in which case the Coombs test is not suitable.

The serum used for a Coombs test contains an anti-human-globulin antibody which is produced in rabbits by injecting them with human globulin. Any human globulin will combine with this antibody and neutralize it, but in erythroblastosis the human globulin that combines with it is the anti-Rh antibody which is attached to the baby's Rh-positive red blood cells. To make certain that the reaction is due only to this attached antibody, the red blood cells of the baby are thoroughly washed in physiologic saline to remove all of the baby's serum. If agglutination of red cells occurs after this washing it is then assumed to be due to the antibody which is attached to the cells, and the Coombs test is considered positive.

Other significant laboratory findings that aid in diagnosis and that give an indication of the degree of cell destruction are determinations of the hemoglobin level and the red blood cell and nucleated red cell count. The more severe the destruction of cells, the lower the hemoglobin and red blood cells and the higher the number of immature cells.

Other evidence of the disease, especially if treatment is not instituted immediately, includes the early appearance of jaundice and a rapidly rising serum bilirubin level.

Since erythroblastosis may be due to maternal sensitization to blood factors other than the *D* antigen, the nurse must always be alert to the early appearance of jaundice and report it to the doctor immediately. If jaundice appears earlier or is more severe than would seem to be normal for a physiologic jaundice (pp. 588–89), blood studies are necessary to rule out erythroblastosis. Normal babies are usually not jaundiced within 24 hours nor do they have over 5 or at the most 10 mg of bilirubin per 100 ml of blood during the first 24 hours of life. Jaundice, therefore, within the first 24 hours should be considered abnormal and may be a sign of erythroblastosis.

**Treatment.** Prompt care at the time of birth is the most important factor in the treatment of erythroblastosis fetalis and especially in the prevention of kernicterus. When the disease is anticipated from the past history and from studies made during pregnancy, it is essential (1) to have laboratory facilities available at the time of the baby's birth in order to do blood studies immediately, (2) to have blood available in case an immediate transfusion is indicated, and (3) to have an adequate staff and sufficient equipment ready to do the transfusion.

Blood transfusion is the only specific treatment known. The blood may be given in multiple small transfusions, as necessary to combat anemia, or as an *exchange,* or *replacement, transfusion,* a procedure by which most of the infant's Rh-positive blood is replaced by Rh-negative donor blood. Repeated small transfusions may be satisfactory for some infants, especially the mild cases, but exchange transfusion is the treatment of choice, particularly when used for more severe cases. It quickly restores the blood to a more normal picture and even more important it greatly improves the baby's chances of escaping kernicterus.

Small transfusions correct the anemia, but do not remove the baby's own cells which will still be hemolyzed; an exchange transfusion replaces these cells and immediately decreases the hemolytic process. Small transfusions increase the blood volume; this may be undesirable. With an exchange transfusion the anemia can be corrected more quickly than with small transfusions, and the blood volume can be controlled. By using 500 ml of blood for an exchange transfusion, which represents approximately twice the blood volume of a newborn infant, there is a 90 to 95 per cent exchange of blood. This removes from the baby's blood a large percentage of coated Rh-positive cells, many free antibodies, approximately one-third of the bilirubin, and possibly other products of red cell destruction. An exchange transfusion will prevent a large accumulation of bilirubin, and although it is not known how much bilirubin contributes to the cause of kernicterus it is known that there is a close relationship between the bilirubin level and kernicterus.

For maximum benefit from an exchange transfusion it must be done as soon after birth as possible. Jaundice is better controlled by immediate transfusion than by one done several hours later. This does not mean, however, that an exchange transfusion should not be done even after 24 to 48 hours after birth if it has not been performed earlier.

The decision to do an early exchange transfusion will rest upon the findings present at birth. The clinical manifestations of the disease are an indication for replacement of blood. An exchange transfusion is apt to be done even in the absence of signs of disease, provided that the Coombs test is positive and laboratory findings and past history indicate that some destruction of red blood cells is present or will occur, with the result that evidence of the disease appears later. Thus some of the indications for a replacement of blood besides the clinical evidence of the disease are the findings of a positive Coombs test in the presence of one of the following conditions: (1) a past history of erythroblastosis, (2) immaturity of the baby, (3) a maternal antibody titer of 1:16 or above, (4) a cord blood hemoglobin below 15 gm per 100 ml of blood, (5) a red blood cell count below 4,500,000 cells per microliter, and (6) the presence of many nucleated red blood cells. If an exchange transfusion is not done immediately after birth, appearance and rapid increase of jaundice and increase in bilirubin level to over 15 mg per 100 ml of blood are indications for a delayed transfusion. A serum bilirubin level is done daily or more frequently on these infants until there is a definite decrease.

Jaundice usually does not appear or is much less severe in babies that have been treated by replacement transfusion than in untreated infants, but if it does appear and seems to increase or if the serum bilirubin level increases to between 15 and 20 mg per 100 ml of blood, a second exchange transfusion may be given in approximately 24 hours.

The baby's blood must be carefully checked for anemia over a period of several weeks. Anemia ordinarily does not increase during the first week following an exchange transfusion, but it may develop to a greater degree during the next two or three weeks. The hemoglobin and erythrocyte blood levels may not become low enough to necessitate treatment; if they do become quite low a small transfusion is often given. Infants who have not had an exchange transfusion must be carefully observed for anemia for at least three weeks; a hemoglobin determination should be done daily for the first week and then twice a week for the next two weeks. If the hemoglobin falls below 9 gm per 100 ml during this time a small transfusion may be indicated. Blood is administered through a vein which can be entered quite easily, this frequently being a scalp vein. The amount of blood that is given is usually determined on the basis of 10 ml of blood per pound of body weight.

To perform an exchange transfusion several routes or technics may be used. The umbilical vein is preferred and can usually be used for the first three to four days; thereafter the extent of the thrombosis present in the vein makes it unavailable. If an exchange transfusion is done later than the third or fourth day it is usually necessary to use the femoral vein. A polyethylene catheter is introduced into the umbilical vein for a distance of 5 to 7.5 cm (2 or 3 in.) or it may be inserted far enough to reach the inferior vena cava. This catheter is attached to a stopcock, and blood is then withdrawn and injected with syringes. Ten to 20 ml of the infant's blood is alternately withdrawn and replaced with an equal amount of donor blood until 500 ml have been exchanged over a period of approximately one and one-half hours. If the venous pressure is high the amount of blood injected may be slightly less than that removed for the first few times or until the venous pressure is normal, but the deficit should not be over 80 to 100 ml. Since the blood may clot in the syringes and cause the barrel to stick in the plunger a sterile solution of heparin in saline (1 ml of heparin to 100 ml of physiologic saline solution) should be available for frequent rinsing of the syringes.

Rh-negative blood, preferably of the same group as the baby's or a group *O* if necessary, is used; as with any other transfusion it must be crossmatched for compatibility. Whole blood is usually used although blood concentrated by the removal of some plasma has been suggested. Blood drawn on the same day that it is used is desirable because it will not undergo as much initial hemolysis as older blood;

if fresh blood is not available, it should not be over four days old.

A small amount of calcium, 5 to 10 ml of a 10 per cent solution of calcium gluconate, is administered in divided doses of 1 to 2 ml after each 100 ml of blood. This is used to overcome any danger of tetany which may result from the large amount of sodium citrate in the donor blood. The nurse assisting with an exchange transfusion should have all the necessary equipment available and must make provisions for keeping the baby warm during the procedure and for the administration of oxygen during this time. Suction must also be available in case the baby is troubled with mucus during the transfusion.

Antibiotics, such as penicillin and streptomycin, are given prophylactically for a few days after a replacement transfusion. Although the procedure is performed under aseptic conditions, considerable manipulation is necessary, and bacteria may enter through the site of injection.

Babies with erythroblastosis are usually given oxygen in a concentration of 30 to 40 per cent before and for approximately 12 to 24 hours after transfusion. It must, of course, be administered with caution to an immature baby. To ensure adequate warmth, proper oxygen concentration, and careful observation these babies may be placed in an incubator for a day or two.

Anti-Rh antibodies are found in the breast milk of sensitized Rh-negative mothers. Although it is questionable that these ingested antibodies can do any harm—it is felt that no large amounts of antibodies are absorbed, unchanged, from the intestinal tract during the first few days of life and none thereafter—some doctors believe that the baby improves more rapidly when he is not breast-fed or at least not breast-fed for the first five to six days of life.

## INFECTIONS

Infections of the newborn infant may be acquired in utero or during passage through the birth canal, or acquired by direct contact with infected personnel and/or supplies. Syphilis and some of the virus infections, such as chickenpox, can be transmitted from the mother to the fetus through the placenta. Infants may develop an infection in utero when the amniotic fluid is infected. A Candida (Monilia) infection (thrush) or gonorrheal ophthalmia may be acquired during passage through the birth canal. Respiratory, gastrointestinal, and skin infections usually develop as a result of postnatal contact and thus appear after the first few days of life. Some infections are peculiar to the newborn infant; some have different manifestations in the newborn than in the older child. Against a few diseases, such as measles, the baby may be protected for a few months if the mother has an immunity to the disease; this protection is through placental transmission of antibodies. Infections of the newborn can be kept to a minimum with early diagnosis and treatment of diseases of the mother and with aseptic technic, sterile supplies, and cleanliness of equipment in the nursery.

## RESPIRATORY TRACT INFECTIONS

Although upper respiratory tract infections are not common in the newborn (this may be because of protection in the nursery), these babies are susceptible to diseases of the upper respiratory tract and they should be protected from exposure to them. Personnel with any evidence of respiratory disease must be excluded from the nursery, and the baby should be kept from contact with the mother if she has an acute cold. Visitors with a respiratory infection should not be allowed in the maternity unit. Babies with respiratory disease must be isolated to protect other infants in the nursery. A cold, by causing the mucous membranes of the nose to swell, may obstruct breathing and thus also make sucking difficult. Nose drops just before a feeding usually make sucking easier. Pneumonia, which is a serious disease of the newborn, has been discussed on pages 773–74.

## EPIDEMIC DIARRHEA OF THE NEWBORN

This is a highly contagious *acute diarrheal infection* occurring in the *newborn period,* which manifests itself by frequent loose stools, rapid loss of weight, dehydration, and acidosis. Severity of the disease varies in different epidemics and from one infant to another in the same epidemic. This is one of the most serious of newborn infections; although there may be no fatalities in some epidemics the average death rate is about 40 per cent of the affected infants. The etiology is rather obscure; it has not been possible to isolate a specific organism as the cause of epidemic diarrhea. Various microorganisms have been identified as the cause, or probable cause in different epidemics; strains of *E. coli* have been recognized as one causative agent. There is strong evidence that the infection may also be caused by viral agents. Epidemics occur in breast- and bottle-fed babies alike and at all seasons of the year. The newborn has no immunity; premature and weak infants are especially susceptible. The incubation period is short, usually just a few days.

**Signs and symptoms** vary considerably, and recognition of the first cases, which may be mild and which occur when an epidemic is not suspected, may be difficult. The recognition of epidemic diarrhea is difficult because the kind and number of stools that are normal for a newborn infant vary considerably; the transitional stools may normally be loose and frequent, and breast-fed babies often have frequent stools. Concern must always be shown over any intestinal disturbance of the newborn, and epidemic diarrhea must be considered if more than one or two infants have loose stools, the cause of which cannot be easily explained.

The onset of the illness may be insidious or rather sudden. With an insidious onset the prodromal signs are a loss of appetite, a stationary weight or a weight loss, listlessness with a feeble cry, and, at times, irritability and restlessness. Vomiting and abdominal distention may occasionally develop. The body temperature usually remains below 37.8° C (100° F); it rarely rises to 38.3° C (101° F). Diarrhea develops; the stools are usually described as watery, yellow in color (later greenish yellow), and acid; they do not contain pus or blood and contain little or no mucus. The first infants affected in an epidemic may not have severe symptoms; the only evidence may be a poor appetite, drowsiness, and increased frequency of loose, not necessarily watery, stools. In severe cases the baby may have from 20 to 30 stools per day which are expelled with explosive force.

As the disease progresses, and this progress may be rapid, weight loss continues and may be marked, dehydration becomes severe, the urine is scanty, acidosis develops, and the baby becomes very toxic. The color becomes ashen, the lips cherry red, the eyeballs and fontanels become sunken, and drowsiness and coma develop. The carbon dioxide combining power of the blood may be as low as 5 meq/L (11 volumes per cent), but it is not necessarily accompanied by very definite clinical evidence of acidosis. Since many newborns have a rather unstable acid-base and electrolyte balance their blood chemistry can very easily be changed to an abnormal state.

The clinical course of the disease may vary from a few days to a few weeks; relapses or exacerbations may occur. Complications of bronchopneumonia, otitis media, or septicemia may develop.

**Preventive** measures are very important. The same precautions that are necessary to prevent infections of any kind in the newborn are preventive measures against epidemic diarrhea. This means that there must be adequate nursery personnel, well trained to use good nursery technic, and adequate space and physical facilities to give good care. Extreme care must be taken to supply food free of pathogenic bacteria; proper sterilization and storage of formula and proper handling of feeding equipment are major factors in reducing the mortality caused by gastrointestinal infections. Individual thermometer technic must be used. Careful hand washing between care of infants and after diaper changing is important. Personnel must be free of respiratory and gastrointestinal disease.

In order to treat sick infants immediately and prevent spread of an infection the nursery personnel must observe all infants' stools and keep a careful record of the number and of their description. In addition, it is important to keep a careful record of feedings and general behavior. With this record it is possible for the doctor to have a picture of any change in the baby. All nursery personnel must be well trained to be alert to any abnormality in the number and character of the stools and in the baby's behavior and must notify the doctor of any deviation from normal. The nurse's observations can be of inestimable value in the early recognition of cases; this is very important for treatment of the sick infant and for the prevention of an epidemic. Any suspicious case of diarrhea must be isolated in a separate nursery, at least until it is proven not to be infectious diarrhea. Babies with epidemic diarrhea must be cared for by a completely separate staff. All other babies in the nursery must be carefully observed for any evidence of illness. New babies should not be admitted into a nursery from which a baby with diarrhea has been removed or cared for by the same personnel. It is thus necessary, in cases of an epidemic, for hospitals to provide three separate nurseries and staffs, or the department may need to be closed to new admissions until the epidemic is over and the nurseries have been thoroughly cleaned. In some instances the latter has been necessary to control the epidemic.

In the **treatment** of epidemic diarrhea restoration of normal fluid and electrolyte balance is important; measured amounts of physiologic fluids, such as physiologic saline, Hartmann's solution, and Ringer's solution, are administered parenterally. Alkali solutions, such as sodium lactate or sodium bicarbonate, are necessary when acidosis is present. When these solutions have been given in the amount that is determined to be necessary daily to restore and maintain the proper electrolyte balance, the remainder of the fluid requirement is supplied by the administration of a 5 per cent glucose solution. After fluid balance is restored, blood transfusion may be given to combat low serum protein levels and anemia. Feedings are withheld for 12 to 24 hours and then resumed in small amounts and increased slowly. Parenteral fluids are continued daily until the baby's fluid requirements can be met by oral intake. If hypocalcemia, with signs of tetany, develops the administration of calcium is necessary. Antibiotic therapy is used to help control any secondary infection; it may or may not be of value in combating the microorganism that is causing the diarrhea.

## IMPETIGO NEONATORUM

Impetigo is a skin infection characterized by the appearance of superficial vesicles. These vesicles are at first tense and then wrinkled; they contain a fluid which is usually clear and thin, but may have a slightly purulent yellowish appearance; they break easily; and they have a reddened base and may be surrounded by a small erythematous area. These blister-like lesions usually appear on moist and opposing skin surfaces—in the groins, axillae, creases of the neck, and on the abdomen under the binder. Lesions may then develop on other parts of the body, probably by contamination with fluid from the broken vesicles. Sometimes the original lesions develop around the fingernails. The etiology of these lesions is unknown; they are believed to be caused by staphylococci or streptococci. The source of the infection is unknown; it is sometimes attributed to a skin infection or an upper respiratory infection in a member of the nursery personnel or in the mother.

These lesions heal quickly in most instances and are not serious, but their appearance always presents a problem in the newborn nursery because of their contagiousness to other infants. The baby should be isolated as soon as the lesions are discovered, and all other infants in the nursery should be observed closely for appearance of vesicles. Treatment with an antibiotic administered intramuscularly and/or locally in the form of an ointment quickly controls the disease. Other local treatment consists of keeping the affected areas clean and dry. The lesions are sometimes opened with a sterile applicator, care being taken that the fluid does not spread to other areas of the skin, and the base is wiped with 60 or 70 per cent alcohol. The affected skin surfaces may be exposed to the air in order to keep them dry, or an antibiotic ointment may be applied to the base of the lesions and the surrounding skin.

### THRUSH

Thrush or oral moniliasis is a mild infection of the mucous membranes of the mouth. White curd-like patches, which resemble milk curds, are seen on the tongue, gums, palate, and inside of the cheeks. These patches do not wipe off easily; if they are loosened there is a raw bleeding area underneath. The infection is usually limited to the mouth and then does not produce systemic symptoms. Thrush is caused by the fungus *Candida (Monilia) albicans;* in the newborn the usual source of infection is a vaginal yeast infection in the mother, also caused by *Candida (Monilia) albicans.* The infection may be spread to other infants in the nursery if feeding equipment is not properly sterilized or properly handled after sterilization.

The nurse should inspect each baby's mouth daily; lesions are often first seen when the baby is five to seven days old. Treatment consists of the application of 1 per cent aqueous solution of methylrosaniline chloride (gentian violet) once or twice daily or aqueous benzalkonium (Zephiran) solution in a 1:1000 to 1:2000 dilution two or three times a day. Treatment is usually given about one hour after a feeding; the mouth is first gently dried of mucus with a sterile cotton applicator. Several days of treatment are sufficient since these lesions heal quickly. Sometimes treatment is given prophylactically if the mother has vaginal moniliasis. Since gentian violet is a dye which gives the baby's mouth a deep violet color the mother must be told to expect the mouth to be stained. The baby usually drools some saliva which stains the clothing with which it comes in contact. If a treatment is given on the day the baby is discharged from the hospital the mother must be warned to protect the baby's clothing until the saliva is no longer colored.

### UMBILICAL INFECTION

Infection of the umbilical area may consist of only a slight redness and slight discharge at the base of the umbilical cord stump, but it can become serious and can result in a generalized body infection since the vessels of the umbilical cord are potential portals of entry for bacteria. Precautions must be taken to avoid any contamination of the umbilical region. The area should be inspected daily for redness and evidence of discharge, and the appearance of such should be reported to the doctor immediately so that appropriate treatment can be instituted.

### INFECTION OF THE EYES

An infection of the eyes usually manifests itself by the appearance of a conjunctival discharge sometime after the second day of life. Silver nitrate often causes a chemical irritation, but signs of this irritation are only present in the first day or two after birth; they may appear within four to six hours. Some babies have considerable edema and redness of the lids and a profuse purulent discharge from the eyes following the instillation of silver nitrate. The inflammation may be quite severe, but it subsides within a day or two and does not leave harmful effects. Gentle cleaning of the lids or irrigation of the eyes with a warm physiologic saline solution is the usual treatment. If there is any suspicion that the inflammation is infectious in nature, an examination of the pus for bacteria is indicated. Any discharge from the eyes after the second day of life is caused by bacterial infection and must be properly identified by smear and culture in order to institute appropriate treatment.

**A gonorrheal conjunctivitis** (ophthalmia neonatorum) is an eye infection caused by the gonococcus which the baby contracts by contact with infected vaginal secretions during passage through the birth canal. It was formerly a common infection of the newborn and one of the greatest causes of blindness, but is not a common disease at present. A gonorrheal infection in the mother can now easily be cured during pregnancy, and state laws require treatment of the eyes at birth as a prophylactic measure against this infection. There is, however, some chance of infection even when prophylactic treatment has been given; occasionally the medication does not get into the conjunctival sac adequately. The disease usually appears on the second or third day of life; the infection may be unilateral at first, but can soon spread to the other eye. The eyelids become reddened and markedly swollen, and there is a discharge from the eyes which is serosanguineous at first, but soon becomes thick and purulent. The conjunctiva is very red and swollen. The disease may run a very rapid course and cause blindness in 48 hours from the time the first signs appear or it may progress more slowly. Ulceration of the cornea is the dreaded consequence of the inflammation as ulcers are followed by scars, and impaired vision or loss of vision is the end result.

Smears and cultures of the pus must be made immediately when there is any question of a gonorrheal conjunctivitis. Treatment with penicillin, given intramuscularly and by instillation into the conjunctival sac, readily cures the disease, but treatment must be instituted early in order to prevent corneal ulceration. The baby must be strictly isolated until the disease has been cured. The eye may be irrigated with a physiologic saline solution while pus is present, and care must be taken to prevent spread of infection to the unaffected eye. Nursery personnel must protect their own eyes also by avoiding contamination with discharge from the baby's eyes or with eye irrigation solution. All persons caring for the baby should wear glasses while giving care, and they should never touch their eyes before they have carefully washed their hands. If the eyes are accidentally contaminated, they should receive appropriate treatment.

A conjunctival infection may be caused by many other organisms among which are viruses, streptococci, staphylococci, and pneumococci or the infection may be mixed. The organisms can frequently be identified by a smear, or both a smear and culture, of the pus. Treatment is with appropriate antibiotic eye drops or ophthalmic ointment.

## CONGENITAL SYPHILIS

Congenital syphilis is an infection caused by the *Treponema pallidum* which is present in the infant at the time of birth; the infection is transmitted from the mother into the fetal blood stream by the passage of spirochetes through the placenta sometime between the fifth month and the end of pregnancy. Congenital syphilis is decreasing; most mothers who receive prenatal care are now tested for syphilis and given adequate treatment. The infant mortality rate due to syphilis has also fallen steadily, and stillbirths due to the disease are not as common as in former years. Prevention of congenital syphilis depends entirely upon preventing transmission of the spirochetes from mother to fetus through detection of the disease in the mother and effective treatment before or during pregnancy (see pp. 254–57).

Congenital syphilis may be difficult to detect at birth, since physical signs are usually absent and the results of a serology test at this time do not prove the presence or absence of the disease. The placenta may show characteristic changes if the infection is present. Although in former years babies often had signs of the disease at birth, the possibility of a child being born with clinical evidence on the skin and mucous membranes is rare in the present day. Signs of the infection are more apt to appear in several weeks or they may not appear until later in childhood when the manifestations are different than in infancy. The presence of signs at birth usually indicates a severe infection. The most frequent signs of early congenital syphilis are snuffles and skin eruptions. Snuffles are due to a swelling of the nasal mucous membrane; this makes breathing and sucking difficult. A profuse purulent nasal discharge, which excoriates the skin with which it comes in contact, soon develops. The mouth and larynx may be infected. The cry may sound hoarse. Skin lesions may consist of eruptions on all or a part of the body; redness, swelling, and peeling of the skin of the palms and soles; and fissures around the mouth, anus, and vulva. The long bones are affected by the disease, and the joints may become swollen and painful. X-rays of the long bones may show bone changes at several weeks of age.

Although a serologic test should be done at birth the disease cannot be detected by this test in the early months; the test becomes accurate sometime between three and six months of age. The test may be negative for a few months even when the baby has the disease because the infant may not yet have developed antibodies; or it may be positive for a few months in the absence of disease because there has been a placental transmission of the mother's antibodies. A positive test may, therefore, reflect the mother's rather than the baby's blood condition; a test done on umbilical cord blood may likewise reflect the mother's blood status. The baby's condition can best be determined by testing the blood in several dilutions once a month or more often over a period of several months; an increasing titer is indicative of the presence of syphilis in the infant, and a decreasing titer indicates absence of the disease, but even then subsequent tests should be obtained at the age of six months and one year.

Penicillin is used for treatment in any phase of congenital syphilis. The decision to treat depends upon the mother's history of disease and treatment (see pp. 255–56), the presence of symptoms, the serology reports, and the x-ray findings. Early treatment is important when there is any evidence of disease. Congenital syphilis can be cured with early recognition and treatment. Whenever actual lesions are seen, spirochetes are present in the discharge; the baby should be isolated, and the persons caring for the baby should wear a gown and rubber gloves for protection since the spirochetes may enter through any breaks in the skin. After several days of treatment the contagiousness of the disease is probably past.

## METABOLIC AND NUTRITIONAL DISTURBANCES

The newborn, and especially the immature infant, develops *acidosis* more easily than the older baby. Acidosis may be caused by functional renal insufficiency in the neonatal period, a low food intake, and a relatively low alkali reserve of the blood. Laboratory studies of the blood, showing a decrease in the carbon dioxide combining power, are necessary for diagnosis, but clinical manifestations of sluggishness or marked restlessness, a disinterest in sucking, a stationary weight or a weight loss, an anxious expression, and evidence of dehydration may point toward the suspected diagnosis. The baby may or may not have hyperpnea. Parenteral administration of alkali in the form of 1/6 molar solution of sodium lactate satisfactorily corrects this condition.

**Edema** may occur in association with certain diseases of the newborn, but it sometimes develops spontaneously in the otherwise normal infant. The edema is apparently due to sodium and chloride retention and is believed to be caused by a temporary deficiency in renal excretion. It may be precipitated by administration of physiologic saline solution to the new infant in an amount even slightly above minimal requirements. If it becomes necessary to administer parenteral fluids to the newborn, this must be done with great caution because the kidneys may not as yet be able to excrete large amounts of water and electrolytes.

**Transitory fever** of the newborn has been discussed in Chapter 21 (p. 591).

**Tetany,** not related to a vitamin D deficiency, may occasionally occur during the first weeks of life. It is characterized by hyperirritability, muscular twitchings, and convulsions. Vomiting, edema, and cyanosis may also be present. It must be differentiated from other causes of convulsions; the diagnosis depends upon finding a low blood calcium level. Laboratory studies show the blood calcium in cases of tetany to be below 7 or 8 mg per 100 ml of blood and the blood phosphorus level to be high.

Tetany may be due to a combination of factors, among which are included transient physiologic deficiency of the parathyroid, the feeding of cow's milk, which has a different ratio of calcium and phosphorus than human milk, and the lowered renal function of early neonatal life.

Tetany is more apt to occur in artificially fed than in breast-fed infants and is apparently the result of the high-phosphorus content of the milk which lowers the calcium in the blood. Cow's milk has approximately equal parts of calcium and phosphorus whereas human milk contains twice as much calcium as it does phosphorus. The phosphorus level of blood plasma is higher and the calcium level lower in artificially fed babies as compared to those fed breast milk. The rise of phosphorus in the blood, with the feeding of cow's milk, is believed by some to depress the calcium. It is mainly in the early days of the neonatal period that this phenomenon occurs.

Calcium gluconate, 5 to 10 ml of a 10 per cent solution, given intravenously will control convulsions. Calcium administration is then continued orally, in the feedings, for about one week. When artificial feedings are used, cow's milk should ordinarily not be fed in higher concentrations than 1 part of milk to 2 parts of water in the early neonatal period. It may be necessary to add calcium gluconate to the feedings to approximate the proportions of calcium to phosphorus in breast milk, this being especially true if it is necessary to feed the baby a formula of a high concentration of milk to water.

## CARE OF THE BABY OF A DIABETIC MOTHER

Although the baby born of a mother who has diabetes may be entirely normal, the incidence of intrauterine and postnatal complications in these infants is rather high. Congenital anomalies occur more frequently, and there is an increase in the stillbirth and neonatal mortality rate. If the mother's diabetes is mild or is well controlled during pregnancy and if she does not have prenatal complications, the baby can be expected to be in good condition at birth; but when the diabetes is difficult to control and complications of pregnancy develop, the baby may die in utero or have difficulty in the immediate postnatal period. The complications which are most apt to occur during pregnancy and which are hazardous to the infant are toxemias of pregnancy, generalized edema and hydramnios, and periods of acidosis. Since the fetal mortality rate is highest during the last few weeks of gestation and especially when complications have developed, these babies are often delivered two to four weeks before term. Delivery may be necessary by cesarean section because conditions may not be satisfactory for induction of labor or for an uncomplicated vaginal delivery. These babies require special care; the complications of prematurity and of birth by cesarean section are added to the handicaps that the baby already has as a result of the mother's condition.

Many babies born of diabetic mothers are overweight; they are obese, have generalized edema, and enlargement of some of the internal organs—especially the liver, spleen, and heart. Their excessive size may make vaginal delivery difficult. Gestational age rather than birth weight must always be considered in determining the degree of prematurity. Respiratory disturbances, especially atelectasis and hyaline membrane disease, are common. Extramedullary hematopoiesis may be excessive, and the baby may have a high number of nucleated red blood cells at birth. Jaundice commonly appears in 24 hours, but it is not accompanied by anemia.

Careful observation and treatment are important at birth and during the first few days of life. The analgesic used during labor should be minimal, and the anesthetic administered for delivery or for cesarean section must be carefully chosen to prevent respiratory depression. Postural drainage and oropharyngeal suction should be used immediately after birth. Drainage of the respiratory passages is continued by elevating the foot of the mattress to a 15- to 20-deg angle for approximately a 24-hour period, and oropharyngeal suction is repeated as fluid accumulates. A gastric aspiration is done as soon as possible after birth to clear the stomach of the large amount of fluid that is usually present in order to prevent regurgitation of stomach contents and subsequent aspiration of this material into the lungs. It is sometimes recommended that the stomach should be aspirated two or three more times at two- to four-hour intervals. Premature care is given to this baby regardless of his size. The baby is placed in an incubator as soon as possible and given prophylactic treatment against respiratory distress for a period of 24 hours, or longer if indicated. Oxygen is administered in a 30 to 40 per cent concentration, and mist is used to increase the humidity in the incubator to 100 per cent. Continued close observation for dyspnea, cyanosis, and accumulation of mucus is important. The baby's position should be changed every one to two hours, and if he is lethargic, skin stimulation may be necessary to make him cry at intervals. Antibiotics are often given prophylactically to prevent respiratory infection.

Blood sugar determinations are often done at birth and at 8, 24, and 48 hours of life. The blood for the first determination may be obtained from the placental end of the umbilical cord immediately after it is severed. The blood sugar values are usually no lower than those of normal newborn infants who also have a relative hypoglycemia and a wide range of blood sugar values. These values usually range from 40 to 75 mg per 100 ml of blood during the first few days of life; there is, however, a slight possibility of a severe hypoglycemia in the baby of a diabetic mother. Parenteral glucose is sometimes given if the blood sugar falls below 30 mg per 100 ml of blood or it may not be administered unless signs of severe hypoglycemia such as muscular twitching, convulsive movements, and shock occur. Whenever the blood sugar level is decreasing the baby must be closely observed for signs of severe hypoglycemia.

All food and fluid are withheld for the first two or three days of life or until the edema has disappeared. There is usually a large urinary output as well as a considerable loss of body weight during the first few days of life while this edema is decreasing (Chart VIII).

The baby's weight is recorded each day, and the nurses may be requested to carefully record the frequency with which diapers become wet during this period of time, since these records will help to determine how rapidly the excess body fluid is lost and when

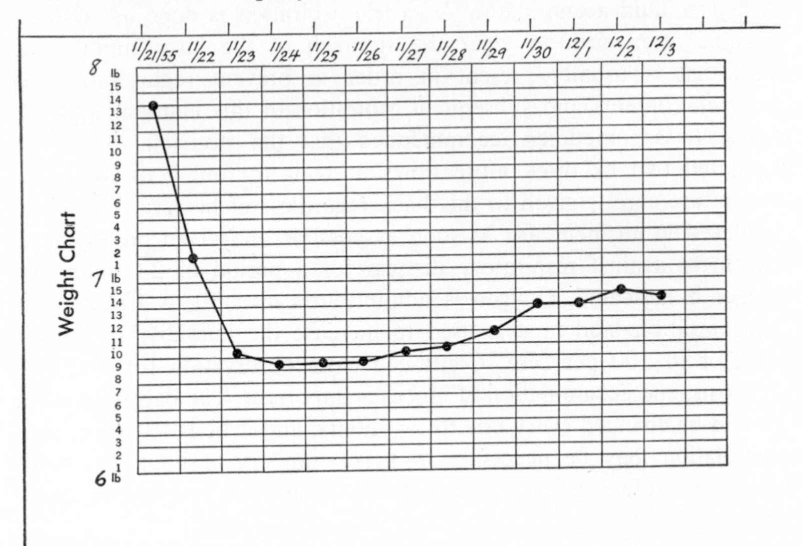


Chart VIII. The weight graph of an infant born at 36-weeks' gestation of a mother with moderately severe diabetes. The excessive weight of this infant, born four weeks prematurely, is characteristic of the baby of a mother with diabetes. The marked weight loss on the first two days of life was due to a decrease in the edema that was present in the baby at birth. A comparison with Chart VII, page 580, will show the difference in weight loss on the first days of life between the normal baby and the one with edema.

this loss levels off. When feedings are begun, the amount and kind of formula and the method of feeding are determined by the gestational age of the infant. After the first few days the subsequent course of the baby's progress is normal for his age.

## POSTMATURITY

There is evidence that babies born after 300 days of gestation may suffer from insufficient functioning of the placenta due to aging. These infants are not large as might be expected, but frequently have a birth weight less than average for full-term infants. They may show wasting of subcutaneous tissue due to lack of adequate nutrition.

There may be some evidence of intrauterine hypoxia; the amniotic fluid and the baby's skin may be meconium stained. These infants must be closely watched for respiratory distress after birth, especially if meconium has been expelled in utero; if meconium is present in the amniotic fluid they may be given prophylactic treatment against respiratory complications by being placed in an incubator in which the oxygen concentration is increased to 30 to 40 per cent and the humidity is increased to 100 per cent by the use of mist.

## BIBLIOGRAPHY AND STUDENT REFERENCES

Association for the Aid of Crippled Children: *Prematurity, Congenital Malformation, and Birth Injury*. The Association, New York, 1953. (Printed by the John B. Watkins Co., New York.)

Battersby, J. S., and Greve, Mary L.: "Modern Treatment of Atresia of the Esophagus," *Am. J. Nursing,* **50**:156–61, (Mar.) 1950.

Bauer, Theodore J., and Shortal, Hazel: "Prevention of Congenital Syphilis," *Pub. Health Nursing,* **42**:81–83, (Feb.) 1950.

Belnap, W. Dean; McKhann, Charles F.; and Beck, Claude S.: "Cerebral Birth Injury in Retrospect," *J. Pediat.,* **37**:326–40, (Sept.) 1950.

Brown, Ivan W.: "Present Status of the Rh Factor," *Am. J. Nursing,* **48**:14–17, (Jan.) 1948.

Bundesen, Herman N.: "Control of Epidemic Diarrhea Is the Hospital's Responsibility," *Mod. Hosp.,* **72**:43–48, (Jan.) 1949, and **72**:66–70, (Feb.) 1949.

Carlson, Earl R.: *Born That Way*. The John Day Co., New York, 1941.

Clifford, Stewart H.: "Fetal Anoxia at Birth and Cyanosis of the Newborn," *Am. J. Dis. Child.,* **76**:666–78, (Dec.) 1948.

Clifford, Stewart H.; Chapple, Charles C.; Cummings, G. D.; Dodd, Katharine; Barbour, Orville E.; and Saltiel, Thomas P.: "Round Table Discussion on Infection in the Newborn Period," *J. Pediat.,* **30**:696–715, (June) 1947.

Clifford, Stewart H.; Cole, Wyman C. C.; and Smith, Clement A.: "Round Table Discussion on Neonatal Asphyxia," *J. Pediat.,* **19**:258–73, (Aug.) 1941.

Committee on Pharmacy and Therapeutics, University of Illinois College of Medicine: "N-allylnormorphine," *Mod. Hosp.,* **79**:106–10, (Sept.) 1952.

Coombs, R. R. A.; Mourant, A. E.; and Race, R. R.: "In-Vivo Isosensitisation of Red Cells in Babies with Haemolytic Disease," *Lancet,* **1**:264–66, (Feb.) 1946.

Darke, Roy A.: "Late Effects of Severe Asphyxia Neonatorum," *J. Pediat.,* **24**:148–58, (Feb.) 1944.

Davidsohn, I.: "The Scientist, the Rh Factor, and Your Baby's Life," *Today's Health,* **33**:20–21 and 42–47, (Oct.) 1955.

Denton, Robert: "Continuous Nebulization Therapy: A Technique for the Treatment of Abnormal Respiration in the Newborn Premature Infant," *Pediat. Clin. North America,* **1**:625–38, (Aug.) 1954.

Diamond, Louis K.: "Replacement Transfusion as a Treatment for Erythroblastosis Fetalis," *Pediatrics,* **2**:520–24, (Nov.) 1948.

Diamond, Louis K.; Allen, Fred H., Jr.; Vann, Dorothea D.; and Powers, John R.: "Erythroblastosis Fetalis—Round Table Discussion," *Pediatrics,* **10**:337–47, (Sept.) 1952.

Drorbaugh, James E., and Fogg, Marguerite F.,: "Respiratory Distress in the Newborn Infant," *Am. J. Nursing,* **56**:1559–62, (Dec.) 1956.

Dunham, Ethel C.: *Premature Infants,* 2nd ed. Paul C. Hoeber, Inc., New York, 1955.

Eastman, Nicholson J.: *Williams Obstetrics,* 11th ed. Appleton-Century-Crofts, Inc., New York, 1956.

Feldman, Felix, and Anderson, James: "Epidemic Diarrhea of the Newborn," *Arch. Pediat.,* **64**:341–49, (July) 1947.

Fischer, Carl C.: "The First Day of Life. The Physician's Responsibility," *M. Clin. North America,* **36**:1561–70, (Nov.) 1952.

Fraser, F. Clarke, and Fainstat, T. D.: "Causes of Congenital Defects," *Am. J. Dis. Child.,* **82**:593–603, (Nov.) 1951.

Gifford, Alice J.; Wright, John J.; Sheps, Cecil G.; and Taylor, Eugene E.: "Congenital Syphilis Can Be Eradicated," *Nursing Outlook,* **1**:28–30, (Jan.) 1953.

Given, William P.; Douglas, R. Gordon; and Tolstoi, Edward: "Pregnancy and Diabetes," *M. Clin. North America,* **35**:659–65, (May) 1951.

Gonce, John E., Jr.: "The Care of the Newborn Baby of the Diabetic Mother," *Nebraska M. J.,* **34**:12–14, (Jan.) 1949.

Goodman, Herman: "Congenital Syphilis," *Am. J. Nursing* **52**:434–35, (Apr.) 1952.

Greenhill, J. P. (ed.): *Obstetrics,* 11th ed. W. B. Saunders Co., Philadelphia, 1955.

Grice, David S.; Williams, Barbara J.; and Macdonald, Mary: "Talipes Equinovarus," *Am. J. Nursing,* **51**:707–12, (Dec.) 1951.

Jeans, Philip C.; Wright, F. Howell; and Blake, Florence G.: *Essentials of Pediatrics,* 5th ed. J. B. Lippincott Co., Philadelphia, 1954.

Kaessler, Henry W., and Ledgard, James J.: "Exchange Transfusion for Fetal Erythroblastosis," *J. Pediat.,* **39**:174–79, (Aug.) 1951.

Laycock, S. R.: "There Must Be No Forgotten Child," *The Crippled Child,* **31**:8–9, (Dec.) 1953.

Little, David M., Jr., and Tovell, Ralph M.: "The Physiological Basis for Resuscitation of the Newborn," *Internat. Abstr. Surg.,* **86**:417–28, (May) 1948.

Lyon, Robert A., and Wallinger, Elgie M.: *Mitchell's Pediatrics and Pediatric Nursing,* 4th ed. W. B. Saunders Co., Philadelphia, 1954.

McDonald, Eugene T.: "Understand Those Feelings," *The Crippled Child,* **32**:4–6, (Oct.) 1954.

MacDonald, Mary: "Nursing Observation of the Infant," *Pub. Health Nursing,* **38**:615–20, (Nov.) 1946.

Miller, Herbert C.; Stern, Curt; Yannet, Herman; and Warkany, Josef: "Congenital Anomalies, A Symposium," *Pediatrics,* **5**:319–36, (Feb.) 1950.

Mollison, P. L.; Mourant, A. E.; and Race, R. R.: *The Rh Blood Groups and their Clinical Effect.* Privy Council Medical Research Council, Memorandum No. 27. Her Majesty's Stationery Office, London, 1952.

Nelson, Waldo E. (ed.): *Textbook of Pediatrics,* 6th ed. W. B. Saunders Co., Philadelphia, 1954.

Pickles, M. M.: *Haemolytic Disease of the Newborn.* Charles C Thomas, Publisher, Springfield, Ill., 1949.

Preston, Mary I.: "Late Behavorial Aspects Found in Cases of Prenatal, Natal, and Postnatal Anoxia," *J. Pediat.,* **26**:353–66, (Apr.) 1945.

Ross, Helen: "The Handicapped Child and His Family," *The Crippled Child,* **30**:8–10, (Feb.) 1953.

Sanford, Heyworth N., and Grulee, Clifford G.: "The Newborn," in McQuarrie, Irvine (ed.): *Brennemann's Practice of Pediatrics,* Vol. I. W. F. Prior Co., Inc., Hagerstown, Md., 1948, Chap. 42.

Shannon, Victoria: "When Children Are Born with Defects," *Children,* **2**:27–31, (Jan.–Feb.) 1955.

Slobody, Lawrence: *Survey of Clinical Pediatrics.* McGraw-Hill Book Co., New York, 1952.

Smith, Clement A., and Cook, Charles D.: "Special Problems of the Newborn. Summary of Round Table Discussion," *Pediatrics,* **15**:348–52, (Mar.) 1955.

Special Committee on Infant Mortality, Medical Society of the County of New York: "Resuscitation of Newborn Infants," *Obst. & Gynec.,* **8**:336–61, (Sept.) 1956.

U.S. Children's Bureau: *Emotional Problems Associated with Handicapping Conditions in Children,* Publication No. 336. U.S. Government Printing Office, Washington, D.C., 1952.

Vaughan, Victor C., III.: "Treatment of Erythroblastosis Fetalis," *Am. J. Nursing,* **52**:320–22, (Mar.) 1952.

West, Jessie Stevenson: *Congenital Malformations and Birth Injuries.* Association for the Aid of Crippled Children, New York, 1954.

# APPENDIX

## The Preparations for Home Delivery

It sometimes devolves upon the nurse to give advice in selecting and preparing the room to be used for a home confinement, to give advice for adequate household assistance, and to help the prospective mother to prepare and assemble adequate equipment for the delivery and for the care of herself and her baby afterward. Under such circumstances the nurse must feel responsible to do all in her power not only to make the home delivery satisfactory, from the standpoint of the patient's happiness and contentment, but from the standpoint of surgical asepsis, efficiency, and economy as well, so that normal cases, at least, may be attended with reasonable safety at home.

Hospital deliveries have increased greatly in recent years, but in spite of this trend toward hospital care for obstetric patients it is as yet impossible for all patients to be delivered in the hospital. There is no doubt that a well-equipped hospital is the safest place in which to have a baby, especially when emergencies arise, but we do know that many women have had their babies safely and with adequate care in the home under the auspices of social agencies such as maternity center associations, the Frontier Nursing Service of Kentucky, and the Catholic Maternity Institute of New Mexico or by efficient doctors and nurses in private practice. This demonstrates the fact that home deliveries may be made relatively safe. Because infection, which is largely preventable, is still one of the chief causes of maternal deaths, it is evident that conscious effort must be put forth to make all home deliveries safe by good aseptic technic. Although the actual procedure in a home varies considerably from that used in a hospital the principles are always the same and without a single exception they all require asepsis—asepsis of equipment and asepsis of technic.

As the first labor is usually longer and more difficult than later ones, and the percentage of lacerations and operative procedures is higher, primigravidas should be delivered in hospitals when possible, as well as all multigravidas presenting any complications or abnormalities. Women who are normal, particularly multigravidas, and these constitute the vast majority of obstetric patients, should be able to remain at home in safety. Ideally a home confinement should only be planned when a normal delivery is expected and where the home setup is such that it can be done with safety and with cooperation from the family. Home deliveries, however, must sometimes be done without this ideal setup, and the doctor and nurse should always be prepared to conduct a delivery where previous plans have not been made. Arrangements should always be made in advance for hospital service in case complications arise.

The nurse assisting with a home delivery must be able to make many adjustments both to the family and to the equipment at hand. She will find that caring for the patient in the home will present many more and different problems than care in the hospital where the patient is relatively isolated from some members of her family and where all equipment is readily available. In the home all members of the family may be present at some time, and the nurse must always take them all into consideration. She should sense their emotional reactions quickly, adjust herself accordingly, and work without upsetting the household (Fig. 204). Also the patient's emotional state will be different in the home due to the closeness of her family and the problems of her home. Besides this she may be concerned about the adequacy of the supplies she has available. The nurse must do what she can to relieve her of any unnecessary worry, get along with what equipment she can find, and make preparation with as little disturbance as possible to the patient and her household. Preparations made with bustle and ostentation are suggestive of inefficiency, are bad for the patient, frequently causing her great alarm, and in the main had better be omitted. The nurse who is able to go into a home quietly and unobtrusively, accept what she finds, and still do aseptic work, is doing better nursing than the one who arranges a faultless room but upsets the patient, and disrupts the household in the process. She will have to learn to improvise and work with what equipment is available and remember that it is possible to do excellent work with meager supplies supplemented with a cool head and ingenuity and training, and, above all, an exacting conscience.

In most instances the patient who is to be delivered at home will

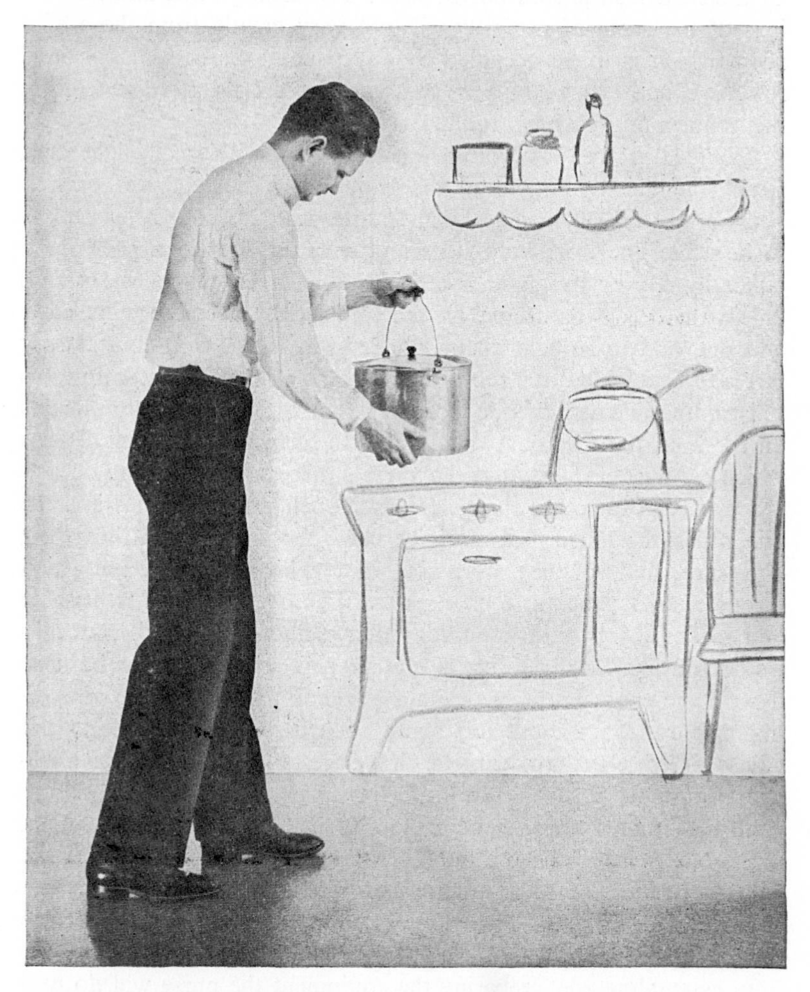

**Fig. 204.** Father helps at home delivery with sterile water and warm things for baby. (Courtesy of Maternity Center Association, Inc., New York, N. Y.)

have to occupy her accustomed room for which there is no alternative. Should there be a choice of rooms, however, one should be selected that is cool and shady, if the confinement takes place during the summer, but bright and sunny for occupancy during most of the year. It should be conveniently near a bathroom if possible or near a source of running water. A room which has recently been occupied by a sick person should not be used. The arrangement and furnishings of the room of necessity will not vary greatly from those of a room which is to be occupied by any patient. Carpets, upholstered furniture, and heavy draperies and curtains are no more suitable in this than in any patient's room.

The ideal is: A room with a washable floor with small, light rugs; freshly laundered curtains at the windows; a single, brass or iron bedstead, about 30 in. high, with a firm mattress, and so placed as to be accessible from both sides and with the foot in a good light, either by day or by night; a bedside table; a bureau; a washstand, unless there is a bathroom on the same floor; a comfortable chair and one or two straight chairs. Barrenness is not only unnecessary but is to be avoided; the room should be as cheerful and comfortable as is compatible with aseptic technic. There is no objection to pictures on the wall, but the room should be free from useless, small articles which are dust catchers, give the nurse unnecessary work, and occupy space needed for other things. Between such a room as this and the one which the nurse finds must be used, there may be a dismaying difference, and so once more she must exercise her ingenuity and resourcefulness; the nurse changes and improves where it is possible and makes the best of conditions that cannot be altered. Much as we should like ideally to equip and prepare every room to be used for a home confinement, we cannot overlook the importance of making preparations without too many changes, and while we do not advise or elect to have carpets, draperies, and upholstery in a delivery room, we know that they need not menace the patient's welfare if all details of the work about the patient herself are aseptic. That is the one point which the nurse must bear constantly in mind, the paramount importance of aseptic work about the patient. The room should be given a thorough housecleaning about two weeks before the expected date of delivery.

In assembling and preparing the equipment the nurse will do well to remember that, although it is possible to use a large number of supplies during labor, it is also possible to manage with a few essentials. The average nurse will wish, usually, to follow a median course in her preparations, having everything at hand that will facilitate the work, be adequately equipped for emergencies, but not burdened with nonessentials.

The doctor and nurse either may carry practically all of the supplies necessary for a home delivery or they may expect the patient to purchase or prepare many of them. It is always well, however, to carry enough equipment to take care of a delivery where no previous preparation has been made. The doctor's and nurse's bags should contain nearly the same equipment so that either one will have at hand everything that is necessary in case of emergency.

The following equipment is usually considered necessary in a home delivery bag used by either the doctor or nurse:

*For examination and preparation of patient:*

Thermometer
Blood pressure manometer and stethoscope
Equipment for testing urine for albumin
Rectal glove and lubricant (soap may be used as a lubricant)
Safety razor and blades
Funnel and rectal tube for enema
Antiseptics, such as tincture of green soap, liquid soap containing hexachlorophene (G-11) 1 to 2 per cent, and benzalkonium (Zephiran chloride) 1:1000 aqueous solution for skin preparation

*For delivery:*

Soap
Hand brushes and orangewood sticks
Caps and masks
Apron
Rubber gloves—several pair, either in sterile packages or to be boiled at the home
Sterile gauze } in sterile glass fruit jars or muslin packages
Sterile cotton balls }
Several packages of sterile towels
Package of sterile perineal pads
Package of sterile sheets }
Package of sterile leggings } if desired
Package of sterile gowns }
Catheter—No. 14 or No. 16 French
2 scissors

4 hemostatic forceps
Ampuls of ergonovine
Ampuls of oxytocin (Pitocin)
Hypodermic syringes and needles
Flashlight—may be desired if a good light is not available
Newspapers

*For care of the baby:*

Jar of sterile bobbin or cord clamps and cord dressings
Alcohol 60 or 70 per cent
Catheter with mucous trap to remove mucus from oropharynx
Ampuls of silver nitrate 1 per cent
Scales and tape for measurements

In addition to the above the doctor will probably wish to include in his obstetric bag:

Anesthetic agent and mask
Morphine and scopolamine
Cardiac stimulants
Plasma expander solution and equipment for administration

*For repair of perineal laceration:*

Catgut
Needles
Needle holder
Tissue forceps

*For operative delivery:*

Obstetric forceps
Retractors
Ring forceps

Besides the supplies mentioned above, the following additional articles will meet the ordinary requirements during a home confinement, and many of these, or adequate substitutes, are to be found in the average household or can easily be obtained:

Soap
Plenty of freshly laundered sheets, pillow cases, towels, washcloths, and nightgowns
Clean cloths—washed and ironed
4 or 6 T binders or a sanitary belt
Perineal pads
Newspapers
2 pieces of rubber sheeting or oilcloth, 1½ x 2 yd
Roll of absorbent cotton

4 to 6 delivery pads
Safety pins
Hot-water bottle
3 or 4 saucepans
Wash basin
Covered pail
Bedpan
Thermometer
1 pt alcohol 60 or 70 per cent
Clothes and crib for baby
Bath equipment for baby

Newspaper delivery pads offer excellent protection and are made of 12 thicknesses of newspaper covered with a piece of freshly laundered muslin or white cotton material, which is folded over the edges and basted in place. These pads may be made virtually sterile by ironing them on the cloth side with a very hot iron, folding the ironed surface inside without touching it, and again ironing on the outside. They should be put in a clean pillow case also recently ironed, and put away in a place protected from dust. Or they may be sterilized according to the method below.

Sterile maternity packs may be provided by local health agencies or maternity centers. The doctor and nurse often carry with them sterile packages of all the necessary equipment. This equipment is wrapped in heavy muslin or heavy Manila paper and sterilized in the autoclave (one hour at 20-lb pressure) at a local hospital or a maternity center.

If the patient is expected to supply the sterile equipment she may either purchase a complete supply of such dressings, sterilized and ready for use, from surgical supply stores or maternity centers, or they may be prepared by the nurse, or by the patient under the nurse's direction. Towels, sheets, gauze sponges, and cotton balls may be put into packages using muslin for wrapping, and sterilized in the patient's home. A pressure cooker, such as is used for home canning, serves as a satisfactory substitute for an autoclave. If a pressure cooker is not available the packages may be baked in an oven for one hour at a temperature of 176.7° C (350° F). If a thermometer is not available to determine the temperature of the oven, the packages may be baked in a slow oven with a large potato and removed when the potato is well done. The packages should be stored in a dry, well-protected place, and the family must be warned not to look inside them after they have been sterilized. It may be desirable to bake some newspapers (a bundle about 12 in. high) in order to have clean papers available for protection of the bed and furniture.

It is usually a good plan for the nurse to advise the patient to have her equipment ready by about the end of the seventh calendar month so as to be prepared in case of a premature delivery. Because they are prepared so early and may become contaminated, all of the dressings should be completely sterilized every four weeks until finally taken out for use at the time of delivery.

As the conditions in the home vary and the wishes and methods of different doctors vary, the articles used must of necessity vary also. It is possible to conduct a delivery with good aseptic technic even with a very small amount of equipment. One essential to remember is that the gloves should be sterile and that nothing but the patient's vulva and the instruments may be touched with them. Sterile sheets and towels to be used for draping are desirable but not absolutely necessary, although a sterile towel or pad beneath the patient's buttocks is usually considered essential.

When the nurse arrives in the home she should immediately try to determine the progress of labor by observing the contractions and by doing a rectal examination and from this decide whether she must hurry in her preparations or whether she may make them without undue haste. She should then get the material together that she will want to use from the supplies in the home, such as newspapers and oilcloth to protect the bed and floor, clean linen to make up the bed, a large pail or basin to be used for waste, and kettles or saucepans from the kitchen for boiling water and the instruments.

During the hours that the nurse is with the patient she must observe the progress of labor carefully, watch closely for any complications, prepare the patient for delivery by giving an enema and shaving the vulva; and prepare the room, the bed, the instruments, and supplies for care of the baby. She must make the same observations on the progress of labor and give the same nursing care in regard to support during labor, rest and activity, observation of temperature, pulse, respirations, blood pressure, and fluid intake and output that she would give to the patient in the hospital.

If there is time the room may be given a final cleaning—the floor washed and the furniture and all small articles wiped with a damp cloth. If there is a carpet on the floor there should be a large canvas or rubber, or an abundance of newspapers, available to protect it, about and under the bed; if the bed is of wood, the side boards and foot should be covered to protect them from damage by soap, water, and solutions which may be spattered or spilled during labor.

In preparing the bed in a patient's home, it is always advisable to make it firm by slipping a board, or several leaves from a dining room table, between the mattress and springs. If the bed is low, the work of the doctor and nurse can be made easier by placing blocks of wood under the bedposts. The bed should be made up with three freshly laundered sheets, the entire mattress being protected by means of a rubber sheet which in turn is covered by the lower sheet, next a rubber draw sheet, covered by one of muslin, or a Kelly pad, while the top sheet or a light blanket should be left free at the foot. A Kelly pad can be made by pinning oilcloth around rolls of newspaper placed at right angles to form three sides of a square or a roll of newspaper which has been bent to form a semicircle. By placing this pad under the patient's hips and arranging it so that it drains to a basin on the floor the bed is well protected.

The unopened packages of sterile supplies, together with the other articles which may be needed during the delivery, should be conveniently arranged on two or three tables, although the top of a bureau and chairs may be used in place of tables (Fig. 205). If possible, a lamp with a bright light should be placed where it will provide good light over the perineal region. If the home is wired for electricity a 100-watt light bulb and extra cord and socket should be secured to provide adequate light.

The instruments, catheter, syringes, and gloves are usually taken to the home in sterile packages. If they are to be boiled in the home they should be arranged in a saucepan which is large enough to give them room to fit down well and to be covered with at least 1 to 2 in. of water. If the gloves are boiled they must be folded in such a way that they can be put on without touching the outside and they must be placed under the instruments to prevent them from floating and therefore from being inadequately sterilized. The instrument pan may be covered with a tight-fitting cover or a large plate; after the water is poured off either the inside of the cover or the pan may be used for an instrument tray. These supplies should not be sterilized until late in the first stage of labor; however, if they are to be boiled on a wood or coal stove it will be necessary to make certain beforehand that there is a good fire. In some areas a Sterno outfit is among the supplies taken to the home in order to have proper facilities available for boiling supplies.

Water to be used for making solutions for the skin preparation

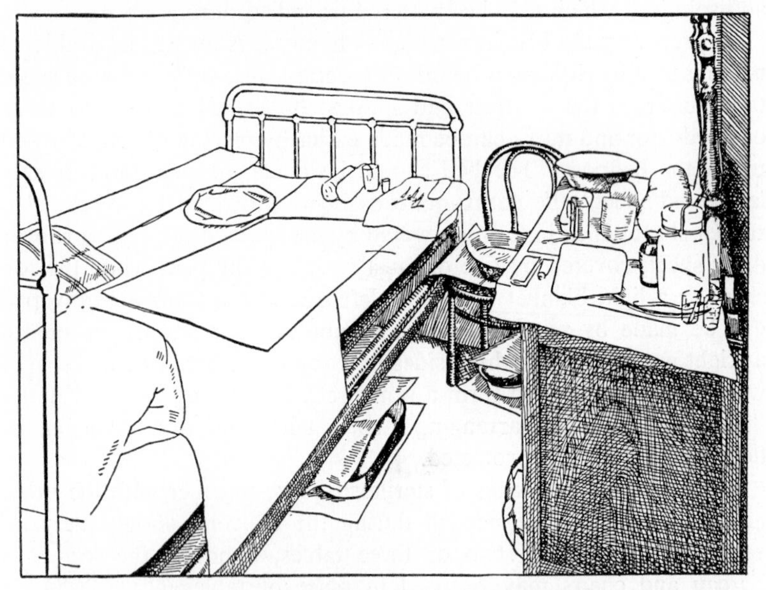

**Fig. 205.** Showing bedroom prepared for home delivery. (Reproduced with the permission of the Maternity Center Association, New York City.)

may be boiled, covered, and set aside to cool. A soup ladle boiled with the water makes a good dipper. Basins in which to make the solutions and to receive the placenta should also be sterilized by boiling water in them. The brushes and orangewood sticks may already be in a sterile package or they may be boiled in a basin; these are placed on a washstand in the bathroom. The rectal glove will have to be cleaned each time it is used and prepared for further use either by washing it with soap and water only or by boiling also if desired. Whenever gloves are boiled they must be wrapped in a small towel to keep them submerged in water.

The baby's bed should be made up, if it is not ready, and a hot-water bottle placed in it for warmth. In addition, the equipment for resuscitation and for care of the eyes, the clothes, bath equipment, and bottles and nipples should be prepared, not only for the initial care of the baby but also for care on the following days. Other members of the family, if present, may be glad to help with preparations for the baby and may at the same time be given instructions for his care.

If time permits, the pitcher with irrigating solution, and the cotton balls for the mother's perineal care on subsequent days should also be prepared.

When the patient has progressed far enough to be prepared for delivery the doctor will scrub his hands and arms, put on sterile gloves, and gown if he wishes, and either he or the nurse should then wash the patient's perineal region with soap and an antiseptic solution. A sterile delivery pad is then slipped under her hips and sterile drapings, if available, are placed over her legs and abdomen. The delivery pads can be changed as they become wet and soiled. If the doctor has prepared the patient he will want to change his gloves for the delivery, and a second pair of sterile ones must be available. The delivery is then conducted in the same manner as it would be in a hospital.

If an operative delivery becomes necessary, many additional preparations must be made. The preparations for operations in hospitals are all so carefully planned and systematized that in the presence of such emergencies the nurse will merely have to carry out the customary procedure, but in a patient's home she may have to exercise a good deal of ingenuity in attempting to meet the needs of the occasion and imitate hospital provisions.

A satisfactory operating table may be fashioned in any one of a number of ways. If the bed is high enough, it may sometimes be made fairly satisfactory by slipping a board, such as a table leaf, under the mattress to make it firm, if this has not already been done. A kitchen table, if it is very secure and firm, may be used. A flat-topped chest of drawers, with the casters removed, makes an excellent operating table, since it is firm, a good height, and about the right size. Or an ordinary bureau may be pressed into service after taking out the casters and removing the mirror by unscrewing its supports. The front and sides of a bureau, or chest of drawers so used, should be protected from the damaging effects of fluids and solutions by being covered with a rubber sheet or newspapers. A pad for the top of the improvised operating table may be arranged by folding a blanket or quilt to the proper size and covering that with a rubber draw sheet and a clean muslin sheet.

Since the operation probably requires that the patient be held in the lithotomy position (on her back with thighs and knees flexed and knees well separated), the doctor's equipment usually includes a strap to hold the legs; if not, one may be improvised from a sheet. The sheet should be folded diagonally, over and over, into a strip about a foot wide, passed over the patient's shoulders and the tapering ends used to tie around her legs, above the knees, to hold them in the desired position. Bandages or tapes are not always satisfactory, because the support is subject to a good deal of strain, and narrow strips sometimes cut painfully into the legs and shoulders. Certainly if tapes or bandages are used, cotton pads or folded towels should be interposed between them and the patient's skin.

In general, the nurse will prepare as for a normal delivery, in each instance adding such details of equipment or preparation as the contemplated operation requires. Rigid asepsis must be observed throughout the preparation and the operation. Sterile gowns for the doctor and sterile sheets, leggings, and towels for draping the patient should be used if possible for an operative delivery. The necessary instruments should be brought to the home in sterile packages.

After delivery the baby is given the usual care to the cord and eyes and is dressed and placed in the warmed crib, and the mother's bed is changed as necessary to make it clean and dry. The nurse must watch the fundus carefully for relaxation and must never leave the home until at least one hour has elapsed since delivery of the placenta. Before leaving, she should again check the baby for any respiratory difficulty or cord bleeding and check the mother's fundus for relaxation and the perineal pads for the amount of vaginal bleeding. She should also leave adequate instructions with the person who will care for the baby and mother. This will include orders concerning the mother's perineal care, breast care, medication, and diet, and instructions for calling the doctor in case of excessive bleeding; instructions must also be left concerning the baby's daily care and feedings and treatment in case of cord bleeding or excessive mucus.

The nurse will either plan to return to the home the next day or for several days to give care to the mother and the baby or teach someone else how to give this care before she leaves. The importance of carefully washing the hands before caring for mother or baby should be stressed. Instructions regarding postpartum care may be similar to those discussed in Chapter 16. It may be necessary to make some changes regarding perineal care during the first few days for lack of equipment that is used in the hospital, but the principles of care remain the same. The perineum may be washed with sterile cotton pledgets and sterile water or sterile soapy water for the first two or three days. The solution may be boiled and put in a boiled pitcher or large glass fruit jar and poured onto the cotton pledgets which are used for washing. The importance of carefully washing the hands before the cotton pledgets and the perineal pads are touched should again be stressed.

While the baby is being bathed, the mother and the person who will be helping her may be instructed in his care. Special emphasis must be made on the importance of keeping the umbilical area clean by using sterile gauze dressings and applying alcohol 60 or 70 per cent until it is well healed.

In addition to instructions for immediate care the nurse must make certain that appointments for subsequent checkup examinations for mother and baby are made and kept.

## BIBLIOGRAPHY AND STUDENT REFERENCES

Burnett, Elizabeth: "A Rural Home Maternity Service," *Am. J. Nursing,* **41**: 1365–72, (Dec.) 1941.

Bookmiller, Mae M., and Bowen, George L.: *Textbook of Obstetrics and Obstetric Nursing,* 2nd ed. W. B. Saunders Co., Philadelphia, 1954.

Children's Bureau: *Prenatal Care,* Publication No. 4. U.S. Government Printing Office, Washington, D.C., 1949.

Davis, M. Edward, and Sheckler, Catherine E.: *DeLee's Obstetrics for Nurses,* 15th ed. W. B. Saunders Co., Philadelphia, 1951.

Frontier Nursing Service, Wendover, Ky.: correspondence.

Goggans, Lalla M.: "Oh Nurse, the Baby Is Coming and the Doctor Isn't Here!" *Pub. Health Nursing,* **35**:559–63, (Oct.) 1943.

Maternity Center Association: "Preparing for a Delivery at Home," *Am. J. Nursing,* **40**:1313–27, (Dec.) 1940. (Material in preparation for "Public Health Nursing in Obstetrics," Part II, by the Maternity Center Association, New York.)

National Organization for Public Health Nursing: *Manual of Public Health Nursing,* 3rd ed. The Macmillan Company, New York, 1939.

Wisconsin State Board of Health: "Delivery and Immediate Postpartum. Basic Principles and Recommendations. Teaching of Home Delivery by Comparison." Hospital Nursing Series No. 3, Bureau of Maternal and Child Health, Wisconsin State Board of Health, Madison, Wisconsin, 1949.

Zabriskie, Louise, and Eastman, Nicholson J.: *Nurses Handbook of Obstetrics,* 9th ed. J. B. Lippincott Co., Philadelphia, 1952.

# GLOSSARY

**ablatio placentae.** *See* abruptio placentae.
**abortion.** Termination of pregnancy before the period of viability or approximately the twenty-eighth week.
**abruptio placentae.** Premature separation of the normally implanted placenta.
**acinus** (of the breast). Secreting cells, circularly arranged about a small duct; in this structure the milk is elaborated from the blood.
**afterbirth.** The placenta and membranes normally expelled from the uterus after the birth of the baby.
**afterpains.** Painful uterine contractions present early in the puerperium, which are caused by the alternate relaxation and contraction of the uterine musculature.
**amenorrhea.** Absence of menstruation.
**amnion.** The inner membrane of the sac containing the fetus and the amniotic fluid.
**amniotic fluid** (liquor amnii). The fluid which is contained in the sac of fetal membranes and which surrounds the fetus.
**amniotomy.** Artificial rupture of the fetal membranes.
**anencephalia.** Partial or complete absence of the cerebral hemispheres and of the cranial bones and the scalp which lie over them.
**anoxia.** Inadequate supply of oxygen, or disturbance of bodily functions resulting from a deficiency of oxygen. Literally means without oxygen.
**antenatal** (prenatal). Existing or occurring before birth.
**antepartum.** Occurring before labor and delivery.
**antepartum hemorrhage.** Bleeding occurring before or during delivery of the baby; usually caused by placenta previa or premature separation of the normally implanted placenta when it occurs in the last trimester of pregnancy.
**anti-Rh antibodies.** Antibodies produced against the Rh factor which are capable of combining with Rh-positive red blood cells to cause hemolysis.
*albumin agglutinins* (blocking antibodies). Antibodies which are capable of producing hemolysis of Rh-positive red blood cells, but do not produce agglutination when the cells are suspended in a physiologic sodium chloride solution; must be tested in an albumin medium.
*saline agglutinins.* Antibodies which produce clumping of Rh-positive red blood cells suspended in a physiologic sodium chloride solution.
**areola mammae.** Circular pigmented area on the breast; surrounds the nipple.
**Aschheim-Zondek test.** A pregnancy test dependent upon the presence of a hormone in the urine of the pregnant woman; made by injecting urine into immature female mice.
**asphyxia neonatorum.** A disturbance in the respiratory system of the newborn developing during or shortly after birth; characterized by slow irregular respiratory movements and cyanosis or an absence of respiration.
**atelectasis** (congenital). An incomplete expansion of the lungs which persists for a longer than normal time postnatally.
**atresia** (of ova). Process by means of which unmatured ova disappear.
**attitude** (of fetus). The position of the fetus in utero.

**autolysis.** Process of self-digestion occurring in tissues under pathologic conditions or in the uterus following delivery.

**bag of waters.** The fetal membranes and amniotic fluid which surround the fetus.

**ballottement.** A rebound to the original fetal position when the head or an extremity of the fetus in utero is given a sudden sharp push from the outside.

**Bandl's ring.** *See* retraction ring (pathologic).

**Bartholin's glands** (vulvovaginal glands). Mucous-secreting glands situated one on each side of the vagina and opening just outside its lateral margins.

**Baudelocque's diameter** (external conjugate). Distance from symphysis pubis to a depression just below last lumbar vertebra.

**biparietal diameter.** The distance between the two parietal eminences of the cranium.

**birth canal.** The channel formed by the uterus and vagina through which the baby passes during delivery.

**bitemporal diameter.** The greatest distance between the temporal bones.

**blastodermic vesicle.** An early stage in the development of the embryo when the cells of the morula are rearranged and fluid forms in a sac.

**bloody show.** A blood-tinged vaginal discharge before or during labor which is caused by tiny lesions that occur in the cervix due to stretching.

**brachial birth palsy.** Partial or complete paralysis of certain muscles of the arm due to trauma to nerve fibers of the brachial plexus, sustained during birth.

**Braxton-Hicks contractions.** Intermittent painless uterine contractions present throughout pregnancy, but which may become painful and occur irregularly at long or short intervals near the end of pregnancy.

**breech.** Buttocks.

**breech extraction.** A procedure in which traction is applied to partially or completely deliver a baby presenting by the breech.

**bregma.** Junction of coronal and sagittal sutures.

**Candida (Monilia) albicans.** A fungus which is sometimes harbored in the vagina and which produces a profuse irritating vaginal discharge; it may cause thrush in the newborn.

**caput succedaneum.** A diffuse swelling, due to edema, in the soft tissues of the scalp that lie over the presenting part of the head.

**carunculae myrtiformes** (carunculae hymenales). Irregular edges of tissue around the vaginal opening due to tears in the hymen.

**caudal anesthesia.** Injection of a local anesthetic agent into the caudal canal to produce anesthesia of the pelvic region.

**cephalhematoma.** A tumor-like swelling caused by an extravasation of blood below the periosteum of any of the cranial bones.

**cervix** (uteri). Neck of the uterus; the lowermost cylindrical part of the uterus.

**cesarean section.** Delivery of a baby through an incision made in the abdominal and uterine walls.

**Chadwick's sign.** The dark bluish or purplish appearance of the vulvar and vaginal mucous membrane during pregnancy due to a great increase in vascularity.

**chloasma.** Brownish or yellowish-brown, irregularly shaped blotches which sometimes appear on the face and neck during pregnancy. Also known as "mask of pregnancy."

**choriocarcinoma.** A highly malignant growth which may develop following an abortion or a normal pregnancy, but more often originates from a hydatidiform mole.

**chorion.** The outer membrane of the sac containing the fetus and the amniotic fluid.

**chorionic gonadotropin.** A hormone produced by the placenta which is present in the blood and urine of pregnant women and which stimulates the gonads in test animals.

**chorionic villi.** Thread-like projections on the surface of the chorion which increase in size and number and soon contain blood vessels. Exchange of food and waste products between fetal and maternal blood takes place through the villi; they serve to attach the embryonic sac to the uterine wall; and those beneath the vesicle enter into the formation of the placenta.

**chromosomes.** Bodies of chromatin material of different size and shape in the nucleus of body cells which carry the hereditary factors that are transmitted to an individual.

**circumcision.** Surgical removal of part or all of the foreskin of the penis.

**cleft lip** (harelip). A congenital fissure of the upper lip due to failure of the embryonic facial processes to fuse.

**cleft palate.** A congenital defect where there is a fissure in the palate due to a failure of the embryonic facial processes to fuse.

**climacteric.** *See* menopause.

**clitoris.** Small projection of erectile tissue at the place where the labia minora join in front; the homolog of the penis.

**colostrum.** Yellowish fluid secreted by the breasts during pregnancy and for the first two to three days after delivery.

**conception.** Fusion of spermatozoon and ovum; marks the beginning of pregnancy.

**congenital anomaly.** A malformation of any part of the body which exists at birth.

**conjugate diameters of the pelvis:**

*diagonal conjugate.* Distance from the lower margin of the symphysis pubis to the promontory of the sacrum.

*external conjugate.* Distance from the symphysis pubis to a depression just below the last lumbar vertebra; also called Baudelocque's diameter.

*transverse conjugate* (of inlet). Diameter joining two most widely separated points of pelvic inlet.

*transverse conjugate* (of outlet). Diameter connecting ischial tuberosities.

*true conjugate.* Distance from the upper margin of the symphysis pubis to the promontory of the sacrum.

*vera conjugate.* Same as true conjugate.

**Coombs test.** A test for the presence of globulin antibodies on the surface of red blood cells. In the newborn it demonstrates the presence or absence of anti-Rh blocking antibodies coating the baby's red blood cells.

**cornua** (of the uterus). Upper angles of the uterine cavity where the fallopian tubes enter the uterus.

**corpus** (of the uterus). The upper triangular part of the uterus above the cervix; also known as the body of the uterus.

**corpus luteum.** A yellow body of cells in the ovary which fills the space left by the rupture of the graafian follicle; produces the hormone, progesterone.

**cotyledon.** Any one of the irregularly shaped lobes or subdivisions of the maternal surface of the placenta.

**craniotabes.** Areas of softening of the skull bones.

**crowning.** That stage in the delivery of a baby's head in which the vulva is greatly distended, and the largest diameter of the head is encircled by the vaginal opening.

**cul-de-sac** (pouch of Douglas). A blind pouch in the peritoneal cavity between the posterior surface of the uterus and the anterior surface of the rectum; formed by a fold of peritoneum.

**cyanosis.** A bluish tinge in the color of mucous membranes and skin due to the presence of excessive amounts of reduced hemoglobin in the capillaries.

**decidua.** The excessively hypertrophied endometrium which lines the uterus during pregnancy.

*basalis* (serotina). That portion directly beneath the embryo which enters into the formation of the placenta.
*capsularis* (reflexa). That part which surrounds and covers the buried embryo.
*vera.* That portion which lines the entire uterus.

**dehydration fever.** A fever that sometimes occurs in the newborn between the second and fourth day of life due to loss of body fluid and low fluid intake.

**diastasis recti abdominis.** A separation of the recti muscles caused by abdominal distention, as with pregnancy.

**dilatation of cervix.** The enlargement of the external os from an orifice a few millimeters in size to an opening large enough to permit the passage of the baby. A cervical opening approximately 10 cm (4 in.) in diameter is usually called complete or full dilatation.

**ductus arteriosus.** A fetal blood vessel connecting the pulmonary artery and the aorta; a temporary structure.

**ductus venosus.** A fetal blood vessel joining the umbilical vein and the ascending vena cava; a temporary structure.

**Duncan's mechanism.** A mechanism of placental separation and extrusion in which separation begins at the margin of the placenta and the raw maternal surface appears at the vaginal outlet first as it is delivered.

**dysmenorrhea.** Painful menstruation.

**dystocia.** Difficult labor.

**eclampsia.** An acute toxemia of pregnancy characterized by convulsions and coma which may occur during pregnancy, labor, or the early puerperium.

**ectoderm.** Outer primitive layer of cells that has arisen from segmentation and differentiation of the inner cell mass.

**ectopic pregnancy.** Gestation outside the uterine cavity (also known as extrauterine pregnancy).

**effacement.** A thinning and shortening of the cervix which occurs during late pregnancy and/or labor. This progresses until the entire canal is obliterated and is continuous with the lower uterine segment.

**embryo.** Baby in utero before third lunar month of development.

**embryonic area.** Cell mass on inner surface of blastodermic vesicle.

**endometritis.** An inflammation of the uterine lining.

**endometrium.** The mucous-membrane lining of the uterine cavity.

**engagement.** Entrance of the fetal head into the superior strait of the pelvis to the extent that the biparietal plane of the fetal head has passed through the area of the pelvic inlet.

**engorgement** (breast). Congestion of the breast, normally sometime between the second and fourth day after delivery, which is due to lymphatic and venous congestion and/or distention with milk.

**ensiform process.** *See* xiphoid process.

**entoderm.** Inner primitive layer of cells that has arisen from segmentation and differentiation of the inner cell mass.

**episiotomy.** Surgical incision of the perineal body beginning at the posterior margin of the vaginal opening. May be performed during second stage of labor to enlarge the vulvar orifice in order to facilitate delivery.

**Erb-Duchenne paralysis.** *See* brachial birth palsy.

**ergonovine.** An alkaloid obtained from ergot which causes uterine muscle contractions.

**ergot.** A fungus parasite upon rye and other grains which can cause powerful uterine muscle contractions and constrict blood vessels.

**erythematous blotches.** Hive-like areas on the skin of the newborn that may appear and disappear at intervals during the first few days following irritation from clothing or after a period of crying.

**erythroblastosis fetalis.** A disease of the blood in late fetal or early neonatal life occurring when there is an incompatibility between the baby's and the mother's blood. Maternal sensitization to antigens present in the fetal cells stimulates production of antibodies in the mother which enter the fetal circulation to destroy red blood cells.

**estrogen.** An ovarian hormone elaborated by the graafian follicle; also elaborated by the placenta.

**exchange transfusion.** A procedure by which 90 to 95 per cent of an infant's blood is replaced with donor blood.

**exstrophy of the bladder.** Partial or complete exposure of the bladder mucosa through an opening in the abdomen due to failure of the abdominal wall and the anterior bladder wall to close.

**extrauterine pregnancy.** *See* ectopic pregnancy.

**fallopian tubes** (uterine tubes). Small tubes, one on each side of the uterus, which convey the ova from the ovaries to the uterine cavity.

**false labor.** Perceptible but nonproductive uterine contractions which continue with some regularity for a few hours; do not increase in intensity, duration, and frequency; and finally subside.

**fertilization.** Fusion of nuclei of spermatozoon and ovum; marks the beginning of pregnancy. This fusion results in a one-celled embryo or zygote.

**fetus.** Baby in utero from third lunar month of development until birth.

**fimbria ovarica.** The longest of the fimbriae of the fallopian tube; is usually attached to the ovary.

**follicle-stimulating hormone.** A hormone elaborated by the anterior lobe of the pituitary gland which stimulates development of the graafian follicle in the ovary.

**follicular fluid** (liquor folliculi). The fluid which surrounds the maturing ovum in the graafian follicle; contains estrogenic hormone.

**fontanel.** Membranous space at junction of cranial sutures in infant; due to incomplete ossification.

*anterior.* Diamond-shaped space where the coronal, sagittal, and frontal sutures meet.

*posterior.* Triangular-shaped space at intersection of sagittal and lambdoidal sutures.

**Foote's sign.** An adder-like, rhythmic protrusion of the tongue.

**foramen ovale.** Opening between atria of fetal heart.

**forceps** (obstetric). An instrument which may be applied to a baby's head for the purpose of extracting it from the birth canal.

**forceps operation.** A procedure by which an obstetric forceps is applied to the baby's head to extract it from the birth canal.

**foreskin** (prepuce). The fold of skin covering the glans penis.

**fornices of the vagina** (*plural*). Divisions of fornix; known as anterior, posterior, right, and left.

**fornix of the vagina.** Space between the outer surface of that part of the cervix that extends into the vagina and the surrounding vaginal wall.

**fossa navicularis.** Depressed space between the hymen and the fourchette.

**fourchette.** Transverse fold of mucous membrane connecting the posterior ends of the labia minora.

**Friedman test.** A pregnancy test dependent upon the presence of a hormone in the urine of the pregnant woman; made by injecting urine into a female rabbit.

**frog test.** A pregnancy test dependent upon the presence of a hormone in the serum and urine of the pregnant woman; made by injecting serum or urine into a male frog.

**fundus** (uteri). The rounded portion of the uterus that is above the place where the fallopian tubes enter the uterus.

**funis.** Umbilical cord.

**gavage.** A feeding given to an infant through a catheter that is passed to the lower end of the esophagus; for adult feedings, the catheter is passed into the stomach.

**genes.** Chromatin particles within the chromosomes which carry the factors that determine the hereditary traits of an individual.
**genotype.** The combination of genes that are carried by the chromosomes of an individual.
**gestation.** Pregnancy.
**gonad.** A sex gland or organ; ovary or testis.
**gonadotropic hormones.** Hormones produced by the anterior lobe of the pituitary gland which influence the gonads; in the female they stimulate the ovary to develop the graafian follicle and the corpus luteum.
**Goodell's sign.** Softening of the cervix early in pregnancy; a probable sign of pregnancy.
**graafian follicle.** A maturing follicle appearing as a blister-like protrusion on the surface of the ovary; contains a maturing ovum and secretes estrogens.
**gravid.** Pregnant. Heavy with child.
**gravida.** A pregnant woman.

**harelip.** *See* cleft lip.
**Hegar's sign.** Softening of the isthmus, or lowermost portion of the body of the uterus; a probable sign of pregnancy.
**hemorrhagic disease of the newborn.** Spontaneous and prolonged bleeding from various sites in the body during the first week of life.
**hot flashes.** Vasomotor symptoms which appear at the menopause, and manifest themselves by flushing of the face and neck, sweating, and flashes of heat which involve the entire body.
**hyaline membrane.** A material which may line the alveoli or plug the alveolar ducts during the first few days of life; it interferes with gaseous exchange.
**hydatidiform mole.** A disease of the chorion in which the chorionic villi become cystic. Many grape-like cysts develop and fill the uterine cavity.
**hydramnios.** Excessive amount of amniotic fluid.
**hydrops fetalis.** Erythroblastosis fetalis with universal edema.
**hymen.** Fold of mucous membrane partially covering the vaginal opening.
**hyperemesis gravidarum.** Severe vomiting of pregnancy; usually in the first trimester. Also called pernicious vomiting of pregnancy.
**hypospadias.** An anomaly in which the urethra does not extend the entire length of the penis, but rather opens on its lower surface behind the glans.
**hypoxia.** A condition in which there is a shortage of oxygen in the blood.
**hysterectomy.** Excision of the uterus.
**hysterotomy.** Incision of the uterus.

**icterus neonatorum.** Physiologic jaundice of the newborn infant which may appear at the second or third day of life and continue until approximately the fourteenth day.
**imperforate anus.** A complete absence of the anus or a persistent membrane over the anal opening.
**impetigo neonatorum.** A contagious skin infection of the infant characterized by the formation of superficial vesicles with a red base.
**impregnation.** *See* fertilization.
**in utero.** Within the uterus.
**inanition fever.** *See* dehydration fever.
**innominate bones** (ossa innominata). The two hipbones which make up the sides and the front of the bony pelvis. Each bone consists of three fused bones—the ilium, the ischium, and the pubis.
**intertrigo.** Chafing which occurs where two moist skin surfaces come together as in the neck, groins, crease between buttocks, and at flexture of joints.
**intervillous spaces.** Areas between the trophoblasts and the decidua which become filled with blood by which the embryo is nourished before the placenta is developed.
**intrapartum.** Occurring any time during labor and delivery.
**introitus** (vaginal). The opening or entrance to the vagina.

**involution** (of the uterus). Return of the uterus, following delivery, to nearly its former size and shape.
**isthmus** (uterine). The lower, narrow portion of the body of the uterus where it meets the cervix.

**jaundice** (icterus). A syndrome characterized by increased amount of bilirubin in the blood and the deposition of bile pigments in the skin and mucous membranes which gives them a yellow color.

**kernicterus.** Jaundice of the nuclear masses of the brain.

**labium** (*plural,* labia). Lip. The folds of integument at the opening of the vulva.
*majus* (*plural,* majora). Heavy ridges of fat, connective tissue, and skin forming the lateral boundaries of the external genitalia.
*minus* (*plural,* minora). Two small cutaneous folds lying between the labia majora on each side of the vestibule.
**labor.** Parturition. Bringing forth of young. The physiologic process by which the fetus and the placenta and membranes are expelled from the uterus.
*first stage* (stage of dilatation). Begins with the onset of labor and ends with complete cervical dilatation.
*second stage* (stage of expulsion). Begins with complete cervical dilatation and ends with delivery of the baby.
*third stage* (placental stage). Begins immediately after the birth of the baby and ends with delivery of the placenta.
**lactation.** The secretion of milk by the mammary glands.
**lactogenic hormone** (prolactin). An anterior pituitary gland hormone which promotes lactation.
**lanugo hair.** A covering of downy hair on the body of the fetus after the fourth month, much of which is lost as full term is reached.
**laparotrachelotomy** (low cervical cesarean section). A cesarean section performed by making an incision through the lower uterine segment.
**let-down reflex.** Expulsion mechanism; the mechanism by which milk is expelled from the breast.
**leukorrhea.** A whitish mucous-like discharge from the female genital tract.
**levator ani.** A broad perineal muscle which extends from the bony wall of one side of the pelvis to the other. It makes up a part of the perineal floor and forms a sling-like structure which helps to support the pelvic organs.
**ligaments** (uterine). Bands of connective tissue formed by folds of peritoneum which hold the uterus suspended in the center of the pelvic cavity.
**lightening.** Descent of the fundus of the uterus near term to the position it occupied at the eighth month of pregnancy; this occurs as the presenting part of the fetus enters the pelvic inlet. The sensation of abdominal distention is decreased.
**linea alba.** White line in middle of abdomen running longitudinally from the sternum to the symphysis pubis.
**linea nigra.** Dark line in middle of abdomen running longitudinally from the sternum to the symphysis pubis; due to pigmentation of the linea alba during pregnancy.
**linea terminalis** (iliopectineal line). A constriction in the pelvis which divides it into the true and false pelvis.
**lineae albicantes** (albicans). *See* striae gravidarum.
**liquor amnii.** *See* amniotic fluid.
**liquor folliculi.** *See* follicular fluid.
**lochia.** Uterine and vaginal discharge during the puerperium.
*alba.* The white or yellowish-white discharge that occurs after approximately the tenth day.
*rubra.* The bloody discharge of the first few days.
*serosa.* The serous discharge occurring after approximately the fourth day.

**lutein cells.** Granulosa cells with a yellow tint which invade the ruptured graafian follicle and form the corpus luteum.
**luteinizing hormone.** A hormone elaborated by the anterior lobe of the pituitary gland which stimulates the development of the corpus luteum in the ovary.

**Mariceau's maneuver.** A method of delivery of the after-coming head in breech extraction. In this maneuver, slight traction and manipulative procedures are used on the baby's body at the same time that suprapubic pressure is applied to the mother.
**maturation.** Developmental changes in the germ cells which reduce the number of chromosomes in the cells to one-half the original number and which prepare the cells for fertilization.
**meconium.** Dark, tarry fecal material, made up of bile pigments, digestive secretions, mucus, desquamated cells, and cast-off hair and vernix caseosa swallowed with the amniotic fluid; found in the intestines of the fetus after the fourth month. This constitutes the first few stools of the newborn.
**membrana granulosa.** The cellular-layer lining of a graafian follicle.
**menarche.** The onset of the menstrual function.
**menopause.** The period of life at which ovarian function stops and menstruation ceases permanently.
**menorrhagia.** An abnormally copious menstrual flow.
**menstruation.** A monthly discharge of blood from the uterus normally recurring during the entire childbearing period except during pregnancy and possibly lactation.
**mentum.** The chin.
**mesoderm.** Middle primitive layer of cells that has arisen from segmentation and differentiation of the inner cell mass.
**metritis.** Inflammation of the uterine musculature.
**metrorrhagia.** Bleeding between the menstrual periods.
**microliter.** A millionth of a liter, or a thousandth of a milliliter. This term replaces the term cubic millimeter as a unit of volume, just as the term milliliter is used to express a unit of volume in place of the previously used term cubic centimeter. Microliter and milliliter are technically more correct terms for units of volume, since a meter is a unit of length.
**milia.** Pin-point white spots beneath the epidermis of the nose and chin of the newborn which are concretions of sebaceous material in the ducts of the sebaceous glands.
**milk leg** (phlegmasia alba dolens). A swelling of the leg following delivery due to a phlebitis of the femoral vein.
**miscarriage.** Termination of pregnancy before the period of viability or approximately the twenty-eighth week. A lay term synonymous with abortion.
**mongolian spots.** Bluish pigmented areas of skin over the back and buttocks in some newborn babies, especially those of the dark-skinned races.
**mongolism.** A congenital malformation in which the child has slanting eyes, a large tongue, a broad short skull, relaxed joints, poor muscle tone, and a severely retarded mental development.
**Monilia albicans.** *See Candida (Monilia) albicans.*
**mons veneris.** A cushion of fat and connective tissue, covered with skin and hair, which lies over the symphysis pubis.
**monster.** A fetus with an abnormal development or superfluity or deficiency of parts.
**Montgomery's tubercles.** Small, shot-like lumps or papillae on the surface of the nipples and the areolae, which are sebaceous glands.
**Moro reflex** (startle reflex). A reaction which occurs with sudden stimulation; the infant draws up his legs and brings his arms forward as in an embrace position. Normally present in the newborn.
**morula.** Mulberry-like mass of cells produced by segmentation of the fertilized ovum.

**mucous plug.** Thick mucus which fills the cervical canal during pregnancy and which is expelled from the vagina sometime early in labor.
**multigravida.** A woman during her second and subsequent pregnancies.
**multipara.** A woman who has given birth to two or more children.
**multiple pregnancy.** One in which the uterus contains two or more fetuses.

**natural childbirth.** Childbirth in a normal physiologic manner in which fear and tension are reduced through education of the mother and through the aid of support during labor.
**neonatal.** Pertaining to the newborn.
**neonatal period.** The first four weeks of life.
**neonatorum.** Pertaining to the newborn.
**nullipara.** A woman who has not had children.

**oöcyte.** An ovum, or germ cell, before the process of maturation, or formation of polar bodies, is completed.
**ophthalmia neonatorum.** Acute conjunctivitis of the newborn; may be caused by the gonococcus unless preventive measures are taken.
**os** (*plural,* ora). Mouth.
**os** (*plural,* ossa). Bone.
**os** (cervical). The orifice of the cervical canal.
*external.* The orifice which opens into the vagina.
*internal.* The orifice which opens into the uterine cavity.
**ossa innominata.** *See* innominate bones.
**ovulation.** Extrusion of a mature ovum from the ovary through the rupture of a graafian follicle.
**ovum.** The female reproductive, or germ, cell.
**oxytocic.** A drug which stimulates contractions of the uterine muscle.
**oxytocin.** A hormone, secreted by the posterior lobe of the pituitary gland, which stimulates the uterine muscle to contract.

**para-.** *See* parous.
**parametritis.** An inflammation of the connective tissue around the uterus.
**paraphimosis.** Retraction and constriction of the prepuce (foreskin) behind the glans of the penis.
**parous** (para-). Having borne a child or children.
**parturient.** A woman in labor.
**parturition.** *See* labor.
**pelvic brim.** Inlet or boundary of the superior strait of the true pelvis.
**pelvimeter.** An instrument used for measuring the diameters and the capacity of the pelvis.
**pelvimetry.** Measurement of distances between certain prominent parts of the pelvis to determine its size.
**pelvis.** Irregular bony cavity resting upon the femurs which contains the reproductive organs, the rectum, and the bladder.
*false.* Shallow expanded upper portion serving mainly as a support for the abdominal viscera and during pregnancy as a support for the enlarged uterus.
*inlet* (superior strait). Brim or upper margin of the true pelvis.
*outlet* (inferior strait). Inferior opening or lower margin of the true pelvis.
*true.* Lower portion; irregularly shaped bony cavity through which the baby must pass at birth.
**perineum.** A pyramidal mass of muscle, connective tissue, and fascia which is situated between the rectum and the vagina and forms the floor of the pelvis.
**pernicious vomiting.** Severe vomiting of pregnancy; usually in the first trimester.
**phimosis.** A tightness of the orifice of the prepuce (foreskin) so that it cannot be drawn back to uncover the glans penis.
**phlegmasia alba dolens.** *See* milk leg.

**Pitocin.** A proprietary name for an extract of the oxytocic principle of the posterior lobe of the pituitary gland.
**placenta** (afterbirth). A flat, round, spongy organ on the wall of the uterus to which the fetus is attached by means of the umbilical cord and by which it receives its nourishment and excretes its waste products.
**placenta previa.** A placenta which is implanted so low in the uterine cavity that it partially or completely covers the internal os of the cervix.
**polar body.** Bodies which are cast off during the process of maturation of an ovum. In this process the number of chromosomes in the mature ovum is reduced to one-half of the original number, and the cytoplasm is divided very unequally with the mature ovum receiving the major portion.
**position** (of fetus). The relation of some arbitrarily chosen point on the presenting part of the fetus to the right or left side of the mother.
**postnatal.** Occurring after birth.
**postpartum.** Occurring after delivery or childbirth.
**pre-eclampsia.** An acute hypertensive disease of pregnancy which may occur in the last trimester; characterized by edema, hypertension, and albuminuria.
**pregnancy.** The condition of being with child. The normal duration of pregnancy in the human is 10 lunar months, or 40 weeks, or 280 days.
**pregnancy test.** A test for pregnancy dependent upon the presence of the hormone chorionic gonadotropin in the serum and urine of the pregnant woman; serum or urine, when injected into test animals, produces changes in their sex glands.
**premature infant.** A baby whose weight is 2500 gm (5 lb, 8 oz) or less at birth.
**premature labor.** Termination of pregnancy after the child is viable, but before maturity is reached.
**premature separation of placenta.** *See* abruptio placentae.
**prenatal.** Existing or occurring before birth.
**prepuce** (foreskin). The fold of skin covering the glans penis. In the female, the hood-like covering over the distal end of the clitoris formed by the joining of the labia minora anteriorly.
**presentation** (of fetus). The relationship of the longitudinal axis of the fetus to the longitudinal axis of the mother.
**presenting part** (of fetus). That part of the baby's body which lies over the brim of the mother's pelvis.
**primigravida.** A woman who is pregnant for the first time. She remains a primigravida during labor and until the baby is actually born.
**primipara.** A woman who has had one child. She remains a primipara until her second child is born. Since no one really calls a woman in labor for the second time a primipara it is best to say she is a multigravida.
**primordial follicle.** An immature follicle consisting of an ovum surrounded by a single layer of cells.
**primordial ovum.** A single immature germ cell found in the connective tissue of the ovary.
**progesterone.** An ovarian hormone produced by the corpus luteum; also elaborated by the placenta.
**promontory** (of sacrum). The body of the first sacral vertebra.
**pseudocyesis.** False or imagined pregnancy.
**puberty.** That period at which sexual maturity develops; the reproductive organs become functional, and secondary sex characteristics develop.
**puerperal infection.** An infection of the pelvic organs due to entrance of pathogenic bacteria before or during labor or during the puerperium.
**puerperium.** The period of time from delivery to complete involution of the pelvic organs; strictly speaking, however, it begins with the onset of labor. A period of five to six weeks after delivery.

**quickening.** The mother's first perception of movements of the fetus.

**racemose glands** (of cervix). Branching glands in the cervix which open into the cervical canal and which secrete a thick mucus.

**rectovaginal septum.** The tissue which forms the partition between the rectum and vagina.

**replacement transfusion.** *See* exchange transfusion.

**retraction ring** (pathologic). An exaggeration of a physiologic retraction ring which normally occurs between the upper and lower uterine segments during labor; there is excessive thinning of the lower segment and more than normal thickening of the upper segment.

**retrolental fibroplasia.** A series of changes that sometimes occurs in the eyes of immature babies after birth, which results in the formation of an opaque membrane behind the lens and complete or partial loss of vision.

**Rh factor.** A term applied to antigens found in red blood cells. Persons whose blood is agglutinated by anti-Rh serum are called Rh-positive (D-positive), and persons whose blood is not agglutinated by this serum are said to be Rh-negative (D-negative).

**Ritgen's maneuver.** Delivery of the baby's head in a slow and controlled manner between uterine contractions by pressure made on the brow or chin through the perineum.

**rooming-in.** A term applied to a hospital arrangement by which the baby is placed in the mother's room so that she has the privilege of caring for him as she wishes.

**rooting reflex.** A reflex present in the newborn which is demonstrated by touching his cheek with any object; he moves his head toward the source of stimulation and opens his mouth for food.

**rugae** (vaginal). Small transverse folds or corrugations in the mucous membrane of the vagina.

**salpingitis.** An inflammation of the uterine (fallopian) tubes.

**Schultze's mechanism.** A mechanism of placental separation and extrusion in which separation begins at the center and the detached area spreads toward the margin; the fetal surface of the placenta appears at the vaginal outlet first as it is delivered.

**secundines.** The placenta and fetal membranes expelled after childbirth.

**segmentation.** The process of cell division by which the fertilized ovum develops into many cells which then become differentiated into layers and go on to further specialization and development.

**show.** *See* bloody show.

**Skene's glands.** Two paraurethral glands in the female with ducts that open on each side of the urethral meatus.

**smegma.** A thick cheesy secretion of the sebaceous glands of the clitoris, the labia minora, and the prepuce.

**spermatozoon.** The male reproductive, or germ, cell.

**sphincter ani.** Bands of circular muscles which control the rectal opening.

**spina bifida.** A developmental defect in the closure of the bony spinal canal; the spinal cord may or may not protrude through the defect.

**stillborn.** Born dead.

**striae gravidarum.** Pink, bluish, and white lines which may be present on the abdomen, thighs, and breasts during and following a pregnancy; caused by rupture and later scarring of elastic tissue fibers of the deep skin layer due to hypertrophic changes and/or tension of the enlarging uterus.

**subinvolution** (of the uterus). Failure of the uterus to return to its usual size and condition at the rate that it normally should following delivery.

**sutures.** Membranous spaces between the cranial bones of the fetus.

*coronal.* Between frontal and parietal bones.

*frontal.* Between frontal bones from anterior fontanel to the proximal end of the nose, located between the orbital cavities.

*lambdoidal.* Between occipital and parietal bones.

*sagittal.* Between parietal bones.

**symphysis pubis.** The place of union of the pubic bones in the front by means of cartilage.

**terminal heating** (of formula). A process by which the entire formula unit (formula, bottle, nipple, and cap) is exposed to a degree of heat which will destroy bacteria, but will not cause nutritive or physical damage to the formula.

**tetanic contraction** (of uterus). An abnormal condition in labor in which the uterine muscle stays continuously contracted instead of relaxing and contracting at regular intervals.

**thrush.** A mild infection of the skin and mucous membranes caused by the fungus *Candida (Monilia) albicans* and characterized by the formation of pearly-white, curd-like lesions. May develop in the mouth of the newborn infant where it appears as white elevated patches which resemble milk curds.

**tongue-tie.** A congenital shortness of the lingual frenum which makes it impossible to protrude the tongue to the normal extent.

**tonic neck reflex.** A postural reflex present in the infant during the first few months of life. As the infant lies on his back and rotates his head to either side, the arm and leg on the side to which the head is turned are partially or completely extended and the opposite arm and leg are flexed.

**toxemia** (of pregnancy). A complication of pregnancy characterized by hypertension, edema, and albuminuria which is due either to the pregnancy itself or to an aggravation by pregnancy of an existing hypertensive disease.

**tracheoesophageal fistula.** A malformation in which the upper part of the esophagus ends in a blind pouch and the lower segment connects to the trachea.

**transitory fever.** *See* dehydration fever.

**Trichomonas vaginalis.** An actively motile, flagellate parasite which is sometimes harbored in the vagina and which may cause a profuse irritating vaginal discharge.

**trophoblasts.** Cells on the outer layer of the vesicle which contains the embryo. These cells have the ability to invade the decidua for implantation, serve to supply the embryo with nourishment and removal of waste, and become the parenchyma of the placenta.

**tubal pregnancy.** Gestation in a uterine (fallopian) tube.

**tubercles of Montgomery.** *See* Montgomery's tubercles.

**umbilical cord** (funis). A cord which connects the fetus with the placenta and which contains blood vessels that carry nourishment to and waste products away from the fetus.

**uterine inertia.** Sluggish and rather ineffective uterine contractions during labor.

**uterine ligaments.** *See* ligaments.

**uterine souffle.** A soft blowing sound which may be heard on auscultation of the lower abdomen during pregnancy and which may be mistaken for the fetal heartbeat. This sound is made by pulsations in the aorta or the greatly enlarged uterine vessels as blood passes through them.

**uterus.** The hollow, muscular female organ of reproduction in which the fetus is developed and from which it is expelled during labor.

**vagina.** Musculomembranous canal leading from the vulva to the uterus.

**variety** (of fetus). The relation of some arbitrarily chosen point on the presenting part of the fetus to the anterior, transverse, or posterior segment of the right or left side of the mother's pelvis.

**vernix caseosa.** A greasy, white, cheese-like material which covers the skin of the newborn at birth. It consists largely of secretion from sebaceous glands and contains some epithelial cells and lanugo hair.

**version.** The turning of the fetus within the uterus so that the part which was presenting at the superior strait of the pelvis is replaced by another part.

*cephalic*. The head becomes the presenting part.
*podalic*. The breech becomes the presenting part.

**vestibule of the vagina.** The triangular space between the labia minora and below the clitoris. The urethral and vaginal orifices open into it.

**vulva.** The external female genitalia.

**Wharton's jelly.** The gelatinous material in the umbilical cord which surrounds the blood vessels.

**xiphoid process** (ensiform process). The pointed piece of cartilage that makes up the lowermost part of the sternum.

**zygote.** The fertilized ovum before cleavage. A cell resulting from the fusion of two sex cells.

# INDEX